THIRD EDITION

Medical Terminology With Case Studies

A Navigated Guide to Learning for Health Care Professionals

THIRD EDITION

Medical Terminology With Case Studies

A Navigated Guide to Learning for Health Care Professionals

Katie Walsh Flanagan, EdD, LAT, ATC
Professor
East Carolina University
Greenville, North Carolina

Routledge
Taylor & Francis Group
NEW YORK AND LONDON

Medical Terminology With Case Studies: A Navigated Guide to Learning for Health Care Professionals, Third Edition includes ancillary materials specifically available for faculty use. Included are Test Bank Questions and PowerPoint slides. Please visit www.routledge.com/9781032955773 to obtain access.

Cover: Tinhouse Design

treasure chest and parrot icons: Memo Angeles/shutterstock.com
skeleton icons: Andreas Meyer/shutterstock.com (pp. 153, 276, 293)
Kadrettin Kahramanlar/shutterstock.com (pp. 61, 332)
Ralf Juergen Kraft/shutterstock.com (p. 246)
Vac 1/shutterstock.com (pp. 30, 38, 54, 402)

First published in hardback 2024

First published in 2023 by SLACK Incorporated

Published 2024 by Routledge
605 Third Avenue, New York, NY 10158

and by Routledge
4 Park Square, Milton Park, Abingdon, Oxon OX14 4RN

Routledge is an imprint of the Taylor & Francis Group, an informa business

Dr. Katie Walsh Flanagan *and* Jill Walker Dale *reported no financial or proprietary interest in the materials presented herein.*

Publisher's Note
The publisher has gone to great lengths to ensure the quality of this reprint but points out that some imperfections in the original copies may be apparent.

Library of Congress Cataloging-in-Publication Data
Names: Flanagan, Katie Walsh, author.
Title: Medical terminology with case studies : a navigated guide to learning for health care professionals / Katie Walsh Flanagan.
Other titles: Medical terminology with case studies in sports medicine
Description: Third edition. | Thorofare, NJ : SLACK Incorporated, [2023] | Preceded by Medical terminology with case studies in sports medicine / Katie Walsh Flanagan. Second edition. [2017]. | Includes bibliographical references and index.
Identifiers: LCCN 2022040163 (print) | ISBN 9781638220510 (paperback)
Subjects: MESH: Terminology as Topic | Problems and Exercises
Classification: LCC R123 (print) | NLM W 18.2 | DDC 610.1/4--dc23/eng/20221104
LC record available at https://lccn.loc.gov/2022040163

ISBN: 978-1-03-295577-3 (hbk)
ISBN: 978-1-63822-051-0 (pbk)
ISBN: 978-1-003-52506-6 (ebk)

DOI: 10.4324/9781003525066

For Product Safety Concerns and Information please contact our EU representative: GPSR@taylorandfrancis.com
Taylor & Francis Verlag GmbH, Kaufingerstraße 24, 80331 München, Germany.

Additional resources can be found at
www.routledge.com/9781032955773

Dedication

This book is dedicated to one of the most forward thinking, creative, passionate, and driven people I know, my dear friend and colleague, Dr. Sharon Rogers Moore. Sharon is an outstanding mother, wife, entrepreneur, researcher, educator, and friend. She is the type of athletic trainer who always finds more efficient ways to protect her athletes and, seemingly effortlessly, seeks out and uses evidence into practice with on-field decision making. Sharon was exceptionally important in my life the past few years, and I would not have been able to write this book and be where I am today without her undying support.

And to my dear husband, Sean Flanagan, who lets me drag him on adventures and brightens my world as does the sun.

Contents

Medical Terminology With Case Studies: A Navigated Guide to Learning for Health Care Professionals, Third Edition includes ancillary materials specifically available for faculty use. Included are Test Bank Questions and PowerPoint slides. Please visit www.routledge.com/9781032955773 to obtain access.

About the Author

Katie Walsh Flanagan, EdD, LAT, ATC, was raised in Carmel, California. She graduated from Oregon State University with a bachelor's degree in Physical Education and from Illinois State University with a master's degree in Athletic Training before embarking on a career in athletic training. She was the head athletic trainer for women and a lecturer at Western Illinois University before leaving to become the head athletic trainer with the men's professional soccer team in Chicago, Illinois, for 3 years. During her 10 years in Illinois, she was active in both the state and District 4 athletic training organizations.

In 1990, Dr. Flanagan was hired as an athletic trainer and lecturer at California State University, Fresno, and she earned a doctorate in Education at the University of Southern California. In 1995, she accepted the position she held for 27 years: Director of Sports Medicine at East Carolina University (ECU) in Greenville, North Carolina. As an athletic trainer, Dr. Flanagan has traveled internationally with both men's and women's US Soccer teams and volunteered at the Pan American and Atlanta Olympic Games. She provided medical coverage for cheerleading and other sports at ECU for 15 years and still works as an athletic trainer helping out with ECU football and other events as needed.

As a dedicated member of the National Athletic Trainers' Association (NATA), Dr. Flanagan is a member of the NATA Board of Directors and represented District 3—the Mid-Atlantic Athletic Trainers' Association from 2015 to 2022. She has been an active volunteer for the national, district, and state levels of NATA and has also served on the Commission on Accreditation of Athletic Training Education, which oversees athletic training education, for 7 years. Dr. Flanagan is an accomplished speaker and has made dozens of international and national presentations and 50 regional/district/state presentations, as well as published dozens of articles and book chapters. Dr. Flanagan is considered an expert in athlete safety policy, especially with environmental and lightning safety. In that area, she is internationally known for her lightning safety policies that govern recreation and sport.

Dr. Flanagan was named the North Carolina College/University Athletic Trainer of the Year in 2000 and 2006 by the North Carolina Athletic Trainers' Association and was inducted into their Hall of Fame in 2013. NATA has recognized her with their National Service Award (2006) and Most Distinguished Athletic Trainer honor (2010).

She is married to Sean Flanagan, and they reside in Greenville, North Carolina, with their two rescue cats, Abby and Tucker.

About the Contributing Author

Jill Walker Dale, MS, ATC, LAT (Appendix B), is currently a Payor Contracts Manager for MaineHealth in Portland, Maine. Following her move from New York to Maine in 2018, she worked as a Quality Specialist at the MaineHealth Accountable Care Organization for 2 years. Prior to this she was a Clinician, Practice Manager, and Owner of Orthopedic & Sports Therapy Associates, LLP, in Elmira, New York, for 30 years. She also worked for Guthrie Sports Medicine doing outreach athletic training to high schools, colleges, and professional athletic teams locally in New York and Pennsylvania. She was an adjunct professor at Corning Community College, where she taught Introduction to Athletic Training for 12 years. Jill served 2 terms on the New York State (NYS) Committee for Athletic Trainers developing the rules and regulations for the NYS Practice Act. She served as Secretary of the New York State Athletic Trainers' Association (NYSATA) for 4 years and chaired the Clinical/Industrial Committee for 6 years. She received her undergraduate degree from SUNY Cortland in Physical Education & Athletic Training and her master's degree in Athletic Training from Illinois State University. She has volunteered for the Board of Certification in exam development since 1996 in many roles, including Test Site Administrator; Examiner Training Program Facilitator; Exam Development Panelist for the practical exam; Chair, Practical Exam Development Committee; and, most recently, Chair, Examination Development Committee from 2008 to 2013.

Jill has received many honors in her career, including the NYSATA's Thomas Sheehan Sr. Award, as well as induction into the NYSATA Hall of Fame (2009). The Board of Certification awarded her with the Dan Libera Service Award in 2004, and the National Athletic Trainers' Association honored her with the Athletic Trainer Service Award in 2012.

Introduction

Welcome to the world of medical terminology! At East Carolina University, we created and teach this class for all types of students, but never found a textbook we really loved, so I wrote this one. Blackbeard the pirate lived and held control over the islands of the Outer Banks of North Carolina, near East Carolina University, which is why our mascot is a pirate. Throughout this book, you will see Skully, the pirate skeleton, leading students through the various islands that relate to different body systems. His helper is Tango, a colorful parrot. He has a huge personality, and I chose him to run through the pages to keep learning interesting.

This is not your typical textbook. It has all the necessary attributes, words, and lessons, but I attempted to keep it more light and not so serious. Learning is an adventure, and I hope your education is a bit easier with Skully and Tango as they travel the islands.

This textbook became a reality due to a chance meeting with Brien Cummings at the SLACK Incorporated booth at a professional meeting. Brien took flight with the idea of this different-from-usual textbook and made it a reality. He became my "handler" and navigated the waters for me as we worked together to merge the SLACK philosophies with my ideas of color and graphics. Brien is a dedicated, driven, and focused individual who made this project easier for me, and along the way became a friend for life. Thank you for your unending patience, support, and professionalism.

I would also like to acknowledge the Pirate athletic training staff and students who have provided ideas, taught us patience, and made an impact in their profession.

Overview

Medical terminology is a way of communicating in medical and allied health worlds. It is largely memorization as this is a new language that uses combinations of word parts to accurately explain a given condition or description of medical issue. This textbook will put a bit of fun in navigating the new language by using Skully who is sailing between his islands (combining forms) to explore the various words and word parts to help students direct their learning. The purpose of this text is to become to become educated and comfortable with medical learning. There are plenty of textbooks that offer more detail in certain chapters. This specific text will launch students with enough information to communicate effectively with medical professionals. It is not intended to be an exhaustive list of medical term (we have medical dictionaries for that), but instead it will get students interested in learning medical language and understanding various word parts. This textbook is not to replace an anatomy and physiology course, nor is it a medical/pathology class. Medical terminology textbooks are primarily dictionaries that are organized in a manner to facilitate learning. Rather than just list words, word components (prefixes and suffixes), and their meanings alphabetically, this textbook is organized in body systems to facilitate learning.

Section I provides the background for the rest of the text. The text begins with an overview of the vast variety of medical professionals that use medical terminology on a daily basis, and may help you find a career in the medical field. Chapter 2 introduces **prefixes**, **suffixes**, and common **combining forms**. A prefix comes before a word root, and a suffix follows it. By learning combining forms (also known as *word roots*), and knowing common prefixes and suffixes, students can begin to dissect words and make sense of them. Chapter 3 provides a refresher on the organization of the body, anatomical directions, and abbreviations. Chapter 4 is an overview of therapeutic and diagnostic terms. The purpose of Section I is to provide a language background that provides the foundation for the rest of the book.

In **Section II**, each chapter corresponds to a body system, and an island is used to help visually characterize the word root that is the basis for the words in that body system. In the cardiovascular chapter, for example, the island is shaped like a human heart (the real human heart, not the Valentine's Day portrayal of one). Gold coins (which a true pirate is never without) are used to depict prefixes and suffixes. Students will learn that prefixes and suffixes (a.k.a. gold coins) can easily be used with most word roots. Each chapter (island) begins with basic and relevant anatomy to that body system, as many medical terms are related to the specific anatomical structure of the body. The chapters continue by introducing combining forms specific to that body system, and by adding the common prefixes and suffixes, students understand the newly created word.

Section III contains appendices for specialized areas that students may be interested in exploring but are not contained in depth in any chapter. Appendix A displays commonly used medical abbreviations, Appendix B pertains to medical coding (putting the right numerical code on a condition or procedure so the technicians/physicians get paid from the insurance company), and Appendix C lists common pharmacological terms.

Answers for each chapter's Learning Activities and Case Study are found in **Section IV**.

Section I

Introduction to Medical Terminology

1

Medical Terminology and the Health Care Professional

This textbook is designed to introduce and teach students a new language—but one that is used throughout the health care profession. If the content of this book is interesting to you, this chapter is perfect to learn more about the health care professionals who use medical terminology at work on a daily basis. Table 1-1 displays the more common specialties for physicians, whereas Table 1-2 dives into nonphysician health care providers. The second table is alphabetical (as are the physician specialties) and also provides the scope of practice, minimum degree for the area, and a URL to the specific profession.

Physician Specialties

Table 1-1 provides a list of medical doctors (MDs) and doctors of osteopathy (DOs) with additional training after their 4-year college degree and an additional 3 to 4 years of medical school. Each of these specialists require focused training and practice in the area prior to taking Boards (exams) qualifying them to practice their craft.

Table 1-1
Physician (MD/DO) Specialties

NAME	PHYSICIAN WHO SPECIALIZES IN
anesthesiologist	Administration of anesthesia
cardiologist	Disorders of the cardiac system
dermatologist	Disorders of the skin
endocrinologist	Disorders of the endocrine system
gastroenterologist	Disorders of the gastrointestinal system
geriatrician	Diagnosis and treatment of aging and older adults
	(continued)

Flanagan KW.
Medical Terminology With Case Studies: A Navigated Guide to Learning for Health Care Professionals, Third Edition (pp 3-10).

Table 1-1 (continued)

Physician (MD/DO) Specialties

NAME	PHYSICIAN WHO SPECIALIZES IN
gynecologist	Disorders of the female reproductive system and breasts
hematologist	Disorders of the blood
internist	Internal organs of the body
neonatologist	Studying and treating disorders of newborns
nephrologist	Disorders of the kidneys
neurologist	Disorders of the nervous system
neuropsychiatrist	Working with the relationship between brain function and psychiatry
neurosurgeon	Operating on the nervous system
obstetrician	Care of women, childbirth, and postpartum care
oncologist	Studying and treating cancer
ophthalmologist	Disorders of the eye
orthopedist	Musculoskeletal conditions
osteologist	Treatment of bone diseases
otolaryngologist	Disorders of the ear and larynx
otorhinolaryngologist	Disorders of the ear, nose, and throat (larynx); also called *ENT*
pathologist	Microscopic examination of tissue
pediatrician	Well-being of children and treatment of childhood conditions
proctologist	Diseases of the rectum and anus
psychiatrist	Diagnosis and treatment of mental conditions
pulmonologist	Diagnosis, prevention, and treatment of the chest, respiratory system, and lungs
radiologist	Translating images from a variety of mediums (eg, magnetic resonance imaging, computed tomography scans, x-rays, positron emission tomography scans)
urologist	Disorders of the urinary system

Health Care Provider Specialties

The following list is an example of the variety of health care providers who are not physicians, and is not inclusive of all medical specialties. Some of these practitioners have a 1-year (or less) program of study, but most require at least a 4-year bachelor's degree, if not post-graduate education and clinical experience. Most have national/state Boards (exams) and state regulations. State practice acts determine the scope of practice for these medical specialists. Regulations such as prescription authority (if they can write a prescription for medications), under whom (if anyone) they must work, and their scope of practice are all determined by individual states.

Table 1-2
Health Care Provider Specialties

NAME	SCOPE OF PRACTICE	MINIMUM DEGREE*	WEBSITE#
athletic trainer (AT)	Specializes in the prevention, assessment, treatment, and rehabilitation of injuries and illnesses	Master's degree	http://www.nata.org
audiologist	Specializes in hearing disorders	Doctorate degree	https://www.audiology.org
chiropractor (DC)	Trained in the manipulation of the spine and joints	Doctorate degree	https://www.acatoday.org
clinical laboratory assistant/technician	Collects body fluid, tissues for analyzing	Bachelor's degree	https://ascls.org
dental assistant	Assists dentist with record keeping, patient aid, x-rays	Associate's degree	https://www.adaausa.org
dental hygienist	Provides routine care of the teeth and gums	Associate's degree to master's degree	https://www.adha.org
dentist (DDS, DMD)	Provides preventative and restorative dental care	Doctorate degree	https://www.ada.org
emergency medical technician (EMT)/paramedic	Responds to emergency calls, treats emergent conditions, and transports to medical facilities	Postsecondary certificate	https://www.naemt.org
genetic counselor	Provides maternal or family assistance regarding risk of genetic conditions	Master's degree	https://www.nsgc.org
health information manager	Organizes and oversees patient health information and data	Bachelor's degree	https://www.ahima.org
health information specialist	Collects, appraises, and tracks patient information, treatments, and follow-up	Postsecondary certificate	https://www.ahima.org
home health care/personal care aide	Monitors and provides daily living assistance for people living at home with chronic/disabling conditions	High school diploma	https://www.nahc.org
massage therapist	Applies touch to manipulate soft tissues and muscles	Postsecondary certificate	https://www.amtamassage.org
medical assistant	Completes clinical and administrative tasks in physician offices, clinics, hospitals and health care facilities	Postsecondary certificate	https://www.aama-ntl.org
medical transcriptionist	Transcribes verbal recordings into written medical record	Associate's degree/certificate	https://www.ahdionline.org
nuclear medicine technologist	Prepares patients and administer radioactive medications for imaging or treatment	Associate's degree	https://www.asrt.org
nurse—advance practice nurse (APN)/nurse practitioner (NP)/nurse anesthetists (NA)/nurse midwife	Has prescription authority	Master's degree	https://www.aanp.org http://www.aana.com

(continued)

Table 1-2 (continued)

Health Care Provider Specialties

NAME	SCOPE OF PRACTICE	MINIMUM DEGREE*	WEBSITE#
nurse—bachelor of nursing (BSN)	Works under the direction of a physician	Bachelor's degree	https://nurse.org/orgs.shtml
nurse—certified/licensed nursing assistant (CNA/LNA)	Provides nonmedical patient care (activities of daily living) for those in hospitals, nursing homes, home care, or hospice. They work under the supervision of a RN or LPN	On-the-job training, or several-month program	https://nurse.org/orgs.shtml
nurse—licensed practical nurse (LPN)/licensed vocational nurse (LVN)	Provides basic nursing care to patients	Postsecondary certificate	https://nurse.org/orgs.shtml
nurse—master of science in nursing (MSN)	Works under the direction of a physician	Master's degree	https://nurse.org/orgs.shtml
nurse—registered nurse (RN)	Coordinates patient care and education	Bachelor's degree	https://nurse.org/orgs.shtml
occupational therapist (OT)	Specializes in rehabilitation of fine motor skills and activities of daily living through everyday activities	Master's degree	https://www.aota.org
occupational therapy assistant (OTA)/aide	Aids patients in regaining and maintaining activities of daily living	Associate's degree	https://www.aota.org
optician	Assists with fitting eyeglasses and filling prescriptions for corrective lenses	High school diploma	https://oaa.org
optometrist (OD)	Diagnoses and treats visual problems, manages ocular diseases and injuries	Doctorate degree	https://aoa.org
orthotist/prosthetist	Measures, fits, designs, and fabricates medical supportive devices for patients	Master's degree	https://www.aopanet.org
pharmacist (RPh, PharmD)	Licensed to fill, sell, and dispense medications and compounds prescribed by physicians	Doctorate degree	https://www.pharmacist.com
pharmacy technician	Assists pharmacist in dispensing prescription medications	High school diploma	https://www.pharmacytechnician.org
phlebotomist	Draws blood for testing, transfusions, or research	Postsecondary certificate	https://www.nationalphlebotomy.org
physical therapist (PT)	Specializes in rehabilitation of neurological and orthopedic conditions	Doctorate degree	https://www.apta.org

(continued)

TABLE 1-2 (CONTINUED)
HEALTH CARE PROVIDER SPECIALTIES

NAME	SCOPE OF PRACTICE	MINIMUM DEGREE*	WEBSITE#
physical therapist assistant/aide (PTA)	Assists physical therapist in helping patients regain movement and activity following injury/surgery	Associate's degree	https://www.apta.org
physician assistant (PA)	Health care provider with prescription authority and who has subspecialties	Master's degree	https://www.aapa.org
podiatrist (DPM)	Treats disorders of the lower leg, ankle, and foot	Doctorate degree	https://www.apma.org
psychiatric technician/aide	Assists and cares for patients with mental illnesses and developmental delays	Associate's degree	https://psychtechs.org
psychologist	Treats various aspects of human behavior	Doctorate degree	https://www.apa.org
radiology technologist	Performs diagnostic imaging on patients	Associate's degree	https://www.arrt.org https://www.asrt.org
recreational therapist (CTRS)	Plans, directs, and coordinates recreational programs for people with disabilities or illnesses	Bachelor's degree	https://www.atra-online.com
registered dietitian (RD)	Assesses nutritional needs of patients	Bachelor's degree and residency	https://www.eatright.org
respiratory therapist (ARRT)	Works under a physician's orders to improve respiratory function	Associate's degree	https://www.aarc.org
sonographer	Using ultrasound, prepares patients, views, and captures images within the body	Associate's degree	https://www.ardms.org
speech-language pathologist	Evaluates, diagnoses, and treats communication and swallowing disorders	Master's degree	https://www.asha.org
surgical technologist	Assists surgeons during patient operations	Postsecondary certificate	https://www.ast.org

*May vary by state; may require internship/fellowships, as well as national and/or state Board exam to practice
#Some health care professions have many organizations (American, North American, National), and the one listed here may be one of many websites available to these specialties.

BIBLIOGRAPHY

Bureau of Labor Statistics. Healthcare occupations. Updated September 8, 2021. Accessed December 28, 2021. https://www.bls.gov/ooh/healthcare/home.htm

Royal PL. *Today's Health Professions: Working Together to Provide Quality Care.* F. A. Davis; 2016.

Notes

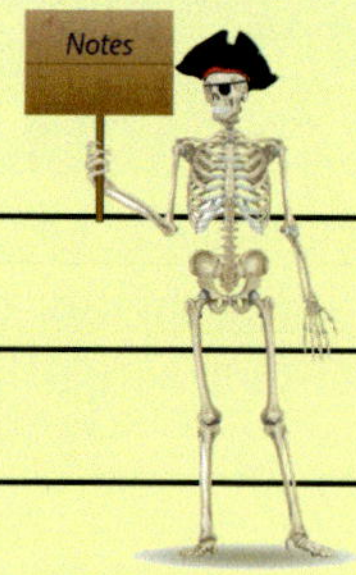

NOTES

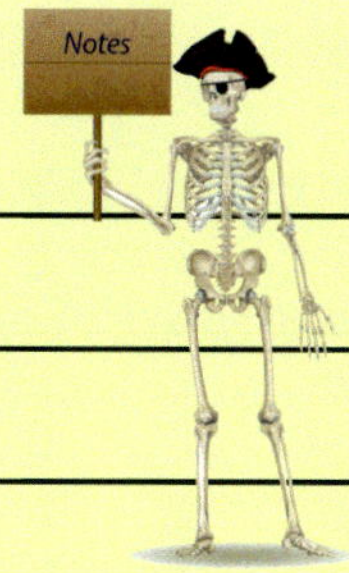

LEARNING ACTIVITIES

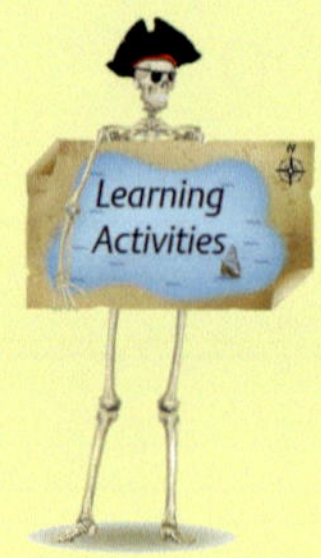

Name:______________________

Medical Terminology and the Health Care Professional

1. List three different areas of health care (either physician and/or health care provider).
   a. ____________________________________
   b. ____________________________________
   c. ____________________________________

Using the area website (or research) determine the following:

2. For each area: Determine the level of education/training one needs to have to practice.

3. For each area: Determine who your client/patient is likely to be using your services?

4. Using the Bureau of Labor Statistics Healthcare Occupations referenced in this chapter, determine the potential growth (or not) in each area.

5. Using the Bureau of Labor Statistics Healthcare Occupations referenced in this chapter, determine the potential annual salary in each area.

6. Using research, find the closest programs (eg, community college, universities, programs of study) to your location. List the educational site and a contact person/email.

2

Word Building

An Introduction to Prefixes and Suffixes

OBJECTIVES

After studying this chapter, you will be able to:

1. Explain the parts of a medical word.
2. Distinguish among prefixes, word roots, and suffixes.
3. Recognize common prefixes, word roots, and suffixes.
4. Create different meaning by adding a prefix or suffix to word roots.

CHAPTER OUTLINE

- Introduction
- Understanding a medical word
- Combining forms
- Common prefixes
- Common suffixes
- Learning activities

Flanagan KW.
Medical Terminology With Case Studies: A Navigated Guide to Learning for Health Care Professionals, Third Edition (pp 11-23).

Introduction

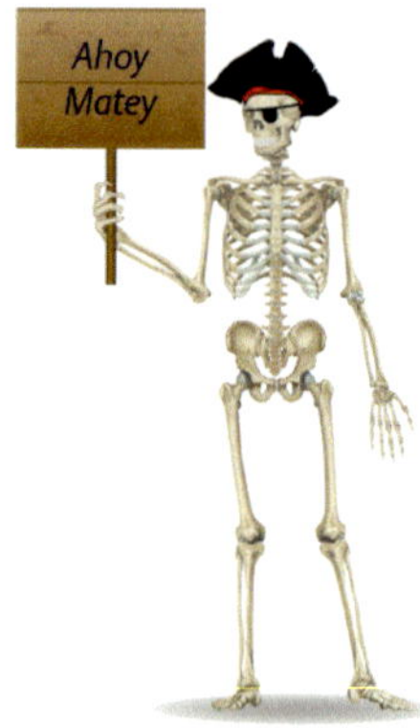

Welcome to the adventure of medical terminology. Please meet Skully, the pirate skeleton who sails from island to island bringing new word elements into your vocabulary. Alongside of Skully is his trusty sidekick parrot, Tango. Tango has a few battle scars, but he is tireless and energetic in his quest to help you understand medical terminology. He can be found throughout the chapters pointing out interesting facts. Both Skully and Tango are your learning companions who will do all they can to make learning a new language fun and interesting. Get ready to set sail into a new world of words and word parts.

Understanding a Medical Word

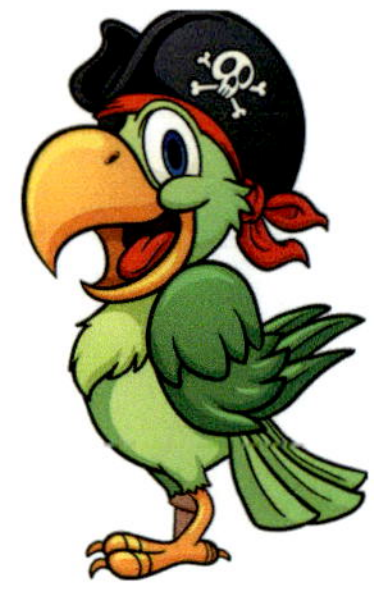

Although medical terminology may look confusing at first glance, it really is merely a series of word parts. Learning how these word parts interact and the meaning of them will make memorizing new terms easier. There are four distinct parts to medical words: the **combining form,** also known as the *word root* (the foundation of the word upon which all else is based), the **prefix** (lies in front of the word root), the **suffix** (found at the end of the word), and the **combining vowel** (typically an o) that combines the word root to either another word root or a suffix. The word root **gastr** means stomach, and its combining form is gastr/o. When the prefix **epi-** (above) is added to **gastr**, it becomes **epigastric** (above the stomach). When the suffix **-itis** (inflammation) is added to **gastr**, the word becomes **gastritis** (inflammation of the stomach); and both a prefix and suffix can be added to a word root to create **epigastritis** (inflammation above the stomach).

Learning medical terminology is best when students begin with the combining form, then look at the other elements of the total word to fully understand the meaning of the combination of the parts. A combining vowel is added to the end of a combining form to join that root to another root or a suffix. The combining vowel is most often *o* but *a*, *i*, and *u* are also used. Sometimes, a medical word can have two combining forms. **Osteoarthritis** is a word having two word roots, **osteo** (bone) and **arthr** (joint), with a combining vowel (o). The suffix **-itis** means *inflammation*; therefore, osteoarthritis pertains to inflammation of the bone and joint. A combining form is a word root with a combining vowel added to it. **Cardi** is a word root for heart and cardi/o is the combining form. When the combining form is added to the suffix **-ology**, the term **cardiology** is created. It means the study of the heart. **Gastr** (word root) added to the combining form gastr/o and the suffix **-logist** creates **gastrologist**, one who studies the stomach.

> Remember to find the combining forms first, then look at the prefix and suffix to fully understand the entire word.

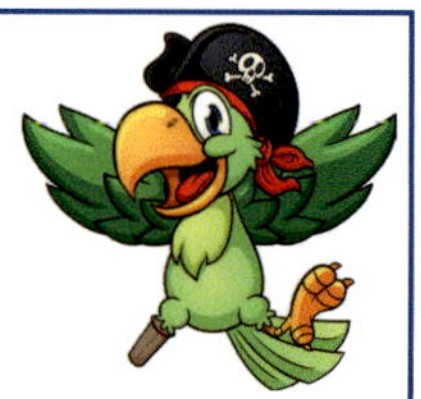

In Section II of this textbook, an island that represents the shape of a main combining form of the chapter is used to provide a visual portrayal of the word root (Figure 2-1). Because combining forms typically mean only one thing (eg, **derm** means skin, **gastr** means stomach), the island shapes are unique. Prefixes and suffixes, however, are not unique and can be combined with a word root to alter the meaning of the word. Skully the pirate and Tango, the parrot will travel from island to island (combining form to combining form) and bring with them gold and silver coins (Figure 2-2). These coins represent prefixes (gold coins) and suffixes (silver coins) as coins can travel and be used anywhere. The combining form (island) is static and does not typically move, whereas the prefixes and suffixes are combined (move from island to island) easily with different word roots.

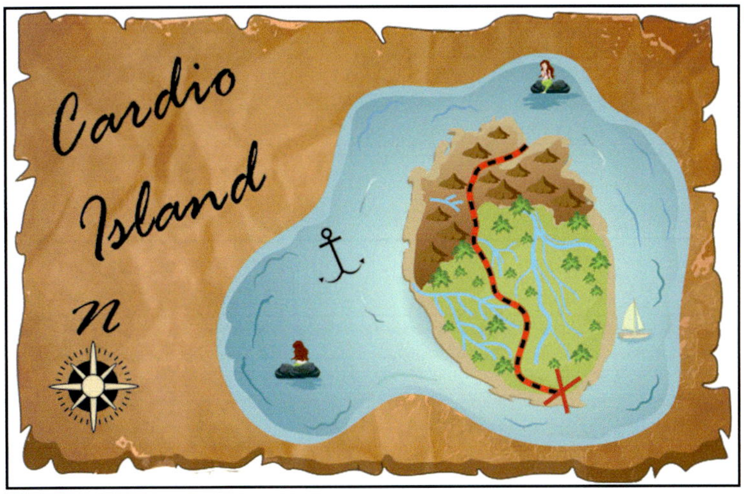

Figure 2-1. Drawing of Cardio Island.

Figure 2-2. Gold coins represent prefixes. (ekle/shutterstock.com)

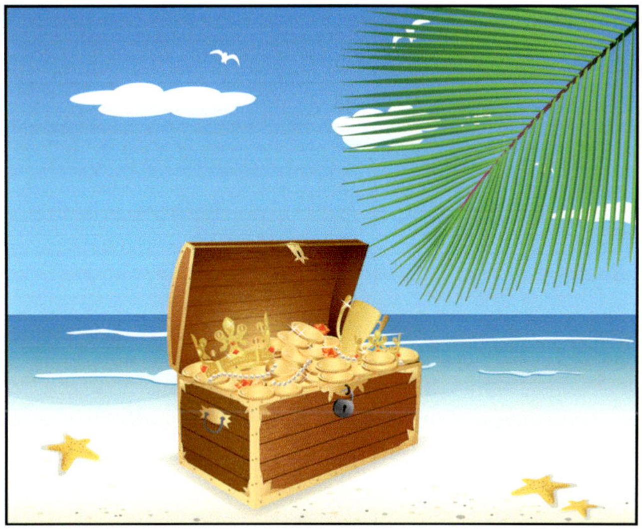

Combining Forms

Tables 2-1 and 2-2 provide simple combining forms that relate to the body. Learning these words will help you understand the whole word when a prefix or suffix is added to it via a combining vowel.

Table 2-1
Combining Forms Relating to the Body

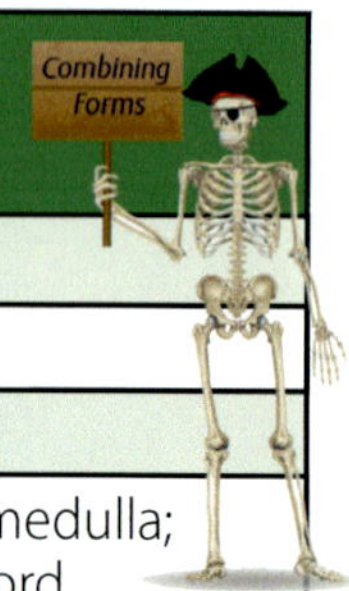

COMBINING FORM	DEFINITION
abdomin/o	abdomen
aden/o	gland
adip/o	fat
angi/o	vessel
arteri/o	artery
arthr/o	joint
axill/o	armpit
blephar/o	eyelid
bronch/o	bronchial tubes (to the lungs)
cardi/o	heart
chondr/o	cartilage
col/o	colon
cyst/o	bladder; sac
dent/o	teeth; dental
derm/o	skin
encephala/o	brain
enter/o	intestines
gastr/o	stomach or abdomen
hem/o	blood
hepat/o	liver
inguin/o	groin
lapar/o	abdomen
laryng/o	larynx
mamm/o	breast
mast/o	breast
my/o	muscle
myel/o	bone marrow; medulla; myelin; spinal cord
nephr/o	kidney
neur/o	nerve
ophthalm/o	eye
orchi/o	testicle; testis
oste/o	bone
ot/o	ear
ovari/o	ovary
phleb/o	vein
pneumon/o	lungs
pulmon/o	lungs
rect/o	rectum
ren/o	kidney
rhin/o	nose
splen/o	spleen
steth/o	chest
test/o	testicle
thorac/o	chest
tonsil/o	tonsils
trache/o	trachea
uter/o	uterus
ven/o	vein

Table 2-2
Other Noteworthy Combining Forms

COMBINING FORM	DEFINITION	COMBINING FORM	DEFINITION
andr/o	male	orth/o	straight; normal
bi/o	life	path/o	disease
carcin/o	cancer	phag/o	eating; swallowing
chem/o	drug; chemical	phot/o	light
chron/o	persisting over time	pnea	breathing
estr/o	female	psych/o	mind
glyc/o	sugar	radi/o	radiation; x-ray
hydr/o	water; fluid	somat/o	body
morph/o	form; shape	ster/o	solid structure
muc/o	mucus	ur/o	urine
necr/o	death		

Common Prefixes

Prefixes precede a word root and alter or add to its meaning slightly. Tables 2-3 through 2-5 contain categories of prefixes that will be used throughout this textbook.

Table 2-3
Prefixes Pertaining to Color

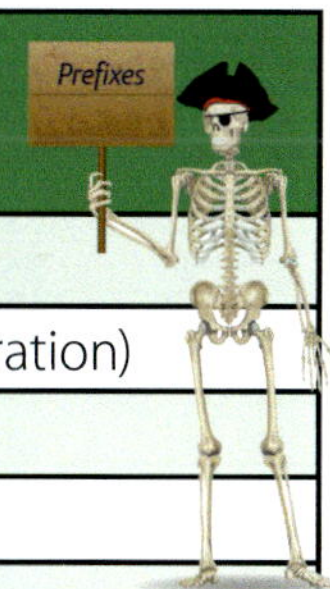

PREFIX	DEFINITION	EXAMPLE
cyan/o-	blue	**cyano**sis (bluish skin discoloration)
erythr/o-	red	**erythro**cyte (red blood cell)
leuk/o-	white	**leuko**cyte (white blood cell)
melan/o-	black	**melano**ma (skin cancer)

Table 2-4
Prefixes Pertaining to Direction or Comparison

PREFIX	DEFINITION	EXAMPLE
a-	without	**a**phasia (without speech)
ab-	away from	**ab**duction (away from the middle)
ad-	toward; near	**ad**duction (move toward the middle)
an-	not; without	**an**oxia (without oxygen)
ante-	before; in front of	**ante**rior (in front)
anti-	against	**anti**biotic (against life)
dextr/o-	right	**dextro**cardia (displacement of the heart on the right side of the body)
dia-	across; through	**dia**rrhea (watery fecal matter)
ec-; ecto-	out; outside	**ecto**pic (outside of usual position)
endo-	in; within	**endo**cardium (lining of the heart chambers)
epi-	above; upon	**epi**gastric (above the stomach)
exo-	away; outside	**ex**cise (to cut out)
hetero-	different	**hetero**graft (a graft of tissue from another species)
homo-	same	**homo**genous (likeness in form or structure)
hyper-	above; excessive; high; increased	**hyper**tension (high blood pressure)
hypo-	below; decreased; deficient; insufficient; low; under	**hypo**glycemia (low blood sugar)
inter-	between; among	**inter**osseous (between bones)
intra-	within; inside	**intra**articular (within the joint)
meso-	middle	**meso**derm (middle layer of skin)
meta-	beyond; change	**meta**tarsals (long bones in the foot beyond the ankle)
olig/o-	scanty; few	**oligo**menorrhea (light menstrual period)
pan-	all	**pan**demic (disease affecting a population)
para-	beside; near; abnormal	**para**denitis (inflammation of tissues around a gland)
per-	through	**per**cutaneous (through the skin)
peri-	around	**peri**carditis (around the heart)
sinistr/o-	left	**sinistro**cardia (displacement of the heart to the left)
sub-	below; under	**sub**dural (below the dura, which is the membrane surrounding the brain)
supra-	above	**supra**clavicular (above the clavicle [collarbone])
sym-; syn-	together; union	**syn**desmosis (membrane in between two bones)
trans-	across; through	**trans**dermal (across the skin)

TABLE 2-5 PREFIXES PERTAINING TO NUMBER		
PREFIX	**DEFINITION**	**EXAMPLE**
bi-	two; twice	**bi**lateral (pertaining to both sides)
dipl/o-	double	**diplo**pia (seeing double)
hemi-	one half	**hemi**sphere (half of a round structure)
mono-	one	**mono**cular (affecting one eye)
multi-	many	**multi**gravida (pregnant more than once)
nulli-	none	**nulli**gravida (person with no pregnancies)
poly-	excessive; many; much; over	**poly**cystic (having many cysts)
prim/i-	first	**prim**ary (first)
quadr/i-	four	**quadri**ceps (a group of four muscles in the thigh)
semi-	half; partial	**semi**permeable (partially permeable [having pores/opening])
tetra-	four	**tetra**paresis (muscular weakness affecting all four extremities)
tri-	three	**tri**ceps (a muscle in the arm with three origins)
uni-	one	**uni**te (to form into one)

COMMON SUFFIXES

Suffixes follow a combining form (or two) and, as with prefixes, alter the meaning of the combining form. Tables 2-6 through 2-8 contain common suffixes that will be used throughout this textbook.

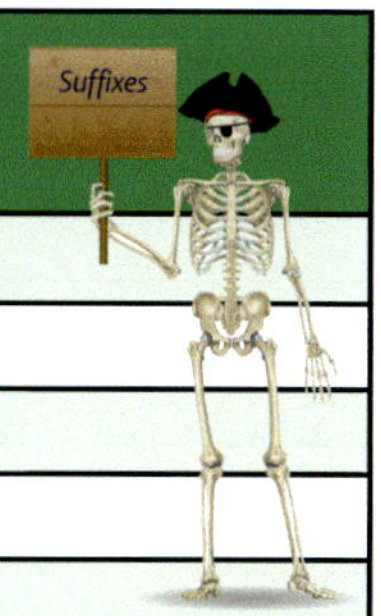

TABLE 2-6 SUFFIXES THAT MEAN "PERTAINING TO" OR "RESEMBLING"	
SUFFIX	**EXAMPLE**
-ac	cardi**ac** (pertaining to the heart)
-al	surgic**al** (pertaining to surgery)
-an	ovari**an** (pertaining to the ovary)
-ar	muscul**ar** (pertaining to muscles)
-ary	axill**ary** (pertaining to the armpit)
-atic	lymph**atic** (pertaining to the lymph)
-eal	epiphys**eal** (pertaining to the growth plate)
-iac	card**iac** (pertaining to the heart)
-ic	neurot**ic** (pertaining to a mental disorder)
-ical	mechan**ical** (pertaining to machines)
-ile	febr**ile** (pertaining to a fever)
-ine	uter**ine** (pertaining to the uterus)
-ior	infer**ior** (pertaining to below)
-oid	disc**oid** (resembling a flat, round shape)
-ory	sens**ory** (pertaining to the senses)
	(continued)

Table 2-6 (continued)

Suffixes That Mean "Pertaining to" or "Resembling"

SUFFIX	EXAMPLE
-ous	ven**ous** (pertaining to a vein)
-ose	varic**ose** (pertaining to a dilated vein)
-tic	therapeu**tic** (pertaining to therapy)
-us	prurit**us** (pertaining to itching)

Table 2-7

Common Suffixes

SUFFIX	DEFINITION	EXAMPLE
-algia	pain	arthr**algia** (joint pain)
-cele	hernia; protrusion; swelling	hydro**cele** (accumulation of water in a sac-like structure)
-cyte	cell	leuko**cyte** (white blood cell)
-dynia	pain	cephalo**dynia** (pain in the head; headache)
-ectasis	dilation; expansion	bronchi**ectasis** (dilation of the bronchi of the lungs)
-gen	that which produces	patho**gen** (that which produces a disease)
-genesis	forming; origin; producing	carcino**genesis** (cancer forming)
-iatry	medical treatment	psych**iatry** (medical treatment for a psychological condition)
-itis	inflammation	cyst**itis** (inflammation of the bladder)
-logist	one who studies	bio**logist** (one who studies life)
-logy	study of	gastro**logy** (study of the stomach)
-lysis	breaking down; destruction; loosening; separating; to loosen or break	hemo**lysis** (destruction of blood)
-malacia	softening	chondro**malacia** (softening of cartilage)
-megaly	abnormally large; enlargement	spleno**megaly** (enlargement of the spleen)
-oma	tumor; mass	carcin**oma** (cancerous tumor)
-osis	condition	lord**osis** (bent-forward condition)
-pathy	disease	osteo**pathy** (disease of the bone)
-phobia	fear	phono**phobia** (fear of sound)
-plasia	growth; formation	hyper**plasia** (excessive growth)
-plasm	formation	cyto**plasm** (the substance of the cell components except the nucleus)
-ptosis	drooping; falling; prolapse	blepharo**ptosis** (drooping eyelid)
-rrhage	bursting forth; excessive flow	hemo**rrhage** (excessive blood flow)
-rrhagia	abnormal flow	cysto**rrhagia** (abnormal flow from the bladder)

(continued)

Table 2-7 (continued)
Common Suffixes

SUFFIX	DEFINITION	EXAMPLE
-rrhea	discharge; excessive flow	rhino**rrhea** (discharge from the nose)
-rrhexis	rupture	entero**rrhexis** (rupture of the intestines)
-sclerosis	hardening	arterio**sclerosis** (hardening of the artery)
-stenosis	narrowing	angio**stenosis** (narrowing of a blood vessel)
-therapy	treatment	thermo**therapy** (treatment with heat)
-trophy	development	hyper**trophy** (excessive development)
-ule	small	ven**ule** (small vein)

Table 2-8
Differences in Singular and Plural Endings

WORD ENDING (SINGULAR VERSION)	WORD ENDING (PLURAL VERSION)	EXAMPLE OF SINGULAR USE	EXAMPLE OF PLURAL USE
-a	**-ae**	vertebr**a**	vertebr**ae**
-ax	**-ces**	thor**ax**	thora**ces**
-ex; -ix; -xy	**-ices**	append**ix**	append**ices**
-is	**-es**	metastas**is**	metastas**es**
-ma	**-mata**	sarco**ma**	sarco**mata**
-nx; -anx; -inx; -ynx	**-nges**	phala**nx**	phala**nges**
-on	**-a**	ganglio**n**	gangli**a**
-um	**-a**	ov**um**	ov**a**
-us	**-i**	fung**us**	fung**i**

Bibliography

Basco R, Allan B. *Medical Language for Modern Health Care.* 5th ed. McGraw-Hill; 2023.
Fremgen BF, Frucht SS. *Medical Terminology: A Living Language.* 7th ed. Pearson; 2019.
Mosby's Dictionary of Medicine, Nursing & Health Professions. 10th ed. Elsevier; 2017.
Shiland BJ. *Mastering Healthcare Terminology.* 6th ed. Elsevier; 2019.
Venes D, ed. *Taber's Cyclopedic Medical Dictionary.* 24th ed. F. A. Davis; 2021.

NOTES

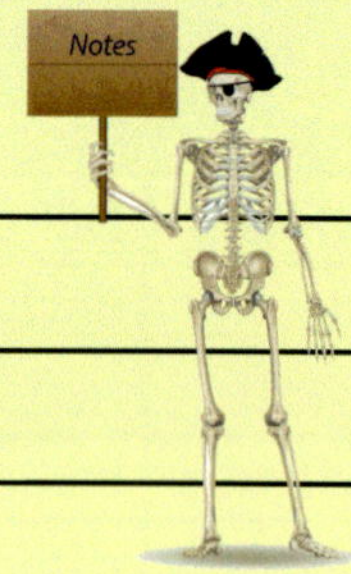

NOTES

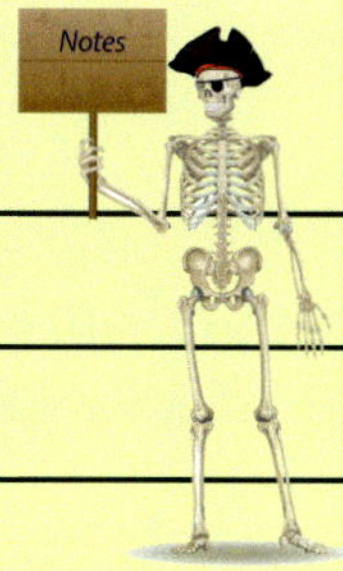

Learning Activities

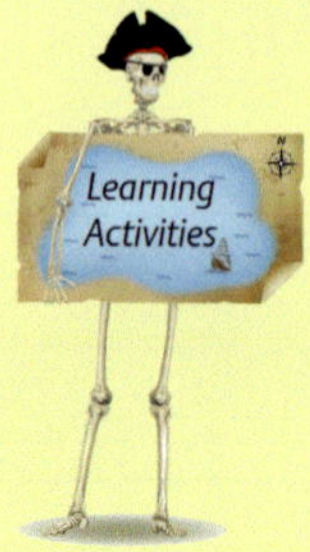

Name:______________________

Word Building: An Introduction to Prefixes and Suffixes

A. Matching: Combining forms.

Match the combining form with its meaning.

1. andr/o_______	a. chest
2. ren/o________	b. female
3. glyc/o_______	c. shape
4. ur/o_________	d. nose
5. somat/o______	e. kidney
6. steth/o______	f. water
7. hydr/o_______	g. male
8. estr/o_______	h. body
9. morph/o_____	i. sugar
10.rhin/o_______	j. urine

B. Matching: Prefixes.

Match the prefix with its meaning.

1. **inter-**________	a. without
2. **tetra-**________	b. within
3. **nulli-**________	c. together
4. **a-**___________	d. four
5. **meso-**_______	e. two
6. **bi-**__________	f. before
7. **intra-**_______	g. three
8. **syn-**_________	h. between
9. **ante-**________	i. middle
10.**tri-**_________	j. none

C. Matching: Suffixes.

Match the suffix with its meaning.

1. **-stenosis**_____	a. enlargement
2. **-algia**_______	b. study of
3. **-megaly**_____	c. fear
4. **-rrhage**______	d. cell
5. **-logist**______	e. narrowing
6. **-itis**________	f. pertaining to
7. **-cyte**________	g. excessive flow
8. **-logy**_______	h. one who studies
9. **-phobia**______	i. pain
10. **-ic**_________	j. inflammation

D. Locate and define the prefix for the following words.

1. pericarditis___________________________
2. hypodermic___________________________
3. tetralogy_____________________________
4. intraarticular_________________________
5. cyanotic______________________________
6. apnea________________________________
7. extrapulmonary______________________
8. supracondylar________________________
9. substernal____________________________
10.epigastric____________________________

2

E. Locate and define the suffix for the following words.

1. hematoma_________________________
2. carditis_________________________
3. chemotherapy_________________________
4. phagocyte_________________________
5. macrocytic_________________________
6. cephalgia_________________________
7. glycolysis_________________________
8. dietary_________________________
9. diarrhea_________________________
10. cytoplasm_________________________

F. For the following words, separate the combining form from the prefix or suffix and write out the meaning.

1. orbitopathy______________________________
2. osteocyte______________________________
3. myalgia______________________________
4. rhinorrhea______________________________
5. periarterial______________________________
6. orthodontic______________________________
7. encephalitis______________________________
8. supraorbital______________________________
9. orchidectomy______________________________
10. ectomorph______________________________

3

Body Organization and Anatomical Directions

Objectives

After studying this chapter, you will be able to:

1. Identify the systems of the body.
2. List the components of the body systems.
3. Translate medical words pertaining to areas of the body.
4. Identify anatomical direction and positions.
5. Label the planes of the body.

Chapter Outline

- Checklist of new combining forms in the chapter
- The systems of the human body
- Body cavities
- Body anatomical position
- Body planes
- Combining forms and terms relating to movement
- Combining forms associated with parts of the body
- Learning activities

Checklist of New Combining Forms in the Chapter

☐ **abdomin/o**
☐ **adip/o**
☐ **anter/o**
☐ **brachi/o**
☐ **bronch/o**
☐ **cardi/o**
☐ **carp/o**
☐ **caud/o**
☐ **cephal/o**
☐ **crani/o**
☐ **crur/o**
☐ **derm/o**
☐ **dermat/o**
☐ **dist/o**
☐ **dors/o**
☐ **femor/o**
☐ **glute/o**
☐ **hem/o**
☐ **hemat/o**
☐ **hist/o**
☐ **infer/o**
☐ **later/o**
☐ **lymph/o**
☐ **medi/o**
☐ **neur/o**
☐ **ocul/o**
☐ **or/o**
☐ **ot/o**

- ☐ **patell/o**
- ☐ **ped/i**
- ☐ **ped/o**
- ☐ **phalang/o**
- ☐ **pod/o**
- ☐ **poster/o**
- ☐ **proxim/o**
- ☐ **pub/o**
- ☐ **pulm/o**
- ☐ **pulmon/o**
- ☐ **super/o**
- ☐ **umbilic/o**
- ☐ **ventr/o**
- ☐ **vertebr/o**

The Systems of the Human Body

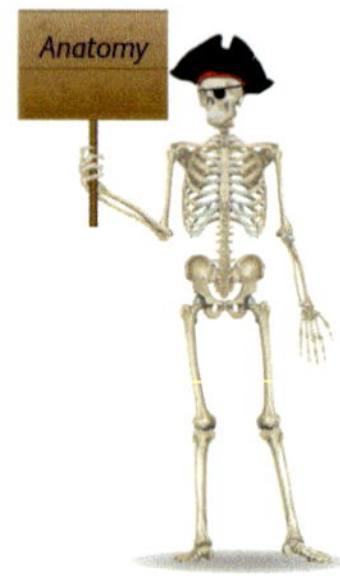

The human body is organized into specialized systems (Figure 3-1). Each system is unique, but interacts with other systems so as to allow the whole body to function properly. Knowing the names, components, and functions of the systems is critical to fully appreciating medical terminology.

Health care providers typically evaluate patients by performing a review of systems (ROS). In a ROS, the health care provider begins the examination at the patient's head and continues by body system (eg, neurological, cardiovascular) through the whole body. Therefore, knowledge of the composition of each system is important to those working in the health care field. Table 3-1 provides a list of the human body systems and the contents of them.

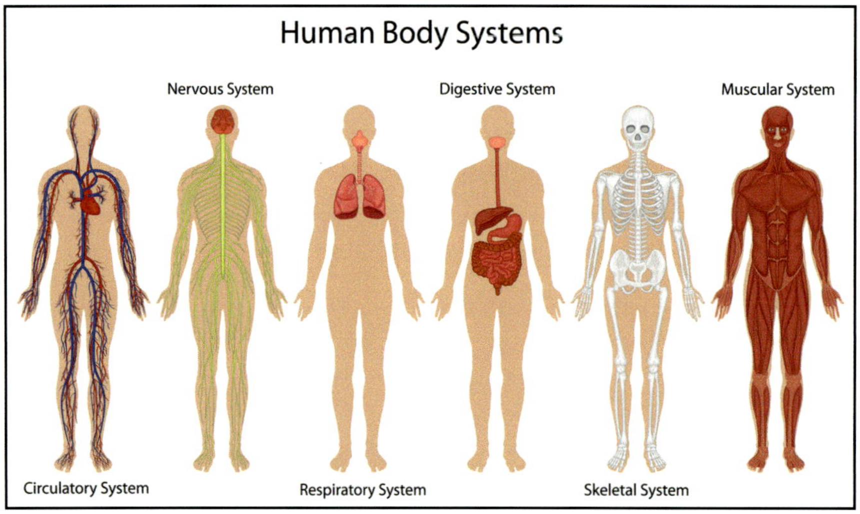

Figure 3-1. Human body systems. (Matthew Cole/shutterstock.com)

Table 3-1
The Systems of the Body and Their Components

SYSTEM	COMPONENTS
musculoskeletal (Chapter 5)	Muscles, bones, ligaments, joints
cardiovascular (Chapter 6)	Heart, blood vessels, lymph nodes and vessels, spleen, thymus, tonsils
respiratory (Chapter 7)	Lungs, pharynx (throat), larynx (voice box), trachea (windpipe)
neurological (Chapter 8)	Brain, spinal cord, nerves
gastrointestinal (Chapter 9)	Mouth, tongue, teeth, esophagus, stomach, intestines, liver, gallbladder, pancreas
integumentary (Chapter 10)	Skin, hair, sweat glands, sebaceous glands
endocrine (Chapter 11)	Thyroid, pituitary gland, adrenal glands, pancreas, parathyroid
urinary (Chapter 12)	Kidneys, ureters, urinary bladder, urethra
reproductive (Chapter 13)	Testes, penis, prostate gland, ovaries, fallopian tubes, uterus, vagina, mammary glands
sensory (Chapter 14)	Nose, eyes, ears

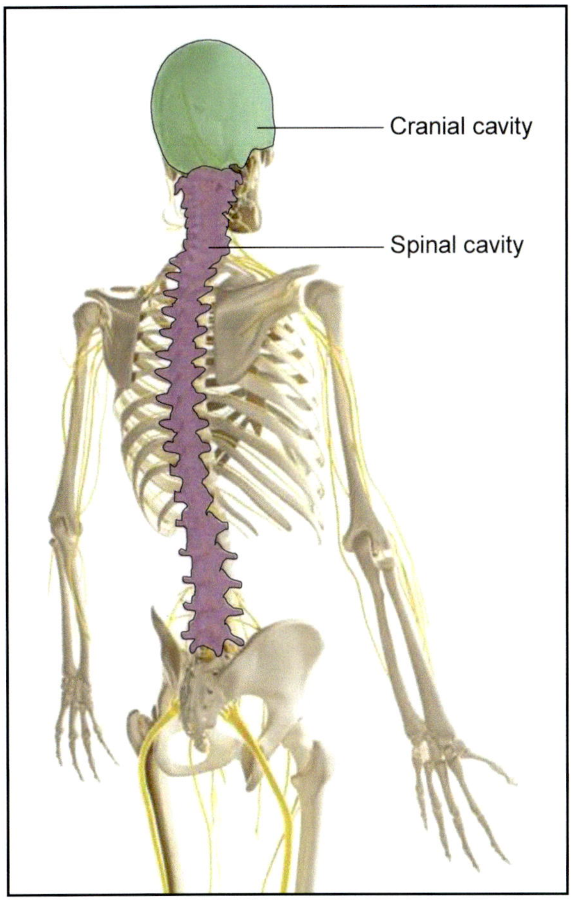

Figure 3-2. Cranial and spinal body cavities lie in the dorsal aspect of the body. (Sebastin Kaulilzki/shutterstock.com)

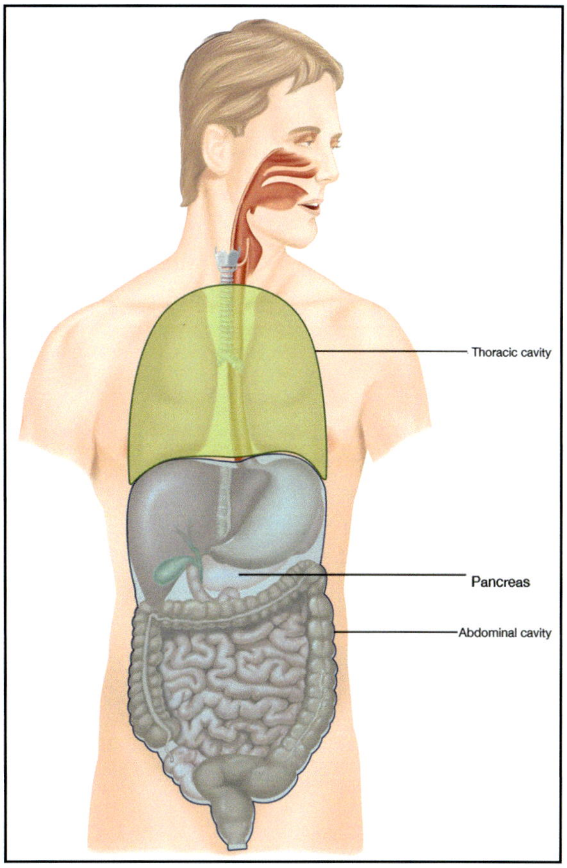

Figure 3-3. Thoracic and abdominal body cavities are found in the ventral (anterior) aspect of the body.

Body Cavities

In addition to body systems, there are specific anatomical regions in the body. These regions relate to the general location of certain body organs. All of these have terms related to them so health care providers can be accurate when describing locations (of pain, swelling, etc) to colleagues. The body has two distinct locations (dorsal and ventral) that are further divided into five body cavities (Figures 3-2 and 3-3; Table 3-2). **Dorsal** (posterior) cavities hold the brain and spinal cord, and **ventral** (anterior) cavities contain most of the rest of the body's organs. If you notice, some organs are not contained within a cavity. The kidneys are two organs that reside in the **retroperitoneal** (**retro-**—behind; peritoneum—the tough membrane that lines the entire abdominal cavity) space and are therefore not within a cavity.

The dorsal and ventral cavities are general locations, whereas the abdominal cavity, for example, is not only divided into four quadrants (Table 3-3; Figure 3-4), but it also has nine identified surface regions (Figure 3-5). Both the quadrants and regions are named for their anatomical location.

Table 3-2
Body Cavities

BODY CAVITY	COMPONENTS	
cranial	• Brain	
spinal	• Spinal cord	
thoracic	• Pleural cavity (lungs) • Mediastinum (heart, thymus, trachea, esophagus)	
abdominal	• Stomach • Spleen • Liver	• Gallbladder • Pancreas • Intestines
pelvic	• Urinary bladder, ureters, urethra, some of the intestines • Prostate • Ovaries, fallopian tubes, uterus, vagina	

Table 3-3
Abdominal Quadrants

ABDOMINAL QUADRANTS	MAJOR COMPONENTS
right upper quadrant (RUQ)	• Gallbladder • Liver • Pancreas* • Small intestine*
right lower quadrant (RLQ)	• Appendix • Right ovary • Right fallopian tube • Right ureter • Small intestine* • Large intestine*
left upper quadrant (LUQ)	• Spleen • Liver* • Pancreas* • Small intestine* • Large intestine*
left lower quadrant (LLQ)	• Left ovary • Left fallopian tube • Left ureter • Small intestine* • Large intestine*

*Indicates that only a portion of the organ lies within the specified quadrant.

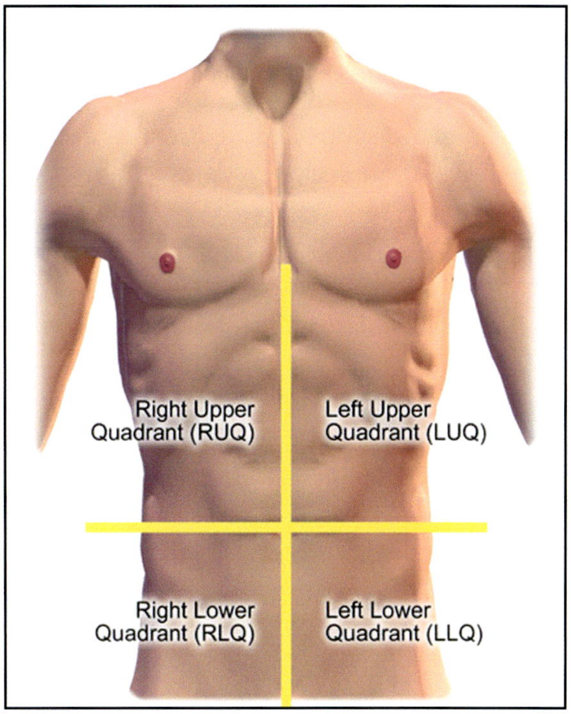

Figure 3-4. Quadrants of the abdomen. (BlueRingMedia/shutterstock.com)

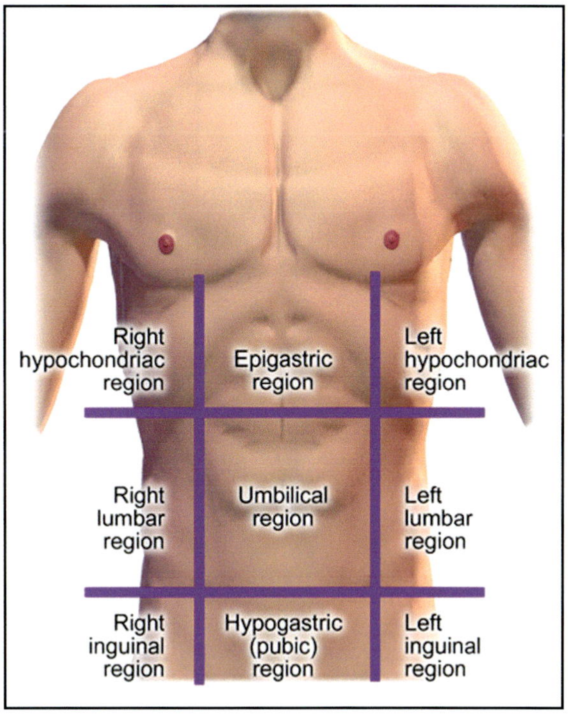

Figure 3-5. The nine regions of the abdomen. (BlueRingMedia/shutterstock.com)

Body Anatomical Position

Anatomical position refers to a person standing with arms at the sides, palms facing forward, and with the head and feet facing forward. It is the position from which anatomical directions begin, and is a reference to describe sites (Figure 3-6).

Figure 3-6. Anatomical position—facing forward with palms of the hands and feet also facing forward. (BioMedical/shutterstock.com)

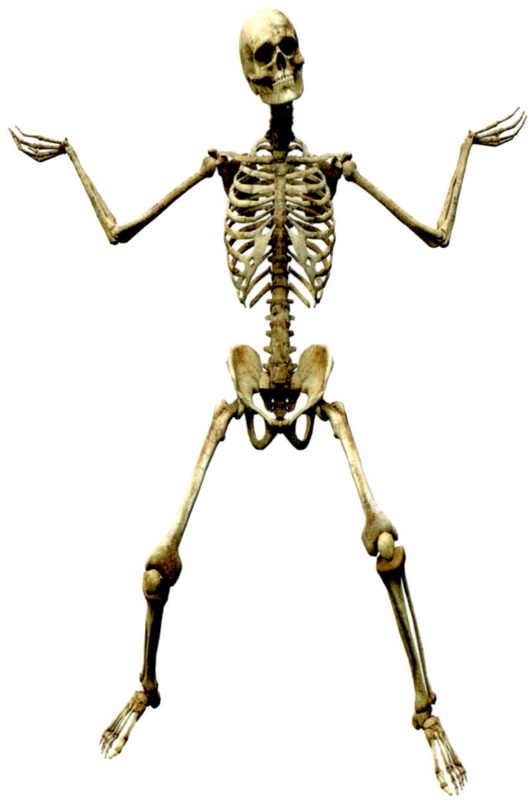

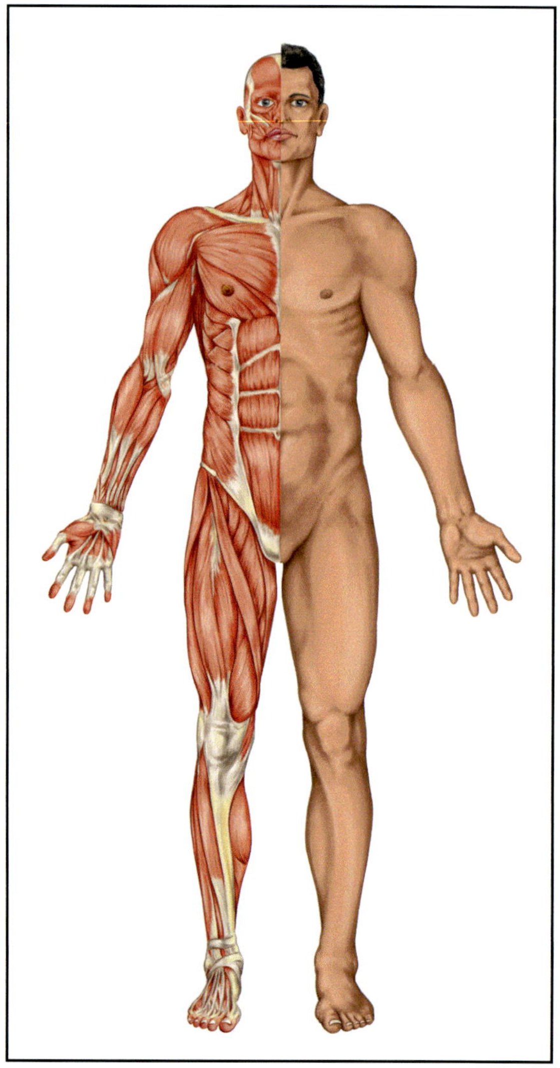

Body Planes

There are three main anatomical planes of the body that assist when describing the location of something or with performing certain tests (eg, x-rays). The **frontal** (**coronal**) plane divides the body into front (anterior) and back (posterior) halves, the **sagittal** plane passes through the body separating the right and left sides, and the **transverse** (**horizontal**) (frontal) plane splits the upper (superior) and lower (inferior) aspects. These planes do not necessarily split in perfect halves and are shown in Figure 3-7.

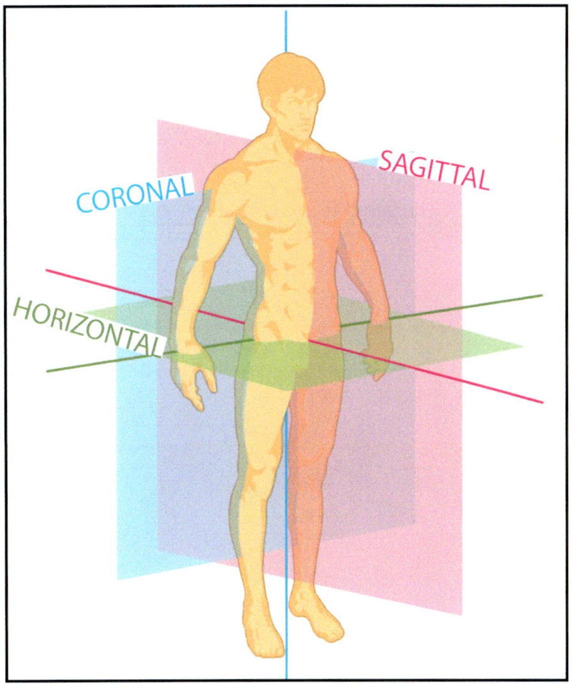

Figure 3-7. Planes of the body. (stihii/shutterstock.com)

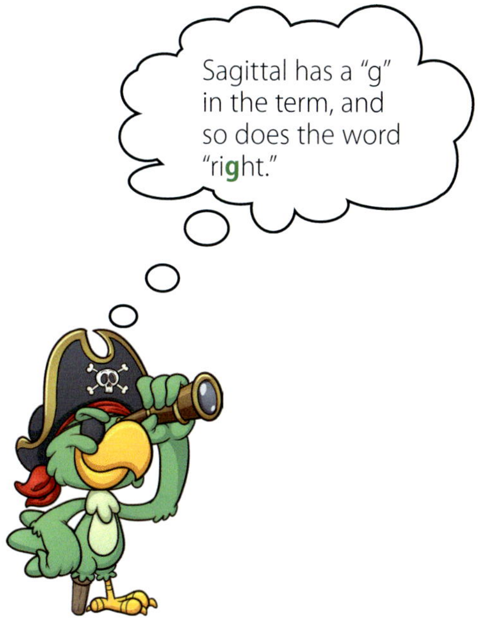
Sagittal has a "g" in the term, and so does the word "right."

3

Combining Forms and Terms Relating to Movement

Table 3-4

Anatomical Directions/Explanations

COMBINING FORM	DIRECTION/DEFINITION
anter/o	Anterior: Pertaining to the front of the body
dist/o	Distal: A farther distance from another body part/main body; the tips of the fingers are distal to the wrist (Figure 3-8)
dors/o	Dorsal: Pertaining to the back of the body (think of the dorsal fin on a shark)
infer/o	Inferior: Below; in relation to another body part
later/o	Lateral: Away from the midline of the body; in relation to another body part
medi/o	Medial: Toward the midline of the body; in relation to another body part
poster/o	Posterior: Pertaining to the back of the body
proxim/o	Proximal: Closer to the main body or point of attachment
super/o	Above: In relation to another body part
ventr/o	Ventral: Pertaining to the front of the body

Figure 3-8. Directional terms. (Sabasatin Kaulitzki/shutterstock.com)

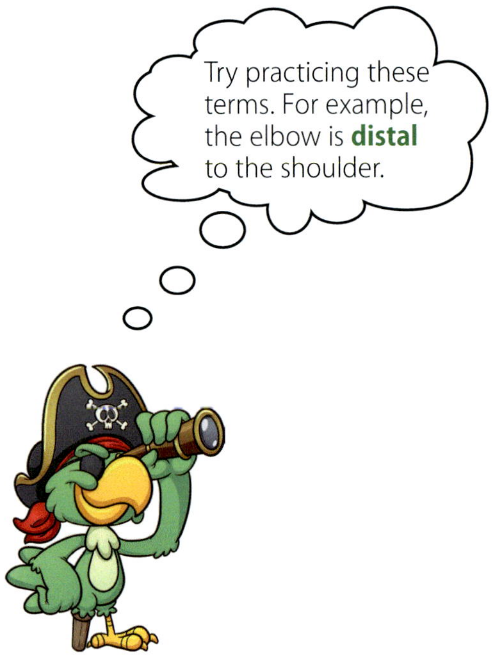
Try practicing these terms. For example, the elbow is **distal** to the shoulder.

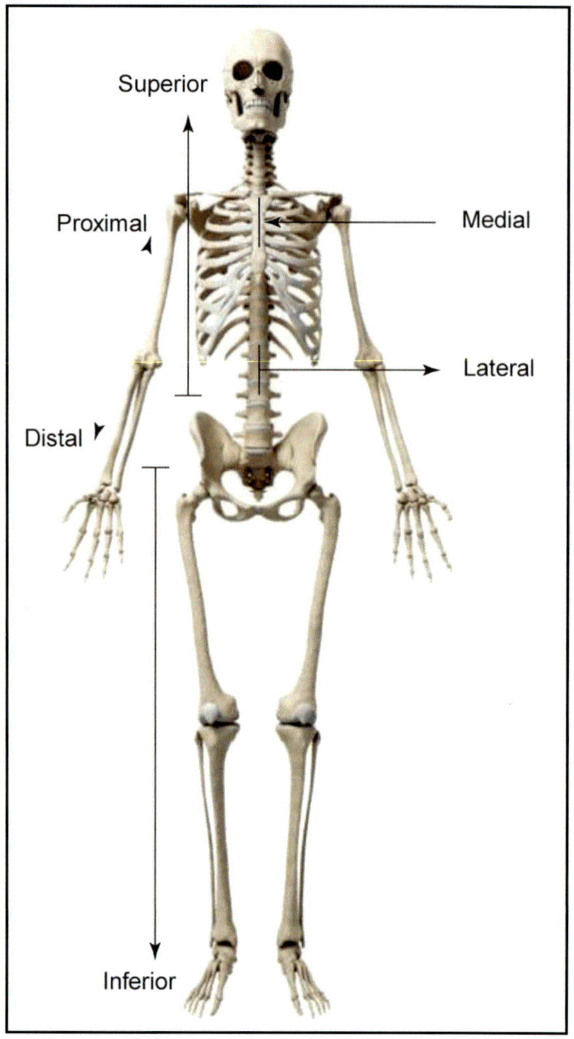

Table 3-5

Terms Relating to Movement of the Body

TERM	DEFINITION
abduction	To move an arm or leg away from the body
adduction	To move an arm or leg closer to the body (to **add** to the body)
extension	To straighten a joint, increasing the angle between two bones
flexion	To bend a joint, moving two bones closer together
lateral bend	To bend the trunk sideways
rotation	To rotate a body part, such as the neck or shoulder; not all body parts rotate; the humerus internally (turns in toward the body) and externally (turns away from the body) rotates

Note that these terms refer to movement from a body in anatomical position (Figures 3-9 and 3-10).

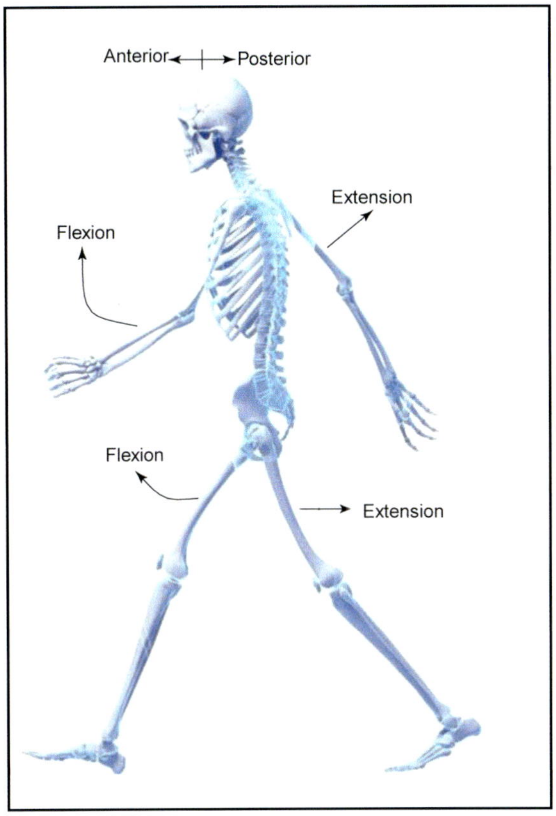

Figure 3-9. Flexion occurs on the anterior aspect of the body; extension occurs on the posterior aspect. (Sebastin Kaulilzki/shutterstock.com)

Figure 3-10. Adduction (to move toward the midline; to "add") and abduction (to move away from the midline) occur at the shoulder and hip joints. (Sebastin Kaulilzki/shutterstock.com)

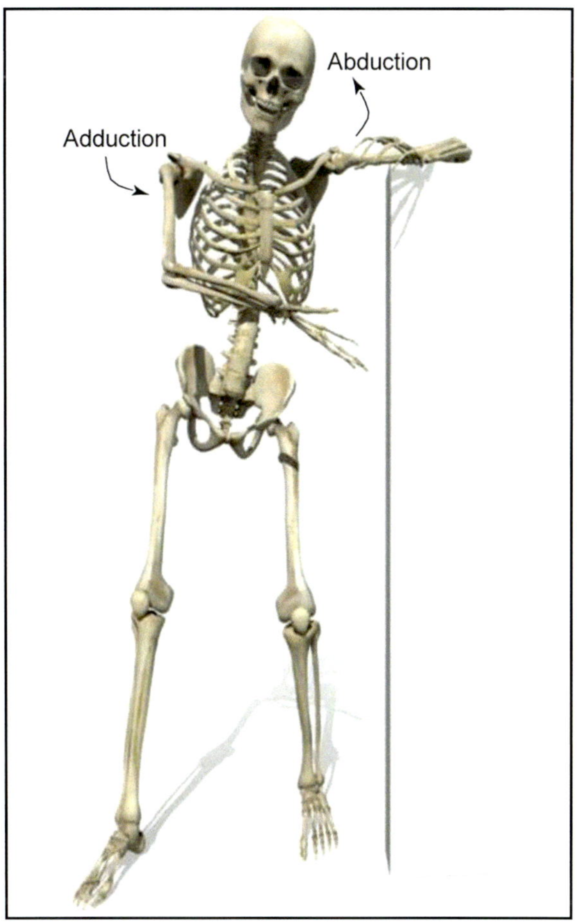

TABLE 3-6 MOVEMENT PERTAINING TO THE LIMBS (FIGURE 3-11)	
MOVEMENT SPECIFIC TO THE ANKLE	
inversion	To turn the ankle by rolling the sole of the foot inward; also invert. Opposite of eversion
eversion	To turn the ankle by rolling the sole of the foot outward; also evert. Opposite of inversion
dorsiflexion	To pull the toes up toward the shin (Figure 3-12)
plantar flexion	To point the toes down

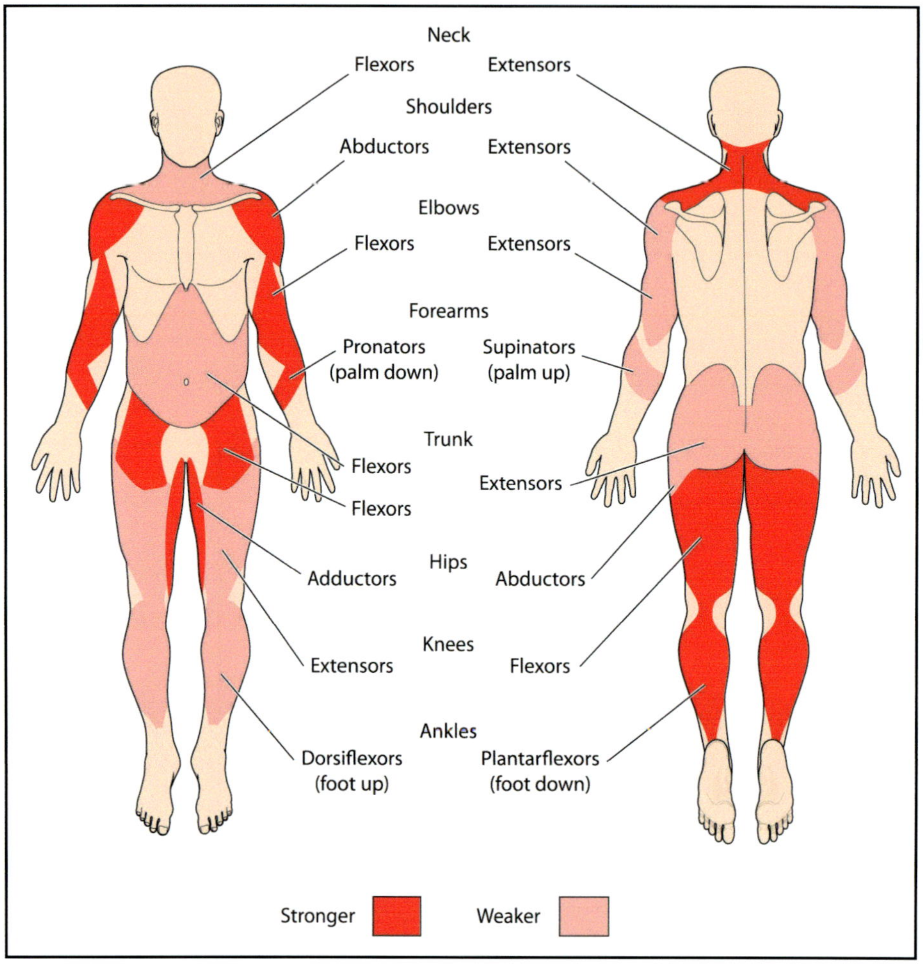

Figure 3-11. Muscles that act on body movement according to function. (Blamb/shutterstock.com)

MOVEMENT SPECIFIC TO THE HANDS AND FEET	
pronation	In the forearm/hand: To turn the palm downward (Figure 3-13) In the foot: To move the sole of the foot outward
radial deviation	To move the thumb side of the wrist away from the body (Figure 3-14)
supination	In the forearm/hand: To turn the hand upward (holding a bowl of soup) In the foot: To roll the sole of the foot inward
ulnar deviation	To move the pinky (5th phalange) side of the wrist toward the body

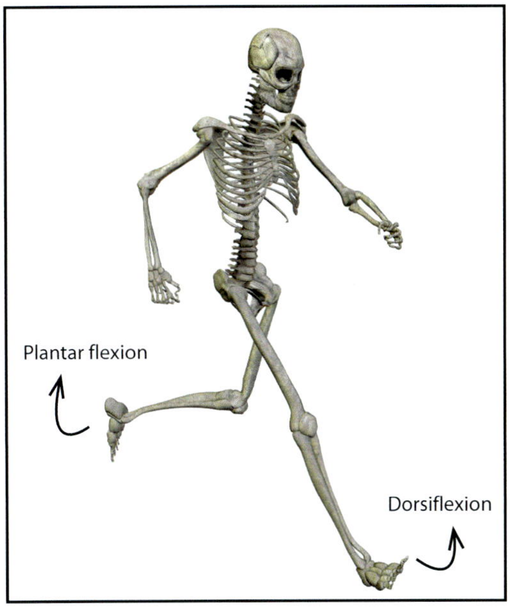

Figure 3-12. Dorsiflexion and plantar flexion. (design36/shutterstock.com)

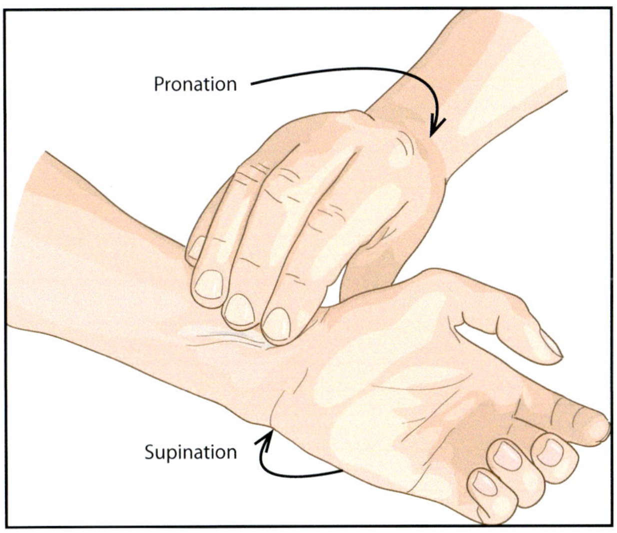

Figure 3-13. Pronation and supination. (grib_nick/shutterstock.com)

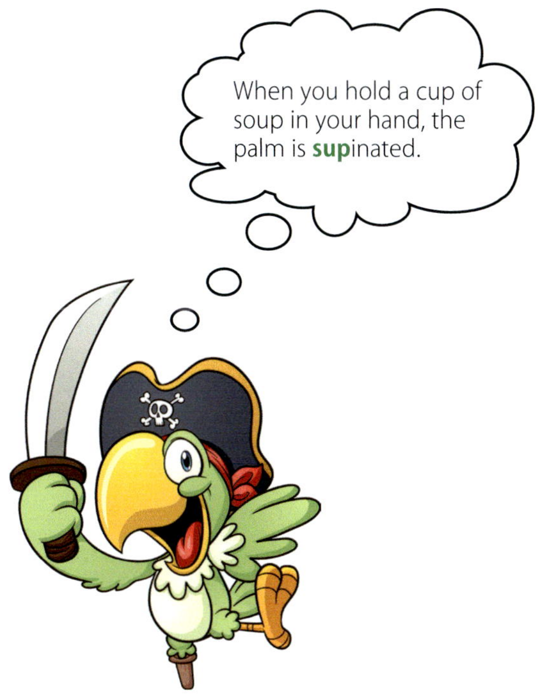
When you hold a cup of soup in your hand, the palm is **sup**inated.

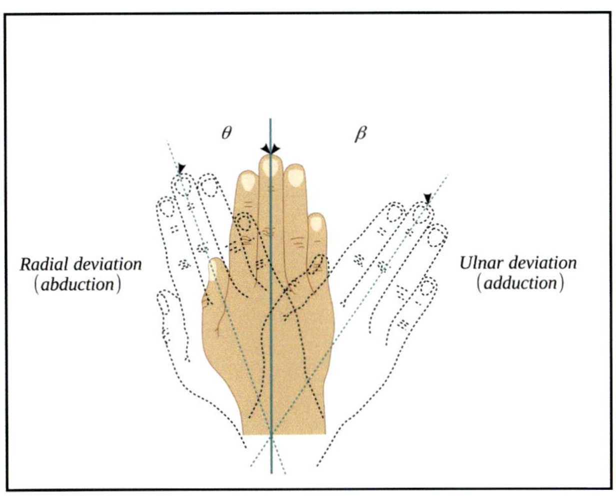

Figure 3-14. Ulnar and radial deviation. (ScientificStock/shutterstock.com)

Combining Forms Associated With Parts of the Body

Table 3-7

Combining Forms Associated With Body Components

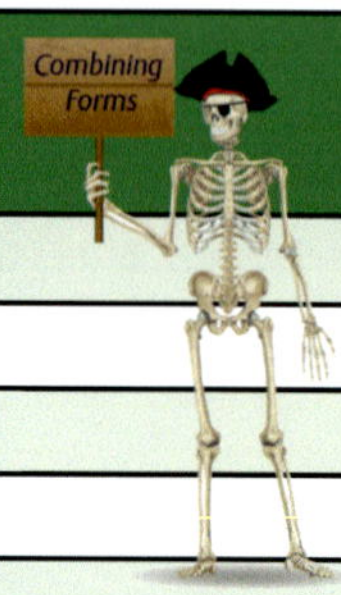

COMBINING FORM	DEFINITION
abdomin/o	abdomen
adip/o	fat
brachi/o	arm
bronch/o	bronchial tubes
cardi/o	heart
carp/o	carpals; wrist bones
caud/o	tail
cephal/o	head; toward the head; pertaining to the head
crani/o	skull
crur/o	leg
derm/o; dermat/o	skin
femor/o	thigh bone
glute/o	buttocks
hem/o; hemat/o	blood
hist/o	tissue
lymph/o	lymph (the watery substance originating in organs and tissues)
neur/o	nerve
ocul/o	eye
or/o	mouth
ot/o	ear
patell/o	kneecap
ped/i; ped/o	foot; child
phalang/o	finger or toe (bones of)
pod/o	foot
pub/o	pubic bone (of pelvis)
pulm/o; pulmon/o	lung
umbilic/o	navel
vertebr/o	vertebra

Table 3-8
Other Terms Associated With the Human Body

TERM	RELATES TO
palmar	The palm of the hand
plantar	The sole of the foot
prone	Lying on the front, the abdomen (Figure 3-15)
supine	Lying on the back facing up (Figure 3-16)
tarsal	Small bones in the ankle

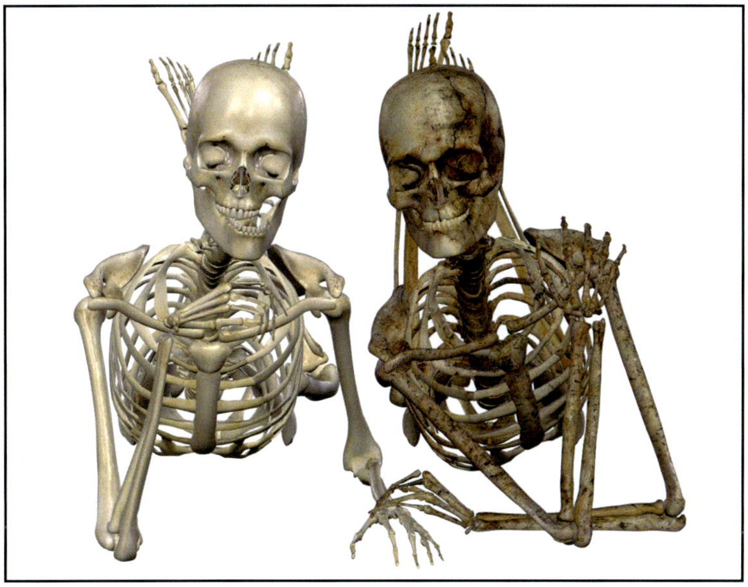

Figure 3-15. Prone position is to lie on your belly. (Andeas Meyer/shutterstock.com)

Figure 3-16. Supine position is to lie face up. (lalilele13/shutterstock.com)

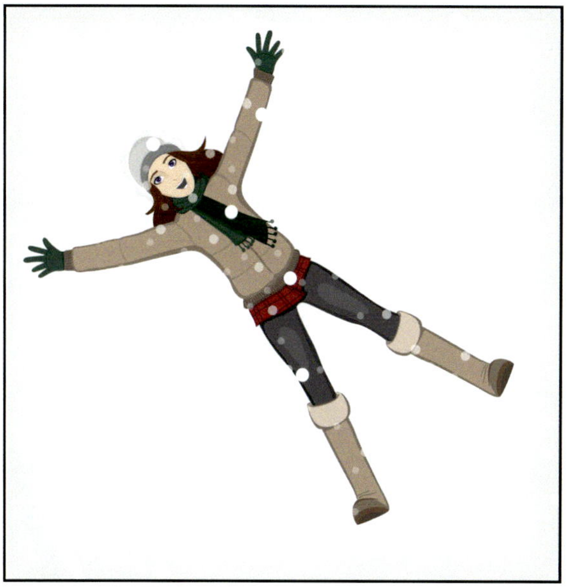

Bibliography

Allan D. *Medical Language for Modern Health Care.* 4th ed. McGraw-Hill; 2019.
Chabner DE. *The Language of Medicine.* 12th ed. Saunders/Elsevier; 2019.
Cohen BJ, Jones SA. *Medical Terminology: An Illustrated Guide.* 9th ed. Jones & Bartlett; 2021.
Fremgen BF, Frucht SS. *Medical Terminology: A Living Language.* 7th ed. Pearson; 2019.
Mosby's Dictionary of Medicine, Nursing & Health Professions. 10th ed. Elsevier; 2017.
Venes D, ed. *Taber's Cyclopedic Medical Dictionary.* 24th ed. F. A. Davis; 2021.

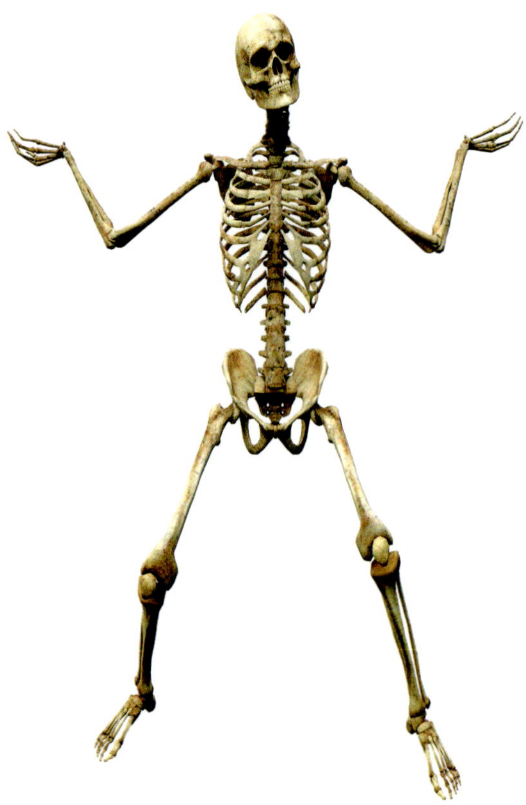

Notes

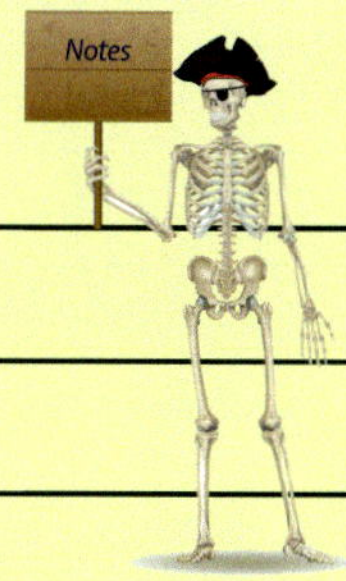

3

NOTES

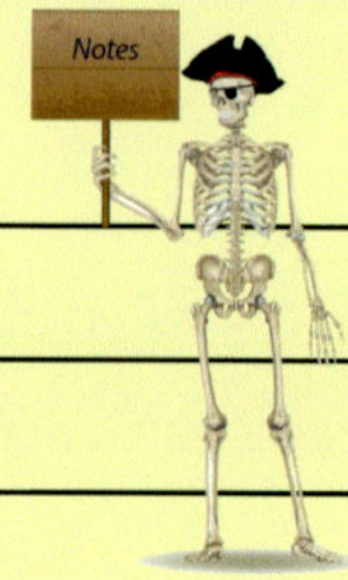

Learning Activities

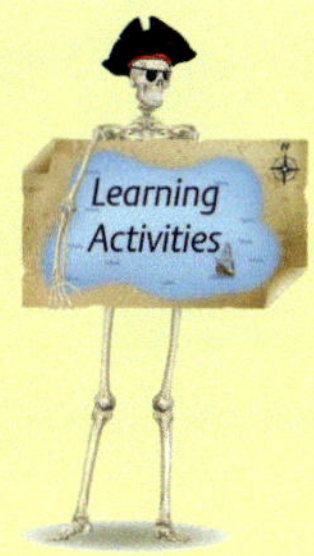

Name:______________________

Body Organization and Anatomical Directions

A. Matching: Combining forms.

Match the combining form with its meaning.

1. brachi/o_____	a. below
2. pod/o_______	b. eye
3. or/o_________	c. ear
4. dors/o_______	d. tissue
5. ocul/o_______	e. fat
6. hist/o_______	f. blood
7. adip/o_______	g. back
8. infer/o______	h. mouth
9. ot/o_________	i. foot
10. hem/o_______	j. arm

B. Match the correct directional terms from the following list.

- anterior
- posterior
- proximal
- distal
- superior
- inferior
- lateral
- medial

1. ______________
2. ______________
3. ______________
4. ______________
5. ______________
6. ______________
7. ______________
8. ______________

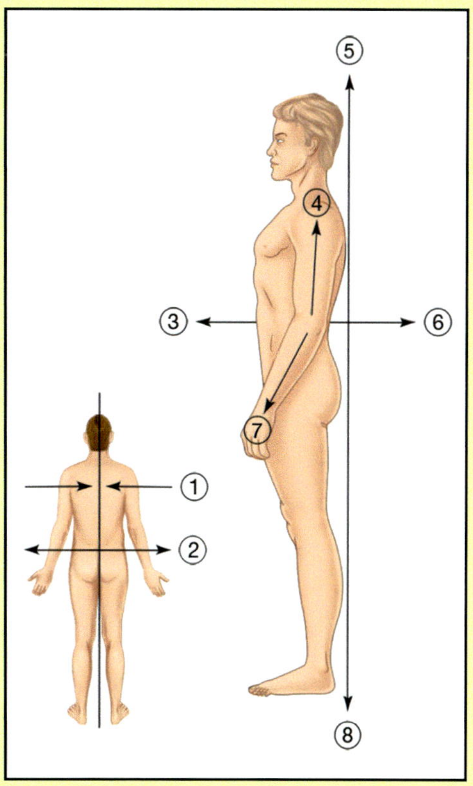

C. Label the correct plane.

1. ____________________
2. ____________________
3. ____________________

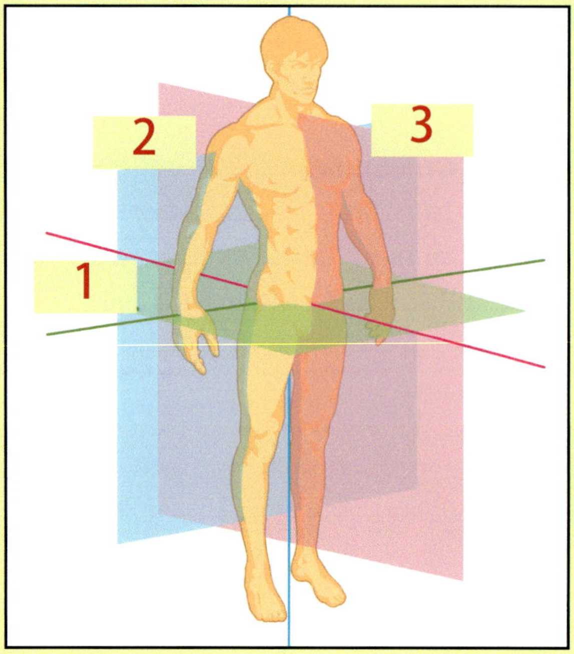

(stihii/shutterstock.com)

D. Using this list, place the tissues in the correct row identified by system. One has been done for you.

Bones, brain, fallopian tubes, gallbladder, hair, heart, kidneys, ligaments, liver, lungs, muscles, nerves, ovaries, pancreas, pharynx, pituitary, prostate gland, sebaceous glands, skin, spinal cord, spleen, thymus, tongue, trachea, ureter, urinary bladder

SYSTEM	TISSUE	TISSUE	TISSUE
endocrine	*thyroid*		
reproductive			
integumentary			
respiratory			
neurological			
gastrointestinal			
urinary			
musculoskeletal			
cardiovascular			

3

E. Separate the combining form from the prefix or suffix and define the following words.

1. neurogenesis *neur/o/genesis: formation of a nerve cell*
2. epicardium__________
3. bronchitis__________
4. cephalgia__________
5. otorrhea__________
6. periumbilical__________
7. extraocular__________
8. erythroderma__________
9. pulmonologist__________
10. hematoma__________

4

Therapeutic and Diagnostic Procedures

Objectives

After studying this chapter, you will be able to:

1. Describe common terms that relate to therapeutic and diagnostic procedures.
2. Differentiate between a sign and a symptom.
3. List categories of therapy.
4. Define common laboratory, therapeutic, and diagnostic tests.
5. Define terms related to disease testing and control.
6. Understand the differences in medical specialties based on the suffix.

Chapter Outline

- Checklist for word parts in the chapter
- Key terms for therapy and diagnoses
- Combining forms
- Therapy categories
- Words relating to medical conditions and therapeutic and diagnostic procedures
- Prefixes
- Suffixes
- Therapeutic and diagnostic procedures
- Learning activities

Flanagan KW.
Medical Terminology With Case Studies: A Navigated Guide to Learning for Health Care Professionals, Third Edition (pp 45-65).

CHECKLIST FOR WORD PARTS IN THE CHAPTER

Prefixes

- ☐ an-
- ☐ anti-
- ☐ epi-
- ☐ hyper-
- ☐ pan-
- ☐ trans-
- ☐ ultra-

Suffixes

- ☐ -centesis
- ☐ -desis
- ☐ -ectomy
- ☐ -er
- ☐ -gram
- ☐ -graph
- ☐ -graphy
- ☐ -ian
- ☐ -iatrical
- ☐ -iatrician
- ☐ -iatrics
- ☐ -iatrist
- ☐ -iatry
- ☐ -ic
- ☐ -ics
- ☐ -ist
- ☐ -meter
- ☐ -metry
- ☐ -ostomy
- ☐ -otomy
- ☐ -pexy
- ☐ -plasty
- ☐ -porosis
- ☐ -rrhaphy
- ☐ -scope
- ☐ -scopy
- ☐ -stomy
- ☐ -tome
- ☐ -tomy
- ☐ -tripsy

Combining Forms

- ☐ aer/o
- ☐ angi/o
- ☐ audi/o
- ☐ bar/o
- ☐ bi/o
- ☐ chrom/o
- ☐ chromat/o
- ☐ cry/o
- ☐ electro/o
- ☐ erg/o
- ☐ fluor/o
- ☐ neur/o
- ☐ orth/o
- ☐ pedi/o
- ☐ phon/o
- ☐ phot/o
- ☐ pod/o
- ☐ radi/o
- ☐ son/o
- ☐ therm/o
- ☐ ultra

KEY TERMS FOR THERAPY AND DIAGNOSES

Prior to discussing therapeutic and diagnostic procedures, a few words need to be added to your vocabulary. These words are commonly used when discussing a specific condition and are relevant when conferring about illness, trauma, injury, or disease.

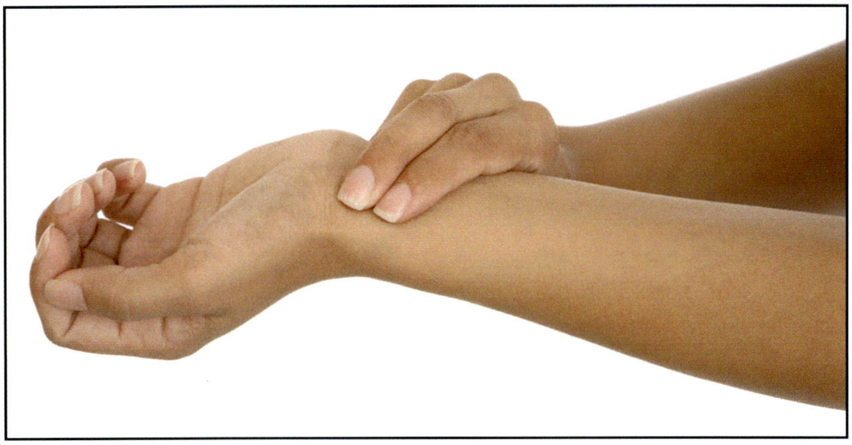

Figure 4-1. Heart rate. Palpate the radial artery to count the heart beats per minute. (caimacanul/shutterstock.com)

- **Sign** Something that is seen and can be verified. Swelling, bruising deformity, rash, and high body temperature are all examples of **signs**.
- **Symptom (Sx)** Something patients tell you they feel or have. Dizziness, nausea, headache, itchy skin, and blurry vision are all symptoms.
- **Acute** Sudden onset. For example, an athlete sustained an acute injury when they sprained their ankle last night at a game.
- **Chronic** Lasting a while (chron/o = time). For example, diabetes is a chronic disease.
- **Diagnosis (Dx)** What the health care provider believes is the medical condition. Diagnosing a condition requires a multistep approach. One method of recording an organized assessment is **SOAP**, which stands for Subjective, Objective, Assessment, and Plan. Briefly, the **Subjective** category contains information the patient tells the health care provider about their main complaint and present illness. **Objective** is what the medical care provider discovers through the medical record, observation, and other measurable tests. **Assessment** is a list of problems/symptoms the patient has, as well as a list of what the condition may be (the differential diagnosis). **Plan** is what the health care provider intends to do to treat the condition or assign further diagnostic tests or referrals to narrow the diagnosis down. A follow-up time period is typically mentioned in the Plan.
- **Differential diagnosis (Dd)** A group of possible diagnoses that have similar presentations or symptoms.
- **Prognosis** The outcome of a given condition.
- **Sequela** (plural is **Sequelae**) The consequences of a given condition, a result of a specific disease or trauma, often a complication. For example, difficulty sleeping may be the sequela of a concussion.

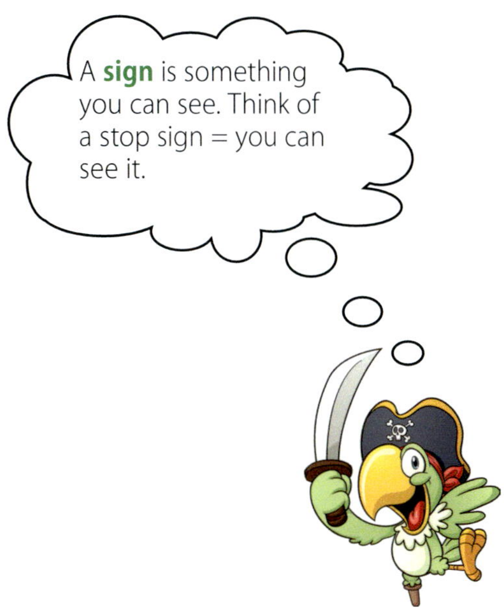
A sign is something you can see. Think of a stop sign = you can see it.

- **Vital signs** (**VS**) Measurements taken and compared to national norms, as well as the patient's normal values. These signs consist of heart rate (**HR**), respiration (breathing) rate (**RR**), blood pressure (**BP**), and temperature (**T**). HR and RR are measured in minutes (Figure 4-1), and BP is measured via a stethoscope and sphygmomanometer (blood pressure cuff) in millimeters of mercury (mm Hg; Figure 4-2). In the United States, temperature is typically measured in Fahrenheit (°F) but is also recorded in a centigrade scale as Celsius (°C; Figure 4-3). It is critical to indicate which unit is being recorded. Together, temperature, pulse, and respiration is abbreviated TPR.

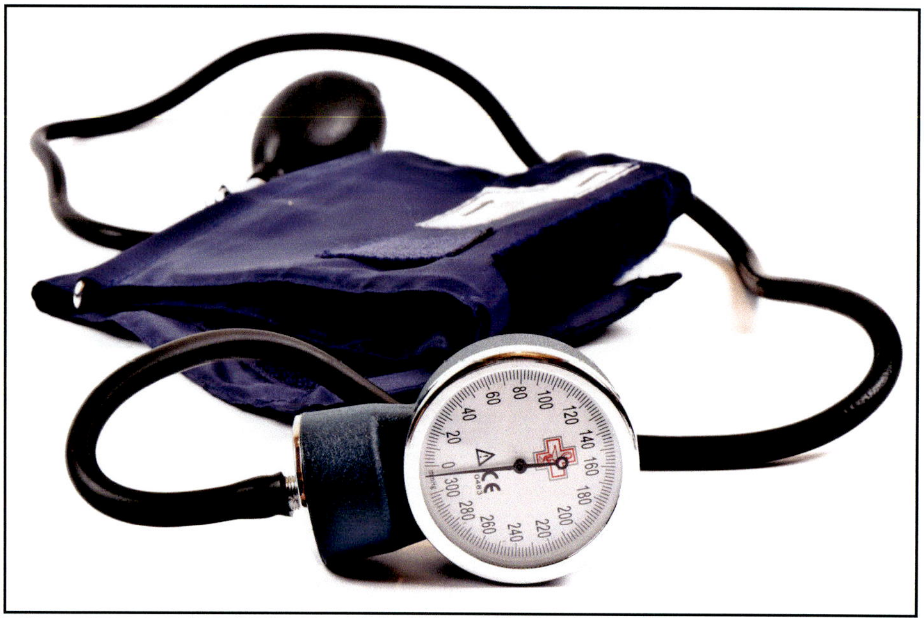

Figure 4-2. Blood pressure. The health care provider uses both a stethoscope and a sphygmomanometer to measure blood pressure. (Uros Zunic/shutterstock.com)

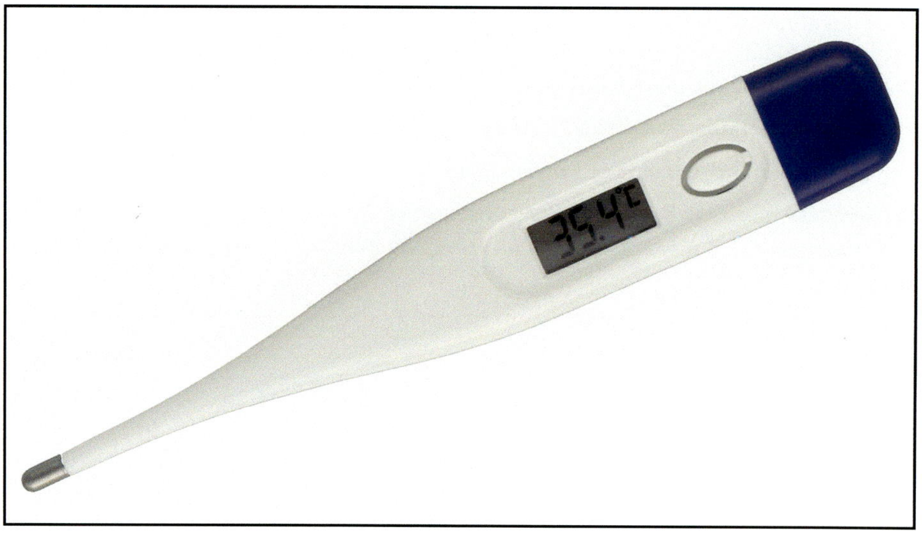

Figure 4-3. An oral thermometer is one way to assess body temperature. (Goh Hock Choon/shutterstock.com)

Combining Forms

The combining forms (Table 4-1) in this chapter pertain mainly to therapy, but they will pop up throughout the textbook. Familiar words such as *aerobic* make more sense when you learn that **aer/o** is the combining form for air; you already know from Chapter 2 that **-ic** is a suffix meaning "pertaining to." Literally translated, *aerobic* means "pertaining to air."

Table 4-1

Combining Forms for Physical Forces

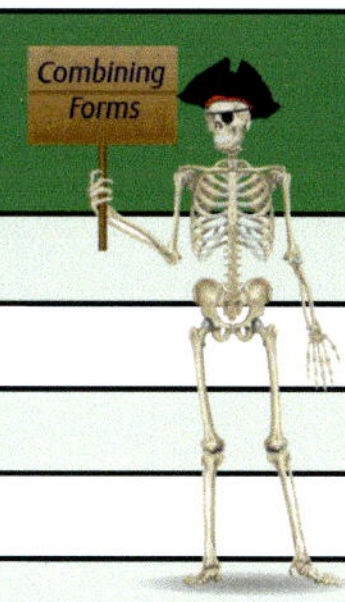

COMBINING FORM	DEFINITION
aer/o	gas; air
bar/o	pressure
chrom/o; chromat/o	color; stain
cry/o	cold
electro/o	electricity
erg/o	work
fluor/o	luminous
phon/o	sound; voice
phot/o	light
radi/o	radiation; x-ray
son/o	sound
therm/o	heat; temperature
ultra	beyond; farther

Therapy Categories

There are seven different forms of therapy commonly used today. Each has benefits and characteristics making it more useful for particular conditions. Acute tendinitis (sudden-onset inflammation of a tendon) responds best to cryotherapy, but chronic tendinitis (occurring over time) reacts better to thermotherapy. Table 4-2 provides a brief overview of the different types of therapy.

Table 4-2

Therapy Categories

THERAPY	EXAMPLES
cryotherapy cry/o (cold)	• Cryokinetics • Compression
thermotherapy therm/o (heat)	• Heat packs • Diathermy
sound	• Ultrasound (**ultra-**—beyond, farther) • Phonophoresis (phon/o—sound)
electricity	• Transcutaneous electrical neuromuscular stimulation (TENS; **trans-**—across; cutan/e—skin; **-ous**—pertaining to; neur/o—nerve) • Electrical muscle stimulation (EMS)
light	• Laser • Ultraviolet (**ultra-**—beyond, farther) • Light emission diode (LED)
mechanical	• Traction • Exercise
oxygen	• Hyperbaric oxygen therapy (HBOT; **hyper-**—excessive; bar/—pressure; **-ic**—pertaining to)

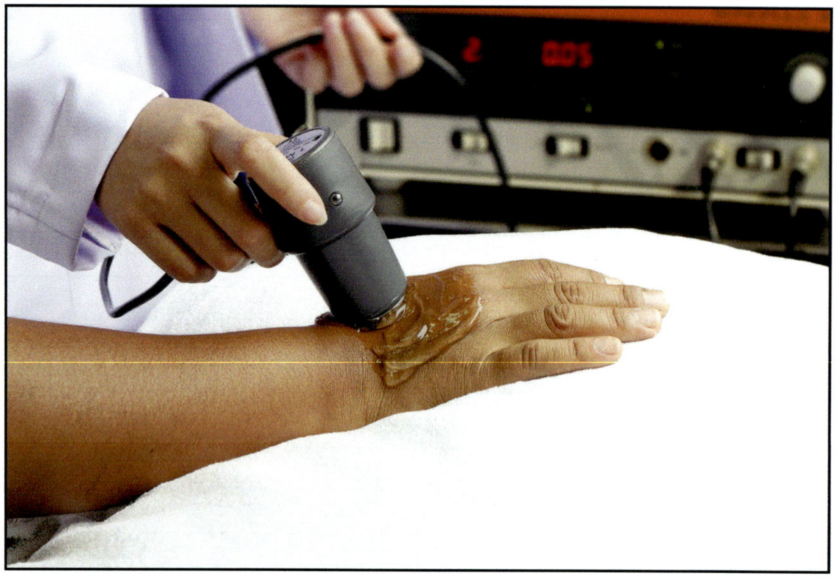

Figure 4-4. Ultrasound used as a therapy. (Praisaeng/shutterstock.com)

Some therapies cross over into more than one type (category). For example, ultrasound is both a sound and thermotherapy. Many forms of therapy can also be used for diagnostic purposes. Depending on the machine and settings, ultrasound can also be either therapeutic or diagnostic (Figure 4-4).

Words Relating to Medical Conditions and Therapeutic and Diagnostic Procedures

Table 4-3 contains words that are used to describe medical conditions, illnesses, and their treatments.

Table 4-3
Words Relating to Medical Conditions and Treatment

WORD	DEFINITION
anesthesia	Absence of all feeling, specifically to pain (**an-**—without)
diaphoresis	Sweating
malaise	Vague, uneasy feeling; often a precursor of a condition/illness
malingering	To fake symptoms; a deliberate attempt to feign a condition or disease
nocturnal	Occurring at night
palliate	To soothe or relieve
palliative treatment	Treatment providing relief but not a cure
pallor	Pale skin color compared to the patient's normal coloring
prodromal	Early symptoms that may indicate the onset of a condition or disease
prophylaxis	Preventing the spread of disease
remission	No sign of a diagnosed disease; lessening of symptoms
staging	Specific process for categorizing malignant (cancerous) tumors
syncope	To faint; a brief lapse in consciousness
syndrome	Specific group of signs and symptoms that indicate a certain disease or condition
triage	Classification of sorting patients for treatment and disposition

Table 4-4 provides a list of words that are usually used in conjunction with treatment or diagnosis of a condition.

Table 4-4

Words Relating to Therapeutic and Diagnostic Procedures

WORD	DEFINITION
auscultation	Act of listening for sounds within the body; most commonly associated with evaluation of the chest or abdomen (Figure 4-5)
biopsy	Removal of a sample of tissue for microscopic examination (bi/o—life)
catheter	Hollow, flexible tube inserted into the body (vessel or cavity) to withdraw or instill fluids
cautery	Tissue purposefully destroyed via heat, chemical, or current
excision	Removal by cutting
fixation	Fastening a structure in a specific position (Figure 4-6)
incision	Cut produced by a sharp surgical instrument
irrigation	Process of washing; cleaning a wound or body cavity
lavage	Process of washing out an organ for therapeutic purposes
ligature	To suture (Figure 4-7)
palpation	To examine by feeling with one's hands
paracentesis	Fluid withdrawn from a body cavity through an incision
percussion	Tapping over cavities to determine characteristics of body organs
resection	Cutting out a significant portion of a structure or organ
sharps	Any sharp item (eg, needle, scalpel) that could cause a wound
speculum	Retractor used to separate walls of a cavity to make visualization possible (Figure 4-8)

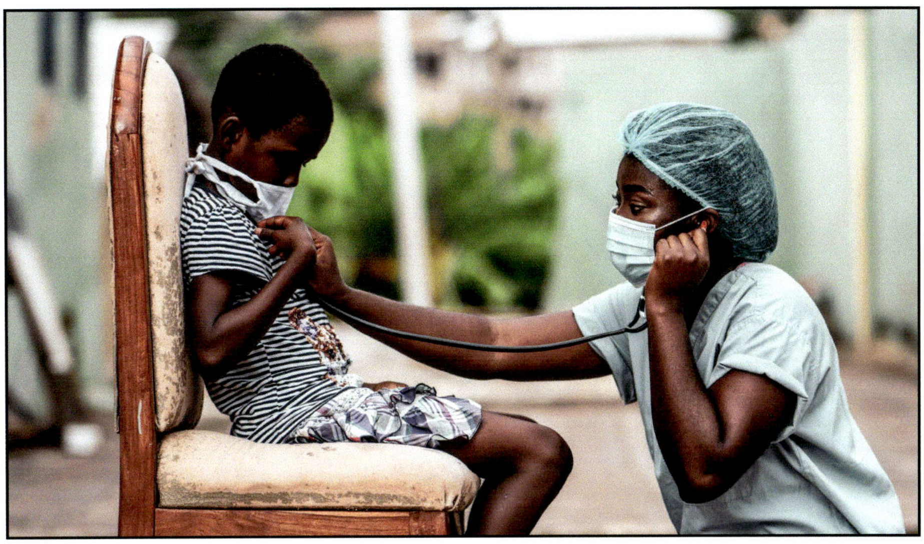

Figure 4-5. Auscultation. Listening to breath sounds through a stethoscope. (Yaw Niel/shutterstock.com)

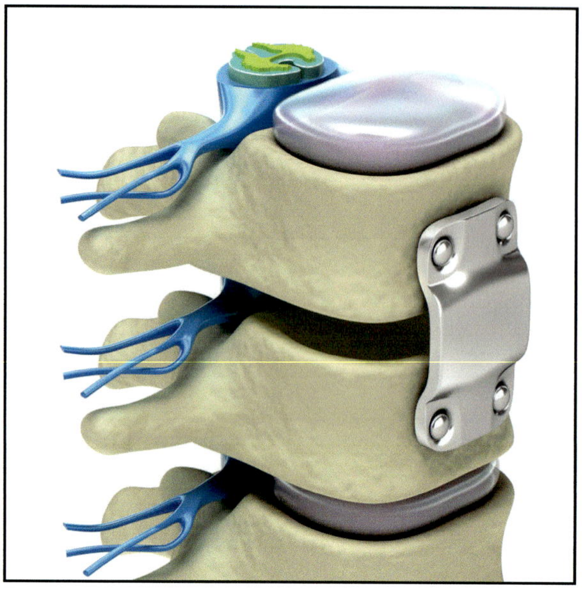

Figure 4-6. Surgical fixation of the lumbar spine with hardware. (Alex Mit/shutterstock.com)

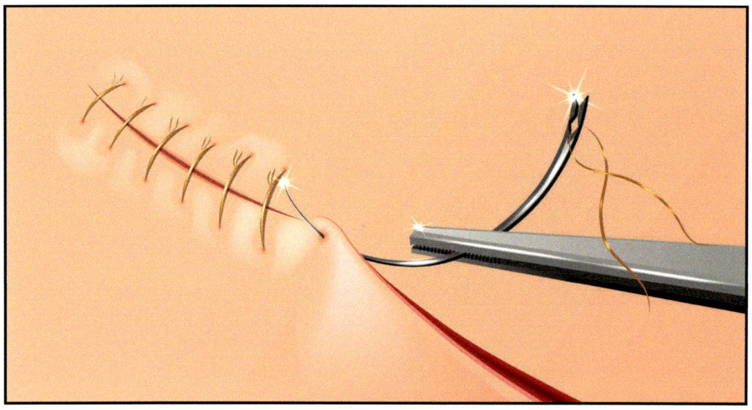

Figure 4-7. A ligature is a suture that is used to close open wounds. (Artemida-psy/shutterstock.com)

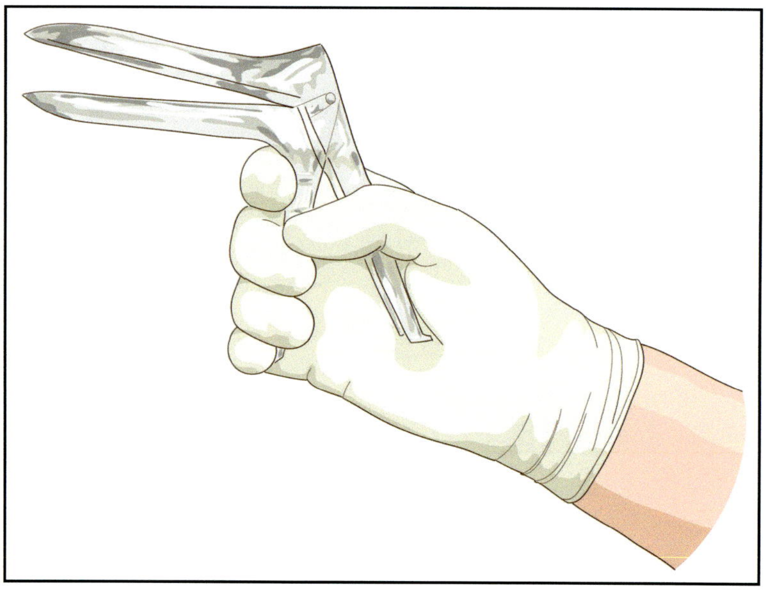

Figure 4-8. A speculum is used to open a cavity to view within it. (grib_nick/shutterstock.com)

Prefixes

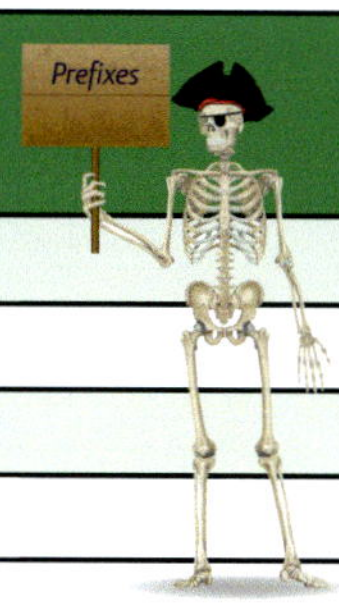

Table 4-5
Common Prefixes in Therapy and Diagnosis

PREFIX	DEFINITION	EXAMPLE
anti-	against	**anti**bacterial
epi-	above; upon	**epi**dermis
pan-	all	**pan**demic

Suffixes

The suffixes listed in Table 4-6 are added to combining words to form terms related to therapy diagnosis of medical conditions. Challenge yourself and see if you can determine the meaning of the words without referring back to Table 2-1 in Chapter 2.

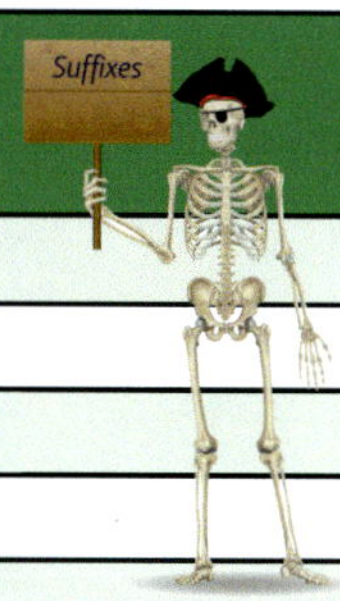

Table 4-6
Suffixes Pertaining to Therapy and Diagnoses

SUFFIX	DEFINITION	EXAMPLE
-centesis	puncture; surgical puncture	arthro**centesis**
-desis	fuse; bind	arthro**desis**
-ectomy	excision; surgical removal	orchi**ectomy**
-gram	a record of	arterio**gram**
-graph	an instrument to record information	electrocardio**graph** (Figure 4-9)
-graphy	process of recording; the act of recording information	broncho**graphy**
-meter	an instrument used to measure	thermo**meter**
-metry	measurement of	sym**metry**
-ostomy	a surgical opening	gastr**ostomy**
-otomy; -tomy	incision; to cut into	thorac**otomy**; phlebo**tomy**
-pexy	surgical fixation of	nephro**pexy**
-plasty	reconstruction; repair; plastic surgery	rhino**plasty**
-porosis	porous	osteo**porosis**
-rrhaphy	suture; surgical repair	hepato**rrhaphy**
-scope	an instrument used to view or inspect	oto**scope** (Figure 4-10)
-scopy	examination of	laryngo**scopy**
-stomy	surgical opening	tracheo**stomy**
-tome	a surgical instrument used to cut	neuro**tome**
-tripsy	crushing	neuro**tripsy**

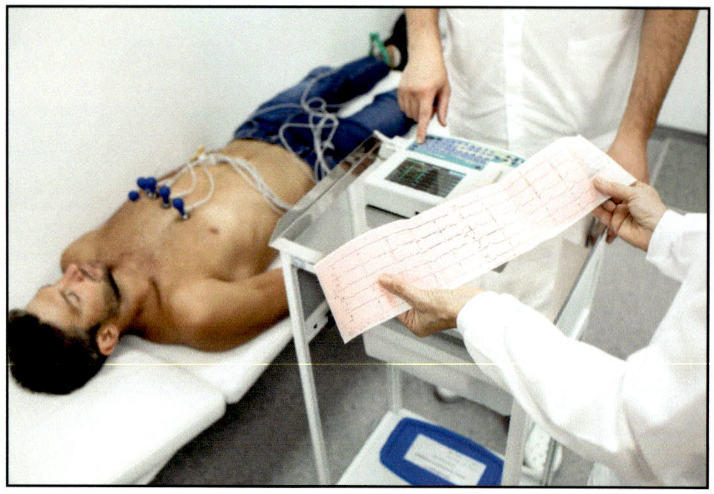

Figure 4-9. An electrocardiograph is an instrument that uses sensors taped over various aspects of the chest and body to record heart activity. (Peakstock/shutterstock.com)

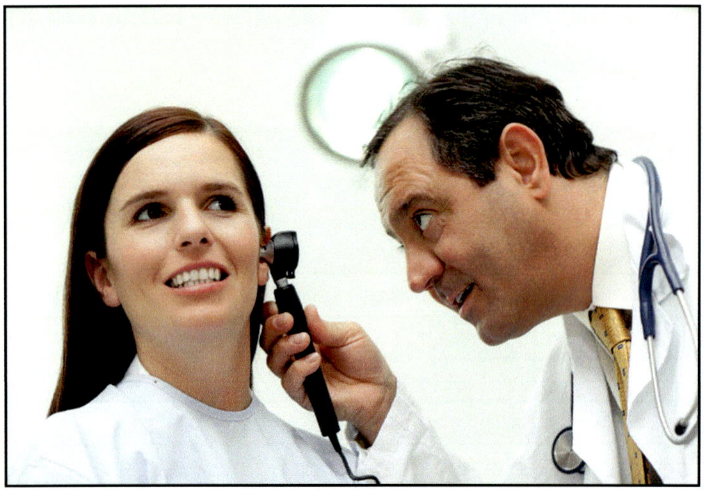

Figure 4-10. An otoscope permits viewing within the ear canal. (wavebreakmedia/shutterstock.com)

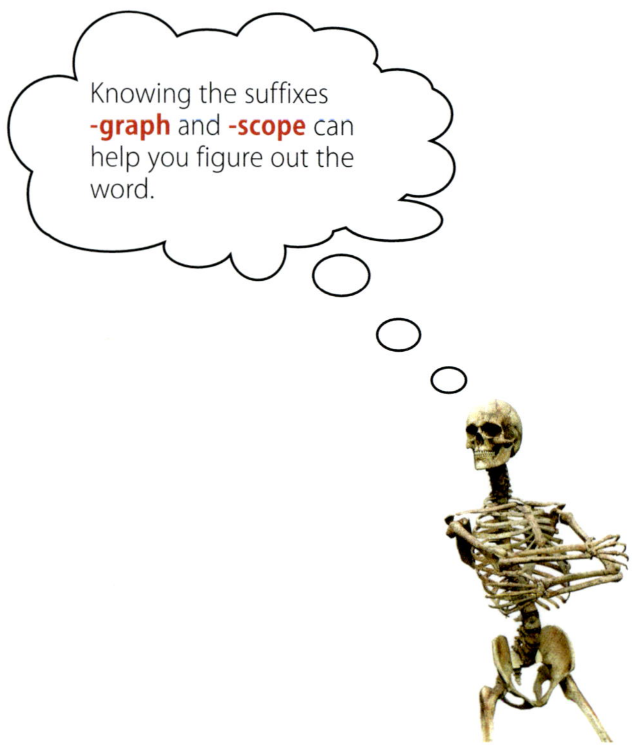

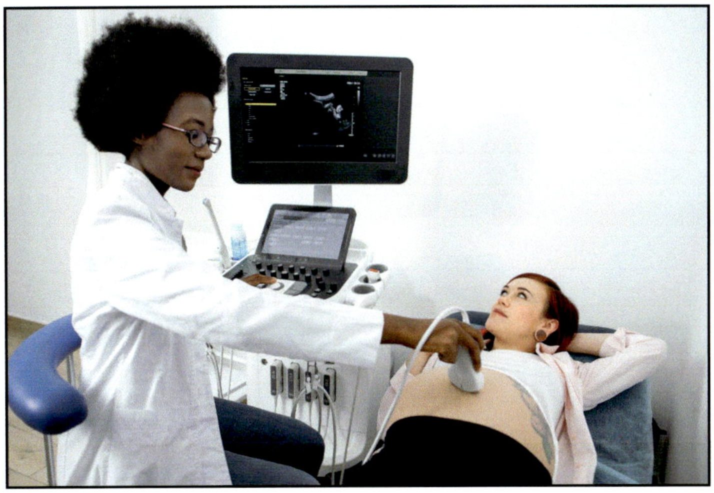

Figure 4-11. Ultrasound utilized as a diagnostic tool through ultrasonography. (SofikoS/shutterstock.com)

Combining word roots learned in Chapter 2 with the suffixes listed in Table 4-6 creates new words:

angiogram (**angi/o**—word root for vessel + **-gram**—a suffix meaning "the record of information" = a record of the blood vessel.)

Specifically, an angiogram is an image of the blood vessel following injection of a dye. The combining forms relating to the body listed in Table 2-1 can be added to the suffixes in Table 4-6 to create new words that pertain to that specific body part. Another example is ultrasonography (**ultra**/**son**/o/**graphy**): **ultra-**—beyond; **son/o**—sound; **-graphy**—process of recording (Figure 4-11).

Therapeutic and Diagnostic Procedures

Laboratory tests (Table 4-7) involve removing something (typically a fluid or tissue sample) from the body for further examination. Most involve a trained specialist in addition to microscopic inspection.

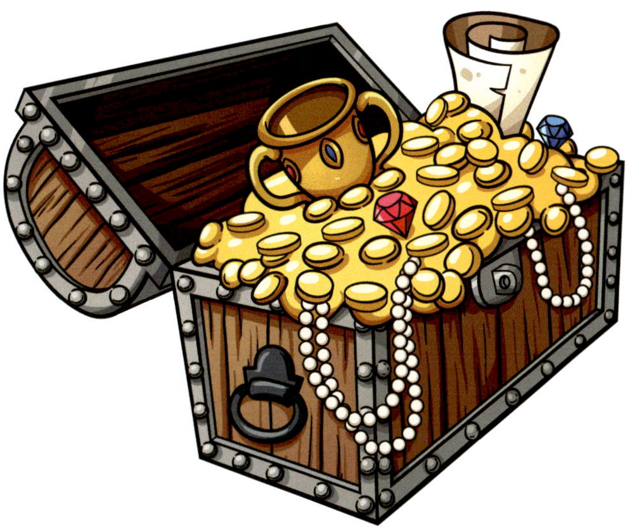

The more you study and learn **prefixes** and **suffixes**, the faster you will understand new terms. Remember that these are like gold and silver coins. Unlike the root part of a word, the prefixes and suffixes (like coins) travel to each island (chapter) and always have the same meaning.

Table 4-7
Laboratory Tests

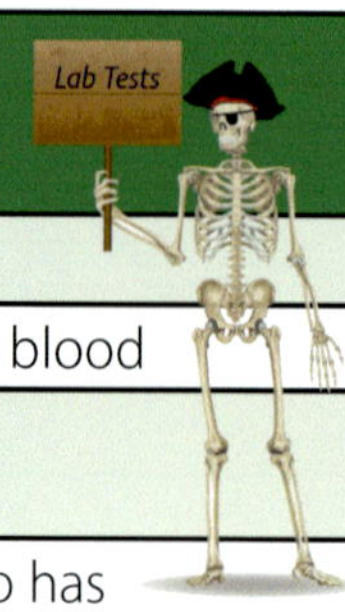

NAME	DEFINITION
blood cholesterol	Blood test measuring the type and quantity of cholesterol (lipids) in the blood
complete blood count (CBC)	Microscopic examination of blood components
fasting blood sugar (FBS)	Blood test measuring the amount of sugar in the blood of a person who has fasted 8 to 12 hours
fecal occult blood test	Examination of fecal matter for presence of blood
HbA1c	Blood test to determine the average blood sugar over 6 to 12 weeks; used for people with diabetes to monitor control of their disease
hematocrit	Blood test determining the packed cell volume of red blood cells (RBCs) in the blood
hemoglobin (Hb)	Blood test determining the amount of protein-iron compound in the blood that carries oxygen
lumbar puncture (spinal tap)	Examination of spinal fluid withdrawn via a needle inserted in between two lumbar vertebrae into the subarachnoid space of the spine (Figure 4-12)
Papanicolaou's test (Pap smear)	Test to examine the superficial layers of the cervix for cervical cancer; performed during a pelvic examination
urinalysis (UA)	Microscopic or chemical examination of the components of urine (Figure 4-13)

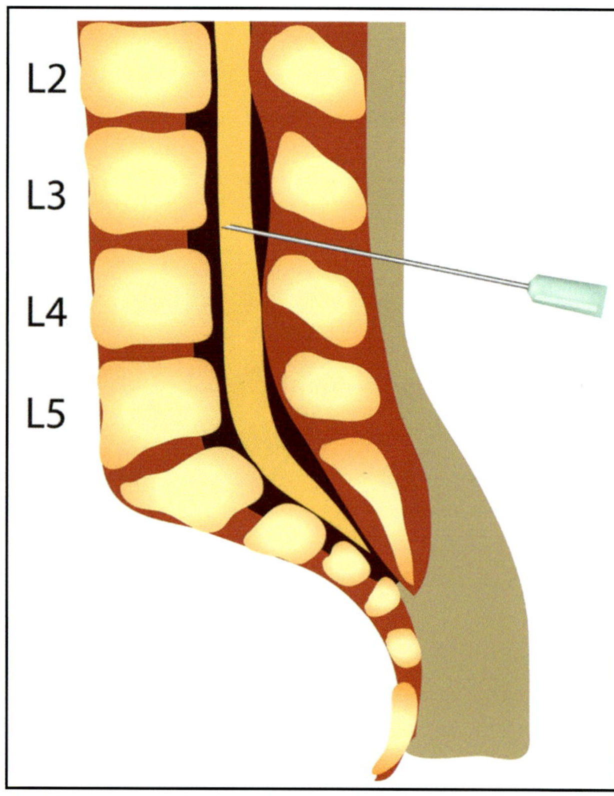

Figure 4-12. A lumbar puncture is used to analyze spinal fluid. (GRei/ shutterstock.com)

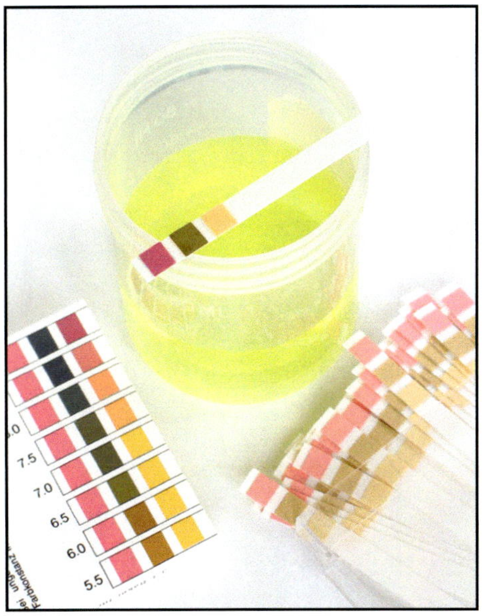

Figure 4-13. A UA involves dipping this sensitive chemical strip into urine. The strip reacts to components of a urine sample and changes color to indicate the various aspects of the sample. (Christina Richards/shutterstock.com)

Procedures that either treat or provide a diagnosis are listed in Table 4-8. Many of these procedures require placing the patient in a specific position, and often medical prescriptions for the procedure involve mention of planes. For example, a prescription for an x-ray may call for "AP lateral," meaning the x-rays should show an anterior-posterior view, and a lateral (side) view. See Figure 3-7 for a review of body planes.

Table 4-8

Therapeutic and Diagnostic Procedures

NAME	DEFINITION
bone scan	Following injection of a radioactive dye, a body part is imaged for uptake of the dye (Figure 4-14)
computed tomography (also termed CT or CAT scan)	Detailed cross-sections of the body using radiation; both hard and soft tissues can be visualized (Figure 4-15)
contrast studies	Radiopaque substance ingested or injected prior to x-ray or scan
endoscopy	Viewing inside a cavity using lighted instruments
fluoroscopy	Process of visualizing; fluor/o (luminous) **-scopy**
magnetic resonance imaging (MRI)	Magnetic radio waves used to provide images of soft tissues and internal structures of the body (Figure 4-16)
oximetry	Noninvasive test using a photodiagnostic method of evaluation to monitor oxygen saturation in the blood; typically performed via an oximeter (Figure 4-17)
positron emission tomography (PET)	Computerized technique using radiographic materials that examine increased metabolic activity in the body
radiography	Radiation is used to produce shadows of hard tissues (mainly bones) as it passes through the body (Figure 4-18)
spirometry	Laboratory evaluation of air capacity in the lungs; performed via a spirometer (Figure 4-19)

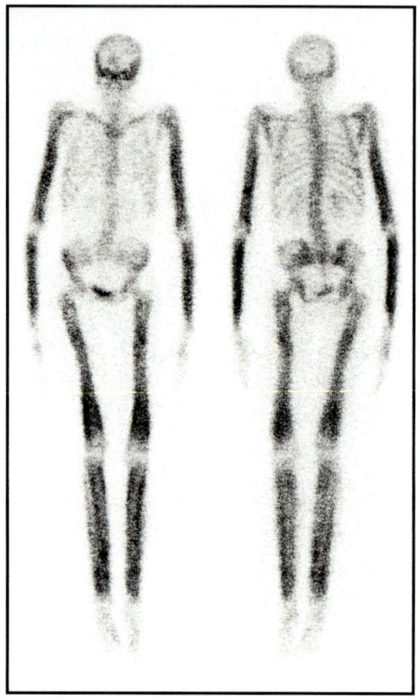

Figure 4-14. A bone scan is often used to determine if there is metabolic activity in a painful area of a bone, which may indicate a stress fracture. (Susan Law Cain/shutterstock.com)

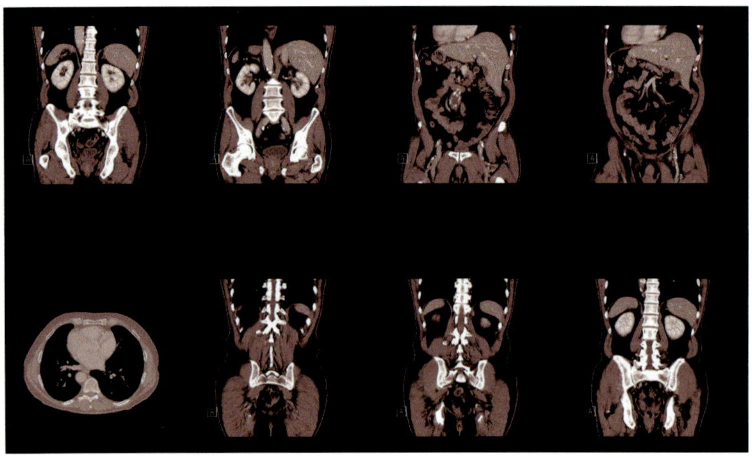

Figure 4-15. A CT scan of the abdomen. (skyhawk/shutterstock.com)

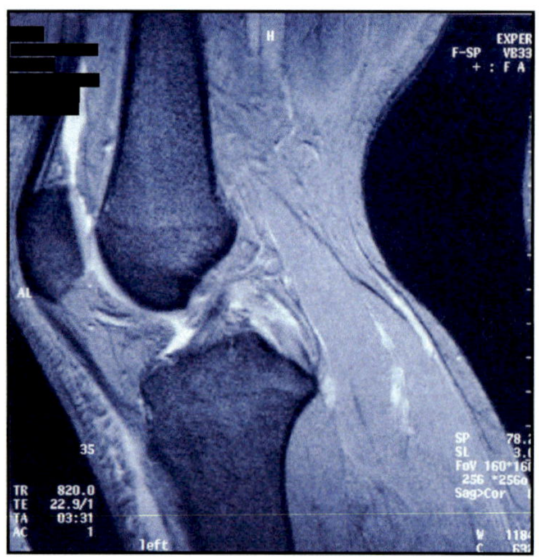

Figure 4-16. An MRI can show soft tissue as well as bone. This is a lateral view of a knee (note the patella [kneecap] and patellar tendon, on the left side of the image). (Kondor83/shutterstock.com)

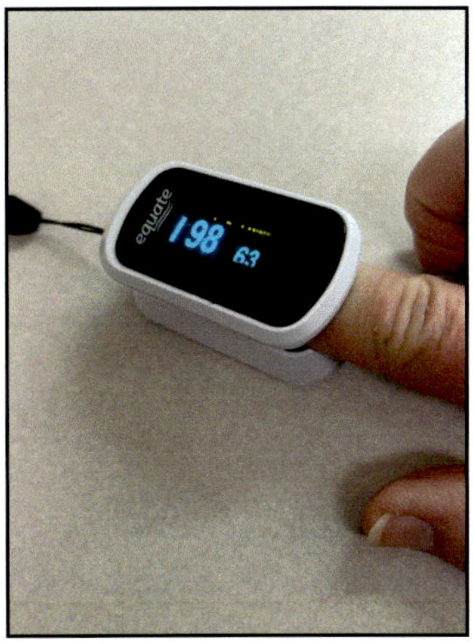

Figure 4-17. A pulse oximeter measures the amount of oxygen in the blood. This pulse oximeter shows a blood oxygen level of 98 and pulse of 63.

Figure 4-18. An x-ray showing a medial view of an ankle. (wonderisland/shutterstock.com)

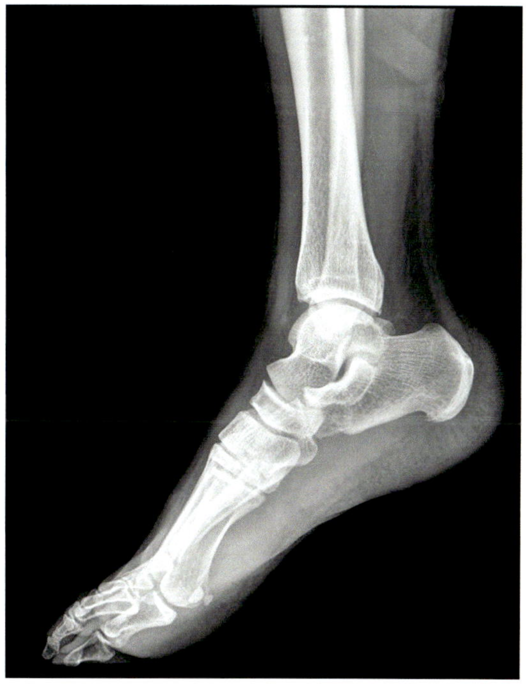

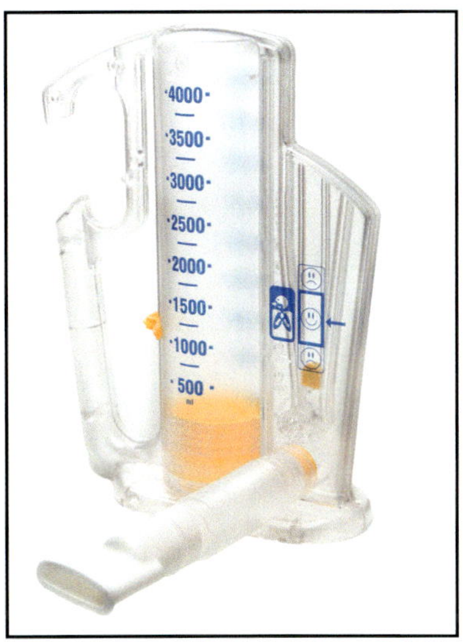

Figure 4-19. A spirometer measures lung capacity. (Rob Byron/shutterstock.com)

Table 4-9
Terms Related to Disease Testing and Control

TERM	DEFINITION
pandemic **pan**- (all)	Exceptionally widespread disease; life-threatening and impacting large percentage of people; typically worldwide
epidemic **epi-** (above; upon)	A disease infecting a large number of people; one that spreads widely within a given population
endemic	A disease found in a specific region/population
antigen test **anti-** (against)	A diagnostic test to determine if the body has been infected or vaccinated against a specific disease.
titer	A blood test to determine if an individual has immunity (antibodies) for a given disease/condition
polymerase chain reaction (PCR) test	Tests for SARS-CoV-2 (the virus that causes COVID-19) infection by analyzing a sample to determine if genetic material from the virus are present; if so, the person is infected with a SARS-related infection

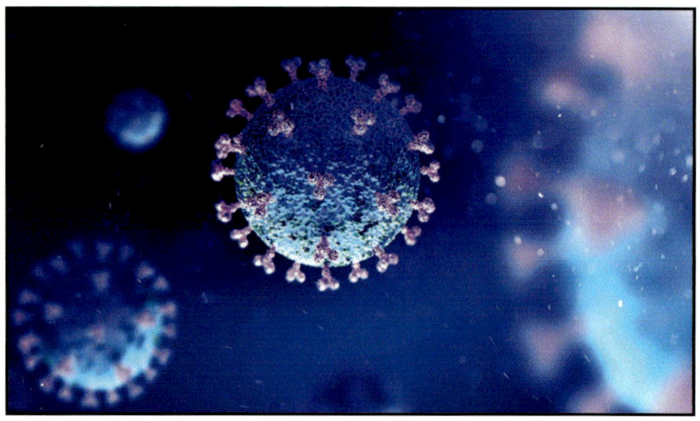

Figure 4-20. COVID-19 was responsible for the pandemic that began in 2020. (Andrii Vodolazhskyi/shutterstock.com)

The word root that precedes the suffix easily identifies medical specialties. An audiologist is a health professional who specializes in hearing disorders (**audi/o**—combining form for hearing; **-ist**—one who specializes in). Table 4-10 is useful to distinguish how a suffix can further delineate the type of practitioner or health care provider.

Table 4-10
Suffixes for Medical Specialties

SUFFIX	DEFINITION	EXAMPLE
-er	one who	sonograph**er** (one who examines via sound)
-ian	a specialist in a particular field	pediatric**ian** (a specialist who treats children—pedi/o)
-iatrics; -iatrical	related to medical treatment	ger**iatrics** (related to treatment of older persons)
-iatrist; -iatrician	one who specializes in a particular treatment	pod**iatrist** (a specialist who treats disorders of the feet—pod/o)
-iatry	medical treatment	psych**iatry** (treatment of mental disorders)
-ics	a medical specialty	orthoped**ics** (a specialty that focuses on bones; orth/o—to straighten)
-ist	one who specializes	psycholog**ist** (a person who helps people with psychological stresses)

Bibliography

Basco R, Allan B. *Medical Language for Modern Health Care.* 5th ed. McGraw-Hill; 2023.
Fremgen BF, Frucht SS. *Medical Terminology: A Living Language.* 7th ed. Pearson; 2019.
Hutton A. *Medical Terminology for Health Care.* 5th ed. Churchill Livingstone; 2017.
Mosby's Dictionary of Medicine, Nursing & Health Professions. 10th ed. Elsevier; 2017.
Rice J. *Medical Terminology for Health Care Professionals.* 9th ed. Pearson; 2018.
Venes D, ed. *Taber's Cyclopedic Medical Dictionary.* 24th ed. F. A. Davis; 2021.

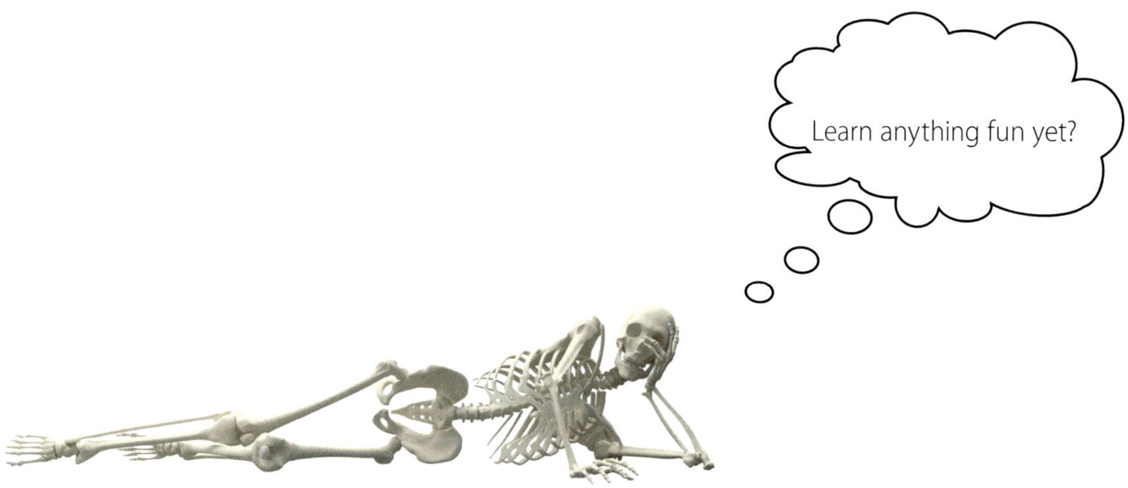

Notes

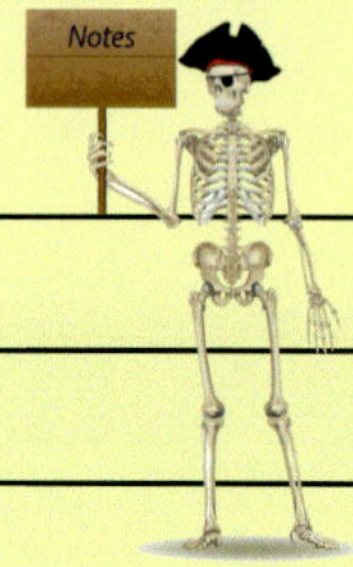

NOTES

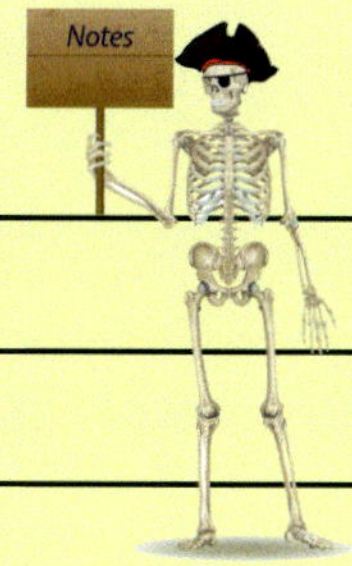

Learning Activities

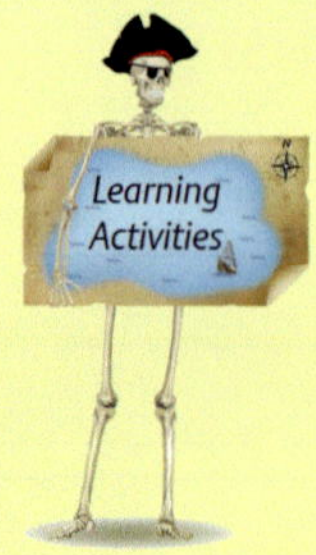

Name:____________________

Therapeutic and Diagnostic Procedures

Note: You may need to refer to earlier chapters to assist with completing these learning activities.

A. Matching.

Recall: Match the medical abbreviation (refer to Appendix A) with the correct meaning.

1. CC______________	a. diagnosis
2. adm______________	b. head of bed
3. Dx______________	c. congestive heart failure
4. Dd______________	d. vital signs
5. DO______________	e. chief complaint
6. CHF______________	f. differential diagnosis
7. HOB______________	g. temperature, pulse, and respiration
8. TPR______________	h. doctor of osteopathy
9. VS______________	i. history of present illness
10. HPI______________	j. admission

B. SOAP notes: Fill in the blanks using medical abbreviations (choose from the list in A). (Review Appendix A to assist with this question.)

The S portion of the SOAP note would include the patient's______________ and__________. The O portion of the note contains ______________and __________. The A portion has a list of _____________.

C. Define the following words/medical abbreviations.

1. thermotherapy__________________________
2. FBS__________________________
3. triage__________________________
4. MRI__________________________
5. lithotripsy__________________________
6. prophylaxis__________________________
7. staging__________________________
8. osteotomy__________________________
9. syncope__________________________
10. CBC__________________________

D. Add the suffix -scope to each of the following combining forms and define the word created.

1. cyst/o________________________________
2. nephr/o________________________________
3. ophthalm/o________________________________
4. end/o________________________________
5. micr/o________________________________

E. Add the suffix -scopy to each of the following combining forms and define the word created.

1. arthr/o________________________________
2. lapar/o________________________________
3. colon/o________________________________
4. laryng/o________________________________
5. bronch/o________________________________

F. Write out the medical word that means the following.

1. to cut out the tonsils________________________________
2. to surgically fixate the ears (so they do not stick out)________________________________
3. a surgical opening in the colon________________________________
4. electrical recording of the brain________________________________
5. using plastic surgery to repair the eyelid________________________________

G. For each of the following conditions, determine if it is a sign or symptom.

1. unequal pupils________________________________
2. nausea________________________________
3. headache________________________________
4. rash________________________________
5. hair loss________________________________
6. cyanosis________________________________
7. itching________________________________
8. swelling________________________________
9. fever________________________________
10. pain________________________________

Section II

Body Systems

5

Musculoskeletal System

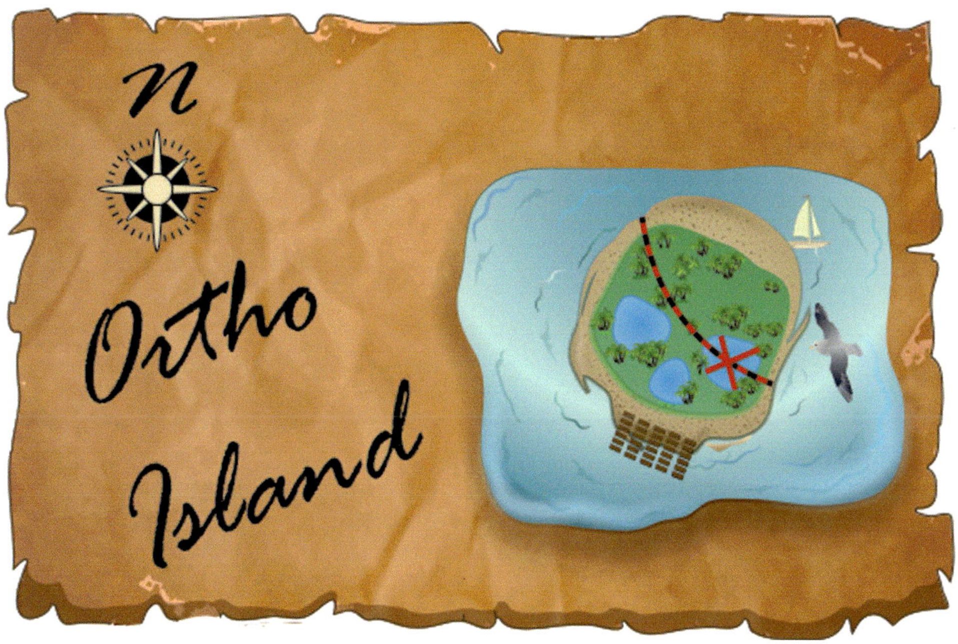

Objectives

After studying this chapter, you will be able to:

1. Locate the major bones and muscles of the body.
2. Describe conditions affecting the musculoskeletal system.
3. Build words associated with the musculoskeletal system.
4. Differentiate between therapeutic procedures based on the word parts used to describe the procedure.

Flanagan KW.
Medical Terminology With Case Studies: A Navigated Guide to Learning for Health Care Professionals, Third Edition (pp 69-110).

Chapter Outline

- Self-assessment
- Checklist for word parts in the chapter
- Checklist of new anatomy
- Introduction
- Word building
  - Prefixes
  - Suffixes
  - Combining forms
- Anatomy
  - Bones
  - Fractures
  - Joints
  - Ligaments
  - Bursae, menisci, and discs
  - Muscles
- Medical conditions
- Tests and procedures
- Learning activities
- Case study

Self-Assessment

Based on what you have learned so far, can you write the definition of these words?

- osteoarthritis____________________
- orthopedic____________________
- myalgia____________________
- osteochondroma____________________
- myositis____________________
- arthroscope____________________
- osteology____________________
- myotomy____________________
- arthroplasty____________________
- myocardial____________________

Checklist for Word Parts in the Chapter

Prefixes

- ☐ a-
- ☐ allo-
- ☐ amphi-
- ☐ auto-
- ☐ brady-
- ☐ con-
- ☐ dia-
- ☐ dys-
- ☐ en-
- ☐ epi-
- ☐ ex-
- ☐ hyper-
- ☐ hypo-
- ☐ infra-
- ☐ inter-
- ☐ intra-
- ☐ mal-
- ☐ non-
- ☐ peri-
- ☐ supra-
- ☐ sym-
- ☐ syn-

Suffixes

- ☐ -al
- ☐ -algia
- ☐ -ar
- ☐ -asthenia
- ☐ -blast
- ☐ -centesis
- ☐ -clasia
- ☐ -clasis
- ☐ -clast
- ☐ -cyte
- ☐ -desis
- ☐ -dynia
- ☐ -ectomy
- ☐ -edema
- ☐ -fida
- ☐ -genesis
- ☐ -gram
- ☐ -graphy
- ☐ -ion
- ☐ -itis
- ☐ -kinesia
- ☐ -lysis
- ☐ -malacia
- ☐ -megaly
- ☐ -occult
- ☐ -oma
- ☐ -osis
- ☐ -otomy
- ☐ -ous
- ☐ -pathy
- ☐ -penia
- ☐ -penic
- ☐ -pexy
- ☐ -plasty
- ☐ -porosis
- ☐ -rrhaphy
- ☐ -rrhexis
- ☐ -scopy
- ☐ -spasm
- ☐ -tomy
- ☐ -tonia
- ☐ -troph
- ☐ -um
- ☐ -us
- ☐ -y

Combining Forms

- ☐ acetabul/o
- ☐ acr/o
- ☐ acromi/o
- ☐ ankyl/o
- ☐ arthr/o
- ☐ axill/o
- ☐ brachi/o
- ☐ bunion/o
- ☐ burs/o
- ☐ calcane/o
- ☐ calci/o
- ☐ carcin/o
- ☐ carp/o
- ☐ cervic/o
- ☐ chondr/o
- ☐ clon/o
- ☐ condyl/o
- ☐ cost/o
- ☐ crani/o
- ☐ dactyl/o
- ☐ derm/o
- ☐ dermat/o
- ☐ fasci/o
- ☐ fibr/o
- ☐ hem/o
- ☐ ischi/o
- ☐ kinesi/o
- ☐ kyph/o
- ☐ lamin/o
- ☐ later/o
- ☐ lord/o
- ☐ maxilla/o
- ☐ menisc/o
- ☐ my/o
- ☐ myel/o
- ☐ necr/o
- ☐ orth/o
- ☐ oss/i
- ☐ osse/o
- ☐ oste/o
- ☐ physis
- ☐ rachi/o
- ☐ rhabd/o
- ☐ sacr
- ☐ scoli/o
- ☐ spin/o
- ☐ spondyl/o
- ☐ stern/o
- ☐ tars/o
- ☐ ten/o
- ☐ tend/o
- ☐ tendi/o
- ☐ tract/o
- ☐ uln/o
- ☐ vascul

Checklist of New Anatomy

Bones—Axial Skeleton

- ☐ Skull
  - ☐ Frontal
  - ☐ Parietal
  - ☐ Zygoma
  - ☐ Mastoid
  - ☐ Nasal
  - ☐ Temporal
  - ☐ Occipital
  - ☐ Maxilla
  - ☐ Mandible
  - ☐ Sphenoid
- ☐ Spine
  - ☐ Cervical
  - ☐ Thoracic
  - ☐ Lumbar
  - ☐ Sacrum
  - ☐ Coccyx
  - ☐ Vertebral body
  - ☐ Transverse process
  - ☐ Spinous process
  - ☐ Lamina
- ☐ Ribs
- ☐ Clavicle
- ☐ Sternum
- ☐ Pelvis
  - ☐ Ilium
  - ☐ Iliac crest
  - ☐ Ischium
  - ☐ Pubis

Muscles—Axial Skeleton

- ☐ Trapezius
- ☐ Sternocleidomastoid
- ☐ Rectus abdominis
- ☐ Internal oblique
- ☐ External oblique
- ☐ Latissimus dorsi
- ☐ Trapezius
- ☐ Serratus anterior
- ☐ Pectoralis major
- ☐ Gluteus maximus
- ☐ Gluteus medius
- ☐ Tensor fasciae latae
- ☐ Adductor magnus
- ☐ Gracilis

Bones—Upper Extremity

- ☐ Scapula
  - ☐ Spine
  - ☐ Acromion
  - ☐ Supraspinatus fossa
  - ☐ Infraspinatus fossa
  - ☐ Glenoid
- ☐ Humerus
  - ☐ Head
  - ☐ Neck
  - ☐ Lateral epicondyle
  - ☐ Medial epicondyle
- ☐ Ulna
  - ☐ Olecranon
  - ☐ Head
  - ☐ Styloid
- ☐ Radius
  - ☐ Head
  - ☐ Styloid
- ☐ Carpals
- ☐ Metacarpals
- ☐ Phalanges
  - ☐ Pollicis (thumb)

Muscles—Upper Extremity

- ☐ Supraspinatus
- ☐ Infraspinatus
- ☐ Trapezius
- ☐ Levator scapula
- ☐ Rhomboid major
- ☐ Teres minor
- ☐ Biceps
- ☐ Triceps
- ☐ Brachialis
- ☐ Deltoid
- ☐ Extensor carpi ulnaris
- ☐ Flexor carpi ulnaris
- ☐ Brachioradialis
- ☐ Extensor carpi radialis longus
- ☐ Flexor carpi radialis longus

Bones—Lower Extremity

- ☐ Femur
- ☐ Head
- ☐ Neck
- ☐ Greater trochanter
- ☐ Lesser trochanter
- ☐ Medial condyle
- ☐ Lateral condyle
- ☐ Patellofemoral groove
- ☐ Patella
- ☐ Tibia
  - ☐ Tibial tuberosity
  - ☐ Medial malleolus
- ☐ Fibula
  - ☐ Head
  - ☐ Lateral malleolus
- ☐ Tarsals
  - ☐ Calcaneus
  - ☐ Talus
  - ☐ Cuneiform I, II, III
  - ☐ Navicular
  - ☐ Cuboid
- ☐ Metatarsal
- ☐ Phalanges
  - ☐ Hallux (great toe)

Muscles—Lower Extremity

- ☐ Sartorius
- ☐ Quadriceps
  - ☐ Vastus medialis
  - ☐ Vastus intermedius
  - ☐ Vastus lateralis
  - ☐ Rectus femoris
- ☐ Hamstrings
  - ☐ Semimembranosus
  - ☐ Semitendinosus
  - ☐ Biceps femoris
- ☐ Gastrocnemius
- ☐ Soleus
- ☐ Tibialis anterior
- ☐ Posterior tibialis
- ☐ Extensor digitorum longus
- ☐ Extensor hallucis longus
- ☐ Flexor digitorum longus
- ☐ Flexor hallucis longus
- ☐ Peroneal longus
- ☐ Peroneal brevis

Introduction

Welcome to Ortho Island! On this island, you will find combining forms for the musculoskeletal system. As mentioned in Section I, prefixes and suffixes are represented as silver and gold coins—they travel with our pirate, Skully, between islands and help local word roots take the meanings specific to the system. You will notice some prefixes and suffixes are quite popular and are in many of chapters, whereas the combining forms are unique to their own island (body system).

The musculoskeletal system is the literal framework of the human body. The skeleton protects and supports the whole body, and muscles are the structures that provide and control movement. In addition to these main attributes, the musculoskeletal system also contains joints, ligaments, cartilage, and other soft tissues such as bursae. With your prior knowledge of anatomical directions (Chapter 3) and word building, this chapter constructs new words pertaining to the musculoskeletal system. This chapter, as with all other body system chapters in Section II, begins with a few tables of word-building terms, then an overview of pertinent anatomy, and finally introduces words and word elements specific to the musculoskeletal system.

Word Building

Table 5-1
Prefixes

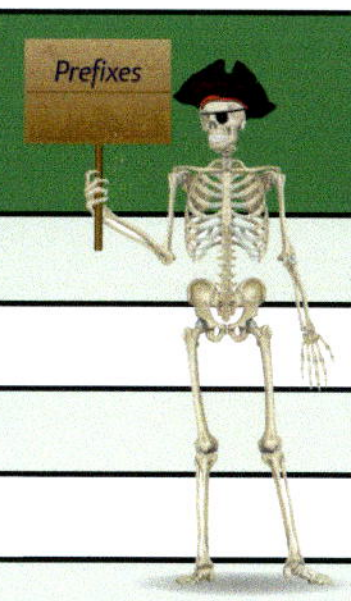

PREFIX	DEFINITION
a-	without
allo-	different; other
amphi-	both sides
auto-	self; own
brady-	slow
con-	together
dia-	across; through
dys-	abnormal; bad; difficult; painful
en-	within
epi-	above; upon
ex-	away; away from; out; outside
hyper-	above; excessive; high; increased
hypo-	below; decreased; deficient; insufficient; low; under
infra-	below
inter-	among; between
intra-	inside; within
mal-	bad
peri-	around
supra-	above
sym-; syn-	union; together

Table 5-2
Suffixes

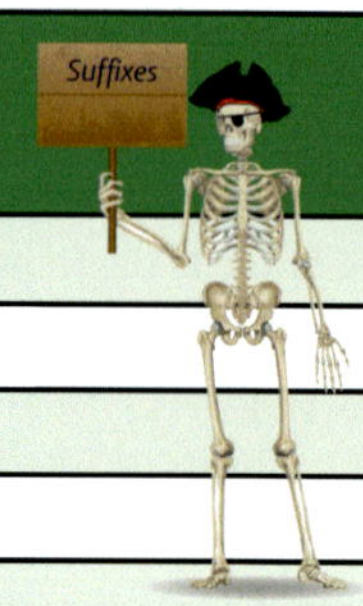

SUFFIX	DEFINITION
-al	pertaining to
-algia	pain
-ar	pertaining to
-asthenia	weakness
-blast	embryonic cell
-clasis; -clasia	to break
-clast	to break
-cyte	cell
-desis	fuse; bind
-dynia	pain
-ectomy	excision; surgical removal
-edema	swelling
-fida	to split
-genesis	forming; origin; producing
-gram	a record of
-graphy	process of recording; the act of recording information
-ion	process; the act of
-itis	inflammation
-kinesia	movement
-malacia	softening
-megaly	abnormally large; enlargement
-occult	hidden
-oma	tumor; mass
-osis	condition
-otomy; -tomy	incision; to cut into
-ous	pertaining to
-pathy	disease
-penia; -penic	decrease; deficient
-pexy	surgical fixation of
-plasty	reconstruction; repair; plastic surgery
-porosis	porous
-rrhaphy	surgical repair; suturing
-rrhexis	rupture
-scopy	examination of
-tonia	tone
-troph	development; growth; nourishment
-um	structure; thing
-us	pertaining to; structure

Remember **-ectomy** means "**e**xcision" (it has an "**e**" in it); **-otomy** and **-tomy** mean "incision" or "cutting into."

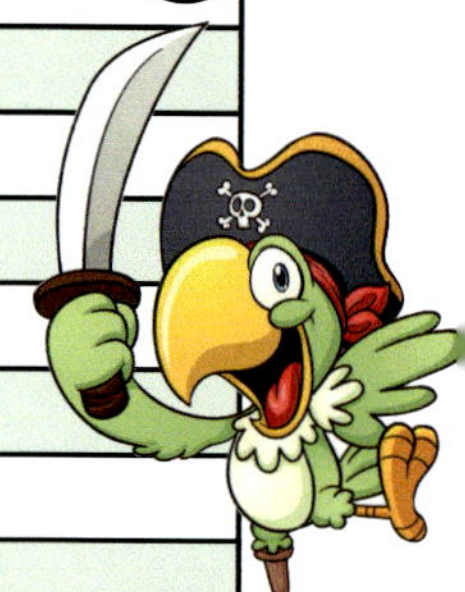

Table 5-3
Combining Forms

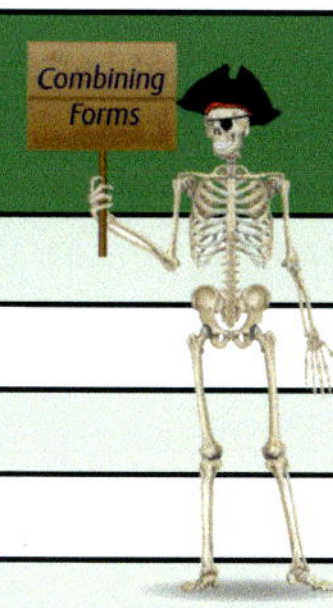

COMBINING FORM	DEFINITION
acetabul/o	acetabulum (hip socket)
acr/o	extremity
acromi/o	acromion (end of the spine of the scapula)
arthr/o	joint
brachi/o	arm
bunion/o	bunion
burs/o	bursa
calcane/o	heel
calci/o	calcium
carcin/o	cancer
carp/o	carpals; wrist bones
cervic/o	neck; cervix
chondr/o	cartilage
condyl/o	condyle (knuckle)
cost/o	rib
dactyl/o	finger; toe
derm/o; dermat/o	skin
fasci/o	fascia
fibr/o	fiber
hem/o	blood
ischi/o	ischium
kinesi/o	movement
kyph/o	bent; hump
lamin/o	lamina (thin plate)
later/o	side
lord/o	swayback
maxilla/o	upper jaw (below the nose)
menisc/o	meniscus
my/o	muscle
myel/o	bone marrow; spinal cord
necr/o	death
orth/o	straight
osse/o; oss/i	bone
oste/o	bone
physis	growth
rachi/o	spine; vertebral column
rhabd/o	rod-shaped

(continued)

Table 5-3 (continued) Combining Forms	
COMBINING FORM	DEFINITION
sacr	flesh; connective tissue
scoli/o	curved
spin/o	spine
spondyl/o	vertebra
stern/o	sternum
tars/o	tarsals (ankle bones)
ten/o; tend/o; tendi/o	tendon
tract/o	pulling; to pull
uln/o	ulna (forearm bone)
vascul	blood vessel

Anatomy

Bones

Bones are critical to support the body and provide other essential functions as well. Bones are formed in the fetus as cartilaginous tissue and continue to grow and solidify (**ossification**; **oss/i** is a combining form for bone) until the late teens to early 20s. Mature bones begin as **osteoblasts** (**oste/o**—bone; **-blast**—embryonic cell), literally, bone cells. **Osteocytes** (**-cyte**—cell) eventually become bony tissue that replaces the cartilaginous tissues. Opposite of osteoblasts are **osteoclasts** (**oste/o**—bone;**-clast**—break). These cells break up and reabsorb bony tissues, and are (as are osteoblasts) active throughout the lifespan. Bones are living tissues and respond to stresses put upon them. They can break under too much stress, and they also adapt and grow under smaller amounts of stress. Healthy bones depend on a regular supply of calcium, phosphorous, and vitamin D. Vitamin D is necessary to help absorb calcium into the bloodstream and is often found in calcium supplements.

There are several types of bones in humans. **Long bones** (found in the thigh, lower leg, and upper and lower arms) are a reservoir for producing **red blood cells** (RBCs), a necessary blood component. Other types of bone are:

- **Short bones**: Small, irregular bones such as those found in the wrist and ankle.
- **Flat bones**: Bones found in the skull, ribs, pelvis, and shoulder blade (scapula).
- **Sesamoid bones**: Small, rounded bones found encapsulated within tendons. They are in the palm, foot, and leg. The most well-known sesamoid is the patella (kneecap).

Long bones are surrounded by a thick fibrous membrane called the **periosteum** (**peri-**—around; **oste**—bone; **-um**—structure, thing). The ends of long bones each contain an **epiphysis** (**epi-**—above, upon; **-physis**—growth), and an **epiphyseal plate,** which is the part of the bone where growth occurs. The length of bone in between the epiphyses is an area termed the **diaphysis** (Figure 5-1). The region of bone where the diaphysis flares out to join the epiphysis is termed the **metaphysis**. There is also **articular cartilage** (also known as **hyaline cartilage**) covering the ends of long bones. This type of cartilage is similar to what is found on the ends of chicken wings; it is tough, white in color, and provides protection between adjoining bones. It is the wearing away of the articular cartilage that causes osteoarthritis (**oste/o**—bone; **arthr/**—joint; **-itis**—inflammation; Figure 5-2). Beneath the periosteum, long bones have a tough outer layer of compact bone that protects the next spongy inner area, called the **cancellous**. The cancellous surrounds the medullary cavity, which is a tube-like center area of long bones. In adults, the **medullary cavity** contains fatty yellow bone marrow. Red bone marrow is found in the cancellous portion of the proximal epiphyses of the humerus and femur, as well as vertebrae, ribs, and the sternum. Red bone marrow is critical to the production and maturation of RBCs and most **white blood cells** (WBCs).

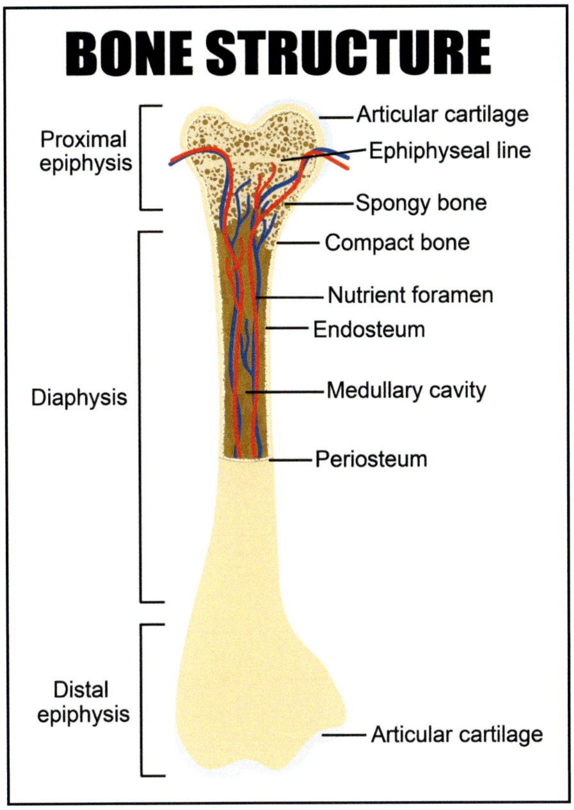

Figure 5-1. Parts of a long bone. (ducu59us/shutterstock.com)

5

Figure 5-2. Osteoarthritis of the knee. (Alila Medical Images/shutterstock.com)

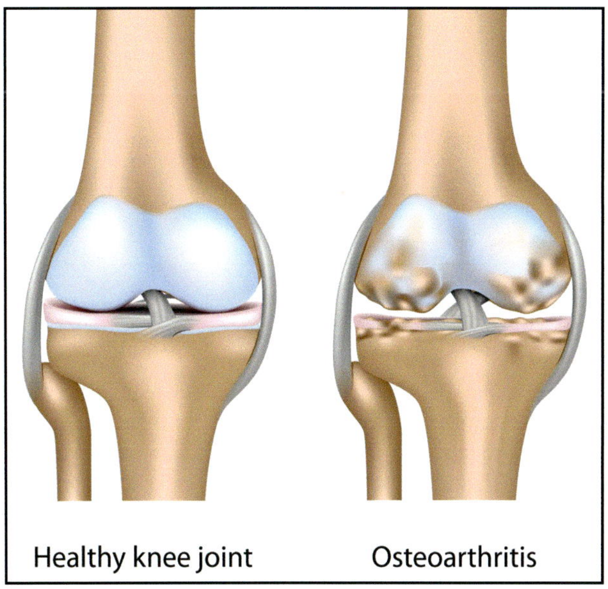

Figures 5-3A through 5-3E show the major bones in the human body, spine, skull, and foot. The spinal column (**vertebra**) is divided into sections (Figure 5-3B). Many of the names are formed from medical word parts you already know; for example, **cervical** in the neck has 7 vertebra, **thoracic** in the trunk has 12 vertebrae (each is attached to a rib), **lumbar** is the low back and has 5 vertebrae, **sacrum** (a fused plate), and **coccyx** (tailbone).

Bones also have bumps and dents (Figure 5-4) that often provide tendon attachments, or spaces for two bones to articulate. Muscles rarely attach directly to bones. Muscles transition to tendons and the tendons attach to specific areas on bones. Most often, these areas are raised sections of bone called a *tubercle* or *tuberosity*. Table 5-4 is a list of the names of the raised or indented areas of bones.

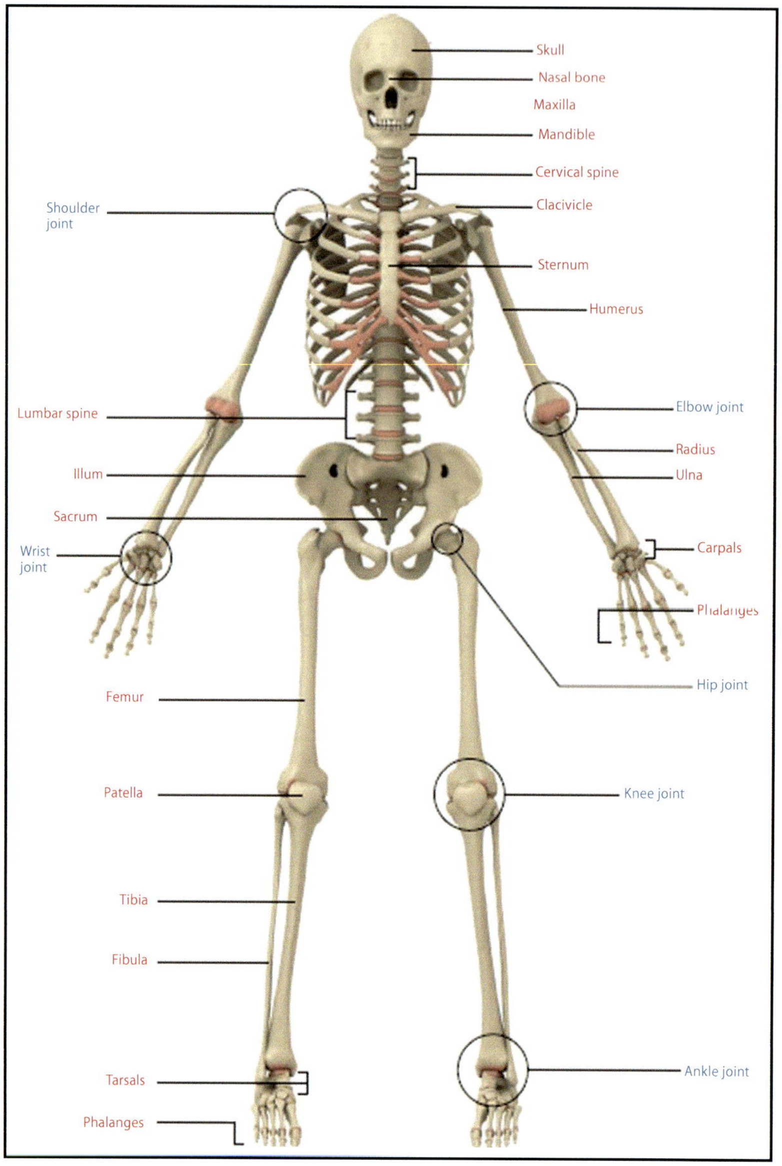

Figure 5-3A. Anterior view of skeleton. (Sebastian Kaulitzki/shutterstock.com)

Figure 5-5 displays a scapula (shoulder blade). If you put together the word parts you already know with your recently acquired knowledge of bones and bony landmarks, you can determine where a given space is on the skeleton. **Infraspinous fossa** of the scapula, for example, is easy to understand if you break the words down. Scapula is the shoulder blade and **infra-** means below, **spin/o** + **-us** means pertaining to the spine, and fossa means a shallow indentation. In this case, the shallow indentation below the spine of the scapula. Likewise, the axillary border of the scapula is the border nearer the armpit (**axill/o**), compared to the vertebral border (nearer the spine).

Fractures

Any crack or break in a bone is termed a *fracture*, although often people are led to believe a "break" is worse than a "fracture." There are several types of fractures, and some even have their own name:

- **Pott's fracture**: A fracture of both bones (tibia and fibula) at the ankle (Figure 5-6)
- **Colles fracture**: A fracture of the distal radius (near the wrist)

Fractures are classified by external and radiographic appearance. Often, groups of similar fractures have a name to organize them. The **Salter-Harris classification** for fractures of the epiphysis is one example of this type of grouping. These types of fractures only occur in immature skeletons (people still growing). In addition, fractures are characterized by how the bone is damaged. Table 5-5 is a list of common types of fractures.

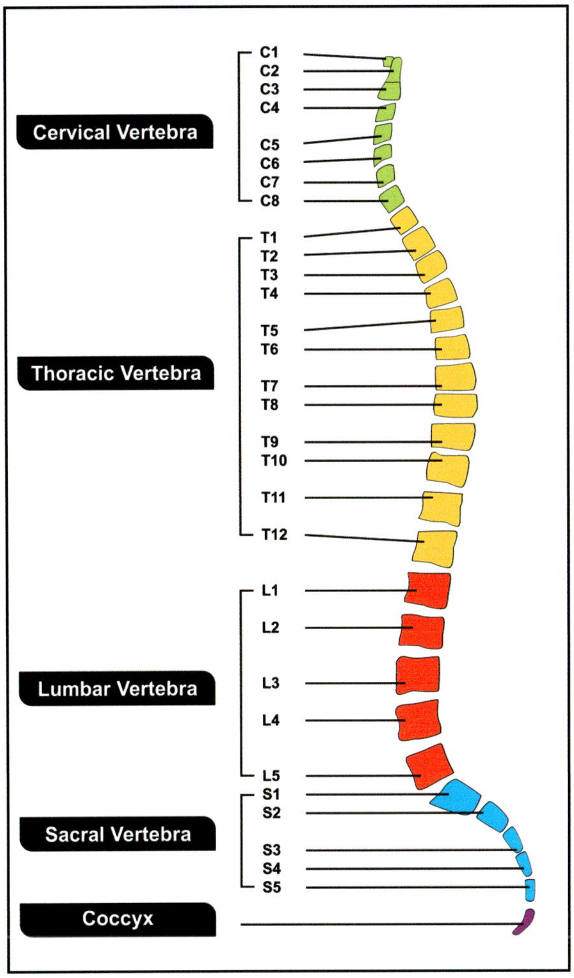

Figure 5-3B. A lateral view of the spine with each section highlighted. (udaix/shutterstock.com)

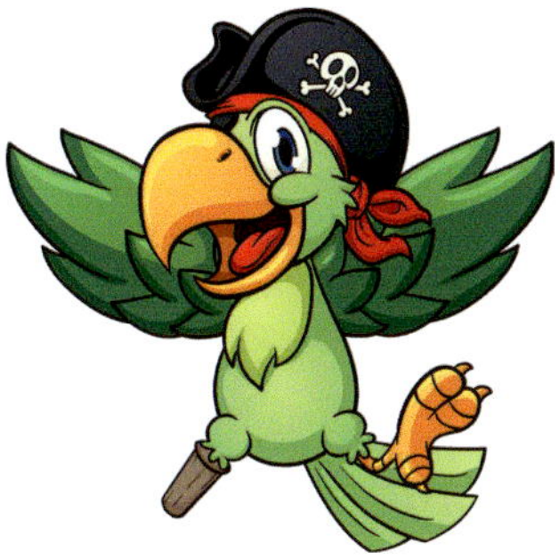

Figure 5-3C. Close-up of the posterior spine. (dream designs/shutterstock.com)

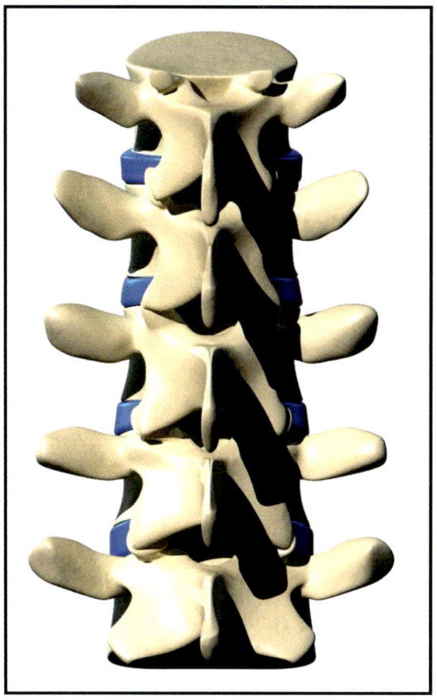

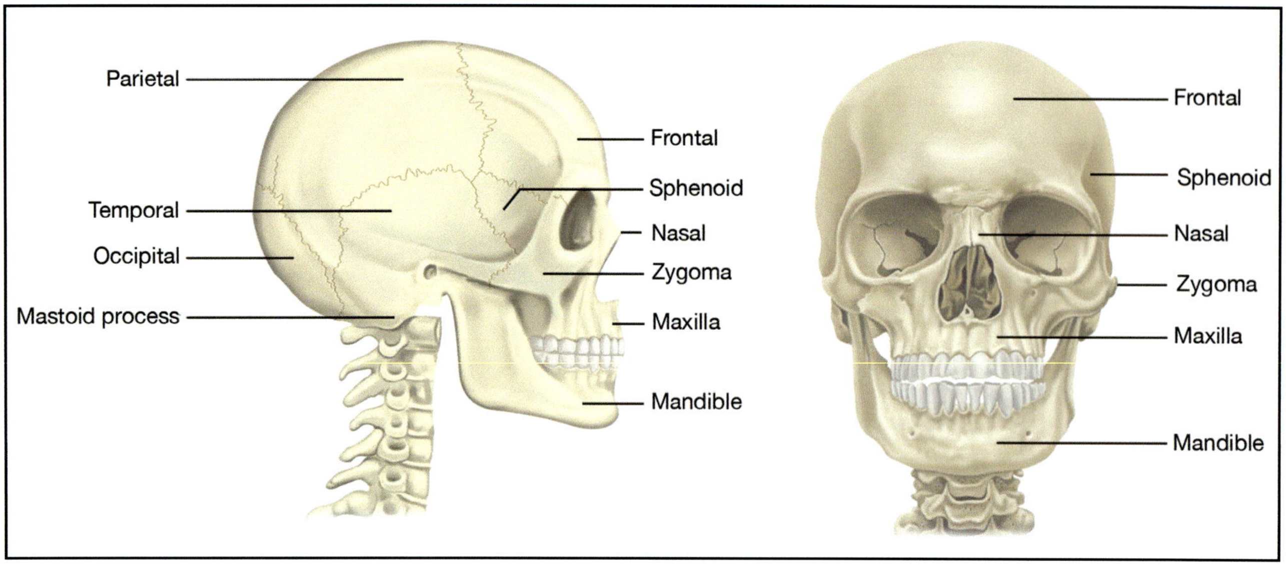

Figure 5-3D. The skull.

Figure 5-3E. The foot. (udaix/shutterstock.com)

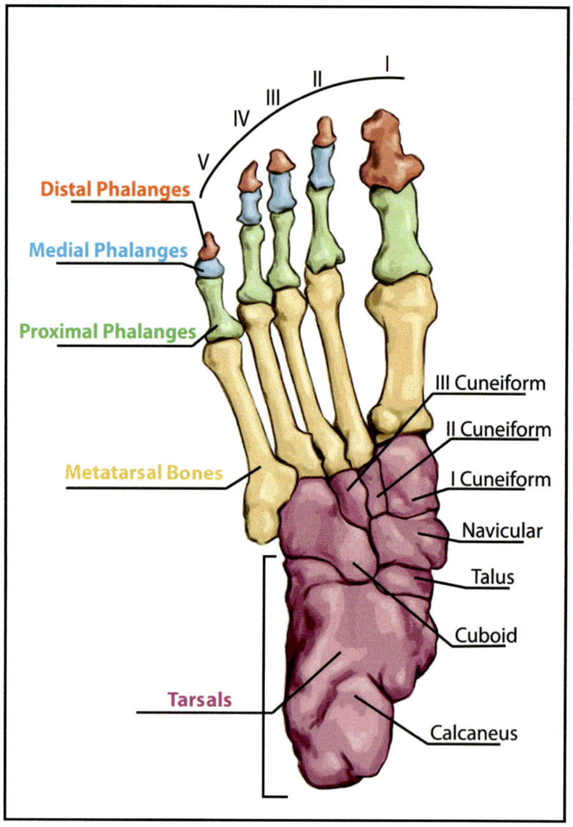

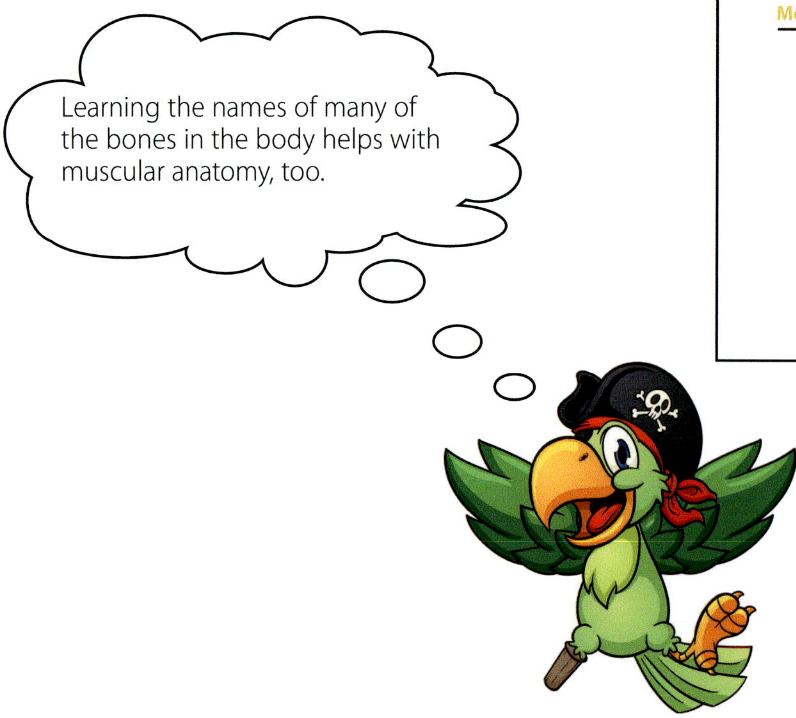
Learning the names of many of the bones in the body helps with muscular anatomy, too.

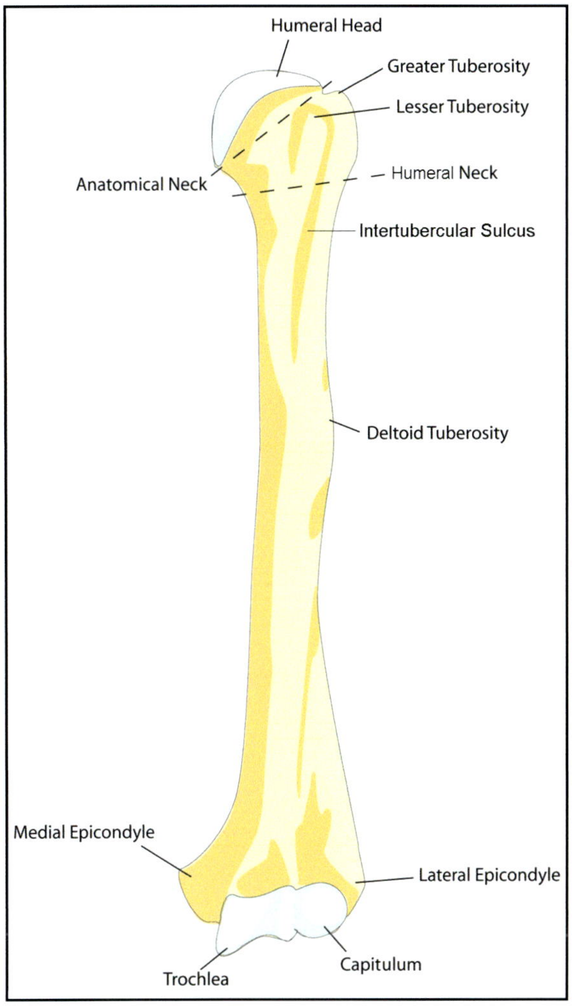

Figure 5-4. Bumps and dents on the humerus. (Morphart Creation/shutterstock.com)

5

Table 5-4
Bumps and Dents in Bones

NAME	DEFINITION	EXAMPLE
condyle	A rounded projection at the ends of long bone	humeral epicondyle
crest	A long, narrow elevated aspect of a bone	iliac crest
foramen	Opening or hole for nerves or blood vessels	vertebral foramen
fossa	Shallow indentation	olecranon fossa
head	Rounded end of a long bone	humeral head
neck	A narrower area of bone between the head and the diaphysis	humeral neck
process	Raised area on a bone where tendons attach	mastoid process
sinus	Hollow cavity within a bone	sinuses within the skull
sulcus	A depression or groove on a bone	intertubercular sulcus on the humerus (the groove between the two tuberosities where the biceps muscles lies)
tubercle/ tuberosity	Round process for tendons; a tuberosity is the same thing in smaller bones	tibia tuberosity

Figure 5-5. The scapula. (Sebastian Kaulitzki/ shutterstock.com)

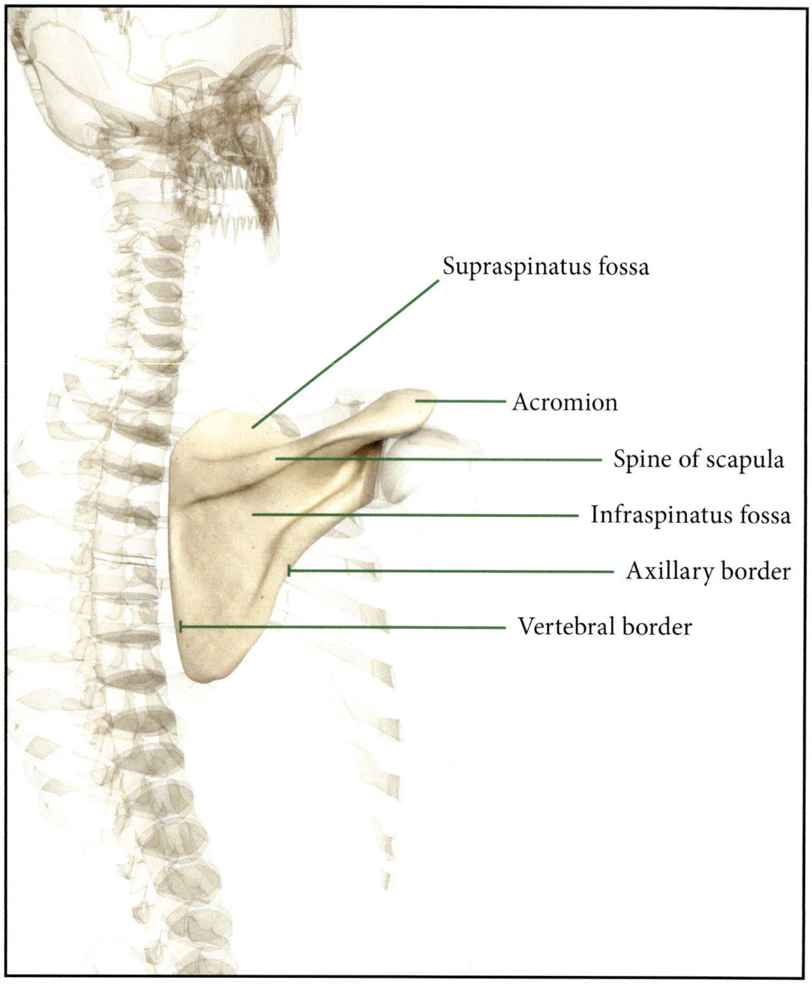

Figure 5-6. Pott's fracture of the ankle. (Alila Medical Images/ shutterstock.com)

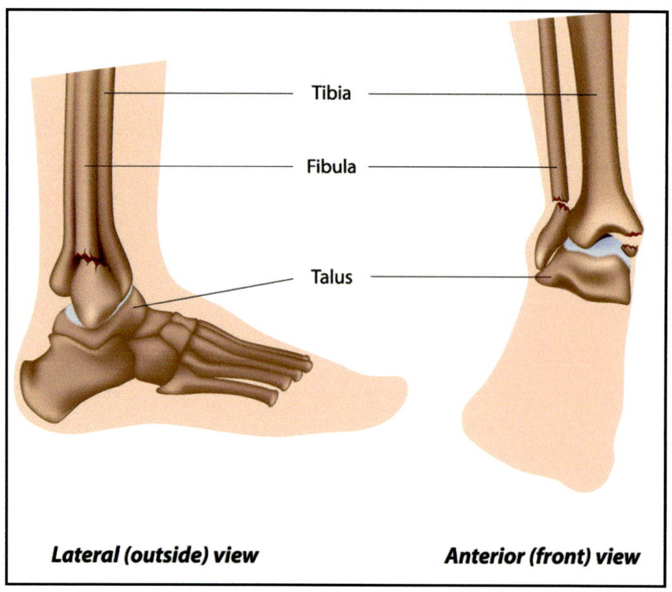

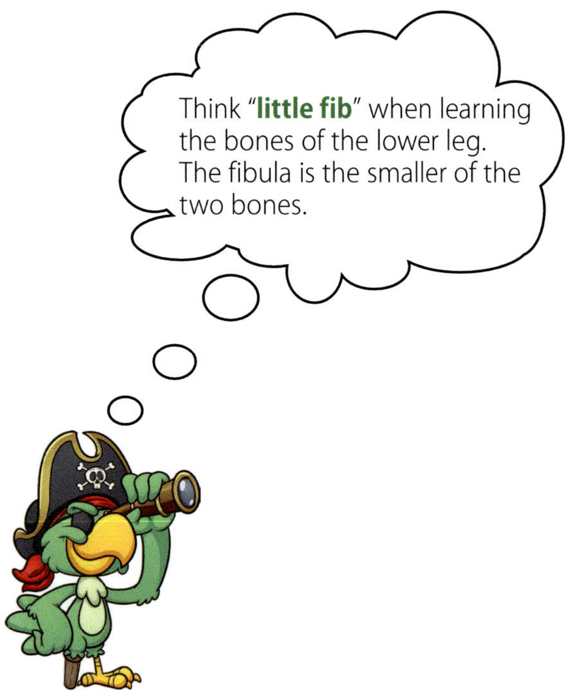

Table 5-5 Types of Fractures (Figure 5-7)	
closed/simple	A fracture that does not break the skin
comminuted	A fracture resulting in a shattered bone in many pieces
compound/open	A fracture that pierces the skin or an underlying organ
compression/impacted	Injured aspect of the bone collapses on itself
greenstick	A fracture that is bent; most common in very young children
hairline/stress	A fracture that does not extend across the whole bone
linear	A fracture in the length (parallel) of a long bone
oblique	A fracture diagonally across the bone
spiral	A fracture that wraps around the bone
transverse	A fracture across the bone, usually at right angles to the bone

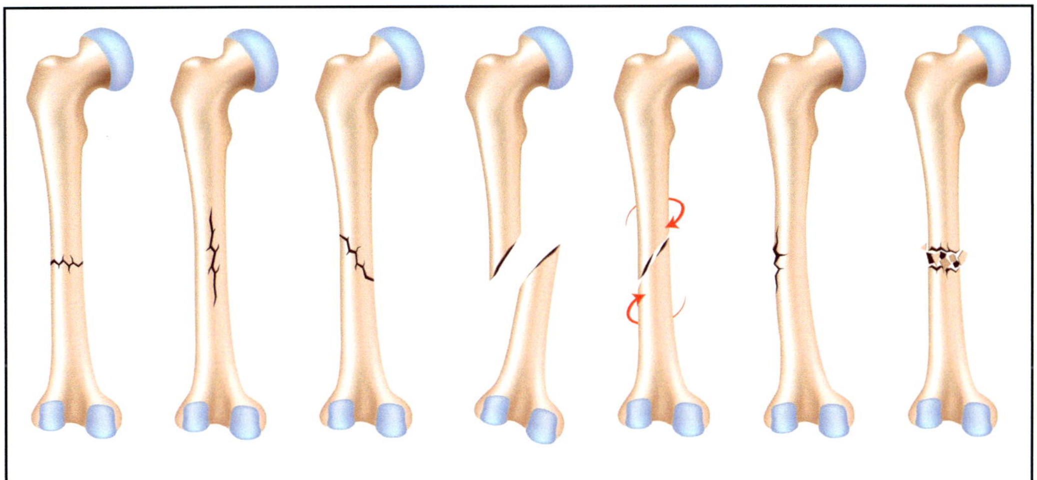

Figure 5-7. Types of bone fractures. (Alila Medical Images/shutterstock.com)

Joints

Bones in the skeleton articulate by several different categories of joints. The three main categories of joints are synarthrosis, amphiarthrosis, and diarthrosis. The **synarthrosis** (**syn-**—union; **arthr/o**—joint), or fibroid, joints are those that do not permit movement, such as sutures, the seam-like lines that connect the majority of the bones of the skull. **Amphiarthrosis** (**amphi-**—both sides) joints allow only slight movement, such as the sternoclavicular joint, which is the connection between the sternum (breast bone) and clavicle (collarbone), symphysis pubis (the joint at the front of the two pelvic bones) joints, and the ulna and carpal (wrist) bones. Amphiarthrosis joints are also called *cartilaginous joints*, as there is usually a fibrocartilage disc in between the bones. But when most people talk of bony joints, they are referring to **diarthrosis** (**dia-**—across, through; **arthr/o**—joint) joints. These articulations, also called *synovial joints*, allow free movement and have synovial fluid in the capsule protecting the joint. The shoulder, elbow, wrist, hip, knee, and ankle joints are all good examples of diarthrosis joints. Figure 5-8 displays the knee and its properties as a diarthrosis joint. There are 6 different classifications of diarthrosis joints in the body, and the motion allowed between the two articulating bones describes each. Table 5-6 provides an overview of synovial joint classifications.

Circumduction is a movement that allows a combination of extension, flexion, abduction, and adduction, but not rotation.

Figure 5-8. The knee is a diarthrosis joint. (Alila Medical Images/shutterstock.com)

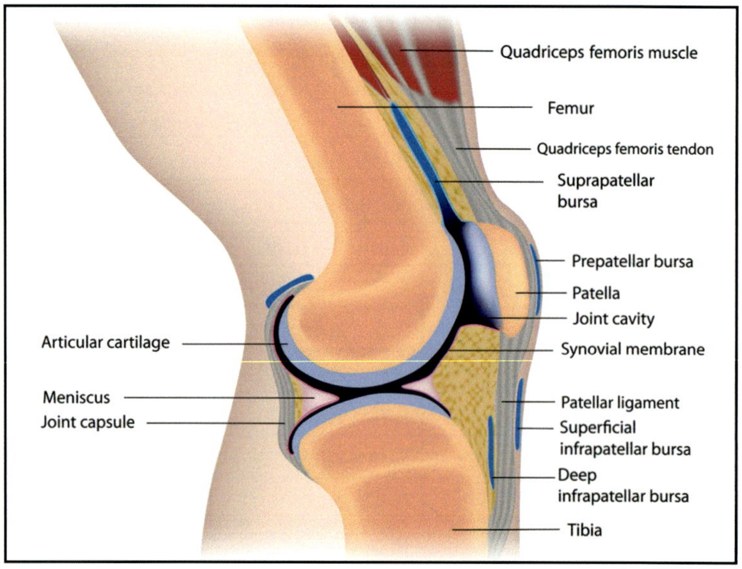

Table 5-6
Synovial Joint Classifications

TYPE	DEFINITION	EXAMPLE
ball and socket	Wide range of motion in all planes (Figure 5-9)	hip or shoulder
condyloid	Permits flexion, extension, abduction, and adduction (together called *circumduction*), but not rotation	wrist
gliding	Limited to gliding between the two articulating bones	wrist and ankle
hinge	Motion in a single plane—usually flexion and extension	elbow
pivot	Limited to rotation	distal elbow where the head of the radius bone rotates via the annular ligament on the ulna bone
saddle	Permits flexion, extension, abduction, and adduction, but not rotation	thumb

Ligaments

Ligaments connect bones together. The fabulous thing about ligaments is that they are almost always named after the two bones to which they attach. If one were to know the names of the bones in the body, then learning the ligament names is easy. For example, the **sacroiliac ligament** joins the sacrum and the iliac bones. Oftentimes, anatomical directions are used in ligament names, such as with the **anterior talofibular (ATF) ligament**. The ATF is the most common ligament injured in an ankle sprain, as it is located in the front of the ankle and joins the talus and the fibula bones (Figure 5-10). Injury to a ligament is called a **sprain**. There are different degrees of ligament sprains, from mild (a stretch of the ligament) to severe (a complete tear/rupture) of the ligament (Figure 5-11). Other commonly injured ligaments are the **anterior cruciate ligament (ACL)** of the knee and the **medial collateral ligament (MCL)**. The word cruciate means "cross," and the ACL crosses from the front of the tibia in the knee to the back of the femur (Figure 5-12). The body has several MCL ligaments, located on the medial aspects of both the elbow and the knee, as well as fingers and toes. Athletes typically have ACL injuries corrected surgically; not everyone who tears (sprains) their ACL needs to have it reconstructed.

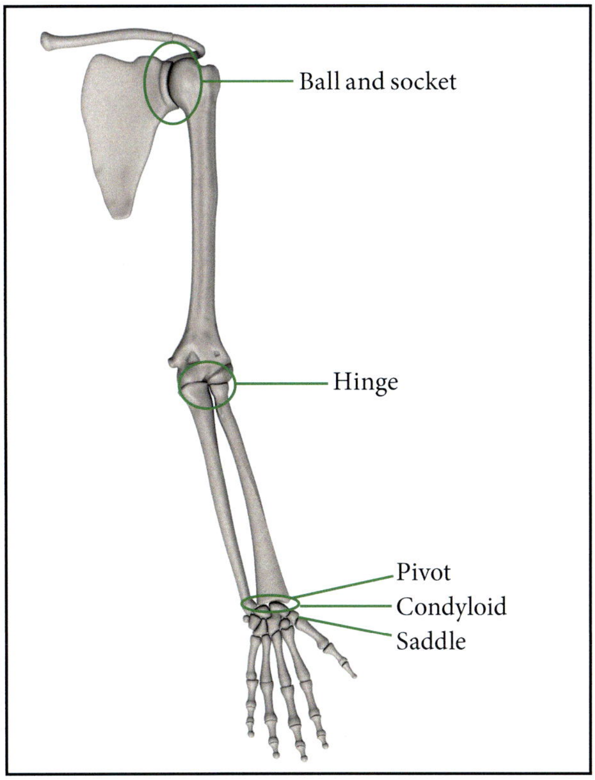

Figure 5-9. Synovial joints of the upper extremity. (3drenderings/shutterstock.com)

Figure 5-10. Lateral ankle sprain of the anterior talofibular ligament. (Alila Medical Images/shutterstock.com)

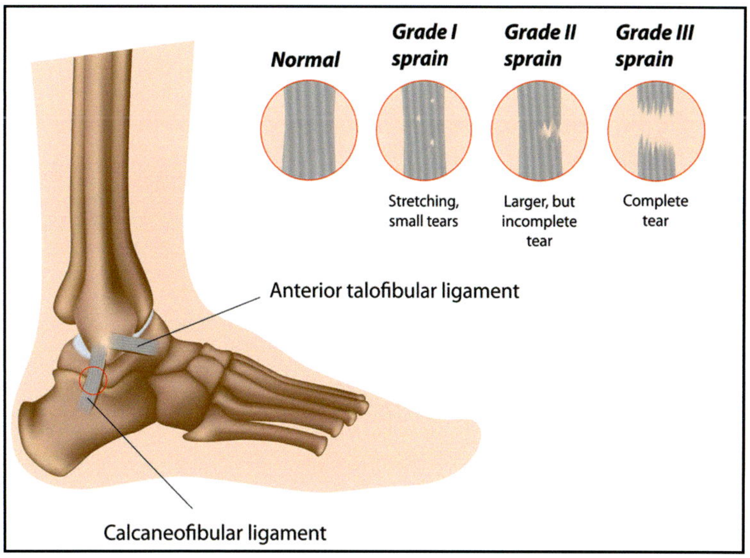

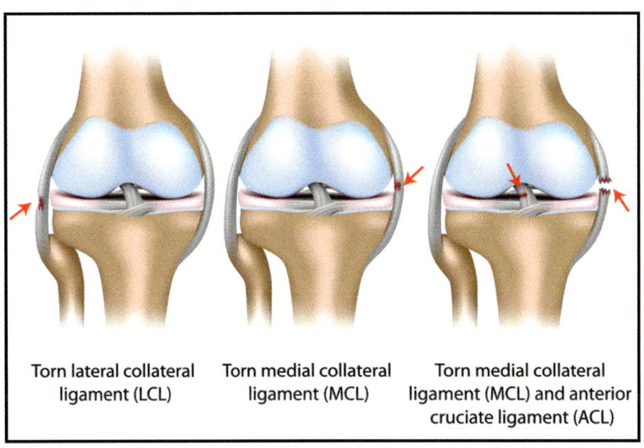

Figure 5-11. Sprained ligaments of the knee. (Alila Medical Images/shutterstock.com)

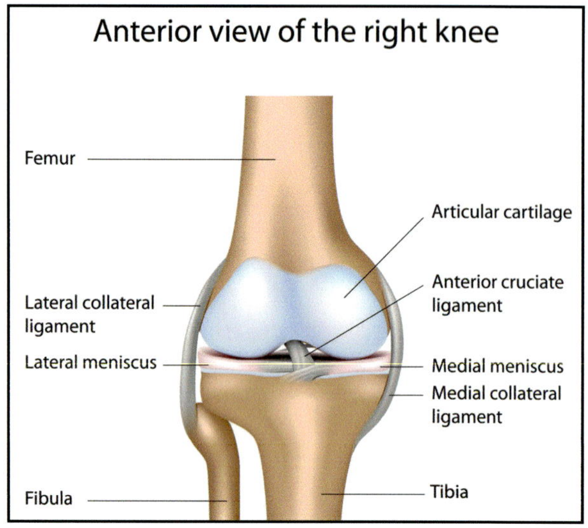

Figure 5-12. Ligaments and cartilage of the knee. (Alila Medical Images/ shutterstock.com)

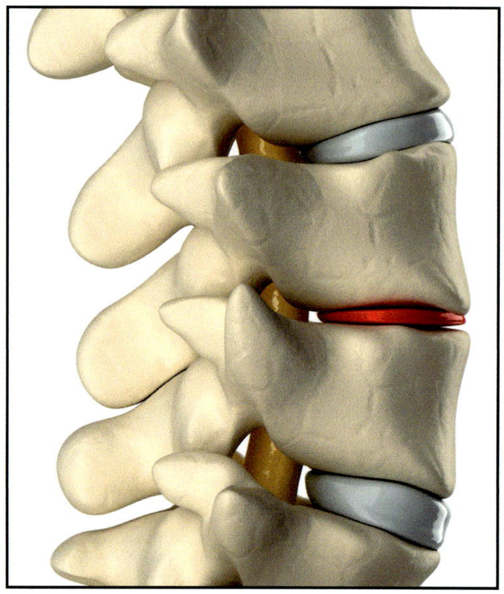

Figure 5-13. Vertebra with protective intervertebral discs. (CLIPAREA I Custom media/ shutterstock.com)

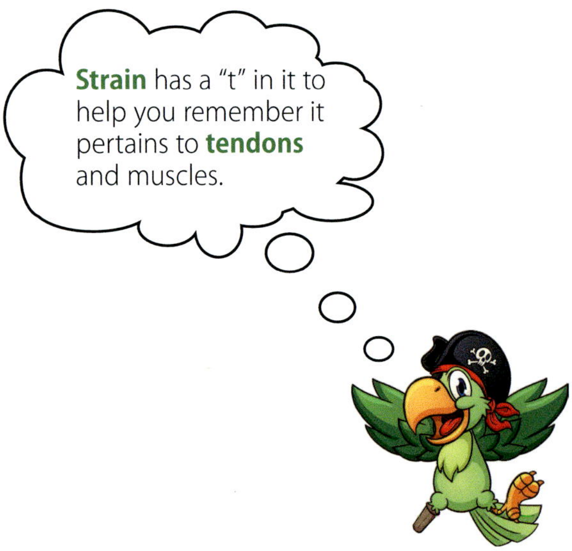
Strain has a "t" in it to help you remember it pertains to **tendons** and muscles.

Bursae, Menisci, and Discs

Other elements of joints are the bursae, menisci, and discs. The function of all of these structures is to protect the joints. Bursae are sacs of synovial fluid that lie in areas (mainly joints) of potential irritation and prevent tendons from rubbing on bones. The bursae are typically small and flexible and move slightly to protect from friction.

When irritated, these sacs can get quite large, inflamed, and infected. **Bursitis** is the term for any inflamed bursa. Common areas for bursitis are in the shoulder, elbow, and knee.

Unlike the articular cartilage that lines the ends of bones, **menisci** (singular—meniscus) are thicker discs of shock-absorbing cartilage. Menisci are solid and are curved to fit perfectly with the articulating bones. Typically, when people refer to a meniscus, they are talking about the protective cartilage in the knee joint between the femur and tibia. Menisci can become damaged with twisting while weight-bearing when they become pinched between the two bones. A **meniscectomy** (**-ectomy**—excision, surgical removal) occurs when a meniscus is surgically excised or removed.

Discs are other protective structures found in joints. Vertebral discs are located in between each vertebra in the back (from the neck to the sacrum; Figure 5-13). Unlike menisci, discs have a semisolid center that creates a shock-absorbing property. Consider the vertebral column as a stack of bricks. If one were to drop the stack, the bricks would most likely shatter. Placing a semi-solid vertebral disc in between the bricks would protect the bricks and likely prevent them from breaking. This concept is the same with the protection the menisci/discs provide in the human body.

TABLE 5-7 WORDS PERTAINING TO THE MUSCULOSKELETAL SYSTEM	
WORD	**DEFINITION**
allograft **allo-**—different	Graft of tissue between two individuals (usually between a person and a cadaver)
aponeurosis	Broad, flat sheets of tissue that act as tendons and attach to bones
apophysitis	Inflammation where a tendon attaches to a bone
autograft **auto-**—self; own	Graft of tissue from the patient's own body
avulsion	Tearing away from a structure
callus	Fibrous mass at a fracture site that is the groundwork for new bone
crepitus	Crackling or crunching sound heard or felt; often associated with a fracture or tendinitis
cyst	Closed sac in or under the skin that contains fluid
debridement	Removal of foreign or damaged tissue to prevent infection and promote healing
deviation	Turning from a straight path; ulnar deviation is to move the hand toward the pinky side
epiphysis	Growth center of long bones
fasciae	Fibrous connective tissue; often separated from other organized tissues
idiopathic	Of unknown cause (this word is not specifically related to the musculoskeletal system)
ligament	Tough fibrous tissue that connects bones together
prosthesis	Artificial body part
retinaculum	Broad, flat tissue that holds tendons close to the bone, such as in the wrist and ankle
sprain	Injury to a ligament
stenosis	Narrowing of a structure
strain	Injury to a tendon or muscle
tendon	End of a muscle as it attaches to a bone
xenograft	Graft of tissue from another species

5

Muscles

There are three types of muscle: striated, smooth, and cardiac (see Figure 5-21). **Striated muscles** also have other common names (voluntary or skeletal) and are what most people are referring to when they speak of muscles. We usually have conscious control over striated muscles. As their name indicates, striated muscles have organized bands (fibrils) and have both fast- and slow-twitch fiber properties. People can train their muscles to adapt and grow based on the demand put upon them. For example, long-distance runners have long, lean muscles that are largely slow-twitch fibers and are critical for activity over time (aerobic). Sprinters have thick, stocky muscles comprised chiefly of fast-twitch fibers that operate best under bursts of activity (anaerobic). Smooth muscles are also referred to as *visceral* or *involuntary muscles*, as they are found in the digestive system, secretory ducts, and blood vessels. **Smooth muscles** are controlled by the autonomic nervous system and not by willing them to move. The fibers of this type of muscle can be found in sheets as they typically wrap around vessels and within organs.

Cardiac muscle is found only in the myocardium (**my/o**—muscle; **card/i**—heart; **-um**—structure, thing) of the heart. This type of muscle has unique fibers that are more similar to striated muscle, but also contains the properties of smooth muscle, as cardiac muscle is not controlled by conscious thought. This chapter focuses primarily on striated muscles. Chapters 6 ("Cardiovascular System") and 9 ("Gastrointestinal System") will discuss cardiac and smooth muscles as they relate to those systems.

Table 5-8
Skeletal and Joint Disorders/Conditions

NAME	WORD PARTS	DEFINITION
acromegaly	acr/o (extremity) **-megaly** (abnormally large; enlargement)	Gradual growth of facial bones due to a chronic metabolic disorder
arthritis (Figure 5-14)	arthr/ (joint) **-itis** (inflammation)	Inflammation of a joint; also called *osteoarthritis* (oste/o—bone)
arthroclasia	arthr/o (joint) **-clasia** (to break)	Surgical breaking of a joint fused due to scar tissue
avascular necrosis	**a-** (without) vascul/ (blood vessel); **-ar** (pertaining to) necr/ (death) **-osis** (condition)	Bone death due to lack of blood
bursitis (Figure 5-15)	burs/ (bursa) **-itis** (inflammation)	Inflammation of a bursa
chondromalacia	chondr/o (cartilage) **-malacia** (softening)	Softening of hyaline (articular) cartilage
costochondritis	cost/o (rib) chondr/o (cartilage) **-itis** (inflammation)	Inflammation where the ribs and cartilage join in the front of the body
dislocation (Figure 5-16)		Situation where two bones are no longer in contact in the normal joint
enchondroma	**en-** (within) chondr/ (cartilage) **-oma** (mass, tumor)	A benign but slowly growing cartilage cell tumor; usually found in long bones, as well as hands and feet
epicondylitis	**epi-** (above; upon) condyl/ (condyle; knuckle) **-itis** (inflammation)	Inflammation above the joint; most often recognized as lateral epicondylitis (tennis elbow)
exostosis	**ex-** (outside) oste/o (bone) **-osis** (condition)	Bone spur (extra bone mass) outside of a normal bone
gout (Figure 5-17)		Genetic form of arthritis causing uric acid crystals to accumulate in a joint (usually the great toe)
hallux valgus	hallux (great toe) valgus (bent)	The great toe is angled away from the midline; toward the remaining toes
hemarthrosis	hem/ (blood) arthr/ (joint) **-osis** (condition)	Blood in the joint
hematoma	hemat/ (blood) **-oma** (tumor; mass)	Bruise; collection of blood

(continued)

Table 5-8 (continued)
Skeletal and Joint Disorders/Conditions

NAME	WORD PARTS	DEFINITION
kyphosis (Figure 5-18)	kyph/ (bent) **-osis** (condition)	Humpback-type curve of the back
lordosis	lord/ (swayback) **-osis** (condition)	Normal curve of the cervical and lumbar spine; can also be abnormal if the curve is excessive (swayback)
malunion	**mal-** (bad) union (together)	Bony break that is not aligned correctly
nonunion	**non-** (not) union (together)	Fracture that is not healing
osteocarcinoma	oste/o (bone) carcin/ (cancer) **-oma** (tumor)	Cancerous tumor of the bone
osteochondritis	oste/o (bone) chondr/ (cartilage) **-itis** (inflammation)	Inflammation of the bone and cartilage
osteomalacia (Figure 5-19)	oste/o (bone) **-malacia** (softening)	Decrease in vitamin D and calcium leading to bony deformities (usually in the legs); in children; termed *rickets*
osteomyelitis	oste/o (bone) myel/ (bone marrow) **-itis** (inflammation)	Infection of the bone marrow
osteopenia	oste/o (bone) **-penia** (decrease)	Decrease in bone mass
osteoporosis (Figure 5-20)	oste/o (bone) **-porosis** (porous)	Abnormal loss of bone tissue
osteosarcoma	oste/o (bone) sarc/ (flesh; connective tissue) **-oma** (tumor)	Cancer (tumor) from connective tissue and bone
polydactyly	**poly-** (many) dactyl/ (fingers/toes) **-y** (process of)	More than five fingers or toes on each hand or foot
scoliosis	scoli/ (curved) **-osis** (condition)	Abnormal lateral curve of the spine
spondylitis	spondyl/ (vertebra) **-itis** (inflammation)	Inflammation of the vertebra
spondylolisthesis	spondyl/o (vertebra) **-listhesis** (slipping)	Forward slippage of one vertebra on another due to bilateral fractures in the vertebra bony ring
spondylosis	spondyl /(vertebra) **-osis** (condition)	Abnormal condition of the vertebra where the joints stiffen

(continued)

5

Table 5-8 (continued)
Skeletal and Joint Disorders/Conditions

NAME	WORD PARTS	DEFINITION
subluxation	**sub-** (under; below) luxation (a dislocated joint)	Partial dislocation
syndactyly	**syn-** (joined) dactyl/ (fingers/toes) **-y** (process of)	Fused digits (fingers or toes)

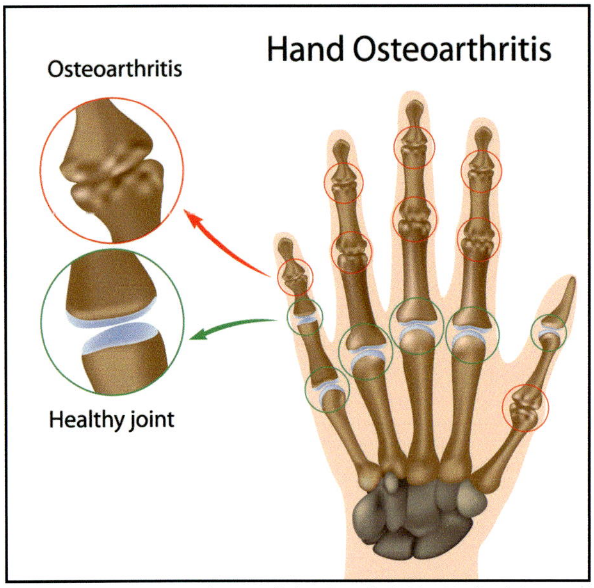

Figure 5-14. Osteoarthritis of the hand. (Alila Medical Images/shutterstock.com)

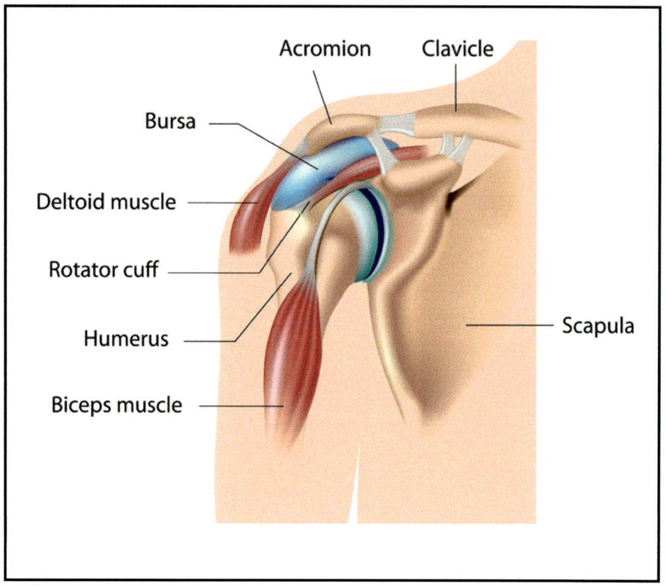

Figure 5-15. Bursitis of the subacromial bursa. (Alila Medical Images/shutterstock.com)

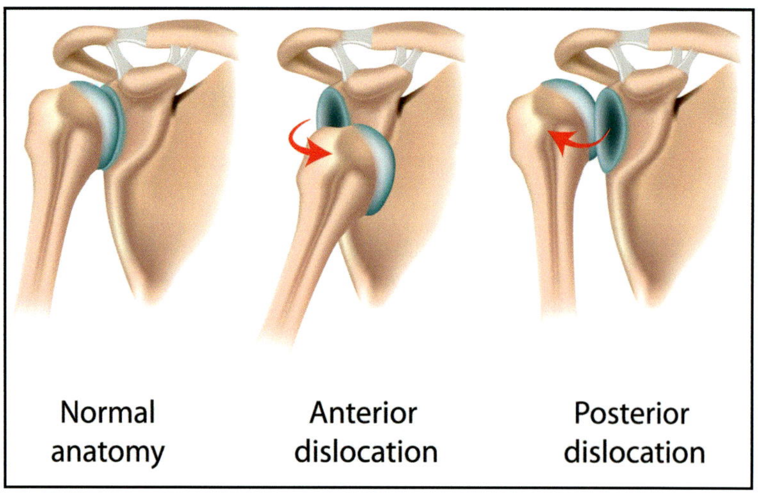

Figure 5-16. Shoulder dislocation. (Alila Medical Images/shutterstock.com)

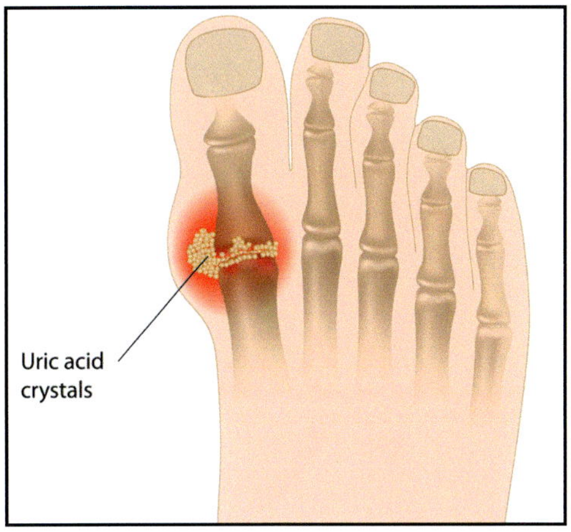

Figure 5-17. Gout of the big toe. (Alila Medical Images/shutterstock.com)

Figure 5-18. Deformities of the spine. (Blamb/shutterstock.com)

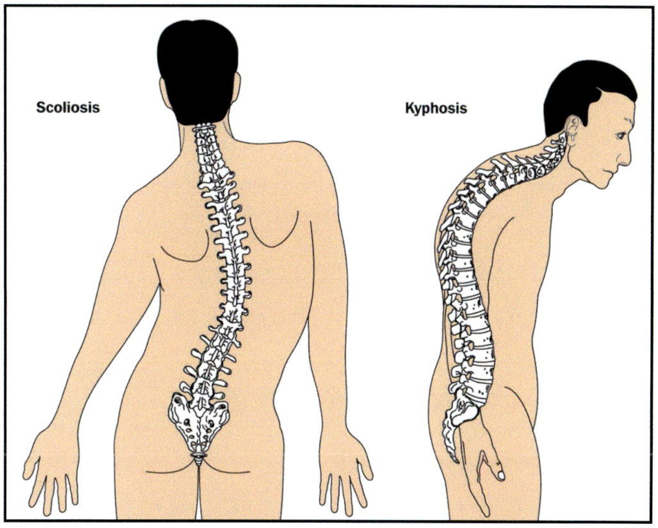

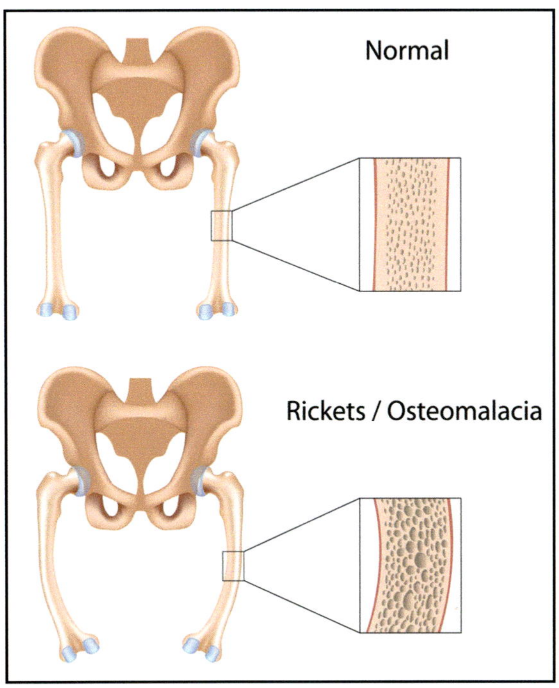

Figure 5-19. Osteomalacia. (Alila Medical Images/shutterstock.com)

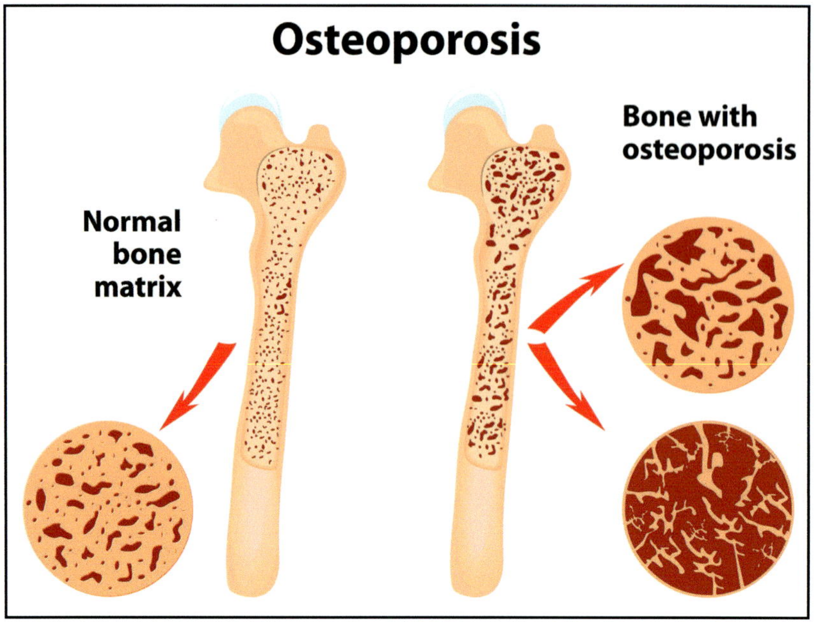

Figure 5-20. Comparison of healthy bone and osteoporosis of the femur. (Ahabska Tetyana/ shutterstock.com)

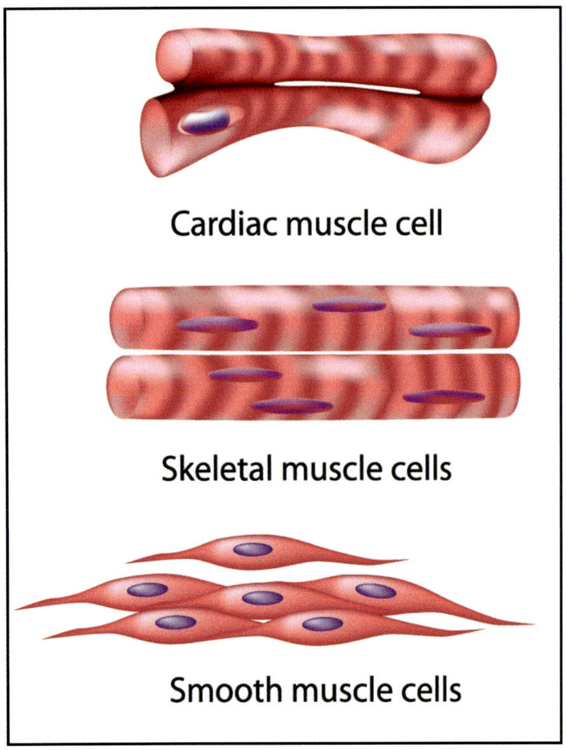

Figure 5-21. Muscle cell types. (Alila Medical Images/shutterstock.com)

Although they may look intimidating at first glance, muscles often have names that coincide with anatomical directions or bones. When looking at a person in anatomical position, it is easier to keep track of the names of the muscles. **Flexor carpi ulnaris**, for example, flexes the **carpals** (**carp/o**—carpals; wrist bones) and is located on the **ulna** (ulnaris) side of the forearm. **Brachioradialis** is easily found on the body, as **brachi/o** means "arm" and the *radialis* aspect of the word tells you that it is connected to the radius bone of the forearm. The forearm muscles are in Figure 5-22. Once you learn the names of the bones (and recall the anatomical directions learned in Chapter 3), there will be few muscles that do not make sense by their names alone.

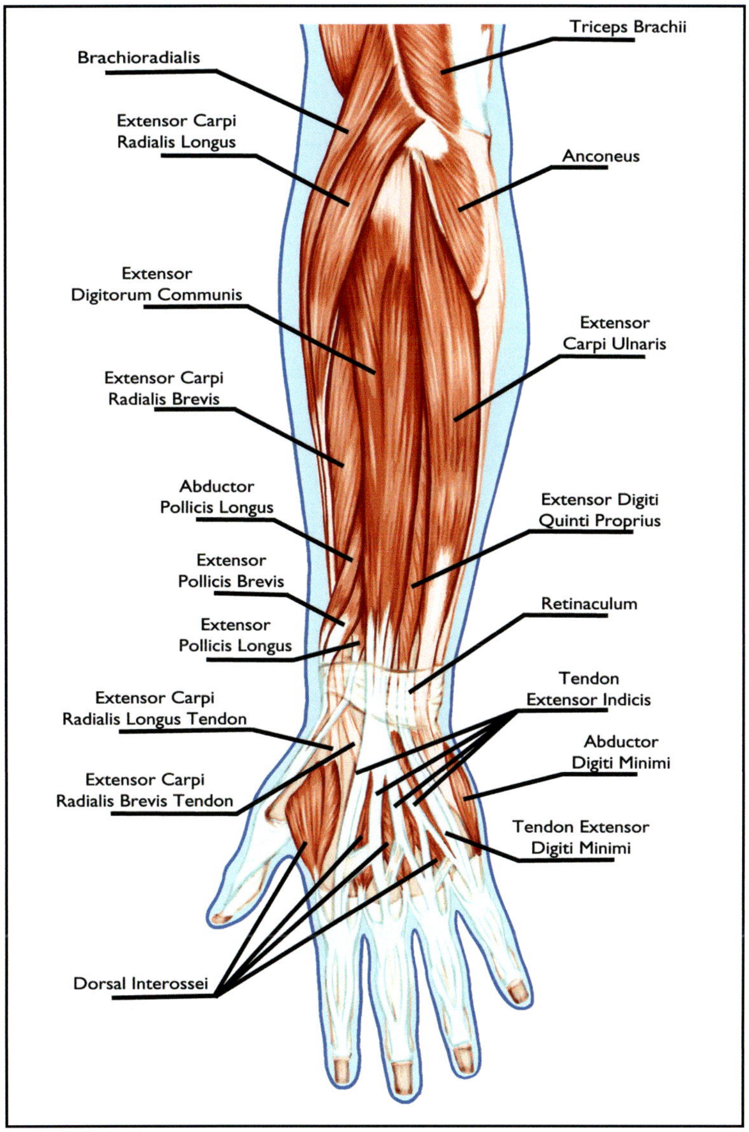

Figure 5-22. Muscles of the dorsal forearm. (stihii/shutterstock.com)

Medical Conditions

This textbook is not intended to be a medical reference nor a pharmacology text, as other books and courses are better geared to pathophysiology and pharmacology of medical conditions. Instead, this book introduces medical words related to each body system and provides a very brief and simple overview of conditions. The focus is learning the words, and relaying how the definition can provide enough information to have a very general understanding of the conditions.

There are many conditions that have names that are not necessarily made up of medical word elements, but are instead unique or named after the person/people who initially diagnosed them. Table 5-10 contains conditions/diseases pertaining to the musculoskeletal system. Some have attributes that cross over systems, but most pertain especially to this system or are first manifested by muscle pain or weakness.

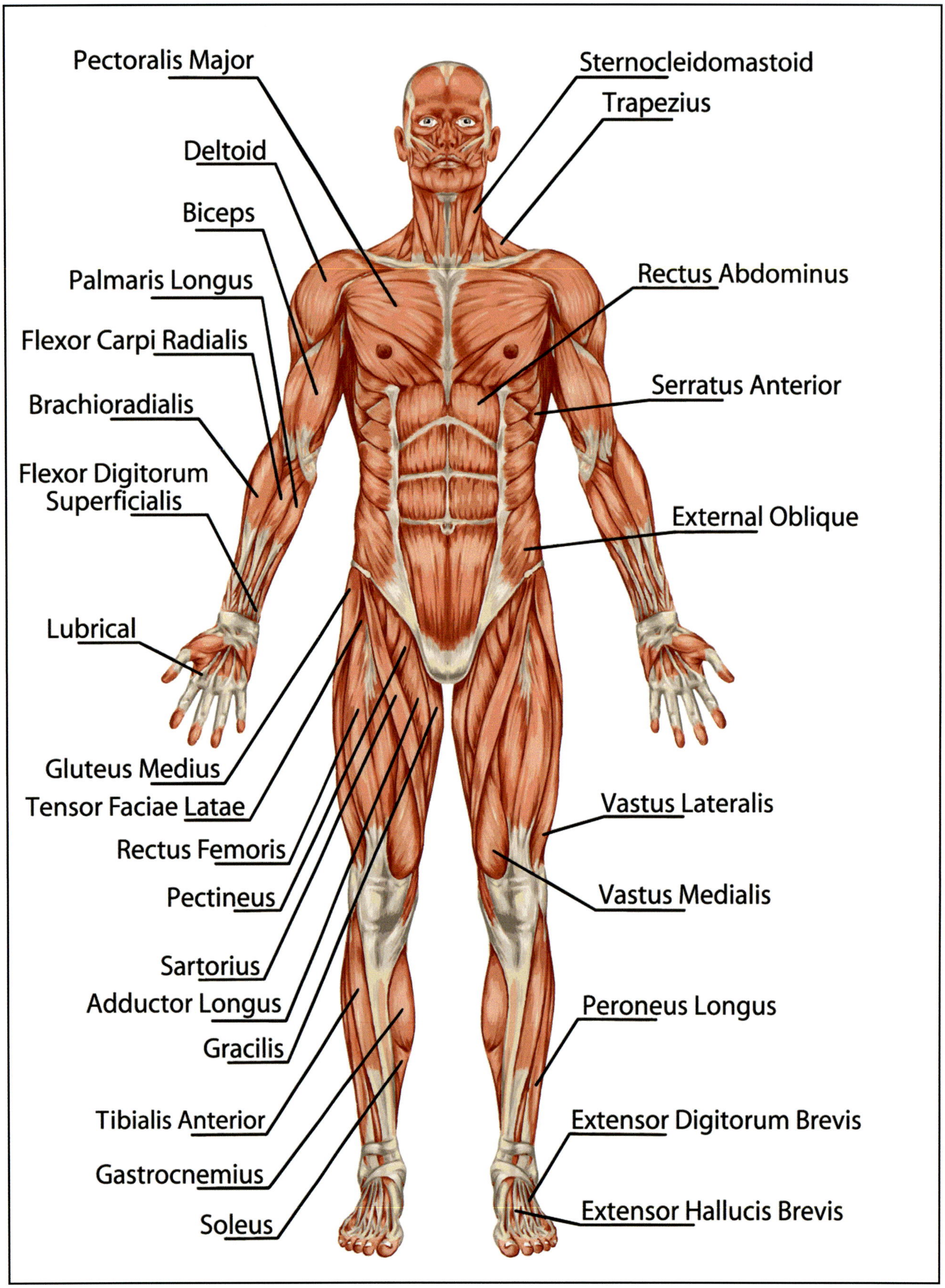

Figure 5-23. Anterior musculature of the body. Note this figure is in anatomical position. (stihii/shutterstock.com)

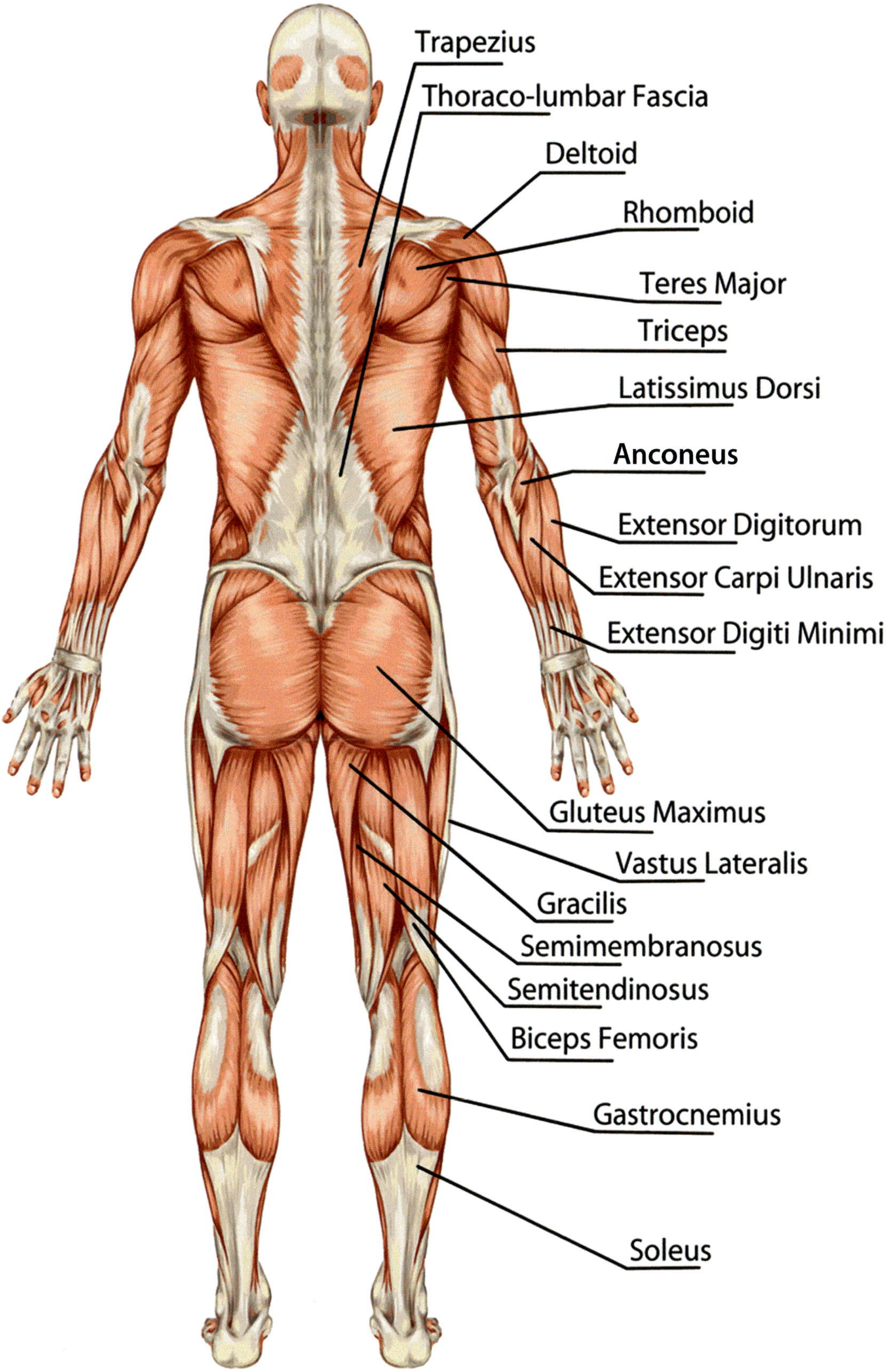

Figure 5-24. Posterior musculature of the body. (stihii/shutterstock.com)

Table 5-9
Muscular Disorders and Terms

TERM	WORD PARTS	DEFINITION
atrophy	**a-** (without) troph/ (development) **-y** (process of)	Wasting away of muscle tissue (usually from disuse, injury, or illness)
bradykinesia	**brady-** (slow) **-kinesia** (movement)	Slow movement
clonic	clon/ (turmoil) **-ic** (pertaining to)	Pertaining to (a muscle spasm) alternating contraction and relaxation of muscles
contraction	**con-** (together) tract/ (to pull) **-ion** (process)	Process of drawing together
dactylospasm	dactyl/o (finger; toe) **-spasm** (involuntary contraction)	Cramp (spasm) in a finger or toe
dermatomyositis	dermat/o (skin) my/o (muscle) **-itis** (inflammation)	Chronic systemic immunological disease involving inflammation of the skin, connective tissue, and muscles
hypertrophy (Figure 5-25)	**hyper-** (excessive) troph/ (development) **-y** (process of)	Excessive muscle tone, excessive development
insertion (Figure 5-26)		Pertaining to muscles, point of attachment (usually distal) where the tendon of the muscle attaches to a bone and causes movement
interosseous	**inter-** (between) osse/ (bone) **-ous** (pertaining to)	Between two bones
origin		Pertaining to muscles, point of origin of attachment (usually proximal) where the tendon of the muscle attaches to a bone and causes movement
rhabdomyolysis	rhabd/ (rod-shaped) my/o (muscle) **-lysis** (breaking down)	Breakdown of striated (skeletal) muscle; potentially fatal condition associated with strenuous exercise, crush injury, and medications
spina bifida occulta	spin/a (spine) **bi-** (two) **-fida** (to split) **-occult** (hidden)	Congenital malformation of the vertebra where the bony ring protecting the spinal cord is not complete; the occulta aspect of this condition indicates the spinal cord is not damaged/ involved
tenodesis	ten/o (tendon) **-desis** (bind)	Surgical binding (tying) of a tendon
torticollis		Muscular spasms in the neck causing neck stiffness

Table 5-10
Conditions of the Musculoskeletal System With Unique Names

NAME	DEFINITION
fibromyalgia	fibr/o (fiber), my/ (muscle), **-algia** (pain); disorder with widespread, chronic musculoskeletal pain and fatigue
Legg-Calvé-Perthes disease	Osteochondrosis of the femoral head in children
muscular dystrophy	**dys-** (abnormal; bad; difficult; painful), **-troph** (development), **-y** (process of); genetic disorder causing progressive atrophy of the skeletal muscles
myasthenia gravis (MG)	Chronic autoimmune disorder where one lacks muscle strength; the primary symptom is increasing weakness with activity, and improvement with rest
Osgood-Schlatter disease (Figure 5-27)	Apophysitis (inflammation of where a tendon meets a bone) in the tibial tuberosity
Paget's disease	Skeletal disease of middle-aged and older adults, characterized by excessive bone destruction and unorganized repair
rheumatoid arthritis (RA) (Figure 5-28)	Disease affecting the connective tissues; chronic, destructive disorder that may have an autoimmune component
Sever's disease (Figure 5-29)	Apophysitis at the attachment of the Achilles tendon on the calcaneus
Sinding-Larsen–Johansson disease	Apophysitis at the distal pole of the patella (and the patella tendon)
systemic lupus erythematosus (SLE)	Autoimmune disorder causing chronic inflammation in many systems of the body

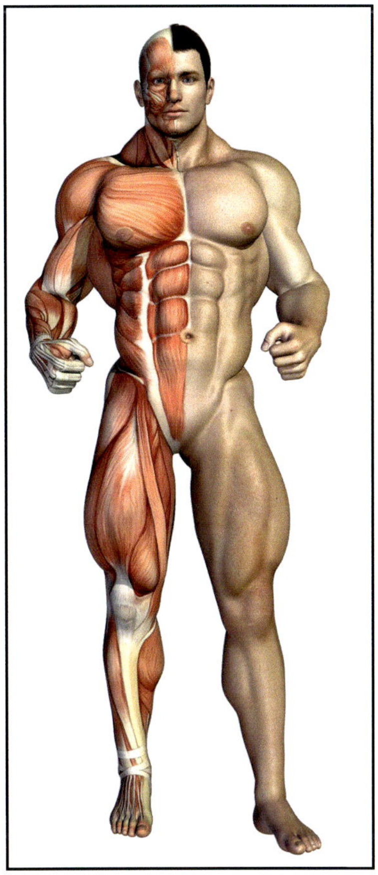

Figure 5-25. Hypertrophy of muscles. (Linda Bucklin/shutterstock.com)

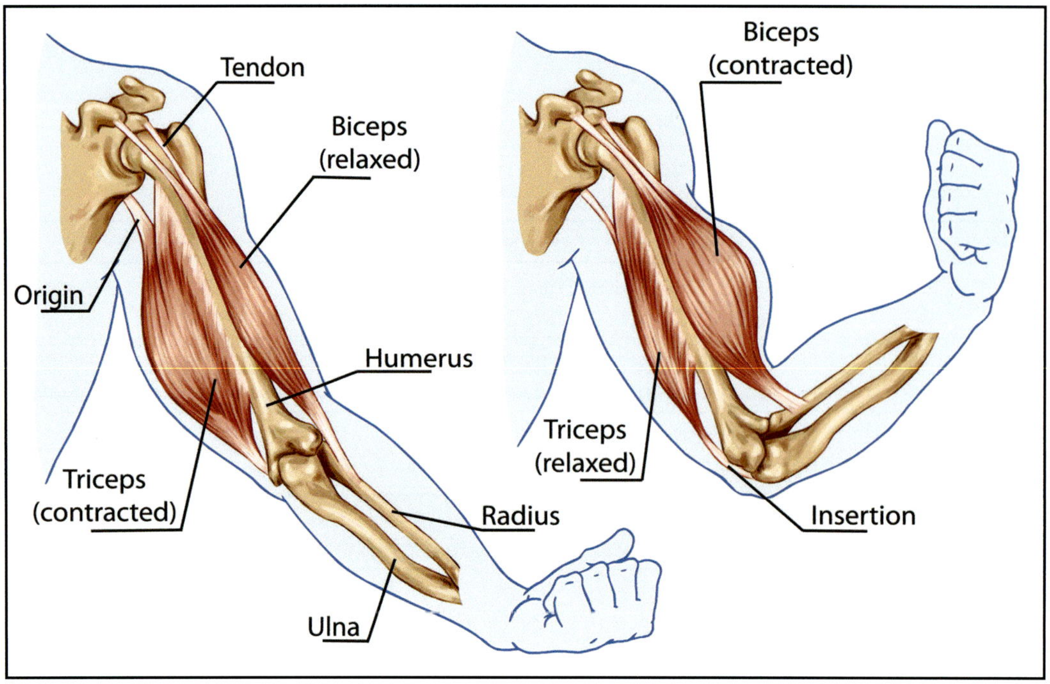

Figure 5-26. Origin and insertions of the biceps and triceps. (stihii/shutterstock.com)

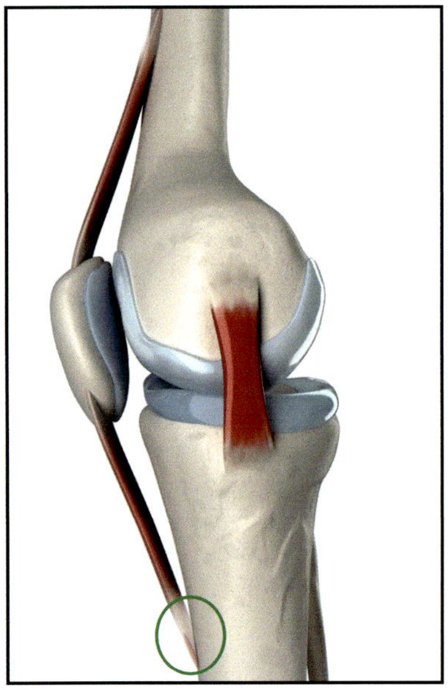

Figure 5-27. In Osgood-Schlatter disease, the patellar tendon pulls on its insertion, the tibial tuberosity (circled). (CLIPAREA I Custom media/shutterstock.com)

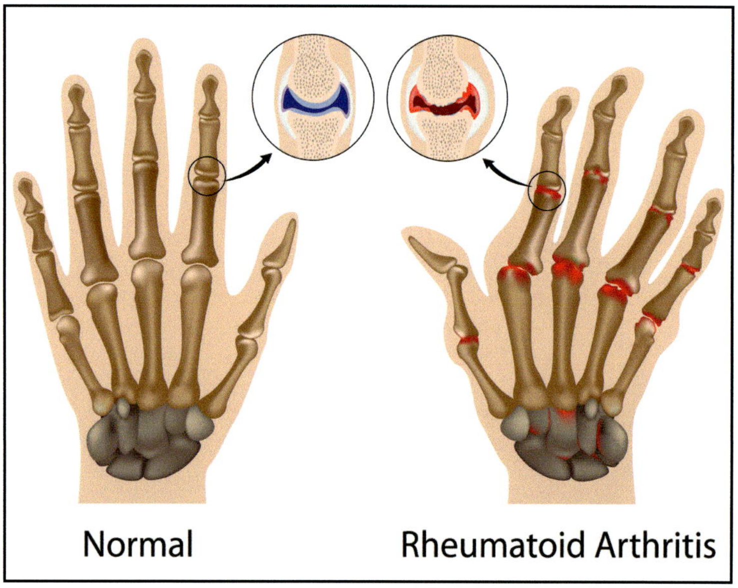

Figure 5-28. Rheumatoid arthritis of hand. (Alila Medical Images/shutterstock.com)

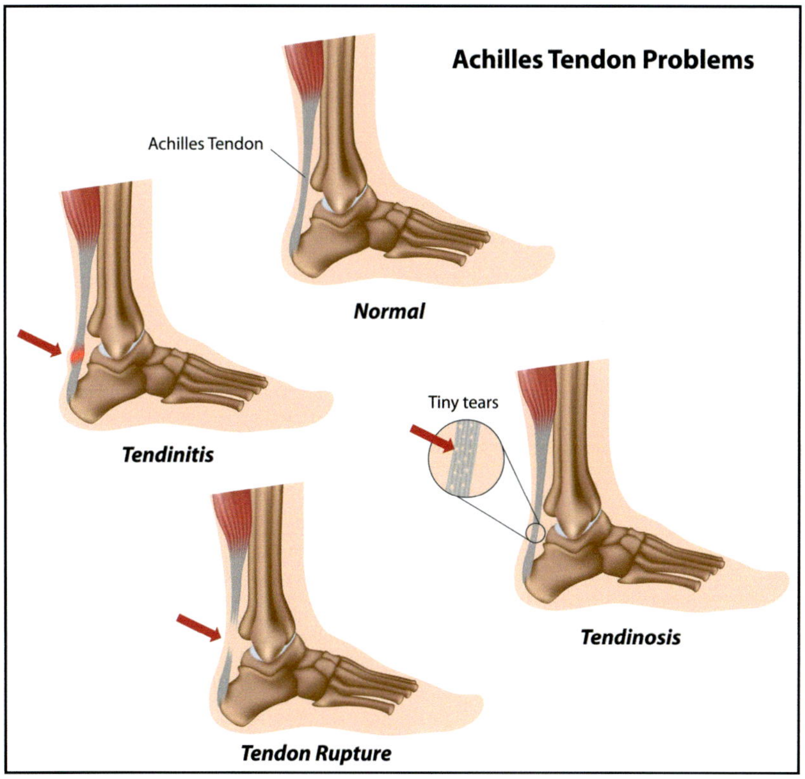

Figure 5-29. Sever's disease is a form of tendinitis. (Alila Medical Images/shutterstock.com)

5

Tests and Procedures

Table 5-11
Tests and Procedures Specific to the Musculoskeletal System

NAME	WORD PARTS	PURPOSE
amputation		Surgical removal of a digit/limb
ankylosis (Figure 5-30)	ankyl/o (bent) **-osis** (condition)	Immobility of a joint; fixation
arthrocentesis	arthr/o (joint) **-centesis** (surgical puncture)	Process used to remove fluid from a joint
arthrodesis	arthr/o (joint) **-desis** (fuse; bind)	Stabilizing a joint via surgery
arthroplasty	arthr/o (joint) **-plasty** (repair)	Surgical repair of a joint
arthroscopy (Figure 5-31)	arth/o (joint) **-scopy** (examination of)	Visual examination of a joint during surgery; often surgical procedures (eg, meniscectomy) are performed during the procedure

(continued)

Table 5-11 (continued)

Tests and Procedures Specific to the Musculoskeletal System

NAME	WORD PARTS	PURPOSE
bunionectomy (Figure 5-32)	bunion/ (bunion) **-ectomy** (surgical removal)	Surgical correction of a bunion
bursectomy	burs/ (bursa) **-ectomy** (surgical removal)	Surgical removal of a bursa
craniotomy	crani/ (cranium) **-otomy** (to cut into)	Cutting an opening in the cranium
discectomy (Figure 5-33)	disc/ (disc) **-ectomy** (surgical removal)	Surgical removal of an intervertebral disc, usually due to disc herniation
fasciotomy	fasci/ (fascia) **-otomy** (to cut into)	Cutting an opening in the fascia, usually to relieve pressure from an injury; typically occurs in the shin or thigh
laminectomy	lamin/ (lamina) **-ectomy** (surgical removal)	Removal of the lamina in the vertebra to provide more room for the spinal cord
meniscectomy	menisc/ (meniscus) **-ectomy** (surgical removal)	Surgical removal of the meniscus in the knee
myelogram	myel/o (spinal cord) **-gram** (a record of)	Following an injection of dye, the spinal canal is x-rayed
myorrhaphy	my/o (muscle) **-rrhaphy** (suturing)	Suture of a muscle
osteoclasis	oste/o (bone) **-clasis** (to break)	Intentional breaking of a bone to reset it in a better anatomical position
rachiotomy	rachi/ (vertebral column) **-otomy** (incision)	Surgical incision into the vertebral column
spondylosyndesis	spondyl/o (vertebra) **syn-** (together) **-desis** (fuse)	Fusion of the spine; done by surgical device (plate/screw), bone graft, or body cast

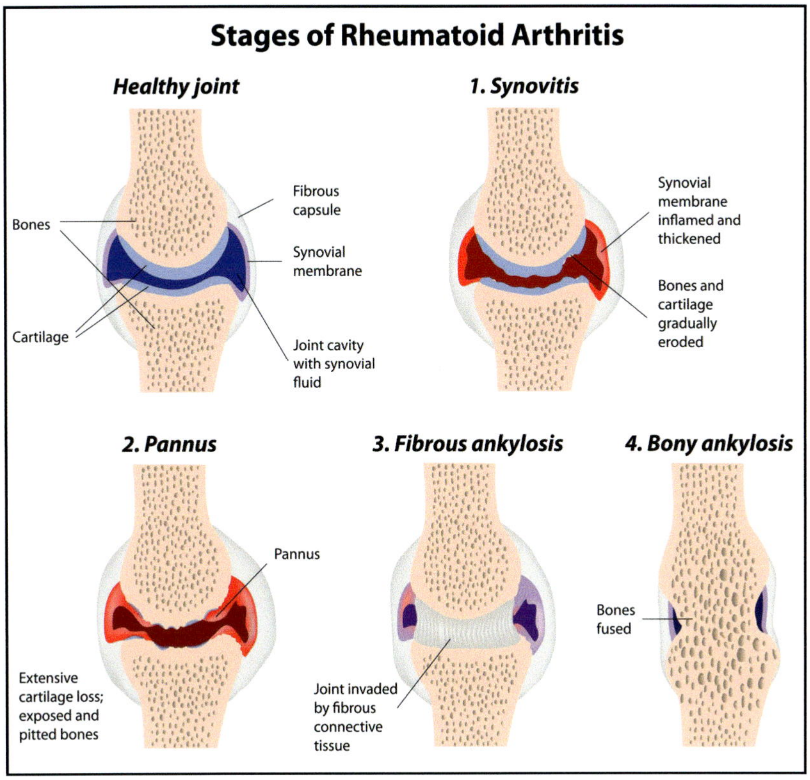

Figure 5-30. A healthy knee and a fused knee. (Alila Medical Images/shutterstock.com)

5

Figure 5-31. Arthroscopy of the knee. (hkannn/shutterstock.com)

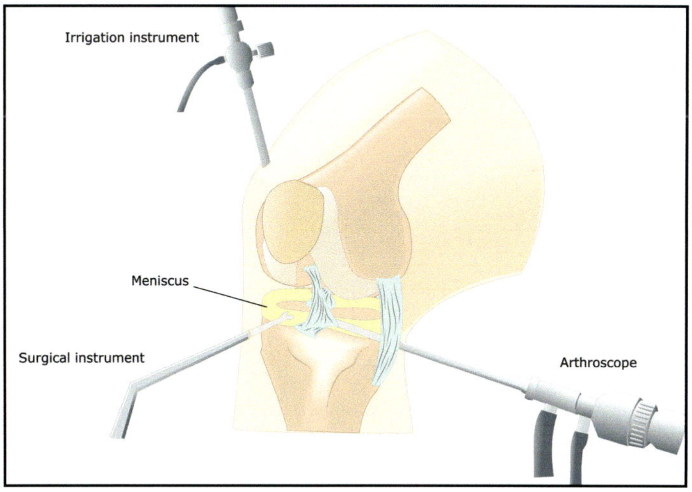

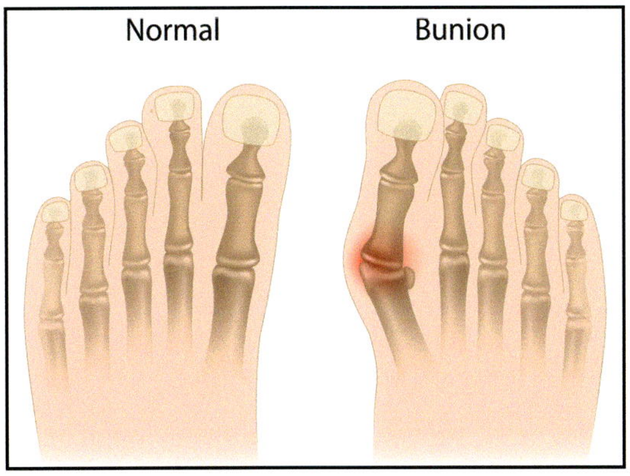

Figure 5-32. A normal foot and a foot with a bunion. (Alila Medical Images/shutterstock.com)

Figure 5-33. A herniated disc can be treated by a discectomy. (CLIPAREA I Custom media/shutterstock.com)

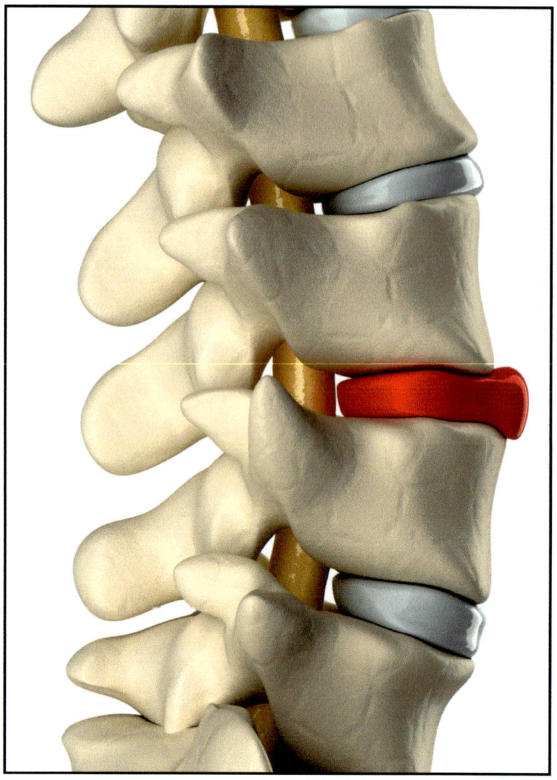

Bibliography

Basco R, Allan B. *Medical Language for Modern Health Care*. 5th ed. McGraw-Hill; 2023.
Fremgen BF, Frucht SS. *Medical Terminology: A Living Language*. 7th ed. Pearson; 2019.
Hutton A. *Medical Terminology for Health Care*. 5th ed. Churchill Livingstone; 2017.
Mosby's Dictionary of Medicine, Nursing & Health Professions. 10th ed. Elsevier; 2017.
Rice J. *Medical Terminology for Health Care Professionals*. 9th ed. Pearson; 2018.
Shiland BJ. *Mastering Healthcare Terminology*. 6th ed. Elsevier; 2019.
Venes D, ed. *Taber's Cyclopedic Medical Dictionary*. 24th ed. F. A. Davis; 2021.

NOTES

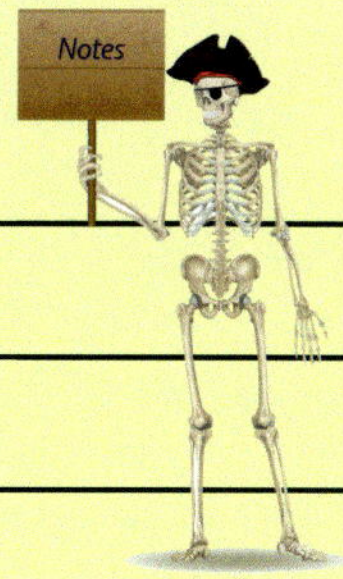

Notes

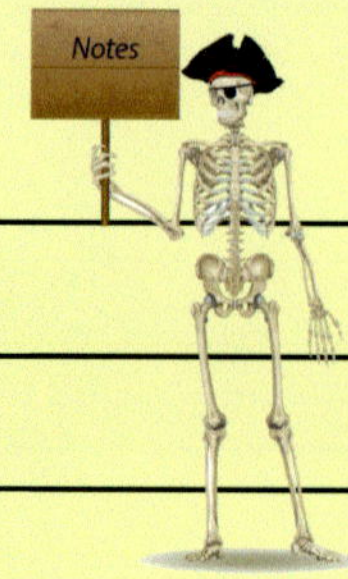

Learning Activities

Name:______________________

Musculoskeletal System

A. Label parts of the joints from the following list.

- synarthrosis________
- amphiarthrosis______
- diarthrosis_________

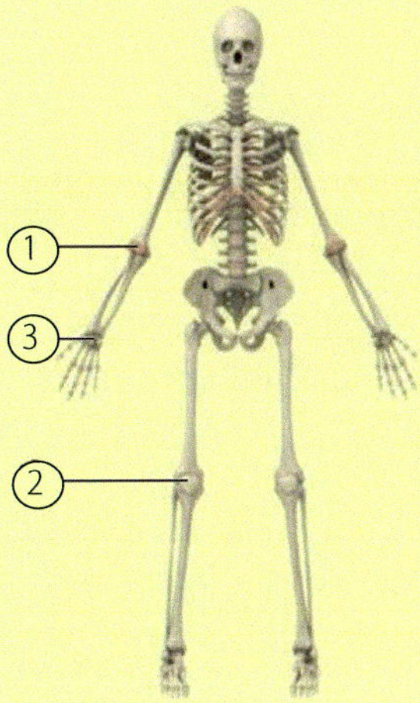

B. Label parts of a long bone from the following list.

- articular cartilage___________
- endosteum________________
- diaphysis_________________
- distal epiphysis_____________
- medullary cavity____________
- periosteum________________
- proximal epiphysis__________
- spongy bone_______________

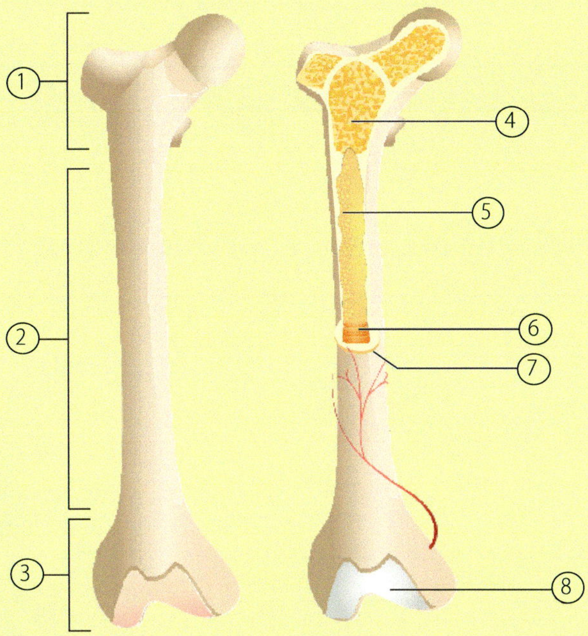

C. Match the word part with its meaning.

1. brachi/o____________ a. pain
2. **syn-**____________ b. split
3. **ex-**____________ c. across; through
4. **-asthenia**____________ d. union
5. myel/o____________ e. arm
6. rachi/o____________ f. flesh
7. **-fida**____________ g. spine
8. sarc____________ h. outside
9. **dia-**____________ i. weakness
10. **-dynia**____________ j. bone marrow; spinal cord

D. Using word parts from previous chapters as well as new ones presented in this chapter, separate the prefix and suffix from the word root and define the following words.

1. intercostal________________________
2. osteomyelitis________________________
3. osteocarcinoma________________________
4. rachigraph________________________
5. periosteoedema________________________
6. radial________________________
7. subcostal________________________
8. atrophy________________________
9. dactylospasm________________________
10. myomalacia________________________

E. Label the bones of the body from the following list.

- sternum____________________
- humerus____________________
- lumbar spine____________________
- cervical spine____________________
- femur____________________
- patella____________________
- ulna____________________
- scapula____________________
- clavicle____________________
- ilium____________________
- mandible____________________
- maxilla____________________

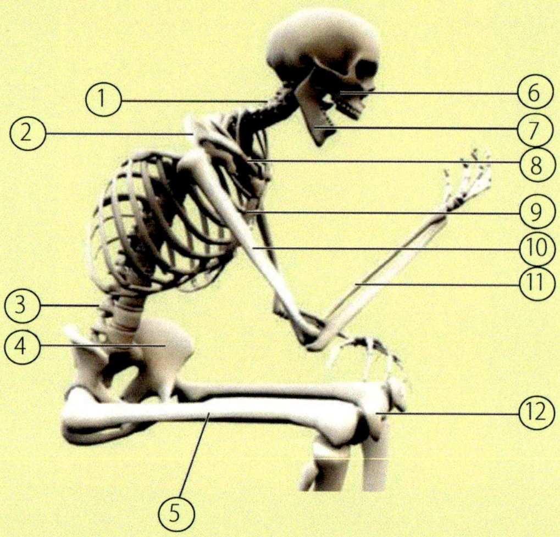

F. Build the word: Using the word root, add the other word element and define the new word created.

1. **arthr/o**
   a. **-centesis**_______________
   b. **-gram**_______________
   c. **-desis**_______________
   d. **-scopy**_______________
   e. **-algia**_______________
2. **chondr/o**
   a. **-oma**_______________
   b. **-malacia**_______________
   c. **-cyte**_______________
   d. cost/ +**-al**_______________
   e. **-clast**_______________
3. **ten/o**
   a. **-rrhaphy**_______________
   b. **-otomy**_______________
   c. **-plasty**_______________
   d. **-itis**_______________
   e. **-pathy**_______________
4. **oste/o**
   a. **-clasis**_______________
   b. **-ology**_______________
   c. **-necrosis**_______________
   d. **-genesis**_______________
   e. **-plasty**_______________

G. Label the muscles of the body from the following list.

- pectoralis major_____
- deltoid_____________
- biceps______________
- rectus abdominis____
- serratus anterior_____
- tensor fasciae latae___
- sartorius___________
- rectus femoris_______
- tibialis anterior______
- gastrocnemius______

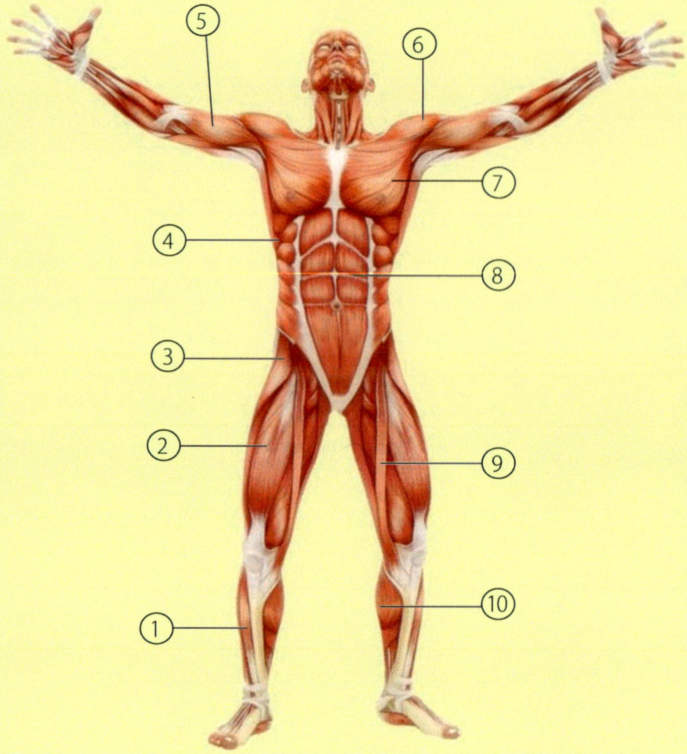

H. Recall: Using the skeleton, label the directions from the following list.

- proximal_________________________
- distal___________________________
- superior_________________________
- inferior_________________________
- anterior_________________________
- posterior________________________

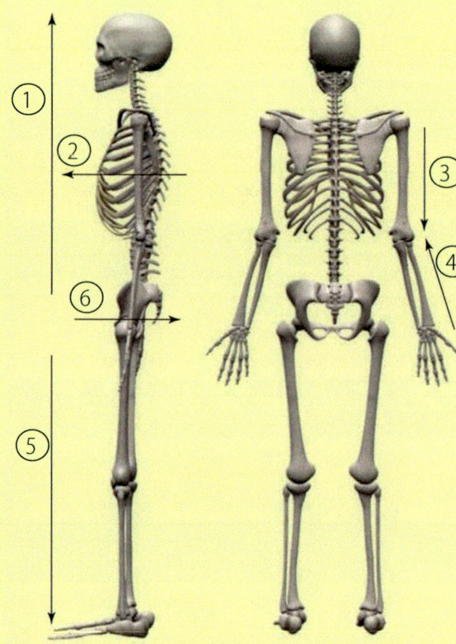

I. Label the skull from the following list.

- frontal______________________________
- parietal_____________________________
- maxilla_____________________________
- mandible____________________________
- nasal_______________________________
- temporal____________________________
- occipital____________________________
- zygoma_____________________________
- mandible____________________________

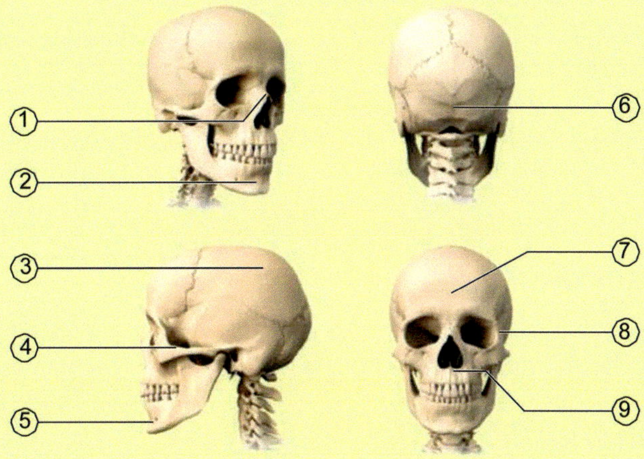

5

J. Recall terms relating to movement and anatomical directions from Chapter 3. Define the following words.

1. adduction_____________________________
2. flexion_______________________________
3. plantar flexion________________________
4. radial deviation_______________________
5. supination____________________________
6. prone_________________________________
7. palmar________________________________
8. extension_____________________________
9. lateral bend___________________________
10. supine________________________________

Case Study

Define the numerical terms (1 to 6) and draw the alphabetical terms (A to D) on the anatomy figure.

History, Chief Complaint

A soccer player complained of injuring her right ankle yesterday while playing in a game. She was unable to continue playing and was carried off the field. By her explanation, it is clear she **inverted** (1) and **supinated** (2) her right ankle.

Evaluation

Athlete has **edema** (3) and **ecchymosis** (4) at her **distal fibula** (A). Upon palpation, she is point tender on her **calcaneofibular ligament** (B) and **ATF ligament** (C), but not her **fibula** (D). She is currently **NWB** (5).

Diagnostic Studies

X-rays confirmed no fracture, and a grade 2 ankle **sprain** (6) is suspected. She was wrapped in an ACE wrap and provided crutches.

Terms

1. ______________________________
2. ______________________________
3. ______________________________
4. ______________________________
5. ______________________________
6. ______________________________

Anatomy

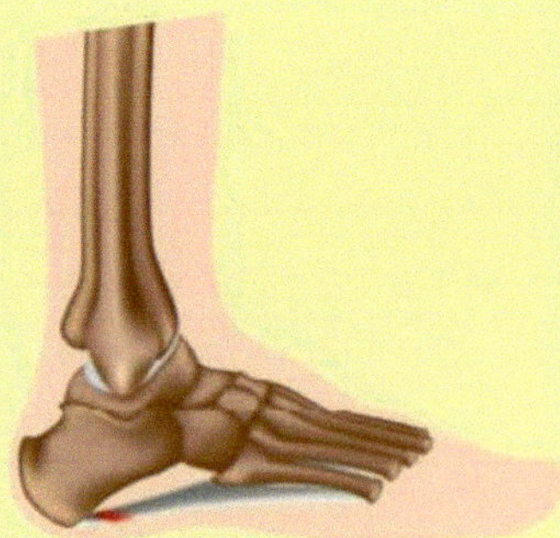

6

Cardiovascular System

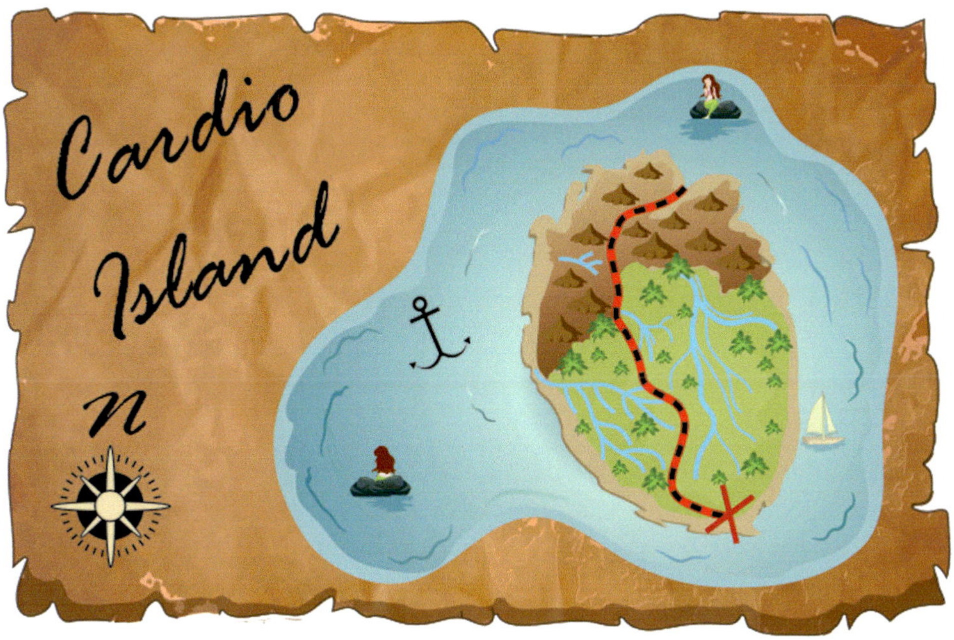

Objectives

After studying this chapter, you will be able to:

1. Locate and name the major components of the cardiovascular system.
2. Identify and build words relating to the cardiovascular system.
3. Describe the relationship between the heart, blood, and lymph components of the cardiovascular system.
4. Explain blood pressure.
5. Describe basic abnormalities or conditions pertaining to the heart, blood, and lymph.
6. Define abbreviations related to the cardiovascular system.

Flanagan KW.
Medical Terminology With Case Studies: A Navigated Guide to Learning for Health Care Professionals, Third Edition (pp 111-149).

Chapter Outline

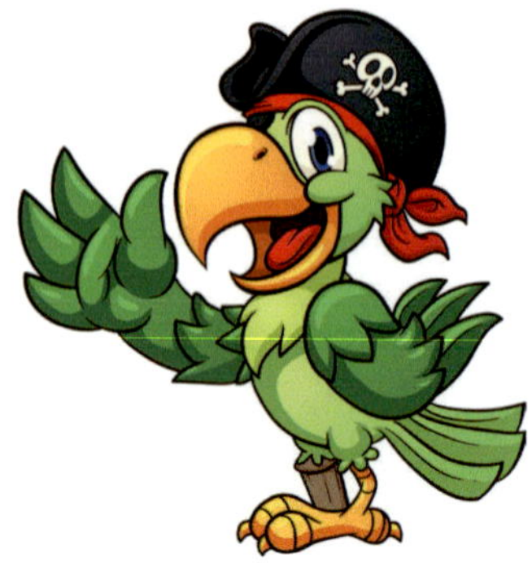

- Self-assessment
- Checklist for word parts in the chapter
- Checklist of new anatomy
- Introduction
- Anatomy
  - Heart
  - Blood vessels
  - Blood
  - Blood pressure
  - Lymph
- Word building
  - Prefixes
  - Suffixes
  - Combining forms
- Medical conditions
- Tests and procedures
- Learning activities
- Case study

Self-Assessment

Based on what you have learned so far, can you write the definition of these words?

- pericardium____________________
- cardiomegaly____________________
- cyanosis____________________
- tachycardia____________________
- myocardium____________________
- arrhythmia____________________
- endocarditis____________________
- erythrocyte____________________

Checklist for Word Parts in the Chapter

Prefixes

- ☐ a-
- ☐ an-
- ☐ auto-
- ☐ brady-
- ☐ dys-
- ☐ endo-
- ☐ extra-
- ☐ home/o-
- ☐ homo-
- ☐ hyper-
- ☐ hypo-
- ☐ inter-
- ☐ intra-
- ☐ mono-
- ☐ per-
- ☐ peri-
- ☐ poly-
- ☐ tachy-
- ☐ tetra-
- ☐ trans-

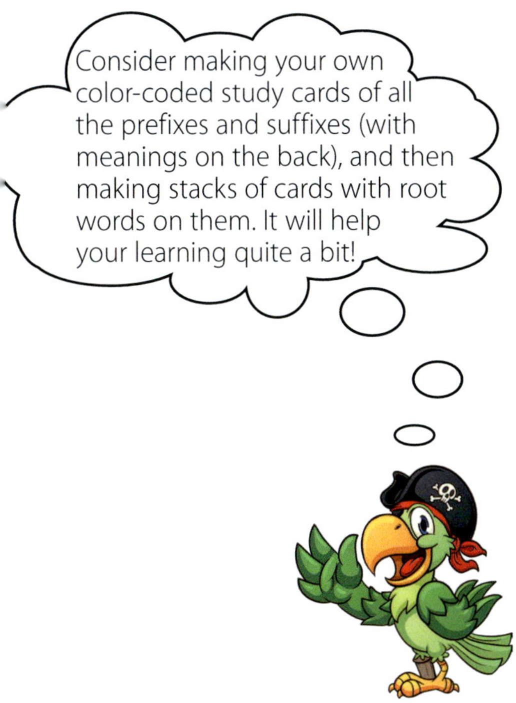
Consider making your own color-coded study cards of all the prefixes and suffixes (with meanings on the back), and then making stacks of cards with root words on them. It will help your learning quite a bit!

Suffixes

- ☐ -ac
- ☐ -al
- ☐ -ar
- ☐ -ary
- ☐ -centesis
- ☐ -cyte
- ☐ -ectomy
- ☐ -edema
- ☐ -emia
- ☐ -gram
- ☐ -graph
- ☐ -graphy
- ☐ -ia
- ☐ -ion
- ☐ -is
- ☐ -ism
- ☐ -itis
- ☐ -lysis
- ☐ -megaly
- ☐ -oid
- ☐ -oma
- ☐ -or
- ☐ -ose
- ☐ -osis
- ☐ -otomy
- ☐ -pathy
- ☐ -penia
- ☐ -penic
- ☐ -pexy
- ☐ -pheresis
- ☐ -phil
- ☐ -plasty
- ☐ -poiesis
- ☐ -ptysis
- ☐ -rrhage
- ☐ -rrhaphy
- ☐ -rrhexis
- ☐ -scope
- ☐ -sis
- ☐ -spasm
- ☐ -stasis
- ☐ -stomy
- ☐ -thelium
- ☐ -tomy
- ☐ -um
- ☐ -us

Combining Forms

- ☐ aden/o
- ☐ angi/o
- ☐ aort/o
- ☐ arter/o
- ☐ arteri/o
- ☐ ather/o
- ☐ atri/o
- ☐ auscultate/o
- ☐ bas/o
- ☐ brachi/o
- ☐ calc/o
- ☐ cardi/o
- ☐ cerebr/o
- ☐ claudicate/o
- ☐ cutane/o
- ☐ cyan/o
- ☐ cyt/o
- ☐ diast
- ☐ dilat/o
- ☐ ech/o
- ☐ electr/o
- ☐ embol/o
- ☐ eosin/o
- ☐ erythr/o
- ☐ gluc/o
- ☐ glyc/o
- ☐ granul/o
- ☐ hem/o
- ☐ hemat/o
- ☐ hemorrh/o
- ☐ home/o
- ☐ homo
- ☐ infarct/o
- ☐ isch/o
- ☐ leuk/o
- ☐ lip/o
- ☐ lipid/o
- ☐ lumin
- ☐ lun/o
- ☐ lymph/o

Combining Forms

- ☐ **mon/o**
- ☐ **my/o**
- ☐ **myel/o**
- ☐ **neutr/o**
- ☐ **nucle/o**
- ☐ **occlus/o**
- ☐ **orth/o**
- ☐ **ox/i**
- ☐ **pector/o**
- ☐ **phag/o**
- ☐ **phleb/o**
- ☐ **phon/o**
- ☐ **plasma**
- ☐ **pulmon/o**
- ☐ **rhythm/o**
- ☐ **sarc/o**
- ☐ **scler/o**
- ☐ **sept/o**
- ☐ **sphygm/o**
- ☐ **splen/o**
- ☐ **static**
- ☐ **sten/o**
- ☐ **stern/o**
- ☐ **steth/o**
- ☐ **syst**
- ☐ **tens/o**
- ☐ **thromb/o**
- ☐ **troph/o**
- ☐ **valv/o**
- ☐ **valvul/o**
- ☐ **varic/o**
- ☐ **vas/o**
- ☐ **vascul/o**
- ☐ **ven/o**
- ☐ **ventricul/o**
- ☐ **vers/o**

Checklist of New Anatomy

Heart

- ☐ Right atrium
- ☐ Left atrium
- ☐ Right ventricle
- ☐ Left ventricle
- ☐ Tricuspid valve
- ☐ Pulmonary valve
- ☐ Mitral valve
- ☐ Aortic valve
- ☐ Sinoatrial node
- ☐ Atrioventricular node
- ☐ Bundle of His
- ☐ Purkinje fibers
- ☐ Myocardium
- ☐ Interventricular septum

Blood and Vessels

- ☐ Tunica externa
- ☐ Tunica media
- ☐ Tunica interna
- ☐ Lumen
- ☐ Erythrocyte
- ☐ Leukocyte
- ☐ Thrombocyte
- ☐ Phagocyte
- ☐ Neutrophil
- ☐ Eosinophil
- ☐ Basophil
- ☐ Lymphocyte
- ☐ Monocyte

Arteries of Note

- ☐ Vena cava
- ☐ Aorta
- ☐ Carotid
- ☐ Brachial
- ☐ Radial
- ☐ Femoral
- ☐ Popliteal
- ☐ Tibialis posterior

Lymph

- ☐ Cervical nodes
- ☐ Axillary nodes
- ☐ Inguinal nodes
- ☐ Thymus
- ☐ Palatine tonsils
- ☐ Spleen

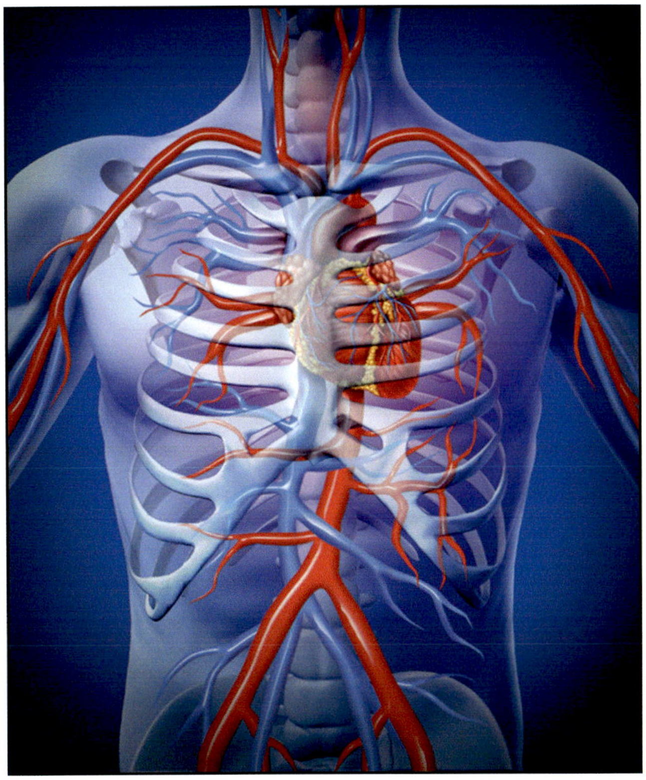

Figure 6-1. Anatomical positioning of the heart. (Lightspring/shutterstock.com)

Introduction

As with the previous chapter, Cardio Island is a separate place and has word roots unique to the cardiovascular system. You will notice many prefixes and suffixes used again, but on Cardio Island, they assist with words relating to the heart, blood, and lymph systems.

The cardiovascular system is divided into two sections: the heart and blood system and the lymph system. The heart is a pump that moves blood through the body, and both blood and lymph circulate to provide nutrients and fight infection. Both the blood and lymph systems carry fluid via vessels throughout the body, but the chief difference between these two systems is that blood is circulated via the heart maintaining a loop; and lymph flow is sporadic and slower, using muscular contractions and gravity to assist in its travel.

Anatomy

Heart

The heart is the central organ to the cardiovascular system. It is a four-compartment, hollow-chambered muscular organ that is the size of a clenched fist and sits at the left side of the chest (Figure 6-1). The ribs and sternum (breastbone) protect the heart. It beats about 70 times per minute in healthy adults. Two small upper chambers, the **atria**, collect blood, and two large, inferior chambers, the ventricles, propel blood. The **ventricles** have a thick **myocardium** (**my/o**—muscle; **cardi/o**—heart; **-um**—structure, thing) and interventricular (**inter-**—among, between) septum that divides the two chambers. A thin membrane, the pericardium (**peri-**—around; **cardi/**—heart; **-um**—structure, thing) surrounds the heart and assist in protecting it.

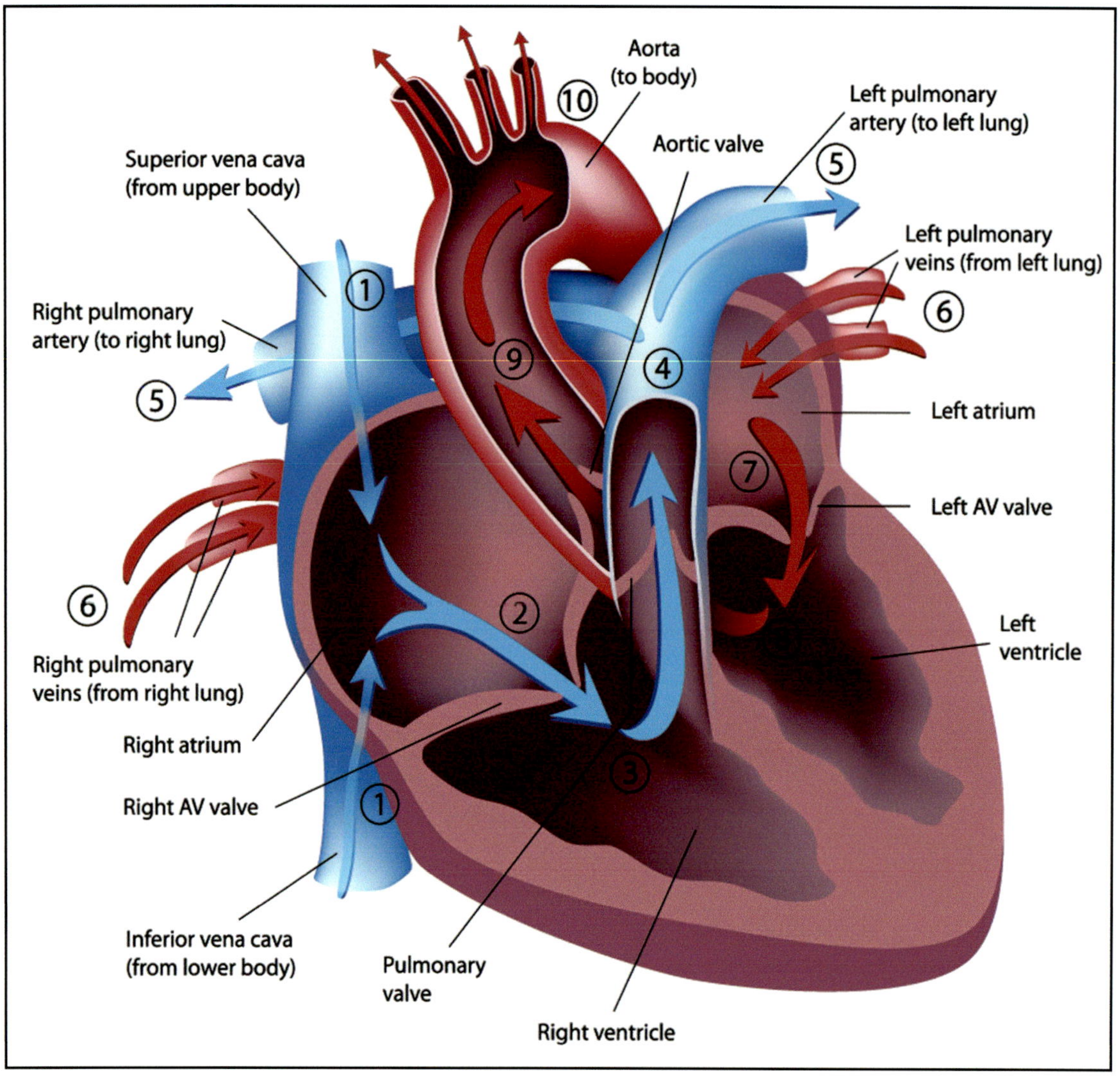

Figure 6-2. Normal blood flow through the heart. (AV = atrioventricular.) (Alila Medical Images/shutterstock.com)

Blood flows through the heart in the following manner (Figure 6-2):

- **Deoxygenated** (without oxygen) blood arrives to the heart via the inferior or superior vena cava veins (1) and enters the right atrium (2), flows through the tricuspid valve into the right ventricle (3), then through the pulmonic valve and right or left pulmonary arteries (4, 5) and lungs (where the red blood cells [RBCs] collect oxygen at the cellular level in the alveoli—smallest area of the lung).
- **Oxygenated** blood then travels back to the heart through the right or left pulmonary veins (6), onto the left atrium (7), mitral valve (also called the *bicuspid valve*), left ventricle (8), aortic valve, aorta (9), and to the rest of the body (10).

All the valves in the heart provide one-way transportation of blood and open and close in synchrony to prevent backflow. A **heart murmur** is heard when blood has an altered pattern through the chambers or when these valves do not close tightly.

A heartbeat is initiated by a pacemaker of nervous tissue in the right atrium called the **sinoatrial (SA) node** that promotes both atria to contract. As this occurs, the **atrioventricular (AV) node** near the septal wall of the right atrium propels the impulses to travel to the **Bundle of His** (also called the *AV bundle*) and extends via the **Purkinje fibers**, which stimulate both ventricles to contract, expelling blood to the arteries (Figure 6-3). **Bradycardia** (**brady-**—slow) is the term for slow heartbeat (less than 60 beats per minute at rest), and tachycardia (**tachy-**—rapid) is a rapid heartbeat (over 100 beats per minute at rest). Whereas bradycardia can represent a serious heart issue, it is common in trained athletes. Endurance athletes typically have a more muscular left ventricle and slower heart rates, which are a byproduct of long-term training.

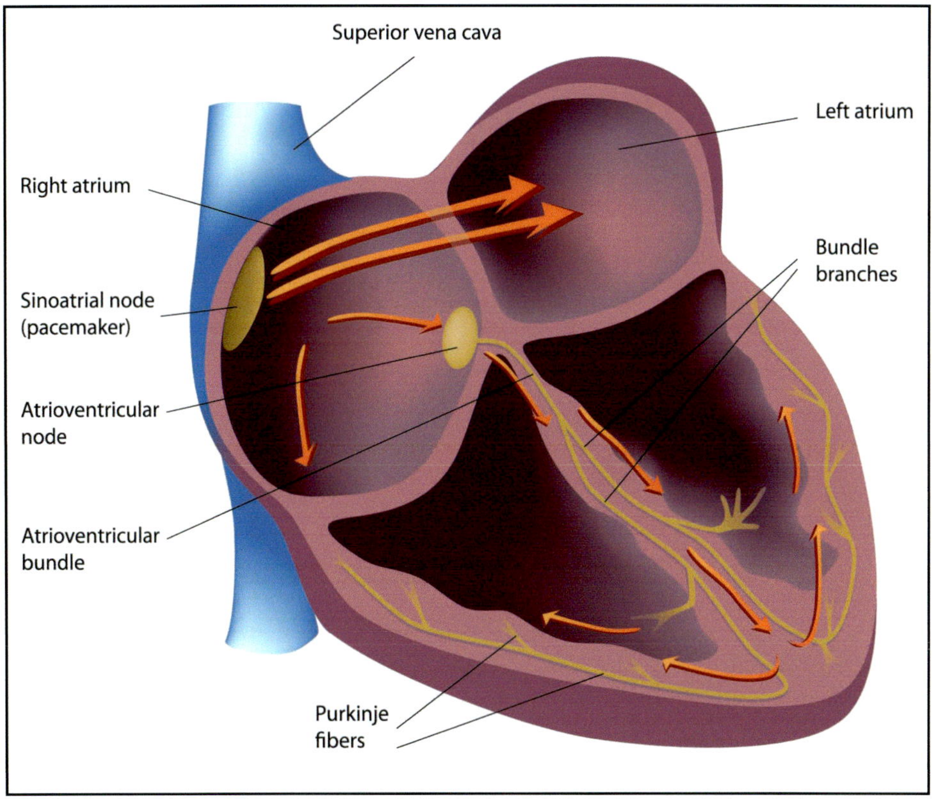

Figure 6-3. Cardiac conduction system. (Alila Medical Images/shutterstock.com)

6

Blood Vessels

Vessels that carry blood are typically called **arteries** (and **arterioles**) if they carry oxygenated blood away from the heart and **veins** (or **venules**) if they carry deoxygenated blood back to the heart. There is one exception to this rule: In the heart, deoxygenated blood leaves the heart via the pulmonary artery traveling to the lungs to leave carbon dioxide and pick up oxygen, then returns via the pulmonary vein to the heart. In this situation, the pulmonary vein is carrying oxygenated blood. Arteries are tough yet elastic to withstand the forces of a strongly beating heart (think of a sprinter). Unlike veins, they have an elastic layer that allows them to dilate and bend. Both arteries and veins are circular tubes with three layers:

1. **Tunica externa** (outermost layer)
2. **Tunica media** (middle layer)
3. **Tunica interna** (internal structure of the tube)

These layers surround the **lumen** (the tube) and its lining, the **endothelium** (**endo-**—in, within; **-thelium**—specialized layer of cells). Although they have the same name for each layer, the structures of the arteries are thicker and more robust than are the like-named aspects of the veins (Figure 6-4). Veins rely largely on peripheral contraction, respiration, and gravity to return blood to the heart. Respiration also plays a role in assisting venous return, and veins have one-way valves that prevent blood from going away from the heart (Figure 6-5A).

Contrary to popular belief (and these drawings), blood in veins is not blue, but darker in color than the bright red blood in arteries (Figure 6-5B). When oxygen from the lungs is added to blood, its color brightens to a more red color. Blood becomes darker in color as tissues absorb oxygen.

Capillaries are the microscopic vessels located where arterioles and venules come together. Unlike arteries and veins, capillaries are so small that they have only a single thin layer of endothelial cells. Exchanges of gases (oxygen and carbon dioxide), fluid, electrolytes, and so on occur easily via the capillary membrane. Figure 6-6 shows the gas exchange of arterioles and venules in the smallest aspect of the lungs (alveoli), which brings oxygenated blood back to the heart for distribution throughout the body.

Figure 6-4. Anatomy of arteries and veins. (Blamb/shutterstock.com)

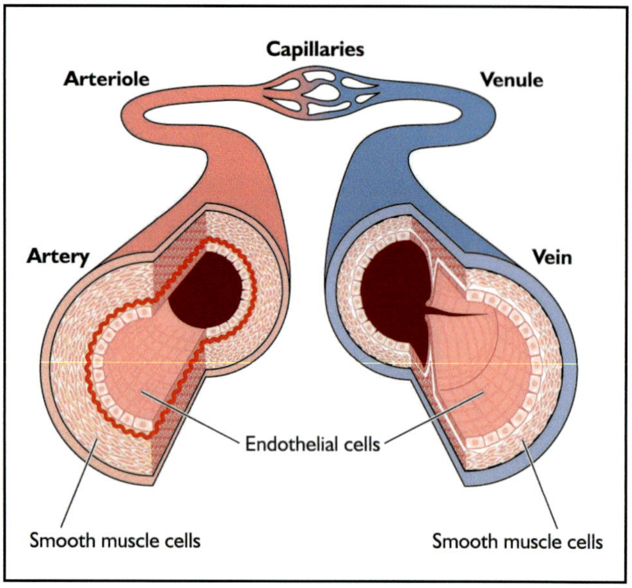

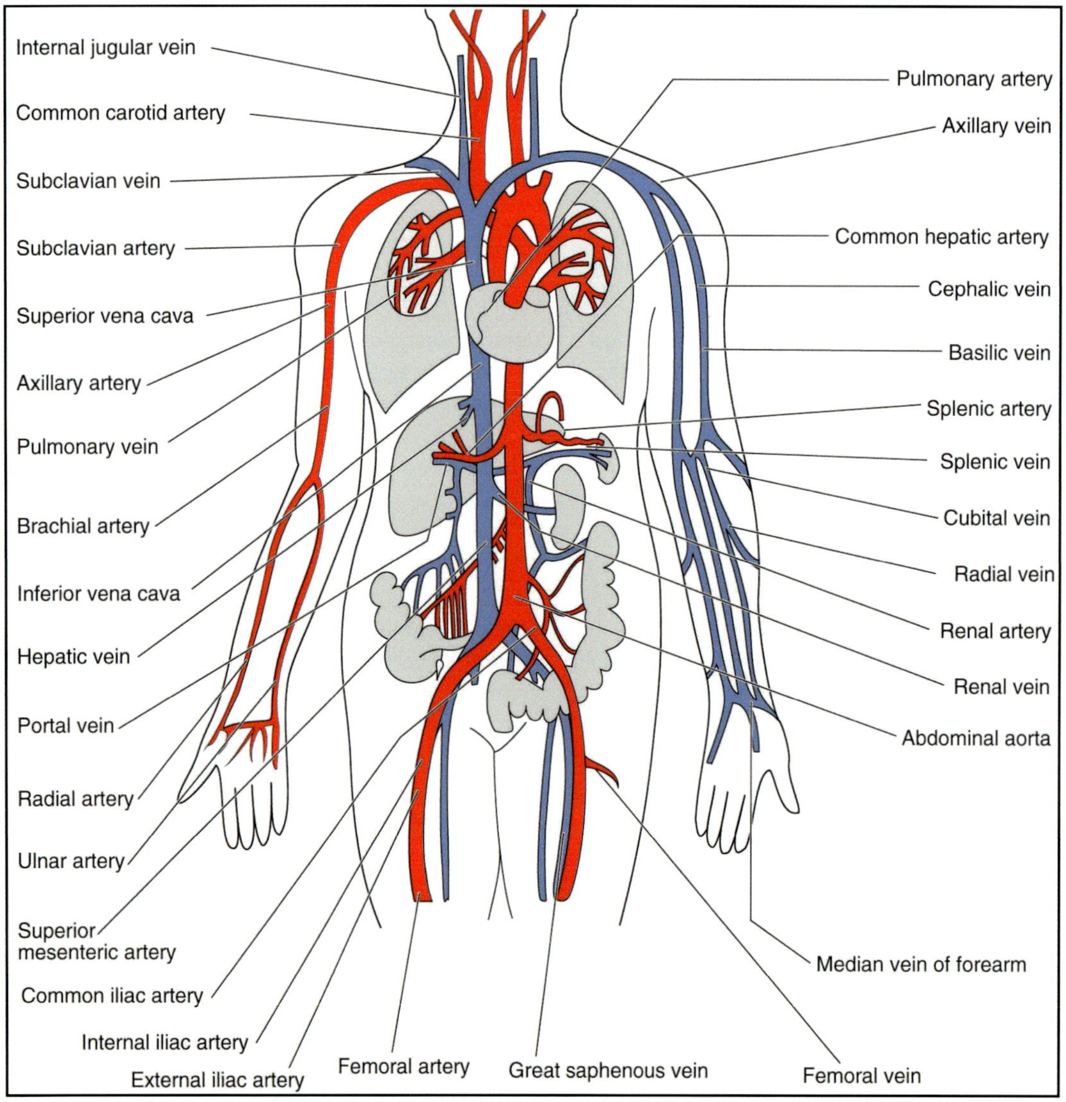

Figure 6-5A. Main arteries and veins of the body. (MikiR/shutterstock.com)

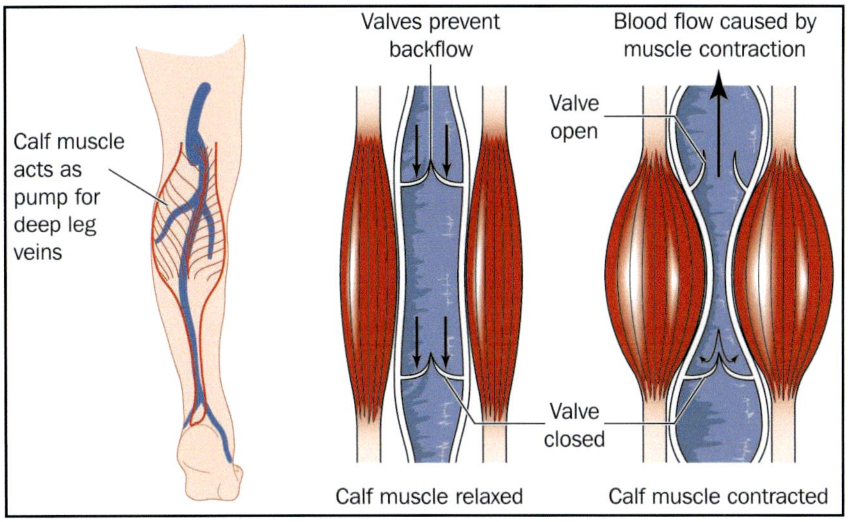

Figure 6-5B. The role of muscles and valves in venous return to the heart. (Blamb/shutterstock.com)

6

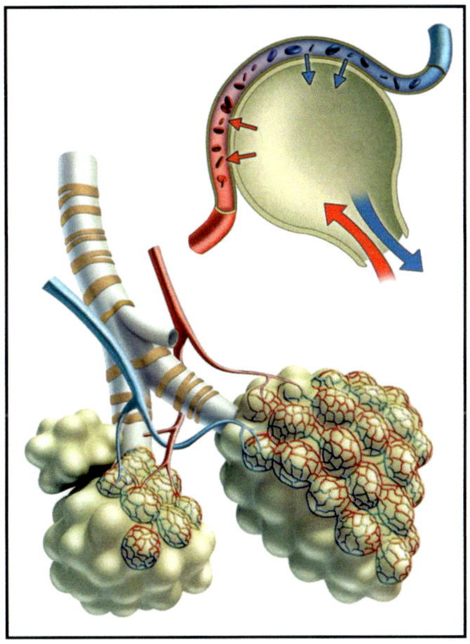

Figure 6-6. Oxygen exchange in the lungs occurs in the aveloi. (Andrea Danti/shutterstock.com)

Blood

Blood contains different types of cells that transport oxygen and nutrients to tissues, fight infection, remove waste, regulate body temperature, and maintain **homeostasis** (**home/o-**—same; **-stasis**—still), which is a consistent internal environment. Blood represents less than 8% of total body weight, and typically humans have about 5 liters (1.3 gallons) of blood flowing through their bodies at any given time. It takes blood about 20 seconds to complete a full systemic cycle (heart → body → heart) through the arteries and veins.

About 45% of blood volume is made up of cells called **erythrocytes** (**erythr/o**—red; **-cyte**—cell; RBCs), **leukocytes** (**leuk/o**—white; white blood cells [WBCs]), and **thrombocytes** (**thromb/o**—clot; platelets). RBCs are biconcave discs whose main function is to transport oxygen to tissues (Figure 6-7). They are generated in the marrow of long bones and live about 4 months (120 days). There are five different types of WBCs, divided into two categories (Table 6-1) that are determined by the presence of granulocytes. The main purpose of leukocytes is to fight infection and support the immune system. They also perform a function known as **phagocytosis** (**phag/o**—eating, swallowing; **-cyte**—cell; **-osis**—condition) as it engulfs and destroys other cells. **Platelets** (literally, "small plate") are the smallest cells in the blood, are disc-shaped, and are formed in red bone marrow. Their chief responsibility is to clot (coagulate) blood. The remaining 55% of blood is watery **plasma**. Plasma contains glucose (sugar), proteins, amino acids, hormones, vitamins, and minerals.

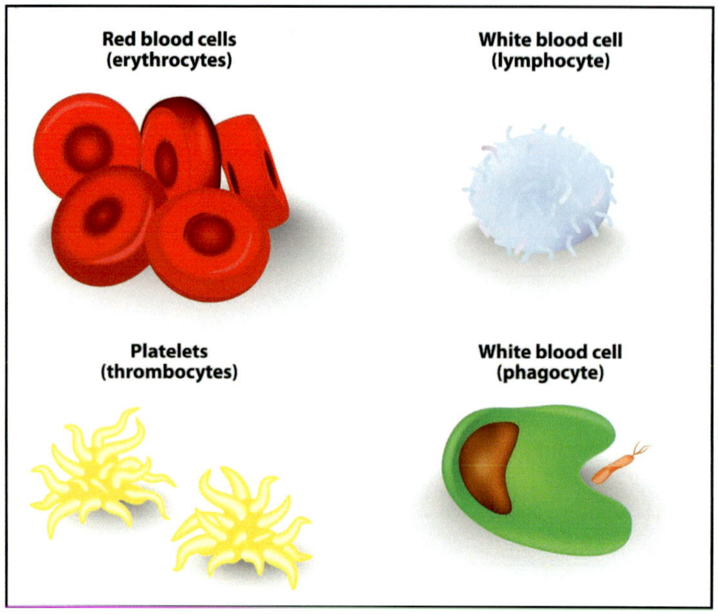

Figure 6-7. Blood cells. (Zhabska Tetyana/shutterstock.com)

Blood Pressure

Blood pressure (BP) is a measure of the force within the arteries at any given time. It is measured in **systole** (the contraction of the heart) and **diastole** (the relaxation of the heart that allows both ventricles to fill with blood; Figure 6-9). Blood pressure is always recorded with the systolic measurement first, then the diastolic measurement. The typical reading is 120/80 (said aloud as "120 over 80"), and it is measured in mm Hg (millimeters of mercury). An instrument called a **stethoscope** (**steth/o**—chest; **-scope**—an instrument used to view or inspect) is used to listen for a heartbeat in an artery (most often the dominant brachial artery [**brachi/o**—arm]). A **sphygmomanometer** (**sphygm/o**—pulse; manometer—pressure meter) is an inflatable cuff with a mercury mechanical reader used to read the pressure exhibited within the artery (Figure 6-10). The term **hypertension** (HTN; **hyper-**—above, excessive, high, increased; **tens/o**—to stretch; **-ion**—process, the act of) refers to patients with systolic readings consistently over 140 and/or diastolic measurements consistently over 90.

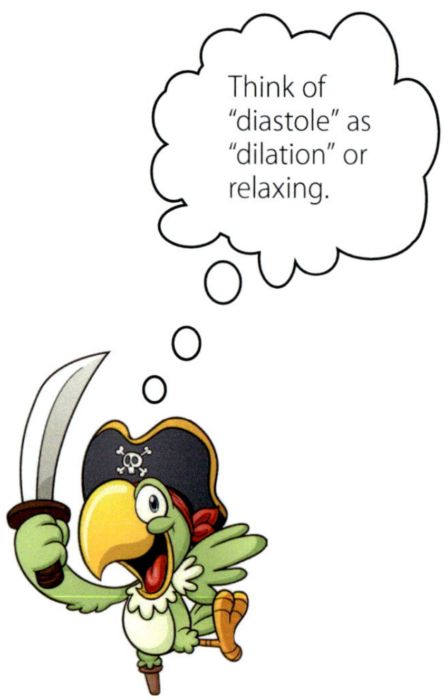

Table 6-1
Types of White Blood Cells (Leukocytes) (Figure 6-8)

CELL TYPE	FUNCTION	NORMAL PERCENTAGE
Granulocytes		
Neutrophil neutr/—neutral **-phil**—to attract	Destroys bacteria, cellular debris, and solid particles	60% to 70%
Eosinophil eosin/o—rose colored **-phil**—attraction	Responds to allergies and some parasite conditions	2% to 4%
Basophil bas/o—base **-phil**—to attract	Releases **histamine** (causes dilation of capillaries) and **heparin** (prevents intravascular clotting)	0.5% to 1%
Agranulocytes **a-**—without granul/o—little grain **-cyte**—cell		
Lymphocytes lymph/—lymph **-cyte**—cell	Maintains immune system **B-cells**: Respond to foreign materials by stimulating the spleen and lymph nodes to produce reactionary cells **T-cells**: Assist B cells in destroying foreign protein and may play a significant role in resistance to production of cancer cells	20% to 25%
Monocytes mon/o—one **-cyte**—cell	Destroys large debris/unwanted materials	3% to 8%

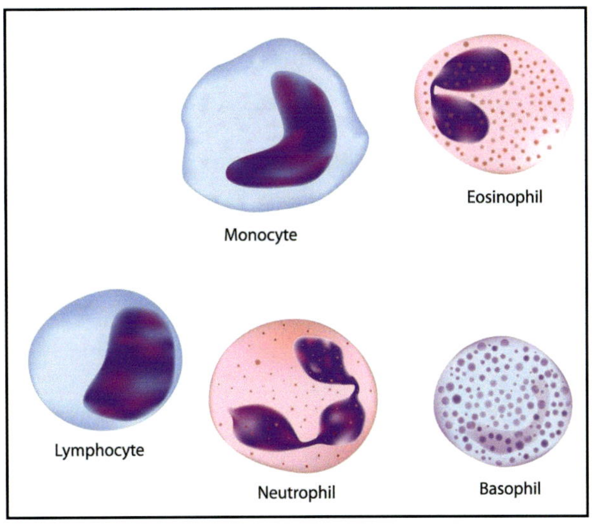

Figure 6-8. White blood cells. (Alila Medical Images/shutterstock.com)

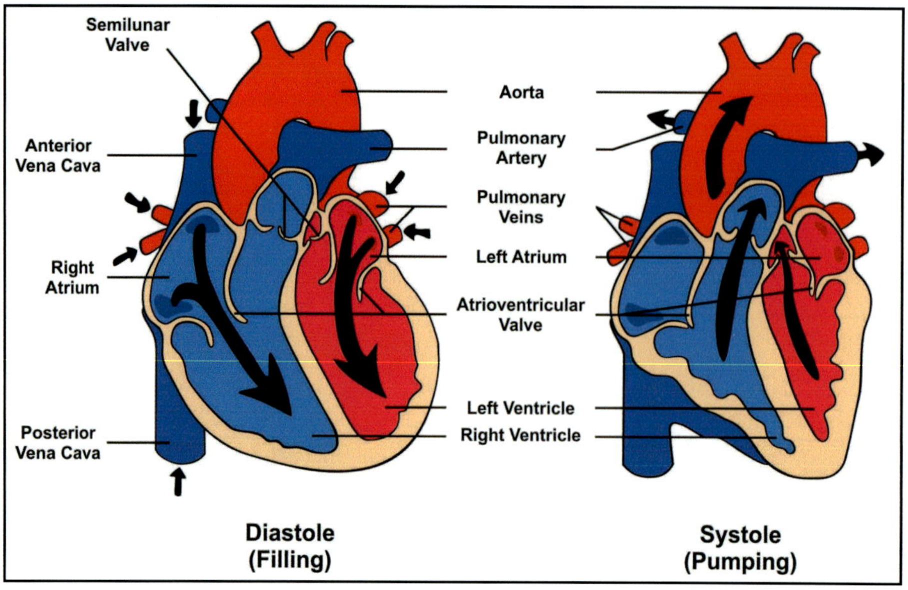

Figure 6-9. Diastole and systole. (udaix/shutterstock.com)

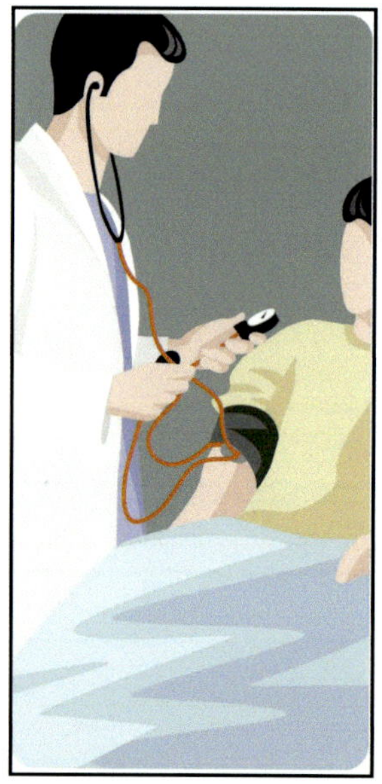

Figure 6-10. Blood pressure assessed via a stethoscope and sphygmomanometer. (Clipart deSIGN/shutterstock.com)

Table 6-2
Surface Pulse Points

ARTERY	ANATOMICAL LOCATION
brachial	Along the upper medial arm
carotid	In the neck on either side of the trachea (windpipe)
femoral	In the groin where the leg attaches to the body
popliteal	Behind the knee in the popliteal fossa
radial	At the wrist, on the lateral (thumb) side on the radius bone
tibialis posterior	Behind the medial malleolus (distal end of the tibia) in the ankle

Lymph

Lymph is a thin, watery fluid that arises from organs and tissues. It circulates throughout lymph vessels and is filtered by various lymph nodes. Lymph contains RBCs, WBCs, and platelets, and is known as *plasma* when cells are removed. The lymphatic system is composed of a network of vessels, ducts, nodes, and glands that move lymphatic fluid through the body. This system is in charge of maintaining internal fluid balance and assisting with immune responses. The lymph nodes are gathered in small kidney-shaped nodules that are usually less than a half-inch to an inch in size. They cluster in the **cervical** (neck), **axillary** (armpit), and **inguinal** (groin) areas of the body and become enlarged when fighting infection. They are connected via ducts and vessels that closely align with the body's arteries and veins (Figure 6-11). Like veins, lymphatic fluid relies on respiration, muscular contraction, gravity, and one-way valves to move the fluid back to the heart (Figure 6-12).

Glands associated with the lymphatic system are the **thymus**, **palatine tonsils** (in the chest and throat), and **spleen** (in the upper left quadrant of the abdomen). The thymus resides above the heart and in between the lungs in the mediastinum. The thymus is bigger in size and activity from age 2 years through puberty, when its function and size begins to decline. Most people refer to the palatine tonsils simply as *the tonsils*. These glands are the first line of defense for inhaled or ingested organisms that may provide danger to the body. The spleen lies behind the protection of the ribs in the upper left quadrant of the abdomen, under the diaphragm. It is most often referred to when one has **mononucleosis**, as the spleen becomes quite enlarged (**splenomegaly**: **splen/o**—spleen; **-megaly**—abnormally large, enlargement) and is in danger of rupturing if injured. All of these glands contain large quantities of WBCs, which are on hand to protect the body and fight infection, becoming swollen in the process. Additionally, a person can survive with little fanfare if any of these glands needs to be surgically removed due to repeated infections (such as in **tonsillitis**) or rupture.

6

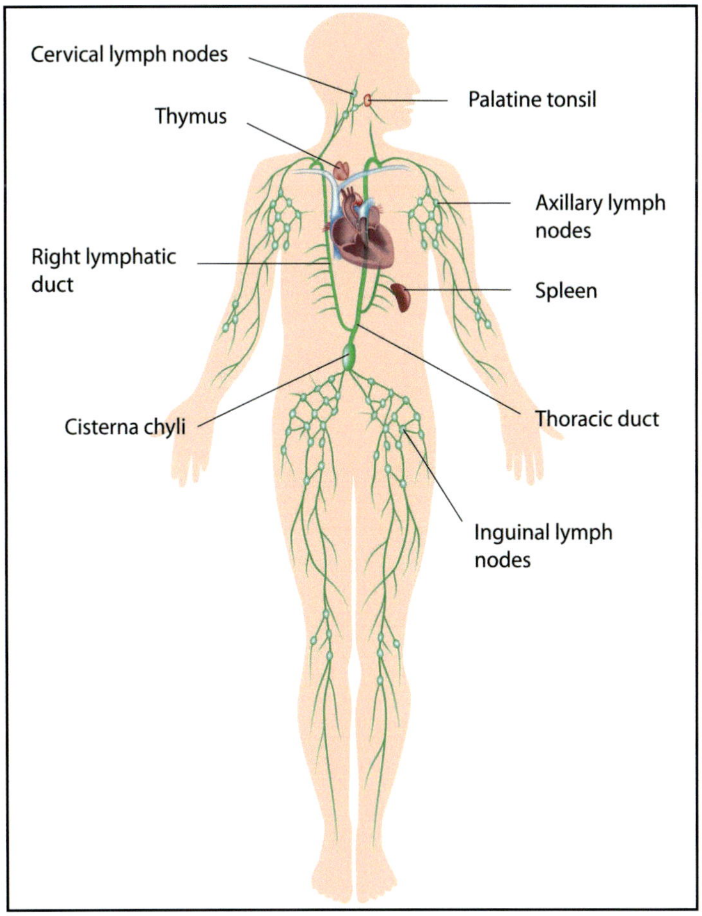

Figure 6-11. The lymphatic system. (Alila Medical Images/shutterstock.com)

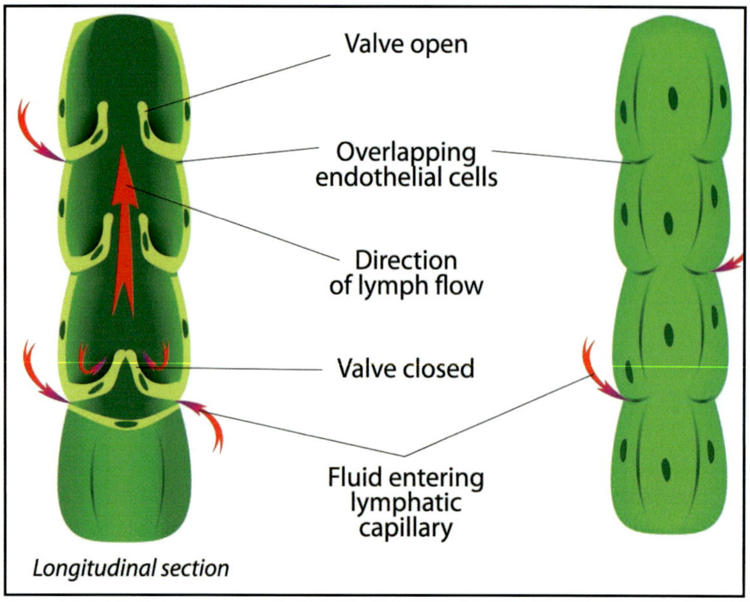

Figure 6-12. Anatomy of a lymph vessel. (Zhabska Tetyana/shutterstock.com)

Word Building

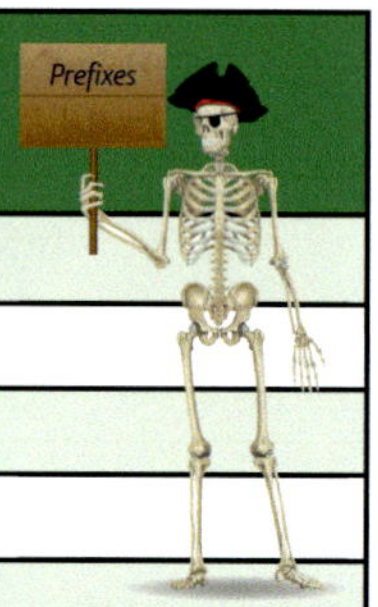

Table 6-3
Prefixes

PREFIX	DEFINITION
a-	without
brady-	slow
dys-	abnormal; bad; difficult; painful
endo-	in; within
home/o-; homo-	same
hyper-	above; excessive; high; increased
hypo-	below; decreased; deficient; insufficient; low; under
inter-	among; between
intra-	inside; within
peri-	around
tachy-	fast; rapid
tetra-	four
trans-	across; through
Some of these you may remember; others are new.	

TABLE 6-4

SUFFIXES

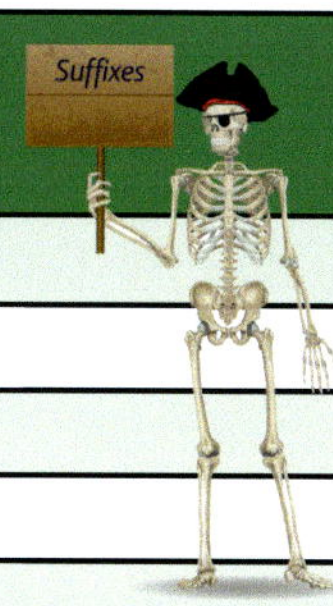

SUFFIX	DEFINITION
-ac; -al; -ar; -ary; -is; -ose	pertaining to
-centesis	puncture; surgical puncture
-cyte	cell
-emia	blood condition
-gram	a record of
-graph	an instrument to record information
-graphy	process of recording; the act of recording information
-ia	condition
-ion	process; the act of
-ism	condition
-itis	inflammation
-lysis	breaking down; destruction; loosening; separating; to loosen or break
-megaly	abnormally large; enlargement
-oid	resembling
-oma	mass; tumor
-osis	condition
-pathy	disease
-penia; -penic	decrease; deficient
-pexy	surgical fixation of
-pheresis	removal
-phil	attraction; an affinity for
-plasty	reconstruction; repair; plastic surgery
-poiesis	formation
-ptysis	to spit
-rrhage	bursting forth; excessive flow
-rrhaphy	surgical repair; suturing
-rrhexis	rupture
-scope	an instrument used to view or inspect
-sis	state of; condition
-spasm	involuntary contraction
-stasis	stopping; still; same
-stomy	surgical opening
-thelium	specialized layer of cells
-tomy; -otomy	incision; to cut into
-um	structure; thing
-us	pertaining to; structure

Some of these you may remember; others are new.

Table 6-5
Combining Forms

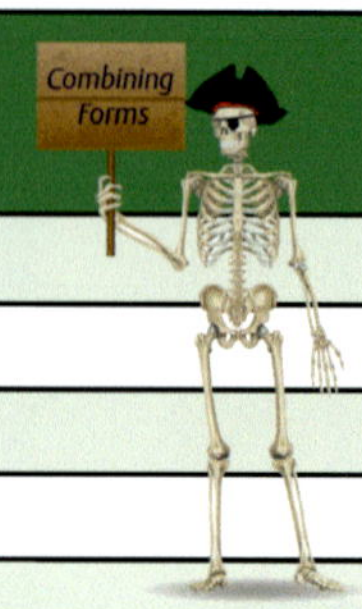

COMBINING FORM	DEFINITION
aden/o	gland
angi/o	vessel
aort/o	aorta
arter/o; arteri/o	artery
ather/o	fatty plaque
atri/o	atrium
auscultate/o	to listen
bas/o	base; bottom
brachi/o	arm
calc/o	calcium
cardi/o	heart
cerebr/o	cerebrum
claudicate/o	to limp
cutane/o	skin
cyan/o	blue
cyt/o	cell
diast	to expand
dilat/o	to widen
ech/o	to bounce sound
electr/o	electricity
embol/o	plug
eosin/o	rose colored
erythr/o	red
gluc/o; glyc/o	sugar
granul/o	little grain
hem/o	blood
hemat/o; hemorrh/o	blood
home/o; homo	same
infarct/o	death of an area
isch/o	to withhold; hold back
leuk/o	white
lip/o; lipid/o	fat
lun/o	moon
lymph/o	lymph (the watery substance originating in organs and tissues)

(continued)

Table 6-5 (continued)
Combining Forms

COMBINING FORM	DEFINITION
mon/o	one
my/o	muscle
neutr/o	neutral
nucle/o	nucleus
occlus/o	to close
orth/o	straight
ox/i	oxygen
pector/o	chest
phag/o	eating; swallowing
phleb/o	vein
phon/o	sound; voice
plasma	the liquid aspect of blood
pulmon/o	lung
rhythm/o	rhythm
sarc/o	flesh
scler/o	hard; hardening; thick; sclera
sept/o	wall
sphygm/o	pulse
splen/o	spleen
static	without movement
sten/o	narrowing
stern/o	sternum
steth/o	chest
syst	contract
tens/o	stretching; pressure
thromb/o	clot
troph/o	development; growth; nourishment
valv/o; valvul/o	valve
varic/o	dilated vein; swollen vein; varicose vein
vas/o	vessel; vas deferens
vascul/o	blood vessel
ven/o	vein
ventricul/o	ventricle; cavity
vers/o	to turn

Medical Conditions

Tables 6-6, 6-7, and 6-8 list some of the more common conditions pertaining to the heart, blood, and lymph.

Table 6-6

Medical Conditions Related to the Heart

NAME	WORD PARTS	DEFINITION
angina pectoris	angi/ (vessel) pector/ (chest)	Chest pain caused by decreased oxygen to the heart
arrhythmia	**a-** (without) rhythm/ (rhythm) **-ia** (condition)	Loss of a heartbeat or irregularity of the heartbeat; also known as *dysrhythmia*
bradycardia	**brady-** (slow) cardi/ (heart) **-ia** (condition)	Abnormally slow heart rate; below 60 beats per minute
cardiomegaly	cardi/o (heart) **-megaly** (enlarged)	Enlarged heart
cardiomyopathy (Figure 6-13)	cardi/o (heart) my/o (muscle) **-pathy** (disease)	Disease of the muscle of the heart
dysrhythmia	**dys-** (abnormal) rhythm/ (rhythm) **-ia** (condition)	Abnormal heart rhythm, usually one of two conditions: tachycardia or bradycardia; also known as *arrhythmia*
endocarditis	**endo-** (in) cardi/o (heart) **-itis** (inflammation)	Inflammation of the inner lining of the heart
hypertrophic cardiomyopathy (HCM)	**hyper-** (above; excessive; high; increased) troph/ (growth) cardi/o (heart) my/o (muscle) **-pathy** (disease)	A cause of sudden death; involves an abnormally enlarged left ventricle

(continued)

HCM is the leading cause of sudden cardiac death in athletes.

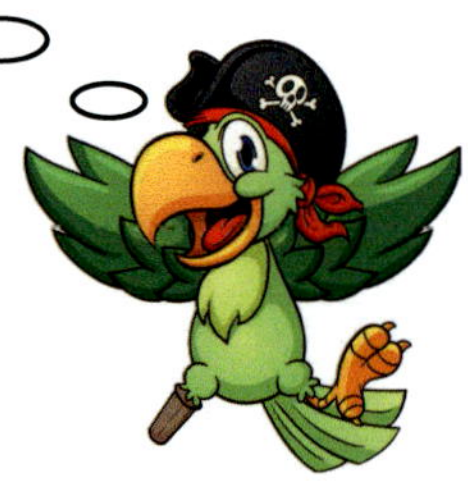

Table 6-6 (continued)

Medical Conditions Related to the Heart

NAME	WORD PARTS	DEFINITION
myocardial infarction (MI) (Figure 6-14)	my/o (muscle) cardi/ (heart) infarct/ (death of an area) **-ion** (process; the act of)	Commonly termed a *heart attack*, it literally means "death of (a part of) the heart muscle"
myocarditis	my/o (muscle) cardi/ (heart) **-itis** (inflammation)	Inflammation of the heart muscle (often from an infection)
orthostatic hypotension	orth/o (straight) static (without motion) **hypo-** (low) tens/ (pressure) **-ion** (the act of)	Abnormally low blood pressure (near fainting) when a patient suddenly stands
pericardiocentesis	**peri-** (around) cardi/o (heart) **-centesis** (surgical puncture)	Surgical procedure that removes fluid from the sack surrounding the heart (pericardium)
pericarditis	**peri-** (around) cardi/ (heart) **-itis** (inflammation)	Swelling in the sac around the heart

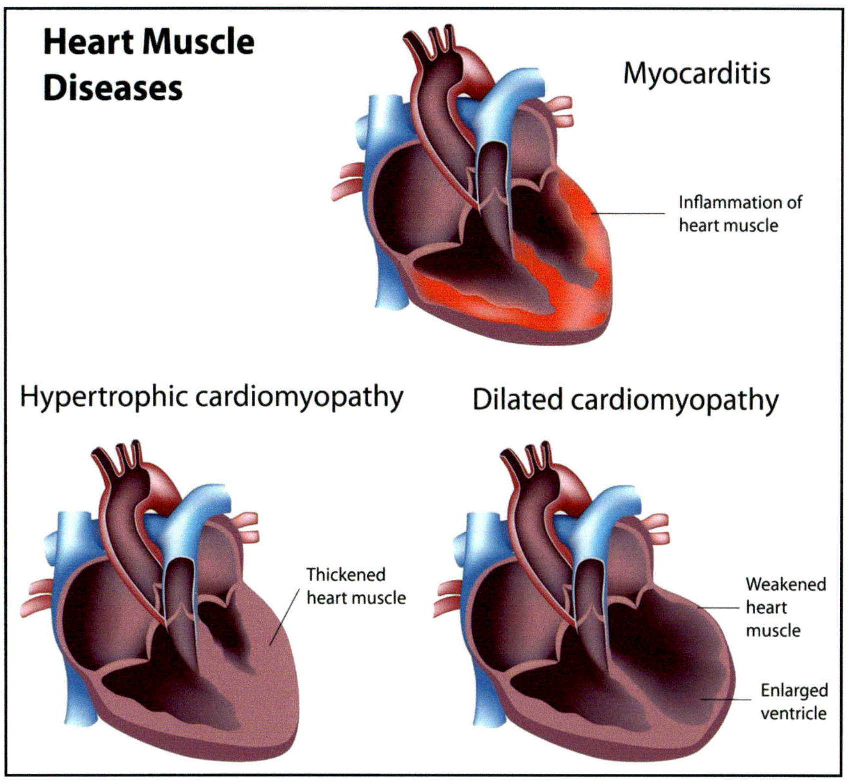

Figure 6-13. Diseases of the heart. (Alila Medical Images/shutterstock.com)

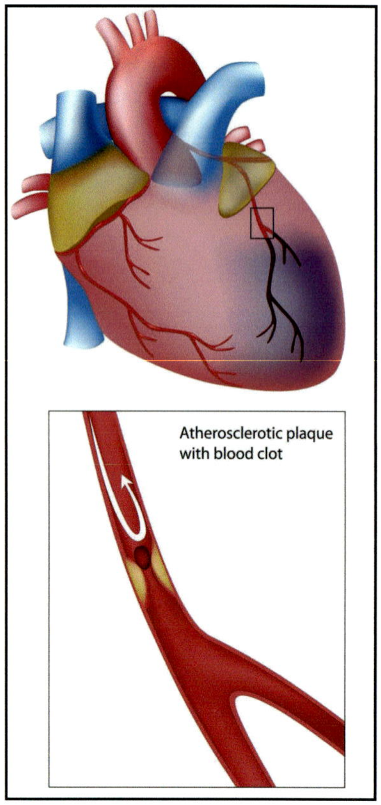

Figure 6-14. Myocardial infarction. (Alila Medical Images/shutterstock.com)

Table 6-7

More Medical Conditions Related to the Heart

NAME	DEFINITION
commotio cordis	Trauma to chest wall that interrupts the electrical impulses to the heart; often fatal
congestive heart failure (CHF)	Ineffective transportation of blood through the heart
coronary artery disease (CAD) (Figure 6-15)	Ineffective delivery of blood to the heart in the coronary arteries (typically due to atherosclerosis)
Marfan syndrome	Genetic connective tissue disorder that can cause a ruptured aorta
mitral valve prolapse (MVP)	When the mitral valve does not close correctly; the most common heart abnormality
murmur	Extra sound in between normal heartbeats heard via a stethoscope; often due to an improper valve closure
rheumatic heart disease	Heart valves damaged and scarred by the streptococcal infection that causes childhood rheumatic fever
syncope	Fainting
tetralogy of Fallot (Figure 6-16)	Congenital malformation involving four distinct heart defects

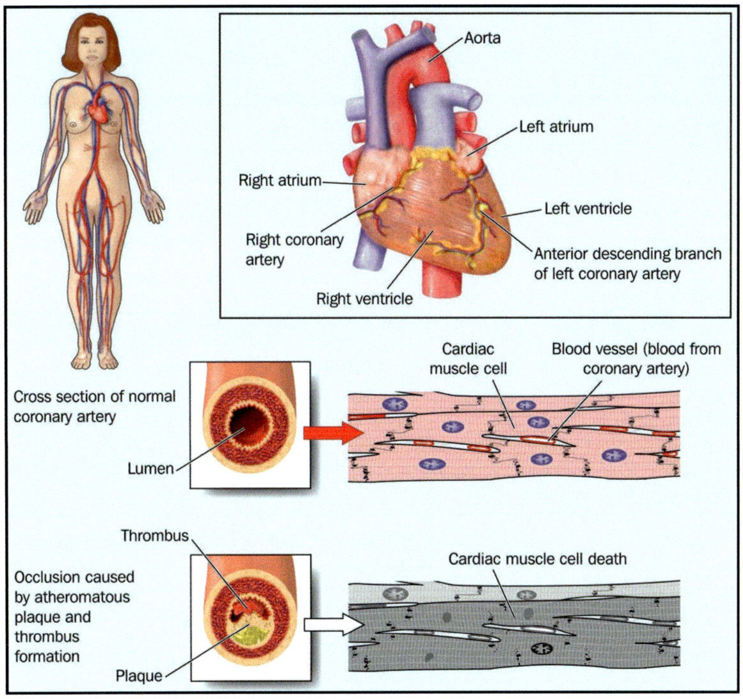

Figure 6-15. Coronary artery disease. (Blamb/shutterstock.com)

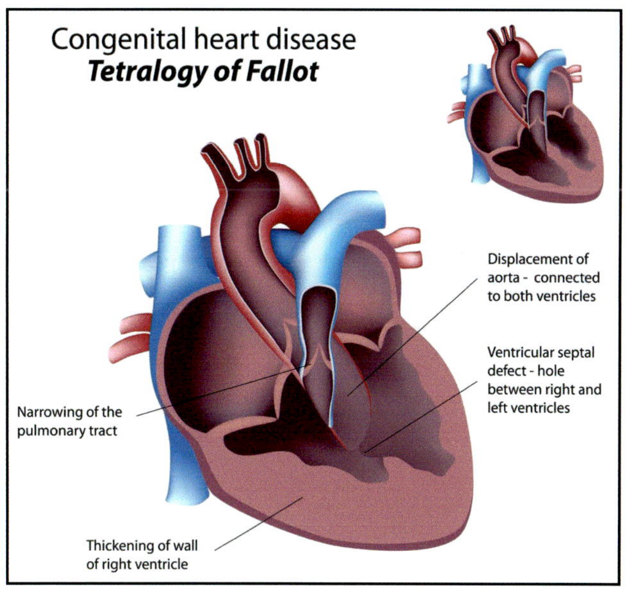

Figure 6-16. Tetralogy of Fallot. (Alila Medical Images/shutterstock.com)

Table 6-8

Medical Conditions Related to the Vascular and Lymph Systems

NAME	WORD PARTS	DEFINITION
acute lymphocytic leukemia (ALL)	lymph/o (lymph) cyt/ (cell) leuk/ (white) **-emia** (blood condition)	Most common form of leukemia for people under age 19; an overabundance of lymphocytes
acute myelogenous leukemia (AML)	myel/o (bone marrow) **-gen** (that which produces) **-ous** (pertaining to) leuk/ (white) **-emia** (blood condition)	Form of leukemia that arises from immature bone marrow cells
anastomosis		Surgical joining between blood vessels
anemia	**an-** (without) **-emia** (blood condition)	Blood condition where there is a decreased number of RBCs or hemoglobin in the blood
aneurysm (Figure 6-17)		Abnormal widening in an arterial wall due to congenital weakening, HTN, or atherosclerosis
angioma	angi/ (vessel) **-oma** (mass; tumor)	Tumor of a blood vessel
angiostenosis	angi/o (vessel) sten/ (narrowing) **-osis** (condition)	Narrowing of a blood vessel
arteriosclerosis	arteri/o (artery) scler/ (hardening) **-osis** (condition)	Hardening of the arteries
atherosclerosis (Figure 6-18)	ather/o (fatty material) scler/ (thick) **-osis** (condition)	Fatty substance attached to the vessel, narrowing the ability for blood to flow through
autoimmune disease	**auto-** (self)	Immune system attacks itself by producing antibodies against itself
cerebrovascular accident (CVA) (Figure 6-19)	cerebr/o (cerebrum) vascul/ (blood vessel) **-ar** (pertaining to)	Blood clot or bleeding in the brain; also known as *stroke*
chronic lymphocytic leukemia (CLL)	lymph/o (lymph) cyt/ (cell) leuk/ (white) **-emia** (blood condition)	An overabundance of immature lymphocytes; most common in middle-aged and older adults

(continued)

TABLE 6-8 (CONTINUED)

MEDICAL CONDITIONS RELATED TO THE VASCULAR AND LYMPH SYSTEMS

NAME	WORD PARTS	DEFINITION
chronic myelogenous leukemia (CML)	myel/o (bone marrow) **-gen** (that which produces) **-ous** (pertaining to) leuk/ (white) **-emia** (blood condition)	Slow-progressing form of leukemia that arises from immature bone marrow cells; most common in middle-aged and older adults
claudication	claudicate/ (to limp) **-ion** (process)	Literally, the process of limping; cramping due to inadequate supply of oxygen (from blood) to the muscles due to constricted arteries
deep vein thrombosis (DVT) (Figure 6-20)	thromb/ (clot) **-osis** (condition)	Blood clot in a vein
edema		Swelling due to lymph fluid accumulating in tissues'
embolism; embolus	embol/ (plug) **-ism** (condition) **-us** (structure)	Blood clot blocking a blood vessel
extravasation	**extra-** (beyond) vas/ (vessel) **-ion** (process)	Fluids escape from the blood vessels into surrounding areas (often seen in improper IV insertion)
granulocytopenia	granul/o (little grain) cyt/o (cell) **-penia** (decrease)	Abnormal decrease in the number of granulocytes (a type of WBCs) in the blood
granulocytosis	granul/o (little grain) cyt/ (cell) **-osis** (condition)	Abnormal increase in the number of granulocytes (a type of WBCs) in the blood; typically in response to an infection
hemangioma	hem/ (blood) angi/ (vessel) **-oma** (tumor)	Blood-filled birthmark or tumor consisting of tightly packed capillaries; also called *strawberry hemangioma*
hemolysis	hem/o (blood) **-lysis** (breaking down)	Intravascular breakdown of RBCs as a result of strenuous physical activity
hemophilia	hem/o (blood) **-phil** (affinity for) **-ia** (condition)	Genetic condition where a person lacks normal blood-clotting properties
hemorrhoid	hem/o (blood) **-oid** (resembling)	Varicose veins near the anus
Hodgkin's lymphoma	lymph/ (lymph) **-oma** (tumor)	Cancer of the lymphatic tissue

(continued)

6

Table 6-8 (continued)
Medical Conditions Related to the Vascular and Lymph Systems

NAME	WORD PARTS	DEFINITION
hypercalcemia	**hyper-** (excessive) calc/ (calcium) **-emia** (blood condition)	Excessive calcium in the blood
hyperglycemia	**hyper-** (excessive) glyc/ (sugar) **-emia** (blood condition)	Excessive sugar in the blood, a sign of diabetes mellitus
hyperlipidemia	**hyper-** (high) lipid/ (fat) **-emia** (blood condition)	High cholesterol (fat in the blood); typically 200 or greater
hypertension (HTN)	**hyper-** (high) tens/ (pressure) **-ion** (process)	Blood pressure that is consistently over 140 (systolic) and/or over 90 (diastolic); normal is 120/80
hypoglycemia	**hypo-** (low) glyc/ (sugar) **-emia** (blood condition)	Low amount of sugar in the blood; can be due to missing meals or diabetes mellitus
hypotension	**hypo-** (low) tens/ (pressure) **-ion** (process)	Low blood pressure
hypoxemia	**hypo-** (deficient) ox/ (oxygen) **-emia** (blood condition)	Deficient amount of oxygen in blood cells; also called *anoxia* or *hypoxia*
infarction	infarct/ (death of an area) **-ion** (process; the act of)	Death of tissue from lack of (or obstructed) blood flow
ischemia	isch/ (to hold back) **-emia** (blood condition)	Lack of blood flow (and oxygen) to a part of the body due to an obstruction or narrowing of a blood vessel
Kaposi's sarcoma (KS)	sarc/ (flesh) **-oma** (tumor)	Malignant tumor of the blood vessels; associated with AIDS
leukemia (Figure 6-21)	leuk/ (white) **-emia** (blood condition)	Cancer characterized by overproduction of leukocytes; found in the blood, lymph nodes, spleen, and bone marrow

(continued)

Table 6-8 (continued)

Medical Conditions Related to the Vascular and Lymph Systems

NAME	WORD PARTS	DEFINITION
leukocytopenia	leuk/o (white) cyt/o (cell) **-penia** (deficient)	Lack of WBCs
lipoprotein	lip/o (fat)	Fat and protein bound together in cholesterol; the two main types are low-density lipoprotein (LDL) and high-density lipoprotein (HDL)
lymphadenitis (Figure 6-22)	lymph/ (lymph) aden/ (gland) **-itis** (inflammation)	Inflammation of a lymph gland
lymphadenopathy	lymph/ (lymph) aden/o (gland) **-pathy** (disease)	Disorder of the lymph glands and vessels
lymphangitis	lymph/ (lymph) angi/ (vessel) **-itis** (inflammation)	Inflammation of the lymph vessels
lymphedema	lymph/ (lymph) **-edema** (swelling)	Swelling due to lymph leaking out of its vessels into the interstitial spaces
lymphoma	lymph/ (lymph) **-oma** (tumor)	Tumor originating in the lymphatic tissue
lymphosarcoma	lymph/o (lymph) sarc/ (connective tissue) **-oma** (tumor)	Tumor in the lymph system, also known as *non-Hodgkin's lymphoma*
mononucleosis	**mono-** (one) **-osis** (condition)	Self-limiting infection of B lymphocytes caused by Epstein-Barr virus
peripheral arterial disease (PAD)	**peri-** (around)	Disease of the vascular system usually brought on by atherosclerosis
phlebitis	phleb/ (vein) **-itis** (inflammation)	Inflammation of a vein
plasmapheresis	plasma (the liquid aspect of blood) **-pheresis** (removal)	Removing (separating) plasma from blood
polycythemia	**poly-** (many) cyt/ (cell) hem/ (blood) **-ia** (condition)	Increased number of RBCs
pulmonary embolism (PE) (Figure 6-23)	pulmon/o (lungs) **-ary** (pertaining to) embol/ (plug) **-ism** (condition)	Blood clot in the lungs; can be fatal

(continued)

6

Table 6-8 (continued)

Medical Conditions Related to the Vascular and Lymph Systems

NAME	WORD PARTS	DEFINITION
Raynaud's disease/phenomenon		Vasospasms causing white/blue fingers and toes Disease: Of unknown origin, but may be triggered by cold, stress, smoking Phenomenon: Usually caused by an underlying condition (eg, atherosclerosis, systemic lupus erythematosus)
septicemia	**-emia** (blood condition)	Bacteria present in the blood
sickle cell anemia (Figure 6-24)	**an-** (without) **-emia** (blood condition)	Genetic defect in the hemoglobin causing decreased RBCs and cells sticking together (so they are unable to carry oxygen)
splenomegaly	splen/o (spleen) **-megaly** (enlargement)	Enlargement of the spleen (also a sign of mononucleosis)
thrombocytopenia	thromb/o (clot) cyt/o (cell) **-penia** (decrease)	Bleeding disorder caused by a reduction in the number of platelets (the cells that clot blood)
thrombophlebitis	thromb/o (clot) phleb/ (vein) **-itis** (inflammation)	Blood clot within a vein
thrombosis	thromb/ (clot) **-osis** (condition)	Development or presence of a blood clot within the vascular system
varicose vein (Figure 6-25)	varic/ (dilated vein) **-ose** (pertaining to)	Enlarged, twisted, distended veins (often when the valves do not work properly)
vasospasm	vas/o (vessel) **-spasm** (spasm)	Spasm of a blood vessel

Other words of note for the cardiovascular system:

Anticoagulant: Anything that prevents normal blood clotting

Diuretic: Drug that promotes urine output, resulting in removal of excess interstitial fluid

Hemoglobin (Hb): Protein–iron compound in erythrocytes that carries oxygen to the body from the lungs and transports carbon dioxide from the cells to the lungs

Vasodilator (vas/o—vessel; vas deferens; dilat/—to widen; **-or**—one who): A medication that widens the blood vessels

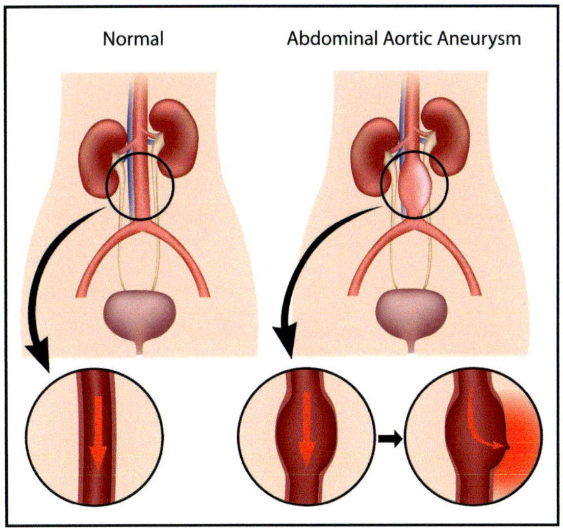

Figure 6-17. Aortic aneurysm. (Alila Medical Images/shutterstock.com)

Figure 6-18. Stages of atherosclerosis. (Alila Medical Images/shutterstock.com)

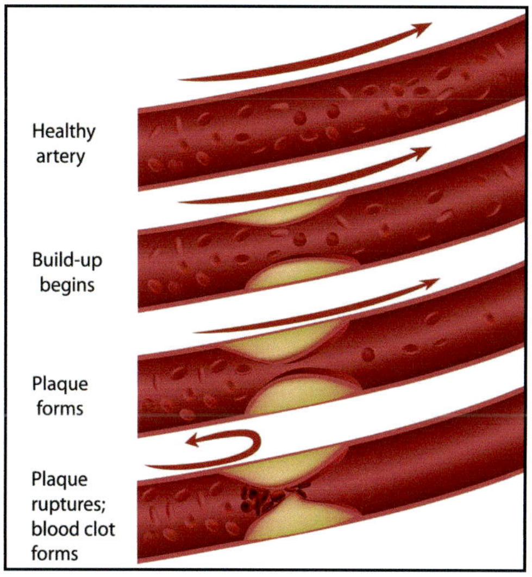

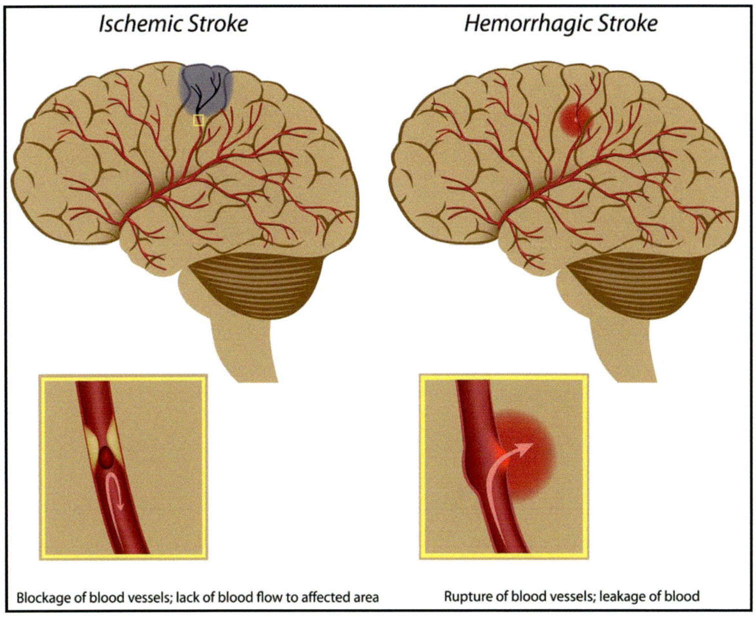

Figure 6-19. Cerebrovascular accident, also known as a *stroke.* (Alila Medical Images/shutterstock.com)

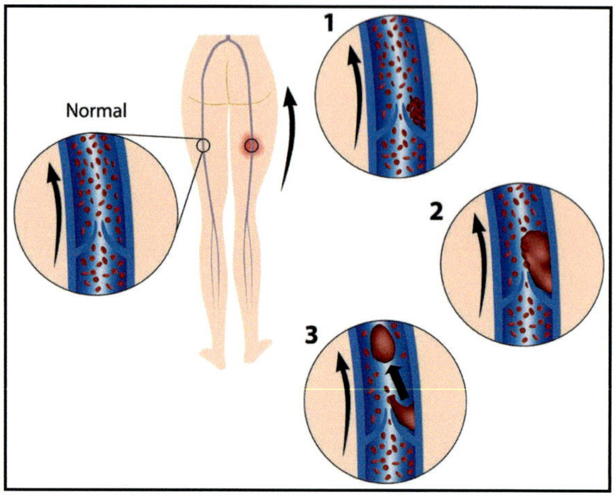

Figure 6-20. Deep vein thrombosis. (Alila Medical Images/shutterstock.com)

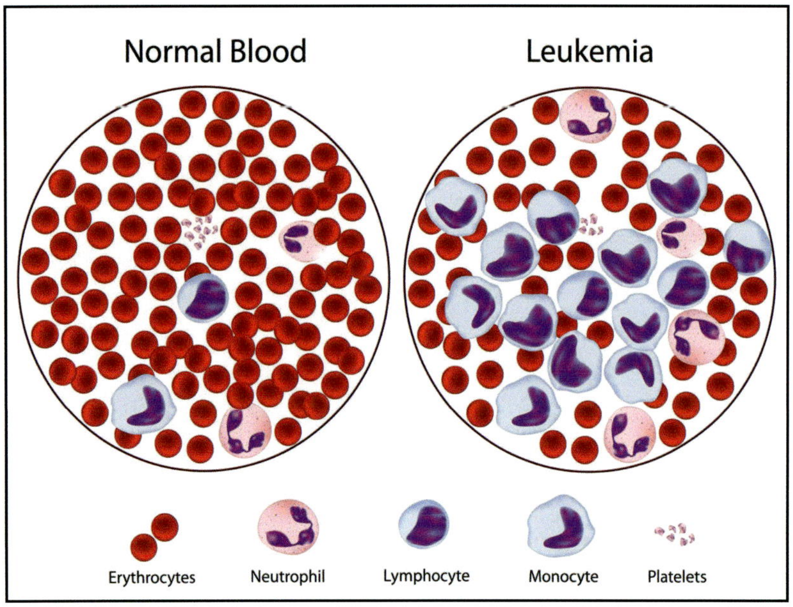

Figure 6-21. Normal blood count vs leukemia. (Alila Medical Images/shutterstock.com)

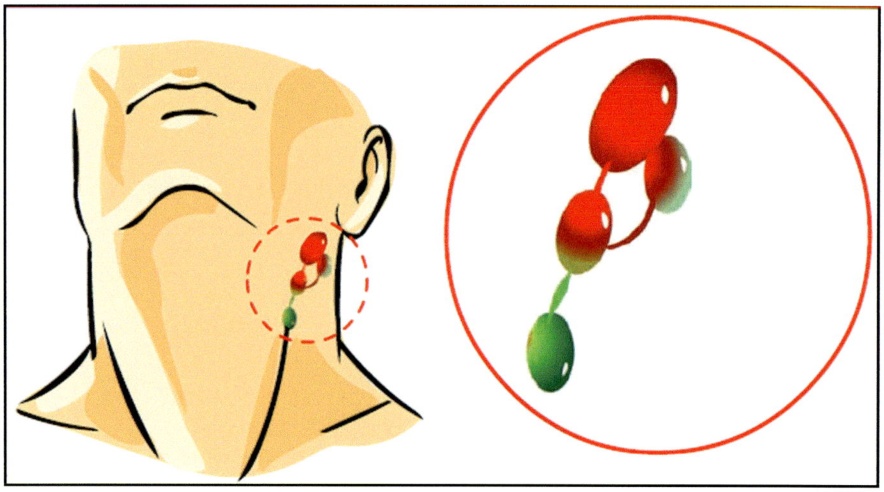

Figure 6-22. Lymphadenitis. (hkannn/shutterstock.com)

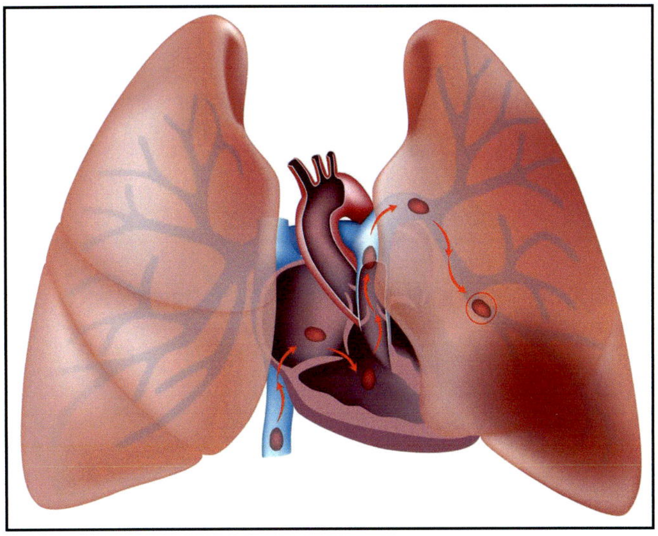

Figure 6-23. Pulmonary embolism. (Alila Medical Images/shutterstock.com)

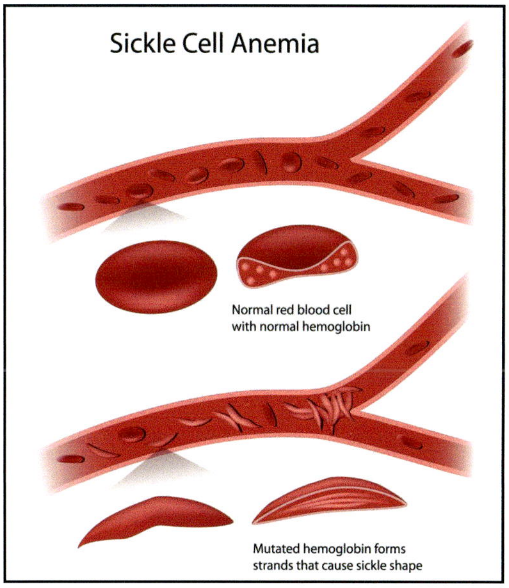

Figure 6-24. Sickle cell anemia. (Alila Medical Images/shutterstock.com)

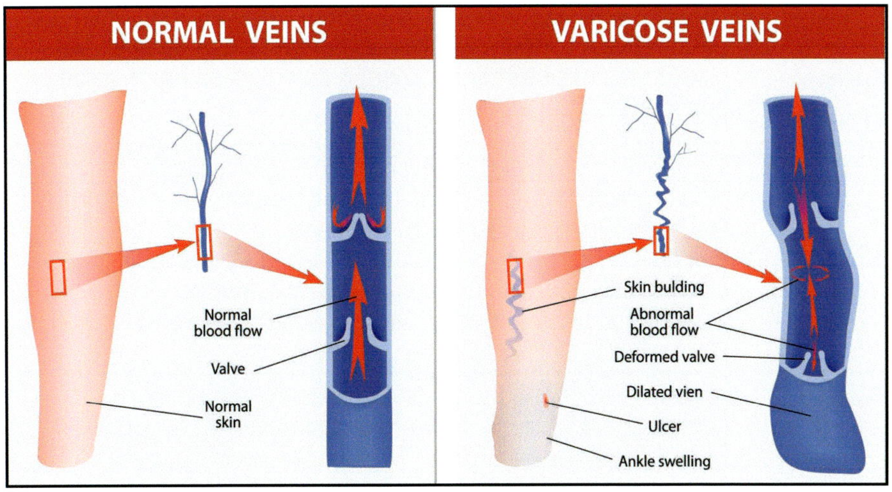

Figure 6-25. Varicose vein vs normal vein. (Zhabska Tetyana/shutterstock.com)

Tests and Procedures

Table 6-9

Tests and Procedures Specific to the Cardiovascular System

NAME	WORD PARTS	PURPOSE
angiocardiography	angi/o (vessel) cardi/o (heart) **-graphy** (process of recording)	Following the injection of radiopaque dye, the process of recording the passage of blood through the heart and vessels using x-rays
angiogram	angi/o (vessel) **-gram** (record)	X-ray recording the heart and blood vessels using radiopaque dye
angioplasty (Figure 6-26)	angi/o (vessel) **-plasty** (repair)	Surgical repair of a vessel; nonsurgical treatment to open a vessel by inserting a deflated balloon and inflating it, opening the passage
basic metabolic panel (BMP)		Series of blood tests that measure certain components of blood, including glucose, calcium, and electrolytes
cardiac catheterization (Figure 6-27)		Using a catheter passing from a vein, a camera is able to view the heart vessels; usually a dye is involved to illuminate the vessels; used to diagnose coronary artery problems and blockage
cardioversion	cardi/o (heart) vers/ (to turn) **-ion** (the act of)	Electrical shock delivered to the heart to reestablish its normal electrical rhythm, typically using an automated external defibrillator (AED), which is an electronic portable electronic devise that can detect an irregular heart beat, and deliver a shock
complete blood count (CBC)		Series of 12 tests performed on blood to determine the number of certain components of the sample (eg, RBC, WBC, Hb)
coronary artery bypass graft (CABG) (Figure 6-28)		Surgical procedure where a healthy vein is used to replace a blocked or damaged coronary artery
echocardiogram	ech/o (to bounce sound) cardi/o (heart) **-gram** (record of)	Noninvasive test using sound waves to record the thickness of the heart, workings of the valves, and other cardiac structures to determine if there is an enlarged heart, valve properties
electrocardiogram (ECG; EKG) (Figure 6-29)	electr/o (electricity) cardi/o (heart) **-gram** (a record of)	Noninvasive method of recording heart activity via electrodes placed on the surface of the chest and extremities to determine arrhythmias of the heart
Holter monitor (Figure 6-30)		Portable ECG test that records activity as the patient goes through activities of daily living to determine arrhythmias of the heart
intracardiac electrophysiology study (EPS)	**intra-** (within) cardi/ (heart) **-ac** (pertaining to) electr/o (electricity)	Invasive procedure consisting of placing catheter-guided electrodes within the heart to evaluate electrical conduction through the heart

(continued)

Table 6-9 (continued)

Tests and Procedures Specific to the Cardiovascular System

NAME	WORD PARTS	PURPOSE
lipid profile		Blood tests measuring different fats in the blood; assists in assessing risks for coronary artery disease
lymphadenectomy	lymph/ (lymph) aden/ (gland) **-ectomy** (surgical removal)	Surgical removal of a lymph gland
mono spot	**mono-** (one)	Test for mononucleosis
percutaneous transluminal inserting coronary angioplasty (PTCA)	**per-** (through) cutane/o (skin) **trans-** (across; through) lumin (light) **-al** (pertaining to) angi/o (vessel) **-plasty** (repair)	Procedure that dilates blood vessels by inflating a balloon in the vessel; usually a treatment for PAD or coronary artery disease
phlebotomy	phleb/o (vein) **-tomy** (incision)	Incision into a vein to draw blood (also called a *venipuncture*)
radiofrequency catheter ablation		Catheter is inserted in a vein (usually the leg) and radio waves are used to destroy tissue that is hyperreactive; used typically to control cardiac arrhythmias
stress test (Figure 6-31)		Typically, a patient walks on a treadmill at various speeds and intensities while attached to an ECG; BP is also monitored; assesses for symptoms (eg, shortness of breath) or signs (on the ECG, BP) of heart disease; also called *exercise challenge test*

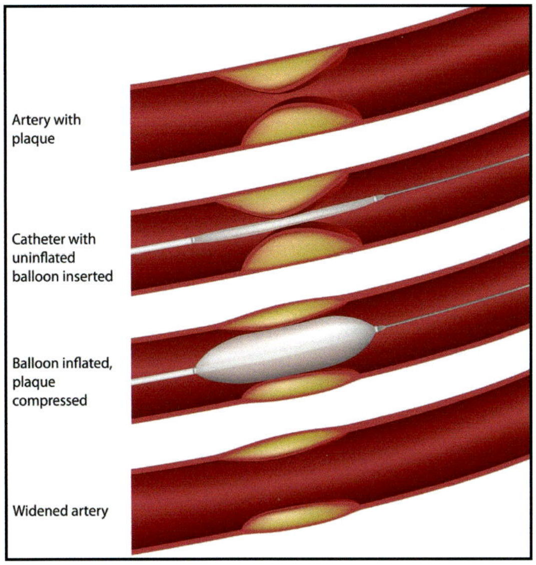

Figure 6-26. Balloon angioplasty. (Alila Medical Images/shutterstock.com)

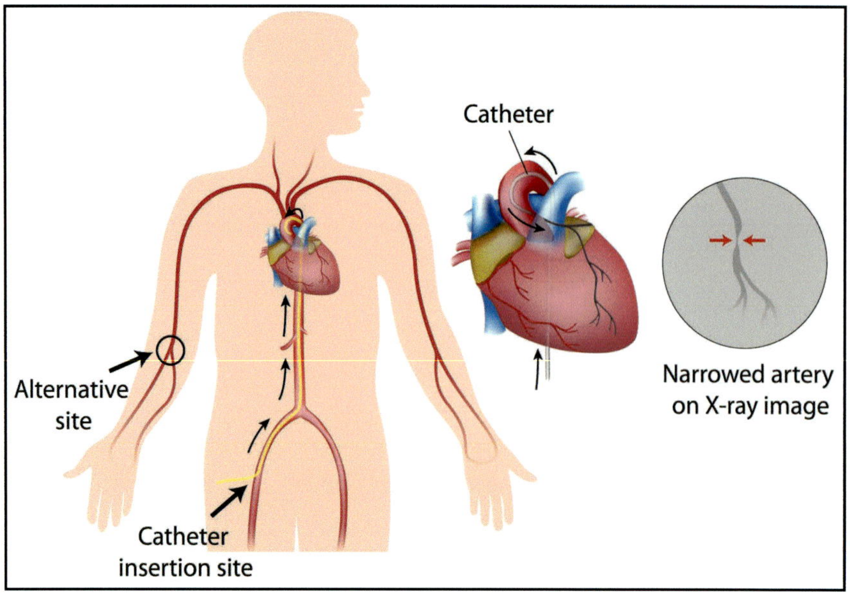

Figure 6-27. Cardiac catheterization. (Alila Medical Images/shutterstock.com)

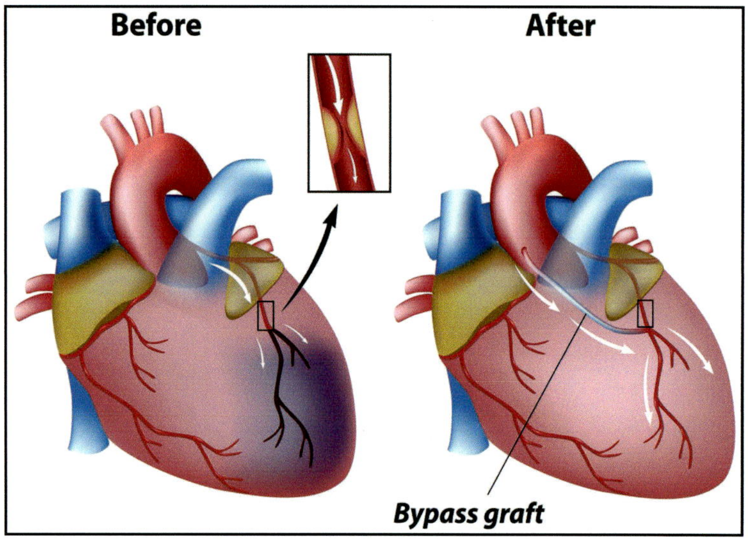

Figure 6-28. Coronary artery bypass surgery. (Alila Medical Images/shutterstock.com)

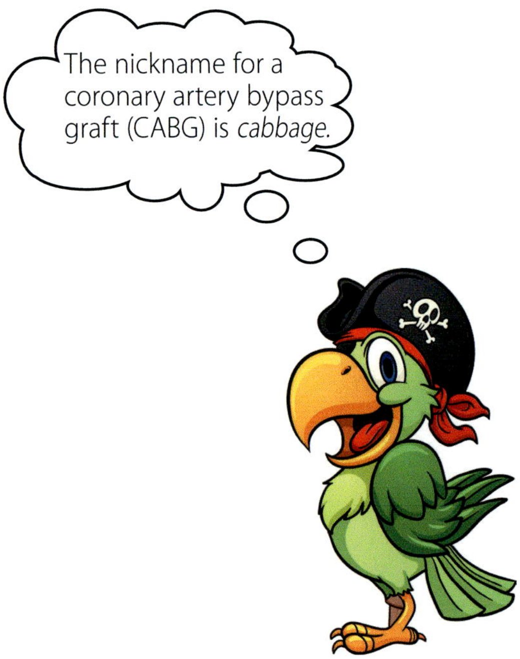
The nickname for a coronary artery bypass graft (CABG) is *cabbage*.

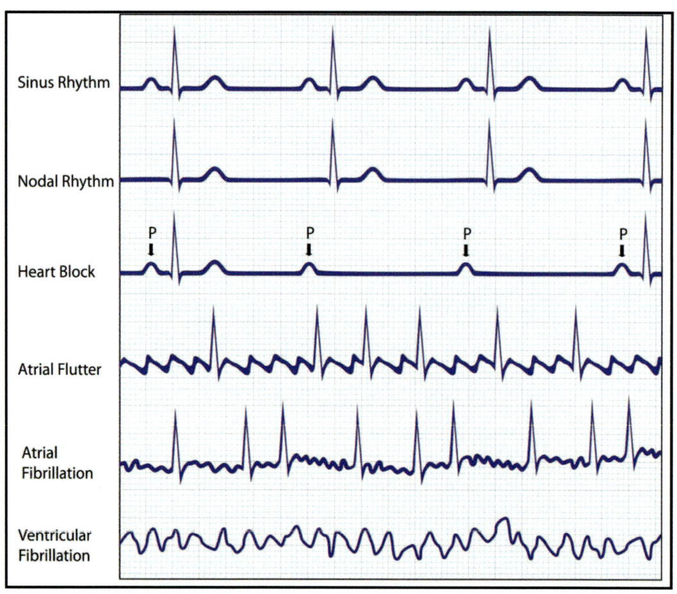

Figure 6-29. Electrocardiogram recordings of normal (sinus) rhythm and other pathologies. (Alila Medical Images/shutterstock.com)

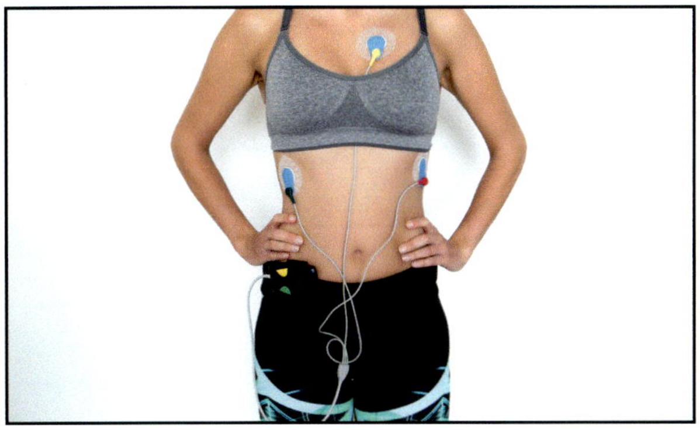

Figure 6-30. Places where electrodes can be taped onto the chest for a cardiac Holter monitor. (Sven Hansche/shutterstock.com)

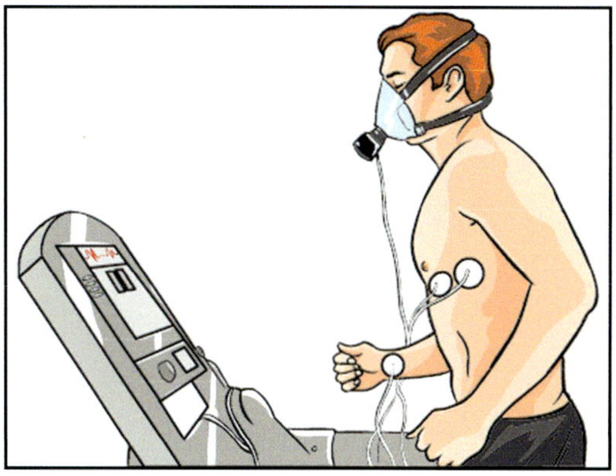

Figure 6-31. Exercise stress test on a treadmill. (hkannn/shutterstock.com)

6

BIBLIOGRAPHY

Flanagan KW, Cuppett M. *Medical Conditions in the Athlete.* 3rd ed. Human Kinetics; 2017.
Mosby's Dictionary of Medicine, Nursing & Health Professions. 10th ed. Elsevier; 2017.
Rice J. *Medical Terminology for Health Care Professionals.* 9th ed. Pearson; 2018.
Shiland BJ. *Mastering Healthcare Terminology.* 6th ed. Elsevier; 2019.
Turley SM. *Medical Language—Immerse Yourself.* 5th ed. Pearson; 2020
Venes D, ed. *Taber's Cyclopedic Medical Dictionary.* 24th ed. F. A. Davis; 2021.

NOTES

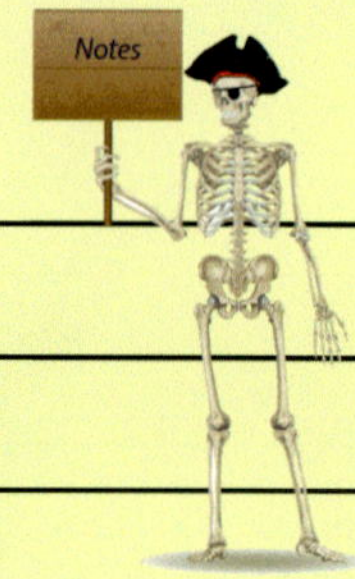

NOTES

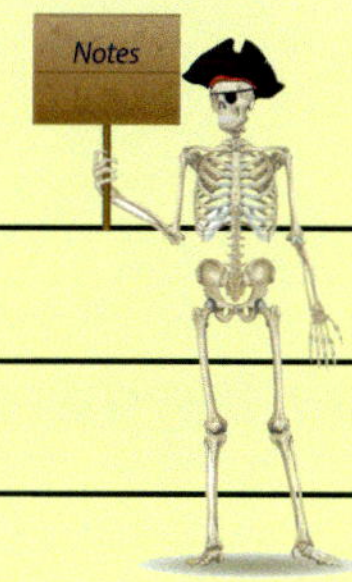

Learning Activities

Name:______________________

Cardiovascular System

A. Label parts of the heart from the following list.

- myocardium__________________
- left atrium__________________
- interventricular septum___________
- left ventricle__________________
- aortic valve__________________
- pulmonary artery______________
- mitral valve__________________
- tricuspid valve________________
- right atrium__________________
- right ventricle________________

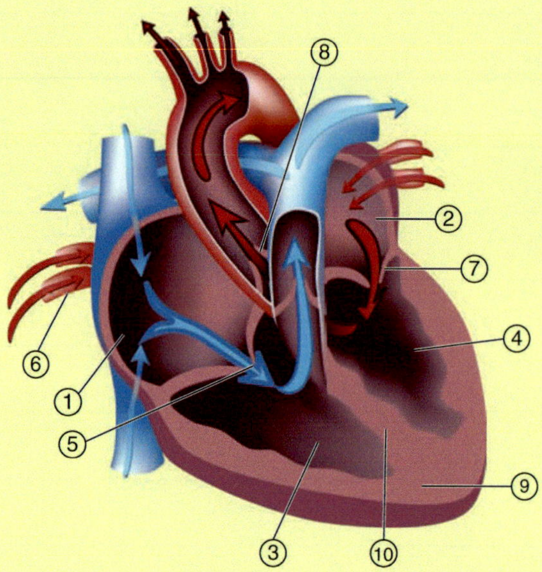

(Alila Medical Images/shutterstock.com)

B. Using the following list, number the anatomical parts of the heart in the correct order that blood flows through the heart.

__________aortic valve
__________right atrium
__________pulmonary valve
__________pulmonary artery
__________mitral valve
__________left ventricle
____1____inferior vena cava
__________aorta
__________tricuspid valve
__________right ventricle
__________left atrium
__________pulmonary vein

C. Define the following medical abbreviations.

1. CAD________________________________
2. MI________________________________
3. CVA________________________________
4. HCM________________________________
5. PAD________________________________
6. HTN________________________________
7. CHF________________________________
8. MVP________________________________
9. DVT________________________________
10. PE________________________________

6

D. Match the medical word part with its meaning.

1. LDL______________	a. four
2. **-osis**______________	b. skin
3. **tetra-**______________	c. a valve problem in the heart
4. AV______________	d. a type of cholesterol
5. glyc/o______________	e. surgical fixation
6. vers/o______________	f. clot
7. cutane/o______________	g. condition
8. **-pexy**______________	h. sugar
9. MVP______________	i. to turn
10. thromb/o______________	j. a node in the heart

E. Build the word: Using the word root, add the other word element and define the new word created.

1. **angi/o**
   a. **-poiesis**________________________________
   b. **-plasty**________________________________
   c. **-oma**________________________________
   d. **-scope**________________________________
   e. **-pathy**________________________________
2. **cardi/o**
   a. vers/o + **-ion**________________________________
   b. **-itis**________________________________
   c. **-rrhaphy**________________________________
   d. **-megaly**________________________________
   e. vascul/o + **-ar**________________________________

3. lymph/o

a. **-cyte**______________________________________

b. aden/o + **-itis**__________________________________

c. sarc/o + **-oma**__________________________________

d. **-edema**______________________________________

e. **-blast**______________________________________

F. Label the glands and nodes of the lymphatic system from the following list.

- cervical nodes__________________________________
- axillary nodes__________________________________
- inguinal nodes__________________________________
- thymus______________________________________
- palatine tonsils__________________________________
- spleen______________________________________

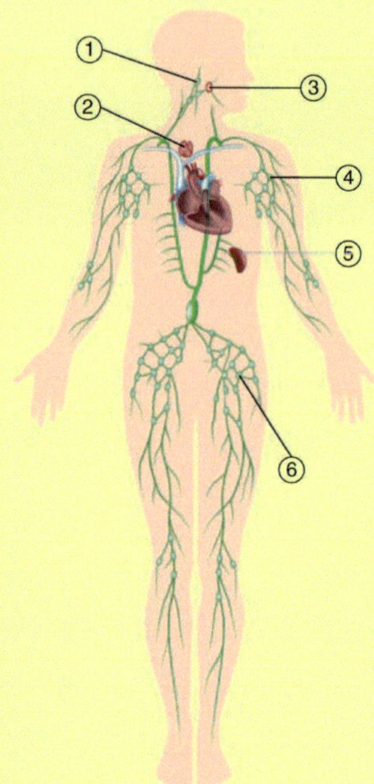

(Alila Medical Images/shutterstock.com)

G. Using word parts from previous chapters as well as new ones presented in this chapter, separate the prefix and suffix from the word root and define the following words.

1. glycopenia______________________________________
2. plasmapheresis__________________________________
3. angiogram______________________________________
4. hemorrhage______________________________________
5. valvotomy______________________________________
6. hemoptysis______________________________________
7. hypocalcemia__________________________________
8. splenopexy______________________________________
9. pericardiocentesis__________________________________
10. phagocytosis__________________________________

Case Study

Define the numerical terms (1 to 14) in the spaces that follow.

History, Chief Complaint

A 19-year-old Black football athlete complained of difficulty breathing while running wind sprints in off-season conditioning. He was just getting over a chest cold, and has a history of asthma. It was a cold and foggy early morning (6:30 am) outdoor conditioning session. He reported a history of rapid heartbeat on and off over the last few weeks.

Evaluation

The athlete had **tachycardia** (1) and **angina pectoris** (2) and had **dyspnea** (3). Other than tachycardia, the athlete had no discernable **dysrhythmia** (4).

Diagnostic Studies

His **systolic** (5) blood pressure was 180 and **diastolic** (6) pressure was 100, which is written as _____ (7). A **lipid profile** (8) determined he had high cholesterol (the total was 280 mg/dL). An **echocardiogram** (9) and **ECG** (10) were performed. Based on these tests, there was no obvious **cardiomyopathy** (11) and an **angiogram** (12) was scheduled. The athlete was diagnosed with **angiostenosis** (13) due to **atherosclerosis** (14). Following an extensive diet change and medication to lower his blood pressure and cholesterol, the athlete returned in the fall to full activity.

Terms

1. ____________________
2. ____________________
3. ____________________
4. ____________________
5. ____________________
6. ____________________
7. ____________________
8. ____________________
9. ____________________
10. ____________________
11. ____________________
12. ____________________
13. ____________________
14. ____________________

7

Respiratory System

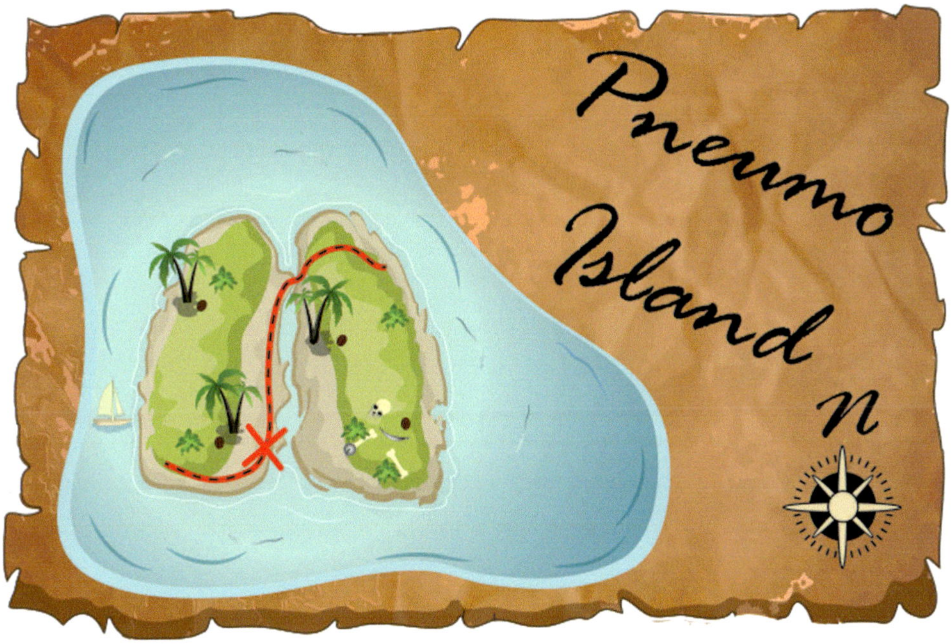

Objectives

After studying this chapter, you will be able to:

1. Identify the major components of the respiratory system.
2. Distinguish between the upper and lower respiratory tract.
3. Build words associated with the respiratory system.
4. Describe medical conditions of the respiratory system based on the word parts.
5. Differentiate between therapeutic procedures based on word parts used to describe the procedure.
6. Identify classifications of medications used to treat respiratory conditions.

Flanagan KW.
Medical Terminology With Case Studies: A Navigated Guide to Learning for Health Care Professionals, Third Edition (pp 151-180).

CHAPTER OUTLINE

- Self-assessment
- Checklist for word parts in the chapter
- Checklist of new anatomy
- Anatomy
  - Upper respiratory tract
  - Lower respiratory tract
  - Sinuses
- Word building
  - Prefixes
  - Suffixes
  - Combining forms
- Medical conditions
- Breathing types and sounds
- Tests and procedures
- Medication classifications
- Learning activities
- Case study

SELF-ASSESSMENT

Based on what you have learned so far, can you write the definition of these words?

- apnea____
- tracheotomy____
- tonsillitis____
- stethoscope____
- pulmonologist____
- bronchoscopy____
- oropharyngeal____
- dysphasia____

Checklist for Word Parts in the Chapter

Prefixes

- ☐ a-
- ☐ an-
- ☐ ana-
- ☐ anti-
- ☐ brady-
- ☐ de-
- ☐ dys-
- ☐ endo-
- ☐ epi-
- ☐ eu-
- ☐ ex-
- ☐ hyper-
- ☐ hypo-
- ☐ meso-
- ☐ pan-
- ☐ para-
- ☐ poly-
- ☐ tachy-

Remember the **prefixes** and **suffixes** never change meaning and are in every chapter.

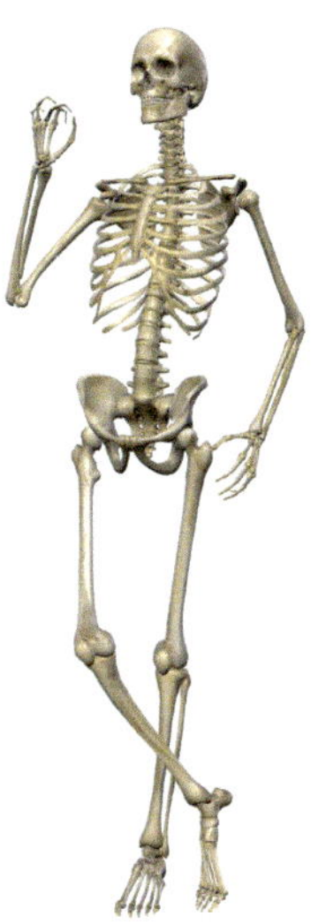

Suffixes

- ☐ -al
- ☐ -ary
- ☐ -algia
- ☐ -ation
- ☐ -atory
- ☐ -capnia
- ☐ -centesis
- ☐ -dynia
- ☐ -eal
- ☐ -ectasis
- ☐ -ectomy
- ☐ -emia
- ☐ -ia
- ☐ -ic
- ☐ -ion
- ☐ -itis
- ☐ -lytic
- ☐ -meter
- ☐ -metry
- ☐ -oid
- ☐ -oma
- ☐ -osis
- ☐ -otomy
- ☐ -phasia
- ☐ -phonia
- ☐ -phylaxis
- ☐ -plasty
- ☐ -pnea
- ☐ -ptysis
- ☐ -scope
- ☐ -scopic
- ☐ -scopy
- ☐ -spasm
- ☐ -sphyxia
- ☐ -stenosis
- ☐ -stomy
- ☐ -thorax
- ☐ -tomy

Combining Forms

- ☐ aden/o
- ☐ alveol/o
- ☐ anthrac/o
- ☐ bronch/o
- ☐ bronchi/o
- ☐ bronchiol/o
- ☐ coni/o
- ☐ cyan/o
- ☐ cyst/o
- ☐ dilat/o
- ☐ epiglott/o
- ☐ fibr/o
- ☐ hem/o
- ☐ laryng/o
- ☐ lob/o
- ☐ muc/o
- ☐ nas/o
- ☐ or/o
- ☐ orth/o
- ☐ ox/o
- ☐ pector/o
- ☐ pharyng/o
- ☐ phas/o
- ☐ phon/o
- ☐ phren/o
- ☐ pleur/o
- ☐ pneum/o
- ☐ pneumon/o
- ☐ pulmon/o
- ☐ py/o
- ☐ sinus/o
- ☐ sphygm/o
- ☐ spir/o
- ☐ steth/o
- ☐ thel/e
- ☐ thorac/o
- ☐ tonsil/o
- ☐ trache/o
- ☐ tuss/o

Checklist of New Anatomy

Upper Respiratory Tract

- ☐ Nasopharynx
- ☐ Oropharynx
- ☐ Laryngopharynx
- ☐ Nares
- ☐ Epiglottis
- ☐ Trachea
- ☐ Glottis
- ☐ Pharyngeal tonsils
- ☐ Adenoids
- ☐ Palatine tonsils
- ☐ Larynx
- ☐ Hyoid bone
- ☐ Thyroid cartilage

Sinuses

- ☐ Paranasal sinuses
- ☐ Maxillary sinuses
- ☐ Frontal sinuses
- ☐ Ethmoidal sinuses

Lower Respiratory Tract

- ☐ Bronchi
- ☐ Bronchioles
- ☐ Alveoli

Chest Cavity

- ☐ Parietal pleura
- ☐ Visceral pleura
- ☐ Pleural cavity
- ☐ Mediastinum

Anatomy

Pneumo Island is home to combining forms unique to the respiratory system. As with your travel to other islands, you will notice many prefixes and suffixes used again, so these gold and silver coins of word parts should be becoming quite familiar to you. Pneumo Island is in the shape of two lungs, and word elements on this island represent aspects of the respiratory system.

The respiratory system can be divided into upper and lower tracts. It primarily consists of the **pharynx** (throat), **larynx** (voice box or Adam's apple), **trachea** (windpipe), **bronchi**, and **lungs** (Figure 7-1). The larynx connects the pharynx to the trachea. The upper respiratory tract is where breathing begins. Air enters the nose or mouth and is warmed and moistened prior to passing into the **pharynx**. Chapter 14 ("Sensory System") will provide a more detailed anatomy and words pertaining to the nose, and Chapter 9 ("Gastrointestinal System") will do likewise for the mouth.

Upper Respiratory Tract

The pharynx is about 5 inches long, begins at the base of the skull, and has several sections. Both air and food pass through the pharynx through its sections. Each section is named according to the structure nearest to it at that location (Figure 7-2):

- **Nasopharynx** (**nas/o**—nose)
- **Oropharynx** (**or/o**—mouth)
- **Laryngopharynx** (**laryng/o**—larynx)

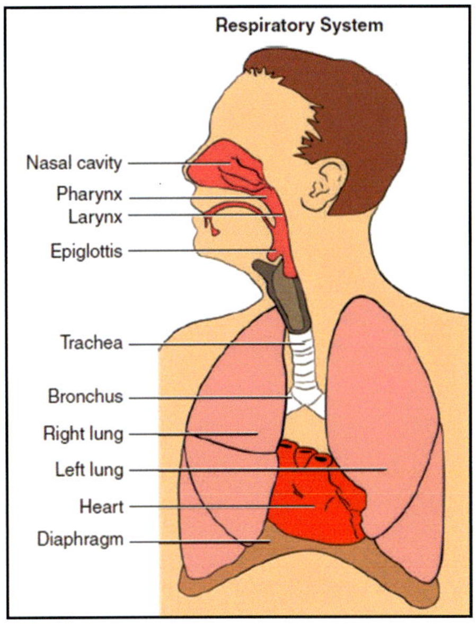

Figure 7-1. Overview of the anatomy of the respiratory system. (Alila Medical Images/shutterstock.com)

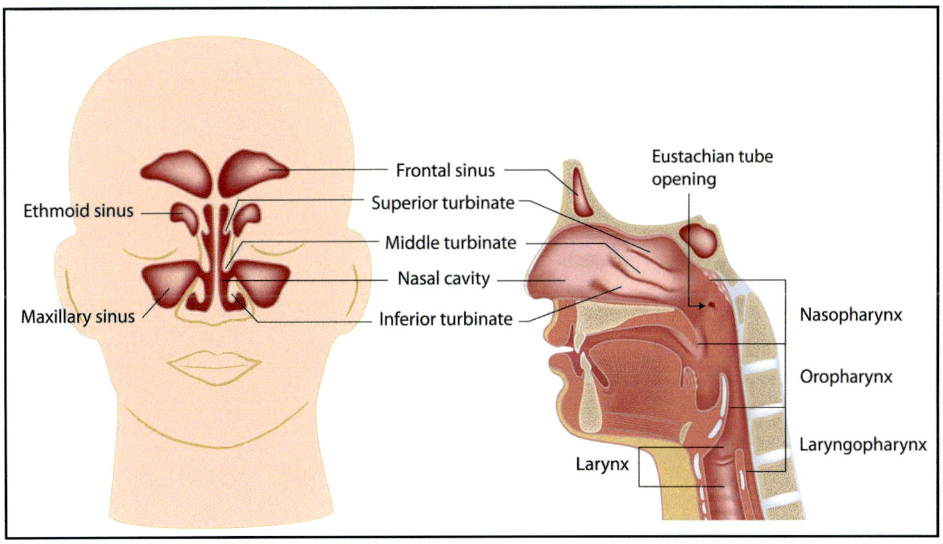

Figure 7-2. Areas of the pharynx and sinuses. (Alila Medical Images/shutterstock.com)

Both **nares** (nostrils from the nose) and both **eustachian** tubes from the middle ear open into the pharynx. This is why some ear infections and allergies that affect the nose can cause reactions in the throat. As the discharge drains into the pharynx, it can trigger a cough or sore throat.

As the pharynx descends down the back of the mouth to the neck, there is a leaf-shaped flap called the **epiglottis** (**epi-**—above, upon) that covers the opening in the **trachea** (the **glottis**) and prevents food or fluid from entering the trachea and lungs (Figure 7-3). Food and liquids pass by the trachea (also known as the *windpipe*), due to the epiglottis covering the trachea, and enter the esophagus to the stomach. The esophagus is a thin, flexible, hollow tube that lies behind the trachea, whereas the trachea is a 1-inch wide and 4.5-inch long hollow tube with smooth muscles and rigid C-shaped rings of cartilage that provide stability and help prevent its collapse. The trachea is visible in most people in the anterior neck.

Also within the upper respiratory tract are small lymphatic tissues that are the first line of defense in protecting the body from inhaled microorganisms. The **pharyngeal tonsils** (**pharyng/**—throat; **-eal**—pertaining to) are located where the back of the nose joins the pharynx (the nasopharynx; **nas/o**—nose), and the tissue most people just call the *tonsils* are actually the **palatine tonsils** and are located further down the larynx in the **oropharynx** (**or/o**—mouth; Figure 7-4). As a group, the tonsils are often referred to as **adenoids** (**aden/o**—gland; **-oid**—resembling). Infections of the upper respiratory tract are grouped under a category called **upper respiratory infections** (**URIs**).

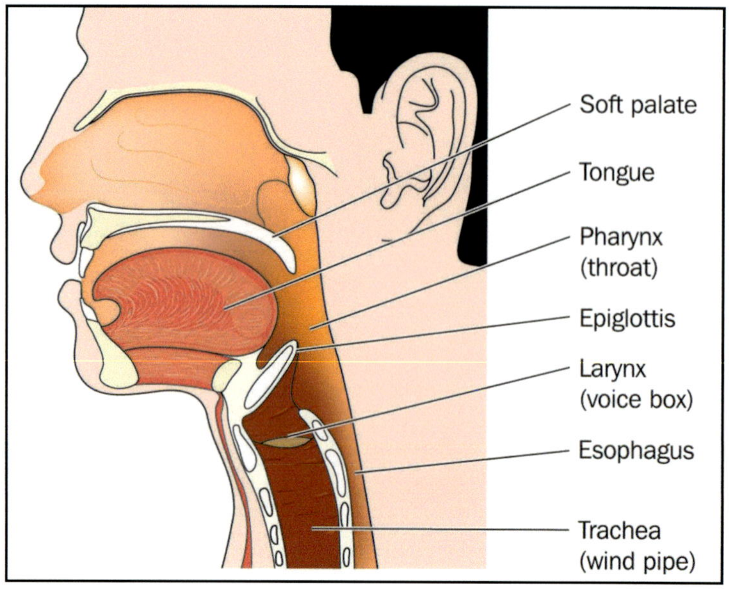

Figure 7-3. Upper respiratory system. (Blamb/shutterstock.com)

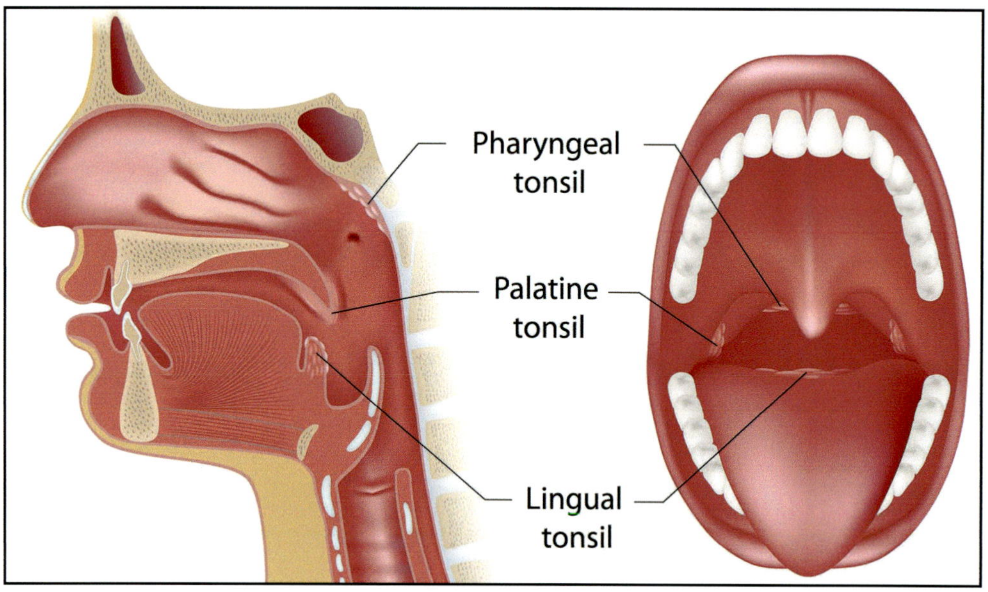

Figure 7-4. The tonsils. (Alila Medical Images/shutterstock.com)

The **larynx** (voice box) is a muscular and cartilaginous structure lined with a mucous membrane that is actually the upper aspect of the trachea. It lies below the root of the tongue and **hyoid bone** (Figure 7-5). The hyoid is a thin, flat bone on top of the larynx and in the front of the throat. The larynx contains the vocal cords, which are tissues that produce sound as air is passed over them. They lie on either side of the glottis. The **thyroid cartilage** (Adam's apple) is a large piece of cartilage in the larynx, said to contribute to the deeper voice in men. After puberty, it is typically more pronounced (visible) in men than in women.

Lower Respiratory Tract

The lower respiratory tract begins as the trachea, divides into two **bronchi** (individually termed *bronchus*), and admits air into the right and left lungs. The bronchi contain the same C-shaped cartilage as the trachea, but the bronchi have both a mucous membrane and tiny hair-like **cilia** to trap any unwanted materials. Anything trapped by mucus or cilia are coughed up and expelled. Consider the shape of the smaller bronchi to be like broccoli; the branches of the main bronchi continue to divide into smaller and smaller sections, ultimately forming **bronchioles**. Bronchioles terminate into **alveoli** (individually called *alveolus*), which is where inhaled air leaves its oxygen as the blood collects it, and receives carbon dioxide from the blood cells as they pass. This gas exchange occurs within the pulmonary capillaries as the blood circulates through the lungs back to the heart, and is then pumped to the rest of the body.

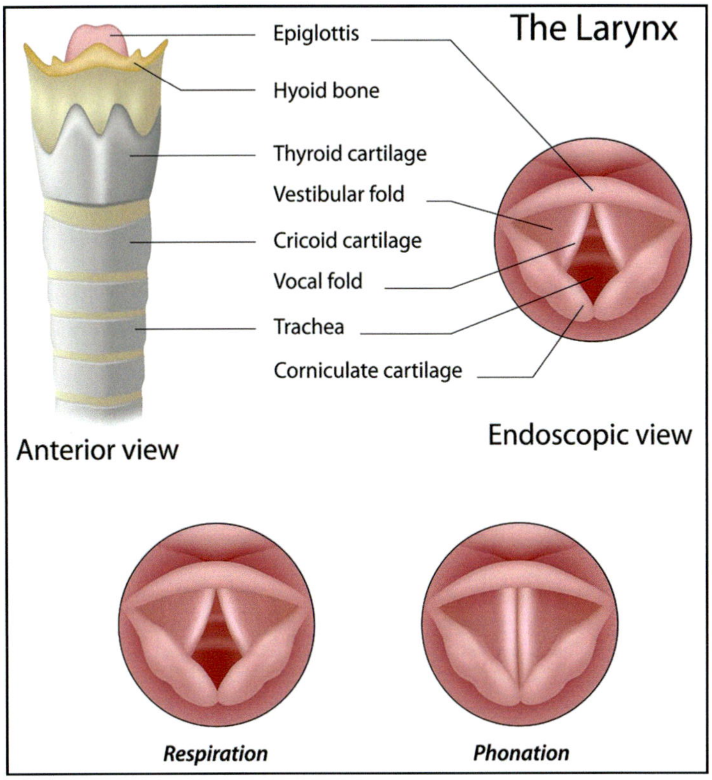

Figure 7-5. The larynx and vocal cords. (Alila Medical Images/shutterstock.com)

The main organ of the respiratory system is the lung. There are two lungs: the right lung has three distinct lobes, whereas the left lung only has two, as the liver butts up against the right lower lobe. The diaphragm is a very tough and muscular divider that separates the thoracic cavity from the abdominal cavity (Figure 7-6). The diaphragm contracts in a downward motion and allows inhalation. This action also enlarges the entire thoracic cavity, as respiration can be easily seen in others. As the diaphragm relaxes, air is expelled (expiration; Figure 7-7).

The **parietal pleura** is a tough membrane that lines the entire thoracic cavity and the **visceral pleura** attaches directly to individual lobes of the lungs. In between these two pleurae is the **pleural cavity**, which also produces small amounts of fluid to allow the lungs to glide easily against the thoracic walls as breathing occurs (Figure 7-8). There is an area, the **mediastinum**, in the chest that is not well defined but is where the two bronchi, heart, aorta, and esophagus reside.

A person usually takes 24,000 breaths a day, or about 12 to 20 times a minute, but that can increase during activity or certain illnesses of the lung. Children have higher breathing rates than adults. Table 7-1 provides a list of words associated with breathing rate.

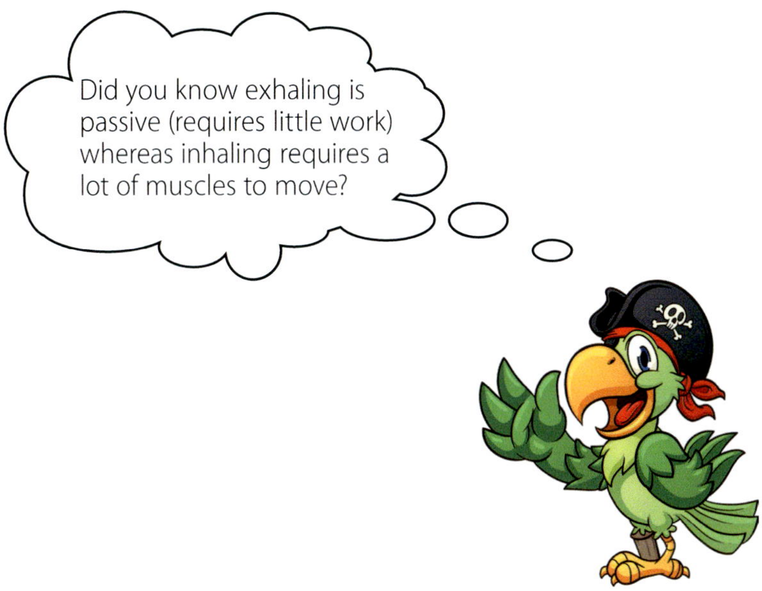
Did you know exhaling is passive (requires little work) whereas inhaling requires a lot of muscles to move?

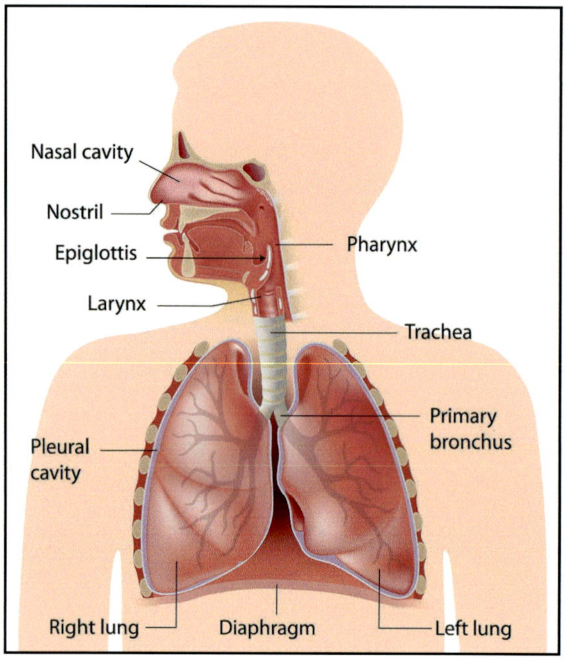

Figure 7-6. The lobes of the lung and diaphragm. (Alila Medical Images/ shutterstock.com)

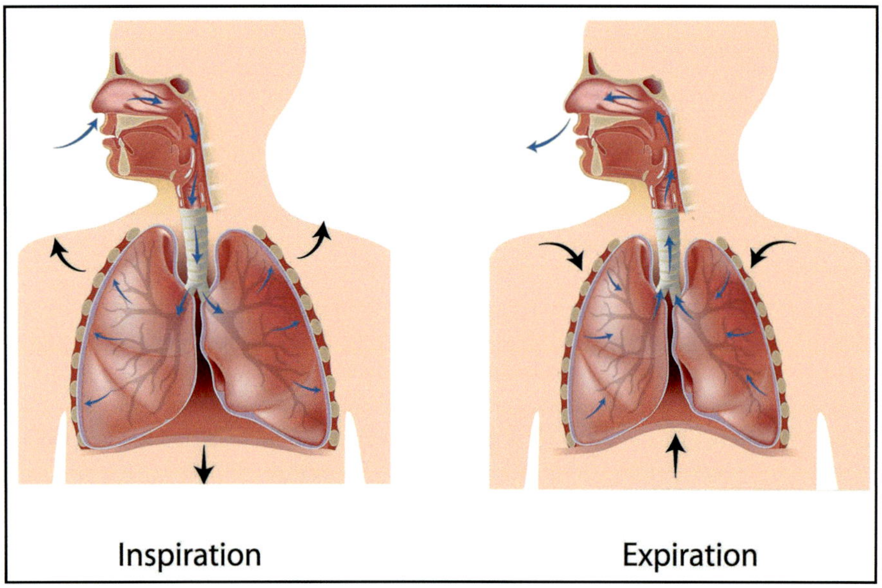

Figure 7-7. Inspiration and expiration and chest movement. (Alila Medical Images/ shutterstock.com)

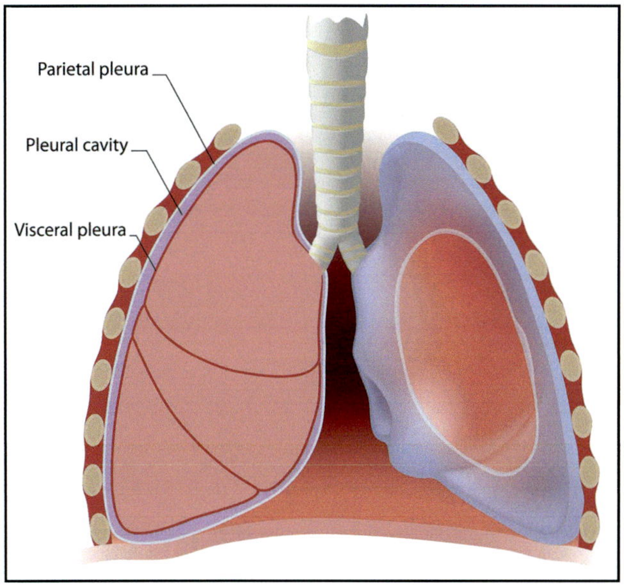

Figure 7-8. The pleura. (Alila Medical Images/shutterstock.com)

7

Table 7-1
Words Pertaining to Breathing Rate (-pnea—breathing)

WORD	WORD PARTS	DEFINITION
apnea	**a-** (without)	No breathing
bradypnea	**brady-** (slow)	Less than 12 breaths per minute
dyspnea	**dys-** (painful)	Painful, labored breathing
eupnea	**eu-** (normal)	12 to 20 breaths per minute
hyperpnea	**hyper-** (above; excessive; high; increased)	More than 20 breaths per minute
tachypnea	**tachy-** (fast)	Very fast breathing

Sinuses

There are four hollow, mucus-lined cavities called *sinuses* that produce mucus and are susceptible to infection (sinusitis). Sinuses are found in pairs and are named according to the bones or structures they reside nearest. Closest to the nasal cavity are the **paranasal sinuses** (**para-**—beside, near; **nas/o**—nose). The **maxillary sinuses** are below the eye under the maxilla bone of the face, and the **frontal sinuses** are above the eyes behind the frontal bone of the skull. The fourth pair of sinuses, the **ethmoidal sinuses**, are located on the base of the cranium (skull), forming the walls and roof of the nasal cavity (see Figure 7 2). Sinuses also assist with the sound of your voice. These hollow chambers are spaces for airwaves to pass through and create your normal voice. Should they get clogged (as with sinusitis), your voice sounds different as air is passing through mucus instead of clear space.

Word Building

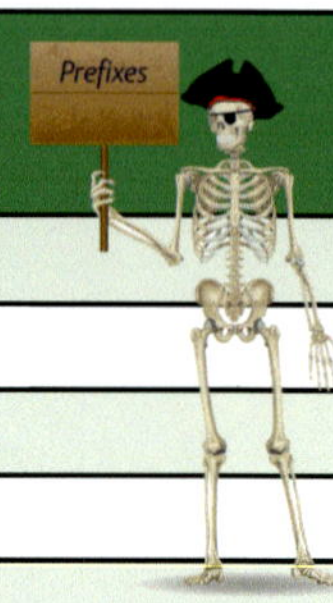

TABLE 7-2 PREFIXES	
PREFIX	**DEFINITION**
a-	without
an-	not; without
ana-	up; apart; away
anti-	against
brady-	slow
dys-	abnormal; bad; difficult; painful
endo-	in; within
epi-	above; upon
eu-	good; normal
ex-	away; away from; out; outside
hyper-	excessive
hypo-	below; decreased; deficient; insufficient; low; under
meso-	middle
pan-	all
para-	beside; near; abnormal
poly-	excessive; many; much; over
tachy-	fast; rapid

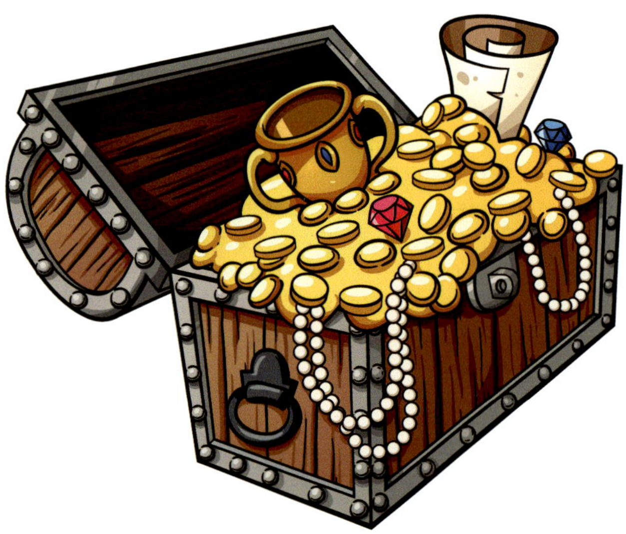

This book has fewer prefixes than suffixes or combining forms, so learning the meaning of these coins that travel to each island (chapter) can save time learning as you go.

TABLE 7-3
SUFFIXES

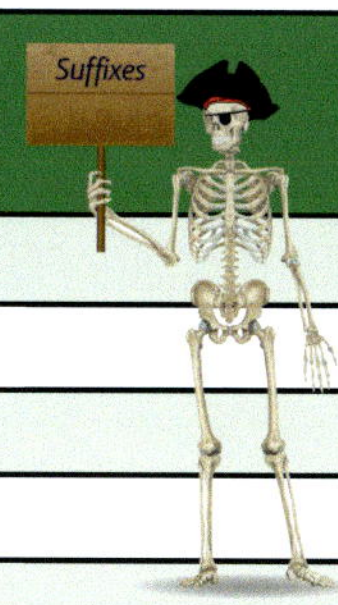

SUFFIX	DEFINITION
-al; -ary	pertaining to
-algia	pain
-ation	process of
-atory	pertaining to
-capnia	carbon dioxide in the blood
-centesis	puncture; surgical puncture
-dynia	pain
-eal	pertaining to
-ectomy	excision; surgical removal
-emia	blood condition
-ia	condition
-ic	pertaining to
-ion	process; the act of
-itis	inflammation
-lytic	destroy
-meter	an instrument used to measure
-metry	measurement of
-oid	resembling
-oma	mass; tumor
-osis	condition
-phasia	speech
-phonia	voice
-plasty	reconstruction; repair; plastic surgery
-pnea	breathing
-ptysis	to spit
-scope	an instrument used to view or inspect
-scopic	pertaining to visual examination (**-ic**—pertaining to)
-scopy	examination of
-spasm	involuntary contraction
-sphyxia	pulse
-stenosis	narrowing
-stomy	surgical opening
-thorax	chest
-tomy; -otomy	incision; to cut into

Table 7-4
Combining Forms

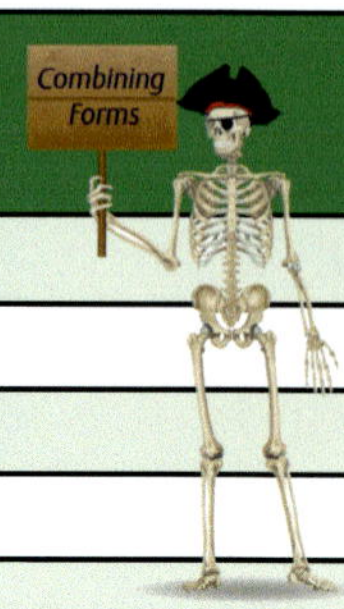

COMBINING FORM	DEFINITION
aden/o	gland
alveol/o	alveoli
anthrac/o	coal; coal dust
bronch/o	bronchus (main tube that carries air to the lungs)
bronchiol/o	large air passage to lung
coni/o	dust
cyan/o	blue
cyst/o	sac; bladder
epiglott/o	epiglottis
fibr/o	fiber
hem/o	blood
laryng/o	larynx
lob/o	lobe
muc/o	mucus
nas/o	nose
or/o	mouth
orth/o	straight
ox/o	oxygen
pector/o	chest
pharyng/o	pharynx (throat)
phas/o	speech
phon/o	sound; voice
phren/o	diaphragm
pleur/o	pleura
pneum/o; pneumon/o; pulmon/o	lung
py/o	pus
sinus/o	sinus
sphygm/o	pulse
spir/o	breathing; breath
steth/o	chest
thel/e	nipple
thorac/o	chest
tonsil/o	tonsils
trache/o	trachea
tuss/o	cough

Medical Conditions

In most body systems, there are pathological conditions that do not have medical word parts associated with them, such as *asthma*. Each chapter will have a table of these terms that you will just have to memorize. Table 7-5 contains medical conditions related to the respiratory system that do not typically have prefixes, suffixes, or combining forms.

7

Table 7-5
Medical Conditions Related to the Respiratory System

NAME	DEFINITION
altitude sickness	Nausea, headache, and dyspnea caused by exposure to low oxygen levels at high elevations
asthma (Figures 7-9 and 7-10)	Respiratory disease marked by constricted breathing
atelectasis	Incomplete expansion of alveoli causing a collapsed lung
chronic obstructive pulmonary disease (COPD) (Figure 7-11)	Chronic, progressive, irreversible respiratory disease that involves diminished inspiratory and expiratory capacity of the lungs
coryza	Common cold
croup	Acute respiratory disease that presents with obstruction of the larynx, cough, dyspnea, and stridor
diphtheria	Acute infection caused by bacteria; immunity is provided to infants via a Tdap (tetanus, diphtheria, and pertussis) vaccine
emphysema (Figure 7-12)	Chronic pulmonary disease damaging the alveoli in the lungs
influenza (nickname: flu)	Acute, contagious respiratory infection
pertussis	Acute infectious disease with a distinctive cough; most receive a Tdap vaccination as an infant preventing this disease; also called *whooping cough*
pulmonary edema	Fluid filling the alveoli and bronchioles
pulmonary embolism (PE) (Figure 7-13)	Blood clot lodged in the vessels of the lung; can be fatal
respiratory distress syndrome (RDS)	Acute lung disease of newborns, occurring most often in premature infants
severe acute respiratory syndrome (SARS)	Highly contagious respiratory infection
tuberculosis (TB) (Figure 7-14)	Chronic infectious disease of the lungs
upper respiratory infection (URI)	Infection in the upper airway in the sinuses

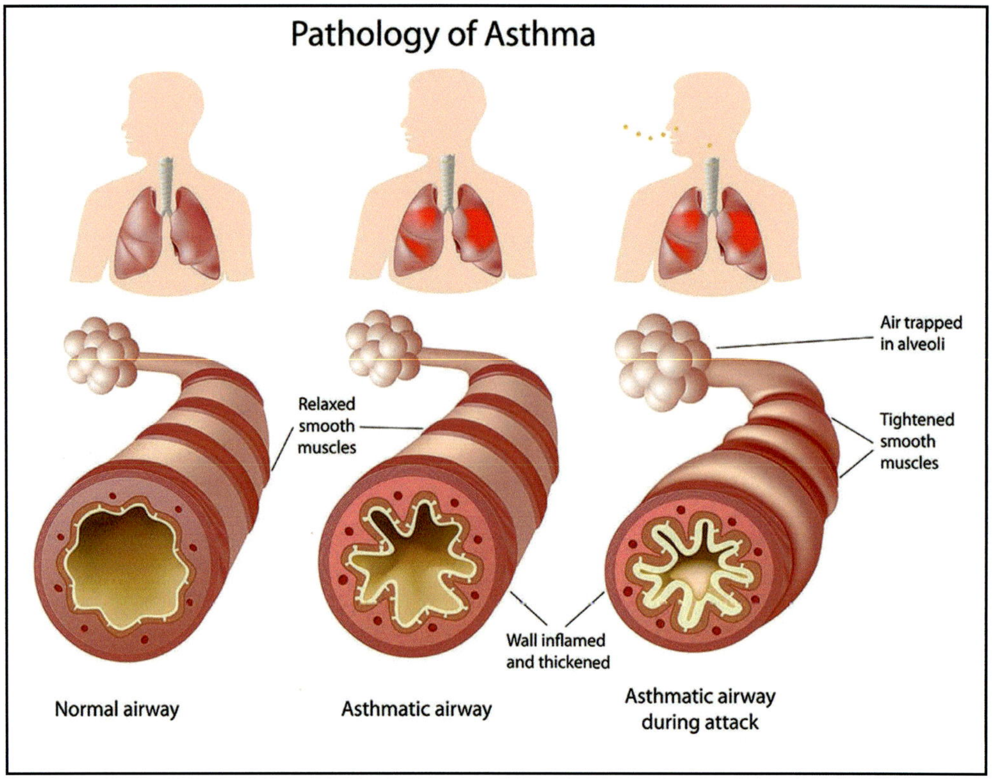

Figure 7-9. Pathology of asthma. (Alila Medical Images/shutterstock.com)

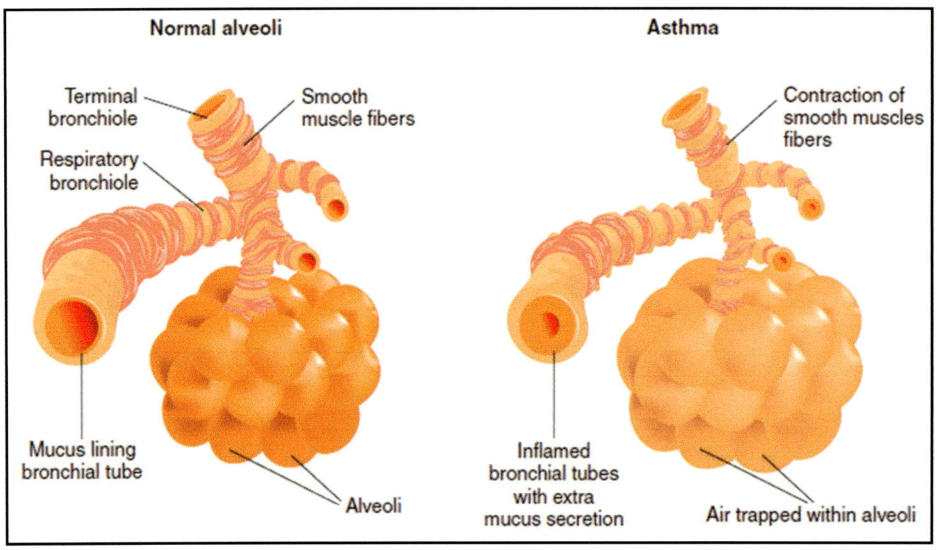

Figure 7-10. Alveoli response to asthma. (Blamb/shutterstock.com)

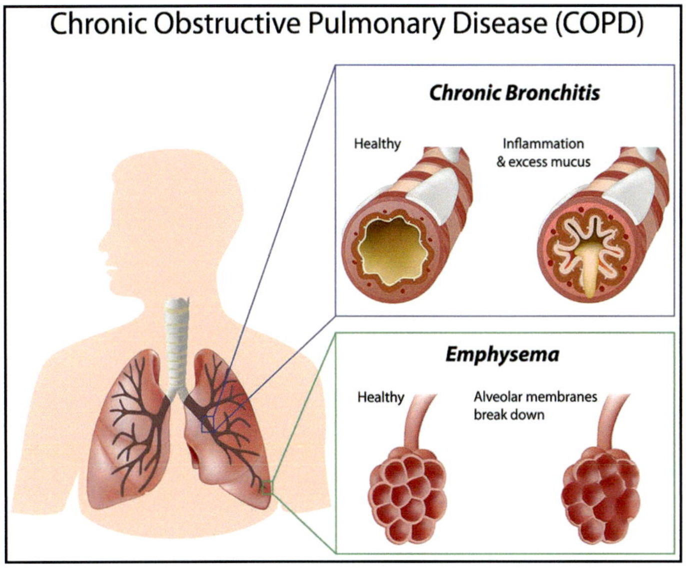

Figure 7-11. Two of the more common culprits of chronic obstructive pulmonary disease. (Alila Medical Images/shutterstock.com)

7

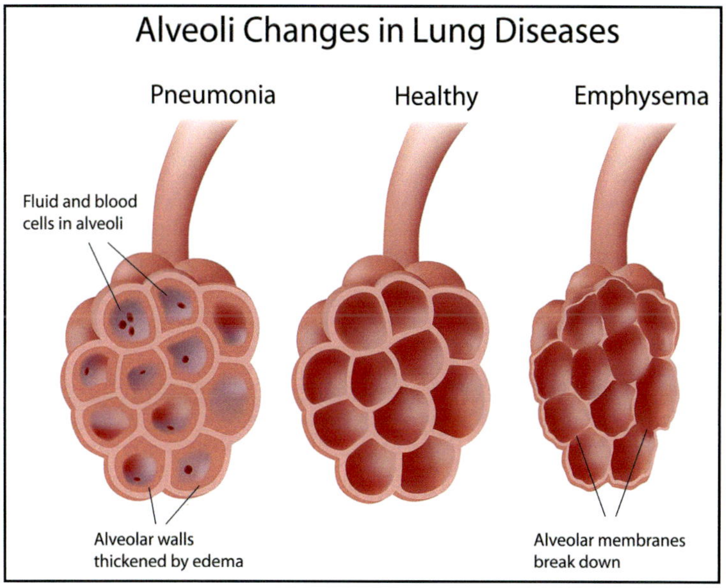

Figure 7-12. Alveoli changes in emphysema and pneumonia compared to normal. (Alila Medical Images/shutterstock.com)

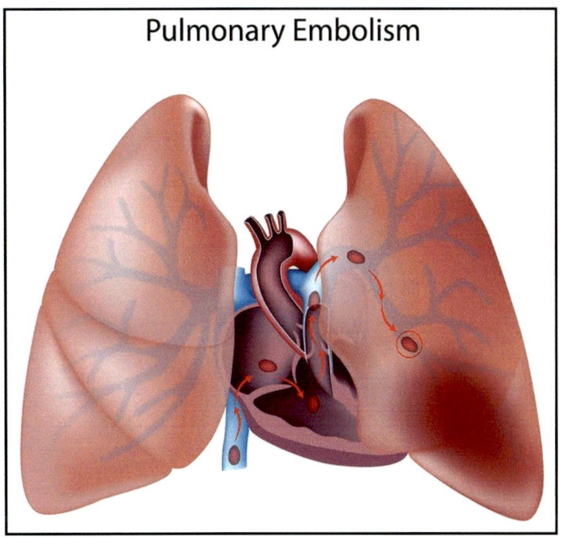

Figure 7-13. A pulmonary embolism can cause death of a portion of the lung or be fatal. (Alila Medical Images/shutterstock.com)

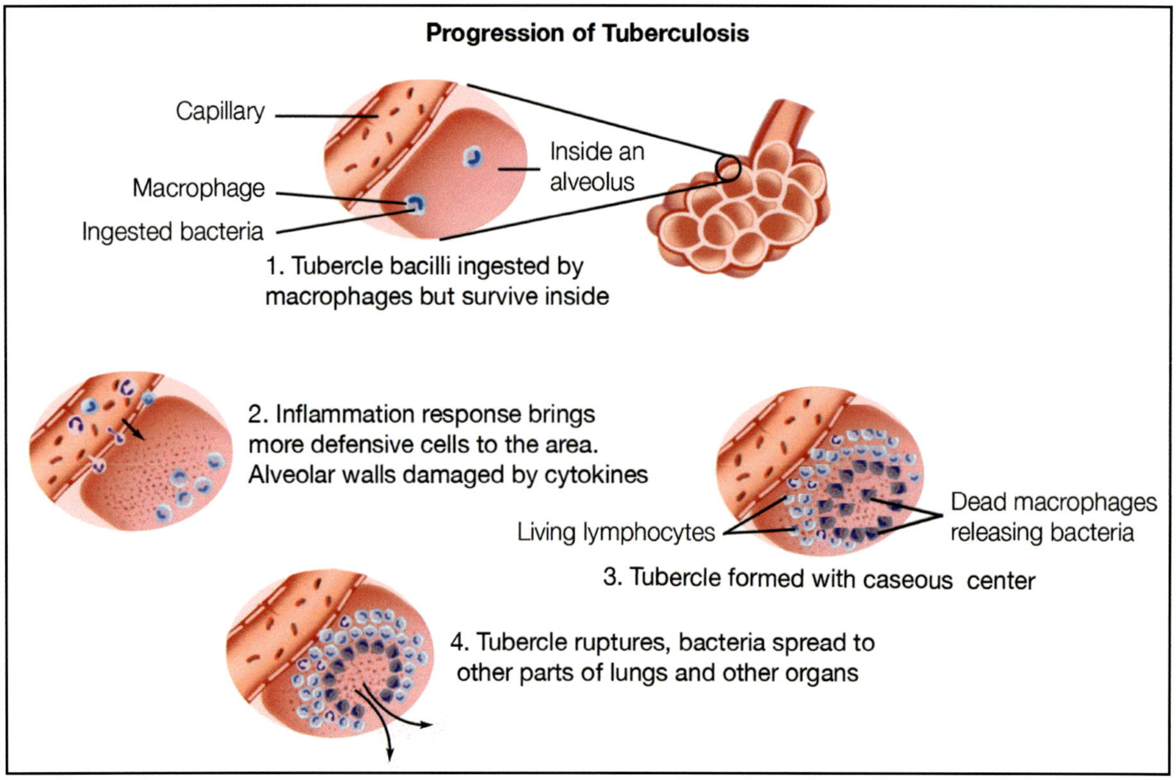

Figure 7-14. Tuberculosis. (Alila Medical Images/shutterstock.com)

Table 7-6
Other Medical Conditions Related to the Respiratory System That Contain Word Elements

NAME	WORD PARTS	DEFINITION
anaphylaxis (Figure 7-15)	**ana-** (up) **-phylaxis** (protection)	Exaggerated allergic response that includes constriction of the airways and hives; can be fatal
anthracosis	anthrac/ (coal) **-osis** (condition)	Condition caused by inhaling coal dust; also known as *black lung*
aphasia	**a-** (without) phas/ (speech) **-ia** (condition)	Inability to speak
apnea	**a-** (without) **-pnea** (breathing)	Temporary cessation of breathing
bronchiectasis	bronchi/ (bronchi) **-ectasis** (dilation)	Irreversible dilation of the bronchial walls; can be genetic or caused by infection, tumor, or foreign body
bronchitis	bronch/ (bronchi) **-itis** (inflammation)	Inflammation of the bronchi

(continued)

Table 7-6 (continued)

Other Medical Conditions Related to the Respiratory System That Contain Word Elements

NAME	WORD PARTS	DEFINITION
cyanosis	cyan/ (blue) **-osis** (condition)	Lack of oxygen in the blood resulting in bluish-looking skin, fingernails, and membranes
cystic fibrosis (CF) (Figure 7-16)	cyst/ (sac) **-ic** (pertaining to) fibr/ (fiber) **-osis** (condition)	Genetic disease affecting the whole body characterized by scarring (fibrosis) in tissues; progressive and often fatal
dysphonia	**dys-** (difficult) phon/ (voice) **-ia** (condition)	Hoarseness, difficulty speaking
hemoptysis	hem/o (blood) **-ptysis** (to spit)	Spitting up blood
hypercapnia	**hyper-** (excessive) **-capnia** (carbon dioxide in the blood)	Excessive carbon dioxide in the blood
hypoxia	**hypo-** (deficient) ox/ (oxygen) **-ia** (condition)	Deficient amount of oxygen reaching the tissues
laryngitis	laryng/ (larynx) **-itis** (inflammation)	Inflammation of the larynx
mesothelioma	**meso-** (middle) thel/ (nipple) **-oma** (tumor)	Malignant tumor of the pleura (mesothelium) associated with exposure to asbestos
nasopharyngitis	nas/o (nose) pharyng/ (pharynx) **-itis** (inflammation)	Inflammation of the nose and pharynx
orthopnea	orth/o (straight) **-pnea** (breathing)	Inability to breathe unless standing up
pharyngitis	pharyng/ (pharynx [throat]) **-itis** (inflammation)	Inflammation of the pharynx; sore throat
pleurisy	pleur/ (pleura)	Inflammation of the lining of the lungs (pleura) due to infection, injury, or disease (also called *pleuritis*)
pleuritis	pleur/ (pleura) **-itis** (inflammation)	Inflammation of the pleura
pleurodynia	pleur/o (pleura) **-dynia** (pain)	Pain in the lining of the lung (pleura)

(continued)

Table 7-6 (continued)

Other Medical Conditions Related to the Respiratory System That Contain Word Elements

NAME	WORD PARTS	DEFINITION
pneumoconiosis	pneum/o (lung) coni/ (dust) **-osis** (condition)	Abnormal condition of the lung caused by inhalation of dust particles
pneumonia	pneumon/ (lung) **-ia** (condition)	Inflammation of the lung caused by chemical irritant, fungi, viruses, or bacteria
pneumothorax (Figure 7-17)	pneum/o (lung) **-thorax** (chest)	Collection of air in between the lung and wall, causing the lung to collapse
pyothorax	py/o (pus) **-thorax** (chest)	Pus in the chest cavity
sinusitis (Figure 7-18)	sinus/ (sinus) **-itis** (inflammation)	Inflammation of a sinus
trachealgia	trache/ (trachea) **-algia** (pain)	Pain in the windpipe (trachea)

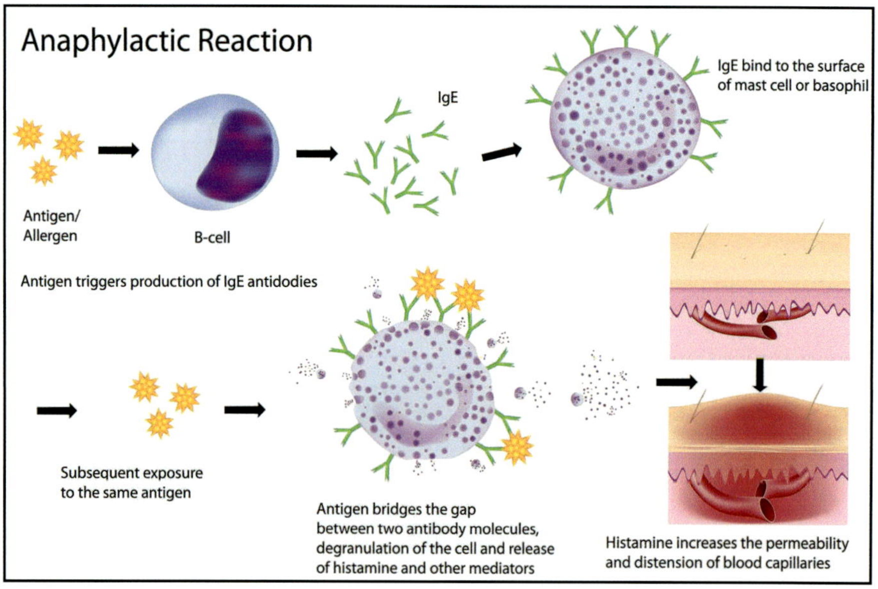

Figure 7-15. The physiology behind an anaphylactic reaction. (IgE=immunoglobulin E.) (Alila Medical Images/shutterstock.com)

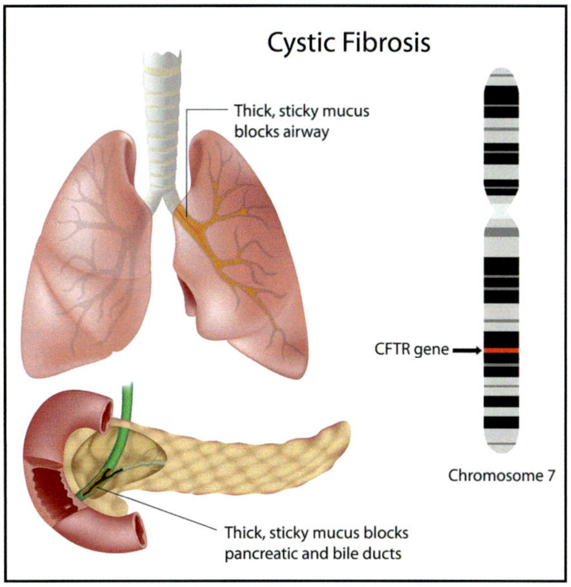

Figure 7-16. Cystic fibrosis is inherited via a gene. (Alila Medical Images/shutterstock.com)

7

Figure 7-17. Pneumothorax. (Alila Medical Images/shutterstock.com)

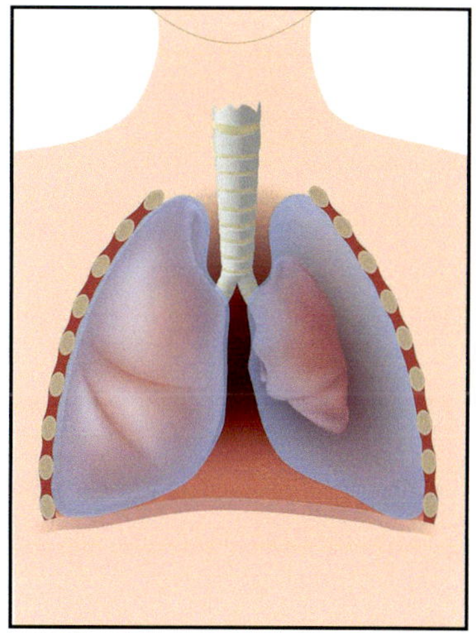

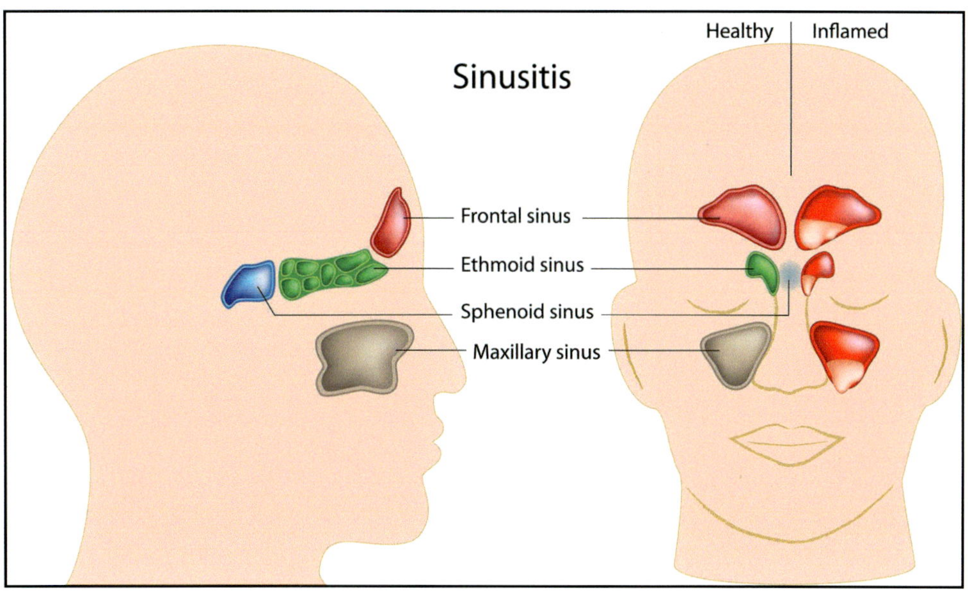

Figure 7-18. Sinusitis. (Alila Medical Images/shutterstock.com)

Breathing Types and Sounds

Table 7-7 Breathing Types and Sounds	
NAME	**DEFINITION**
Cheyne-Stokes	Cyclic breathing pattern of gradual increase in breathing, followed by apnea (cessation of breathing), then gradual increase in breathing repeated
crackles (rales)	Hissing or whistling noises while breathing
dyspnea	Difficulty breathing (**dys-**—difficult)
stridor	High-pitched sound caused by a partial airway obstruction
wheezing	Audible whistling sound while breathing

Tests and Procedures

Table 7-8 Tests and Procedures Specific to the Respiratory System		
NAME	**WORD PARTS**	**PURPOSE**
aspiration		Process of drawing food, liquid, or foreign body from the nose, throat, or lungs; a suction device or syringe is used for the procedure; not necessarily specific to respiratory system
bronchoscope	bronch/o (bronchial tubes) **-scope** (an instrument used to view or inspect)	Flexible scope used to visualize the larynx, trachea, and bronchi
continuous positive airway pressure (CPAP) (Figure 7-19)		Use of continuous positive pressure to keep an airway open; typically used for people who have breathing problems
intubation		Tube inserted into a hollow organ, such as the trachea (**endotracheal** intubation)
laryngoscope (Figure 7-20)	laryng/o (larynx) **-scope** (an instrument used to view or inspect)	Flexible scope used to visualize the larynx
lobectomy	lob/ (lobe) **-ectomy** (surgical removal)	Surgical removal of a lobe of a gland or organ (lung)
pulmonary function test (PFT)		Tests that measure lung function
pulmonectomy	pulmon/ (lungs) **-ectomy** (surgical removal)	Surgical excision of the lung, or a portion of the lung

(continued)

TABLE 7-8 (CONTINUED) TESTS AND PROCEDURES SPECIFIC TO THE RESPIRATORY SYSTEM		
NAME	**WORD PARTS**	**PURPOSE**
spirometer (Figure 7-21)	spir/o (breath) **-meter** (an instrument used to measure)	Instrument used to determine lung volume on inhalation and expiration; also called *pulmometer*
thoracentesis	thorac/ (chest) **-centesis** (surgical puncture)	Removal of fluid by puncturing the chest wall
thoracoplasty	thorac/o (chest) **-plasty** (repair)	Surgical repair of the chest wall
thoracotomy	thorac/o (chest) **-tomy** (incision)	Incision into the chest wall
tonsillectomy (Figure 7-22)	tonsil/ (tonsils) **-ectomy** (surgical excision)	Surgical removal of the tonsils
tracheolaryngotomy	trache/o (trachea) laryng/o (larynx) **-tomy** (incision)	Incision into the trachea and larynx
tracheostomy (Figure 7-23)	trache/o (trachea) **-stomy** (surgical opening)	Cutting a new opening into the trachea

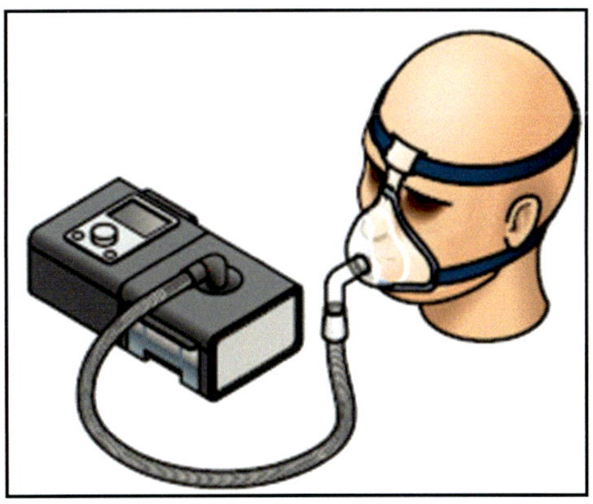

Figure 7-19. A continuous positive airway pressure machine is worn at night to maintain continuous breathing and prevent sleep apnea. (Zern Liew/shutterstock.com)

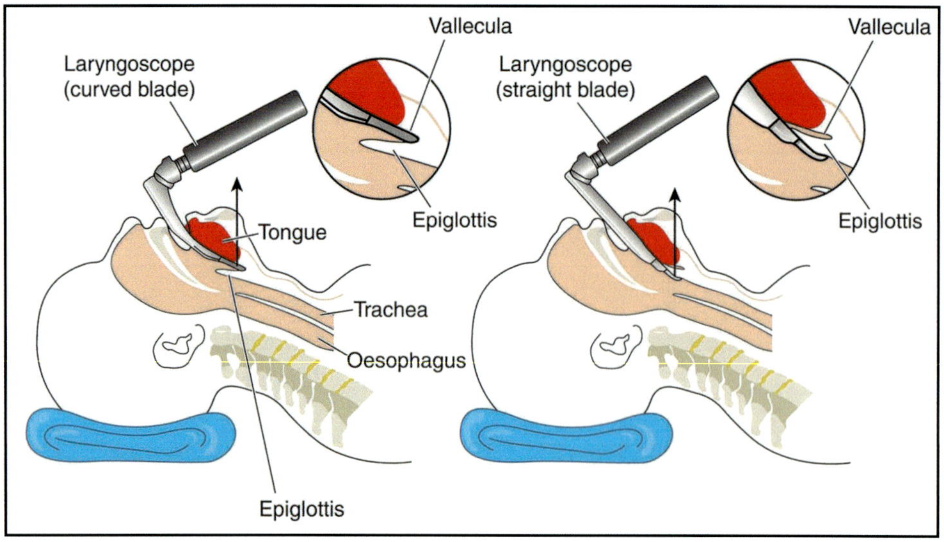

Figure 7-20. Laryngoscope insertion. (Blamb/shutterstock.com)

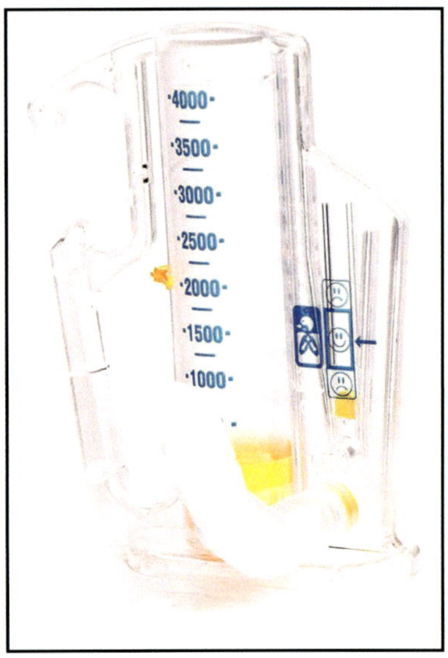

Figure 7-21. A spirometer. Patients breathe into a tube and their volume of air expired is measured. (Renewer/shutterstock.com)

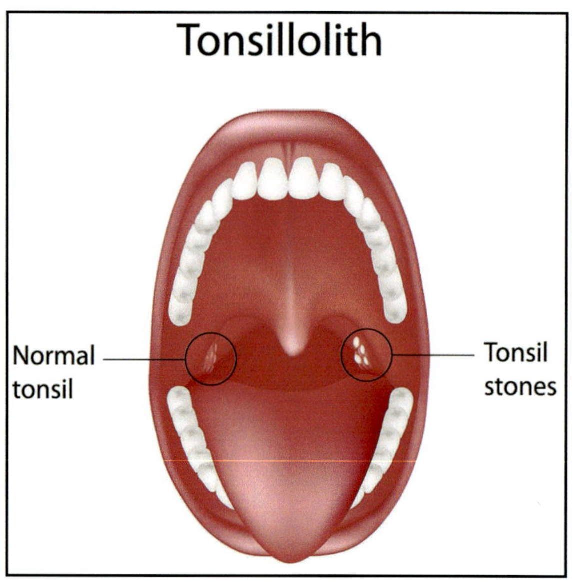

Figure 7-22. Sometimes, tonsils can form stones (-lith), a condition called *tonsillolith.* (Alila Medical Images/shutterstock.com)

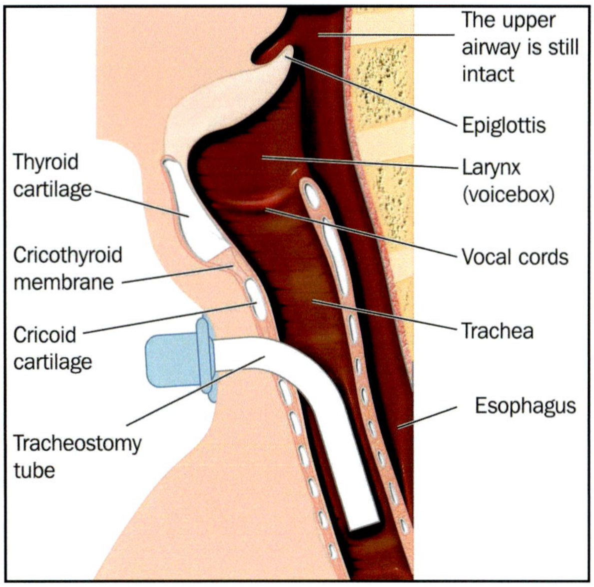

Figure 7-23. A tracheotomy with a breathing tube. (Blamb/shutterstock.com)

Medication Classifications

Table 7-9
Medication Classifications Used in Treatment of Respiratory Conditions

CATEGORY	WORD PARTS	WHAT IT DOES
antihistamine	**anti-** (against)	Prevents reactions to histamine; used in allergy treatment
antitussive	**anti-** (against) tuss/ (cough)	Prevents/relieves coughing
bronchodilator (Figure 7-24)	bronch/o (bronchial tubes) dilat/ (to expand)	Dilates the bronchioles to assist in breathing
decongestant	**de-** (without)	Relieves congestion
expectorant	**ex-** (away; away from; out; outside)	Assists in coughing to relieve mucus in the respiratory tract
mucolytic	muc/o (mucus) **-lytic** (destroy)	Loosens mucus

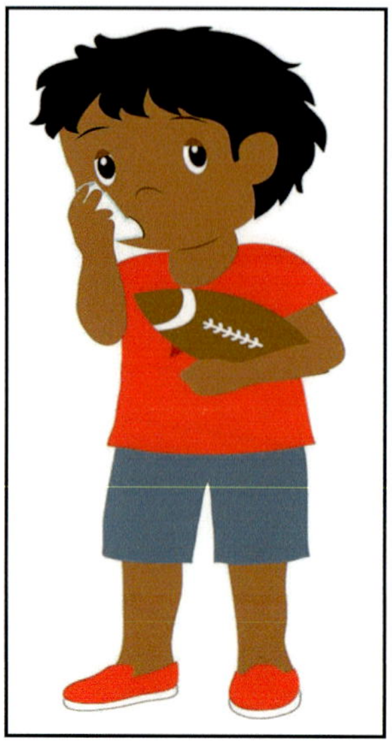

Figure 7-24. Athletes who suffer from exercise-induced asthma can find relief with an inhaler using a bronchodilator. (Rosie Piter/shutterstock.com)

Bibliography

Basco R, Allan B. *Medical Language for Modern Health Care.* 5th ed. McGraw-Hill; 2023.

Flanagan KW, Cuppett M. *Medical Conditions in the Athlete.* 3rd ed. Human Kinetics; 2017.

Hutton A. *Medical Terminology for Health Care.* 5th ed. Churchill Livingstone; 2017.

Mosby's Dictionary of Medicine, Nursing & Health Professions. 10th ed. Elsevier; 2017.

Rice J. *Medical Terminology for Health Care Professionals.* 9th ed. Pearson; 2018.

Shiland BJ. *Mastering Healthcare Terminology.* 6th ed. Elsevier; 2019.

Turley SM. *Medical Language—Immerse Yourself.* 5th ed. Pearson; 2020.

Venes D, ed. *Taber's Cyclopedic Medical Dictionary.* 24th ed. F. A. Davis; 2021.

NOTES

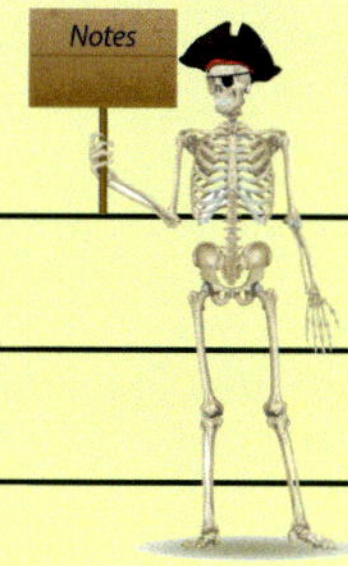

NOTES

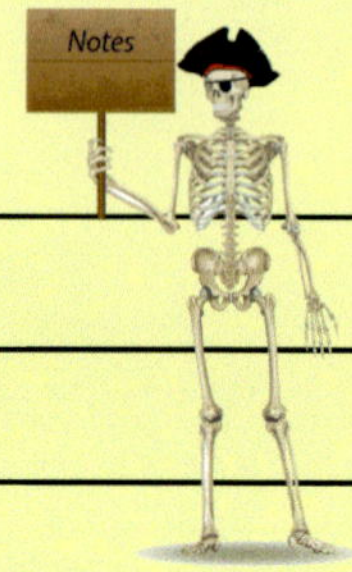

Learning Activities

Name:______________________

Respiratory System

A. Label the upper airway anatomy from the following list.

- nasal cavity_______________
- pharynx_______________
- esophagus_______________
- nares_______________
- epiglottis_______________
- trachea_______________
- tongue_______________
- pharyngeal tonsils__________
- larynx_______________

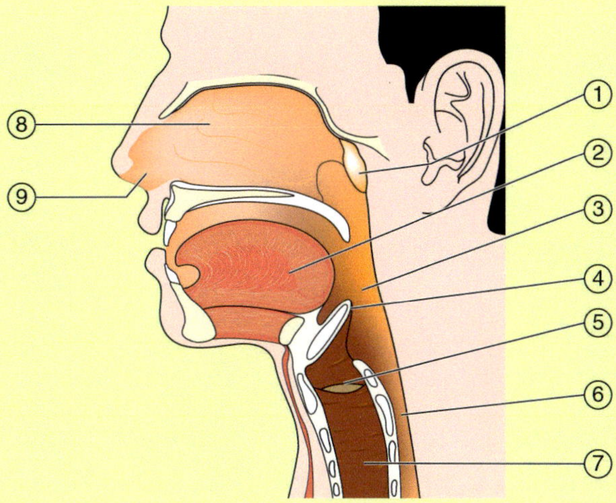

(Blamb/shutterstock.com)

B. Label the aspects of the chest cavity from the following list.

- parietal pleura______
- visceral pleura______
- pleural cavity_______
- mediastinum_______

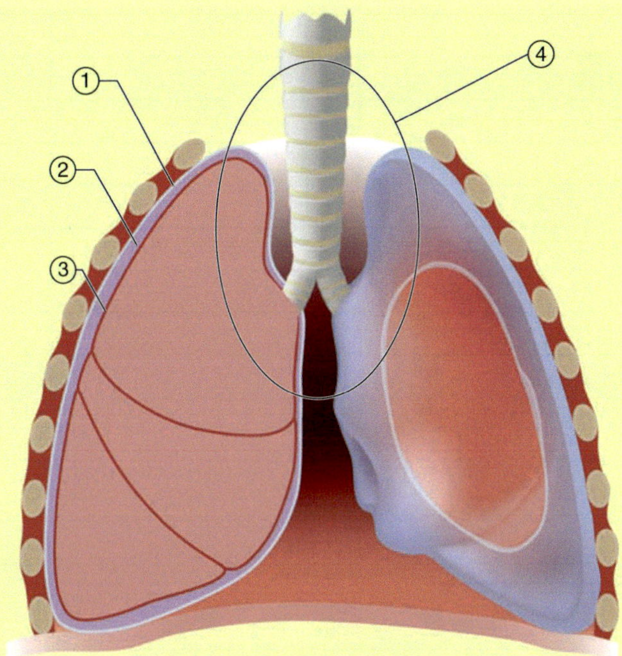

(Alila Medical Images/shutterstock.com)

C. Label the sinuses from the following list.

- maxillary sinuses__________________
- frontal sinuses__________________
- ethmoidal sinuses__________________

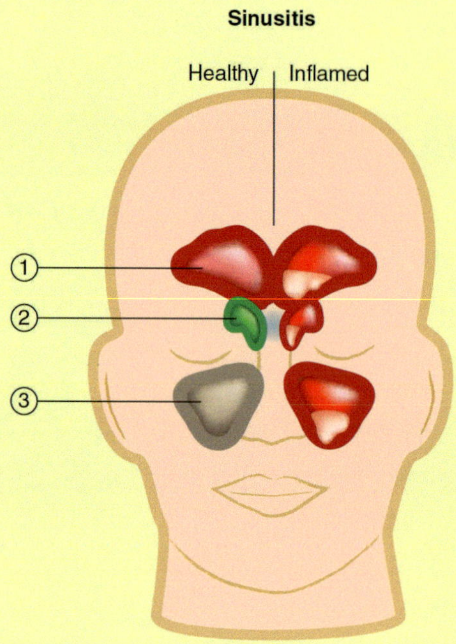

(Alila Medical Images/shutterstock.com)

D. Matching.

1. muc/o____________ a. gland
2. **-stenosis**____________ b. incision
3. **-sphyxia** ____________ c. coal dust
4. **eu-**____________ d. surgical opening
5. or____________ e. sac
6. aden/o____________ f. mouth
7. cyst/o____________ g. good
8. anthrac/o____________ h. pulse
9. **-stomy**____________ i. narrowing
10. **-tomy**____________ j. mucus

E. Fill in the table.

WORD PART	COMBINING FORM	NEW WORD	DEFINITION
tachy-	pnea		
dys-	phonia		
-ptysis	hem/o		
-dynia	pleur/o		
-stenosis	trache/o		
-meter	ox/i		
-otomy	sinus/o		
-ectomy	laryng/o		
hem/o + pneum/o	thorax		
pan- + **-itis**	sinus		

F. Fill in the table with the common name.

MEDICAL WORD	COMMON NAME
thyroid cartilage	
palatine tonsils	
coryza	
influenza	
pertussis	

7

G. Define the following abbreviations.

1. URI____
2. SARS____
3. CF____
4. RDS____
5. PFT____
6. PE____
7. COPD____
8. CPAP____
9. TB____
10. Tdap____

H. Write out the plural forms of the following words.

SINGULAR	PLURAL
alveolus	
pleura	
bronchus	

I. Describe what the following medications do.

1. mucolytic____
2. decongestant____
3. antihistamine____
4. bronchodilator____
5. antitussive____

Case Study

Define the numerical terms (1 to 8) and label the anatomy (A to D) on the figure.
For assistance with medical abbreviations, refer to Appendix A.

History, Chief Complaint

A 45-year old woman was hit by a car as she was riding her bike and thrown to the ground. Although she is conscious and does not appear to have any obvious injuries (bleeding or broken bones), the EMT notes that she presented with dizziness, **dyspnea** (1), and nausea and complained of **HA** (2) and **SOB** (3).

Evaluation

The woman has pain on her right **anterior ribs** (A), but not at the **sternoclavicular joint** (B) or **sternum** (C). She has **hemoptysis** (4) and **hypoxia** (5) according the **pulse oximeter** (6). Her **trachea** (D) has shifted to the left, but she is not **cyanotic** (7).

Diagnostic Studies

An x-ray confirms a **hemothorax** (8) of the right lung.

Terms

1. ______
2. ______
3. ______
4. ______
5. ______
6. ______
7. ______
8. ______

Anatomy

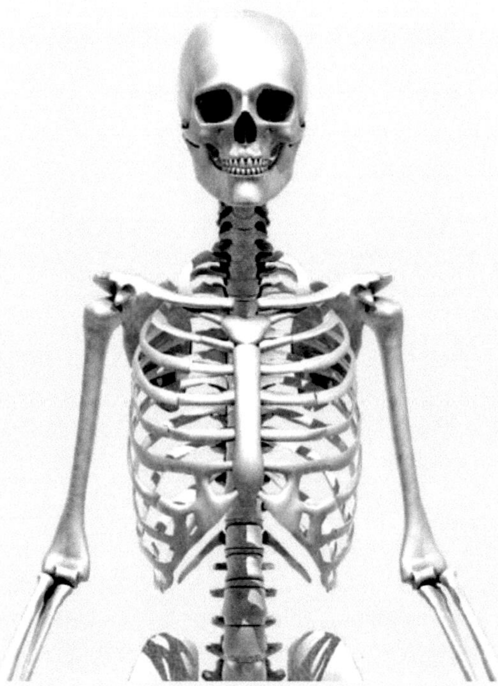

8

Neurological System

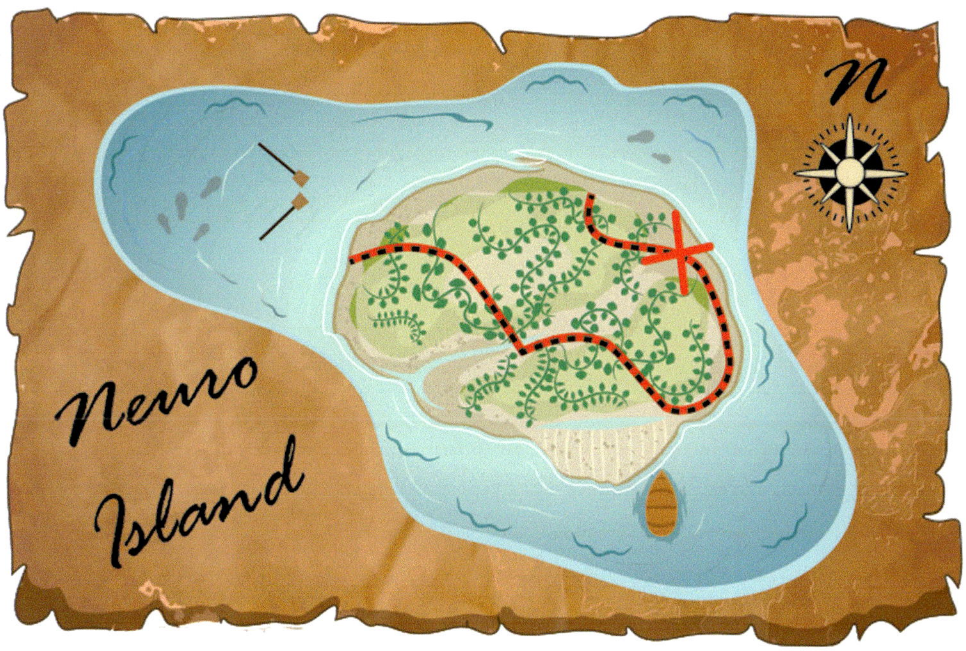

Objectives

After studying this chapter, you will be able to:

1. List the major components of the nervous system.
2. Locate and name various aspects of the central nervous system and peripheral nervous system.
3. Differentiate between the central and peripheral nervous systems.
4. Identify and build words relating to the neurological system.
5. List signs and symptoms of a problem with the nervous system.
6. Describe basic abnormalities or conditions of the neurological system.
7. Identify diagnostic tests and procedures specific to the neurological system.
8. Know the terms associated with mental and behavioral health issues.

Flanagan KW.
Medical Terminology With Case Studies: A Navigated Guide to Learning for Health Care Professionals, Third Edition (pp 181-216).

Chapter Outline

- Self-assessment
- Checklist for word parts in the chapter
- Checklist of new anatomy
- Introduction
- Anatomy
    - The central nervous system
    - The peripheral nervous system
- Word building
    - Prefixes
    - Suffixes
    - Combining forms
- Signs and symptoms
- Medical conditions
- Tests and procedures
- Mental health and behavioral disorders
- Learning activities
- Case study

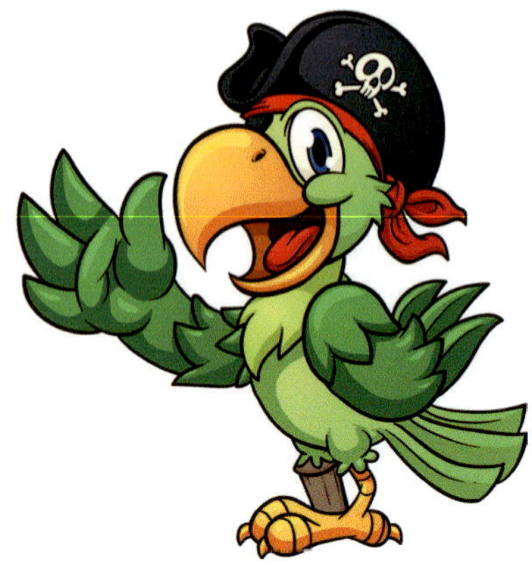

Self-Assessment

Based on what you have learned so far, can you write the definition of these words?

- discectomy____________________
- cerebral atherosclerosis____________________
- neuritis____________________
- craniotomy____________________
- cerebral angiography____________________
- neurology____________________
- echoencephalography____________________
- neuropathy____________________

Checklist for Word Parts in the Chapter

Prefixes

- ☐ a-
- ☐ al-
- ☐ an-
- ☐ de-
- ☐ di-
- ☐ dys-
- ☐ epi-
- ☐ hemi-
- ☐ hydro-
- ☐ hyper-
- ☐ hypo-
- ☐ intra-
- ☐ mono-
- ☐ pan-
- ☐ par-
- ☐ para-
- ☐ poly-
- ☐ pre-
- ☐ sub-
- ☐ tetra-

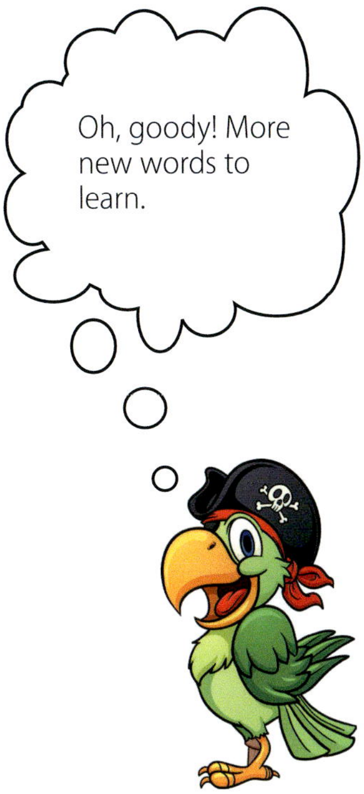

Suffixes

- ☐ -al
- ☐ -algia
- ☐ -ar
- ☐ -asthenia
- ☐ -cele
- ☐ -ectomy
- ☐ -emic
- ☐ -esthesia
- ☐ -gram
- ☐ -graph
- ☐ -graphy
- ☐ -ia
- ☐ -ic
- ☐ -ion
- ☐ -itis
- ☐ -lepsy
- ☐ -lysis
- ☐ -malacia
- ☐ -ology
- ☐ -oma
- ☐ -osis
- ☐ -otomy
- ☐ -paresis
- ☐ -pathy
- ☐ -phagia
- ☐ -phasia
- ☐ -plegia
- ☐ -rrhaphy
- ☐ -stomy
- ☐ -tomy
- ☐ -troph
- ☐ -um
- ☐ -us

Combining Forms

- ☐ alges/o
- ☐ angi/o
- ☐ arachn/o
- ☐ arteri/o
- ☐ arthr/o
- ☐ astr/o
- ☐ ather/o
- ☐ blast/o
- ☐ brachi/o
- ☐ cephal/o
- ☐ cerebell/o
- ☐ cerebr/o
- ☐ cortic/o
- ☐ cran/o
- ☐ crani/o
- ☐ cyt/o
- ☐ derm/o
- ☐ dur/o
- ☐ electr/o
- ☐ embol/o
- ☐ encephal/o
- ☐ fibr/o
- ☐ gangli/o
- ☐ ganglion/o
- ☐ gli/o
- ☐ gloss/o
- ☐ kinesi/o
- ☐ lumb/o
- ☐ lys/o
- ☐ mening/i
- ☐ mening/o
- ☐ ment/o
- ☐ my/o
- ☐ myel/o
- ☐ narc/o
- ☐ neur/o
- ☐ ocul/o
- ☐ opt/o
- ☐ peritone/o
- ☐ pharyng/o
- ☐ phas/o
- ☐ phasi/o
- ☐ plegi/o
- ☐ poli/o
- ☐ praxia
- ☐ psych/o

Combining Forms

- ☐ **quadr/i**
- ☐ **quadr/o**
- ☐ **radic/o**
- ☐ **radicul/o**
- ☐ **scler/o**
- ☐ **somat/o**
- ☐ **somn/o**
- ☐ **spin/o**
- ☐ **taxi/o**
- ☐ **thalam/o**
- ☐ **thromb/o**
- ☐ **vascul/o**
- ☐ **ventricul/o**
- ☐ **vertebr/o**

Checklist of New Anatomy

Central Nervous System

- ☐ Brain
- ☐ Ventricles
- ☐ Cranial nerves
- ☐ Cerebrum
  - ☐ Frontal lobe
  - ☐ Parietal lobe
  - ☐ Occipital lobe
  - ☐ Temporal lobe
- ☐ Cerebellum
- ☐ Diencephalon
  - ☐ Thalamus
  - ☐ Hypothalamus
- ☐ Brainstem
  - ☐ Medulla oblongata
  - ☐ Pons
  - ☐ Midbrain
- ☐ Meninges
- ☐ Dura mater
- ☐ Arachnoid
- ☐ Pia mater
- ☐ Cerebrospinal fluid
  - ☐ Spinal cord
  - ☐ Gray matter
  - ☐ White matter
  - ☐ Cauda equina

Peripheral Nervous System

- ☐ Nerves
  - ☐ Dendrite
  - ☐ Axon
  - ☐ Myelin sheath
  - ☐ Axon terminal
- ☐ Nerve types
  - ☐ Ventral
  - ☐ Dorsal
  - ☐ Afferent nerves
  - ☐ Efferent nerves
- ☐ Ganglia
- ☐ Sensory receptors
- ☐ Autonomic nervous system
  - ☐ Sympathetic nervous system
  - ☐ Parasympathetic nervous system

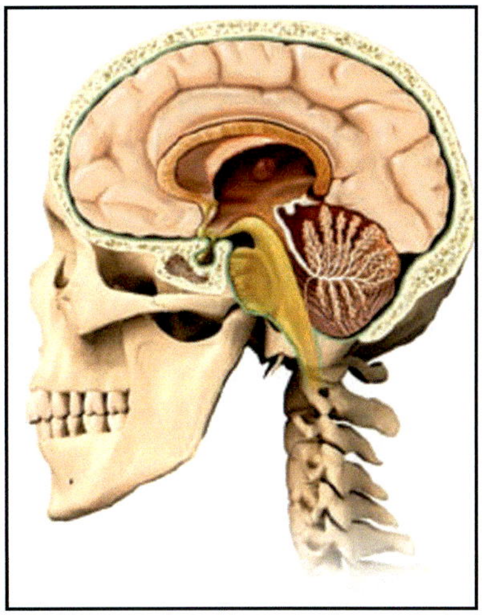

Figure 8-1. The brain is housed within the cranium. (leonello calvetti/shutterstock.com)

Introduction

You have arrived to Neuro Island! On this island you will find combining forms pertaining to the neurological system. Because the brain is the master of the whole body, medical conditions found in this chapter can wreak havoc on many systems. True to the pirate way of life, the neurological system also determines if you will stay and fight (if threatened) or flee (to fight another day) via two subsystems that respond very differently to stress. This chapter discusses terms related to the brain and spinal cord as well as neurological medical conditions, tests, and procedures. It also covers terms used in mental and behavioral health.

Anatomy

The neurological system consists of two distinct sections: the central nervous system (CNS) and the peripheral (outlying) nervous system.

The Central Nervous System

The CNS consists of the brain and spinal cord. Unlike the peripheral nervous system (PNS), the CNS cannot regenerate if damaged, and components of the CNS lie protected within bony structures. The brain is the "command center" of the body and is housed within the skull (Figure 8-1). It has four separate parts: the **cerebrum**, **cerebellum**, **diencephalon**, and **brainstem** (Figure 8-2).

The cerebrum is what most consider the brain and resembles a wrinkled oblong mass. Names of the lobes of the cerebrum correspond with the like-termed sections of the skull (Figure 8-3):

- **Frontal lobe**
- **Parietal lobe**
- **Occipital lobe**
- **Temporal lobe**

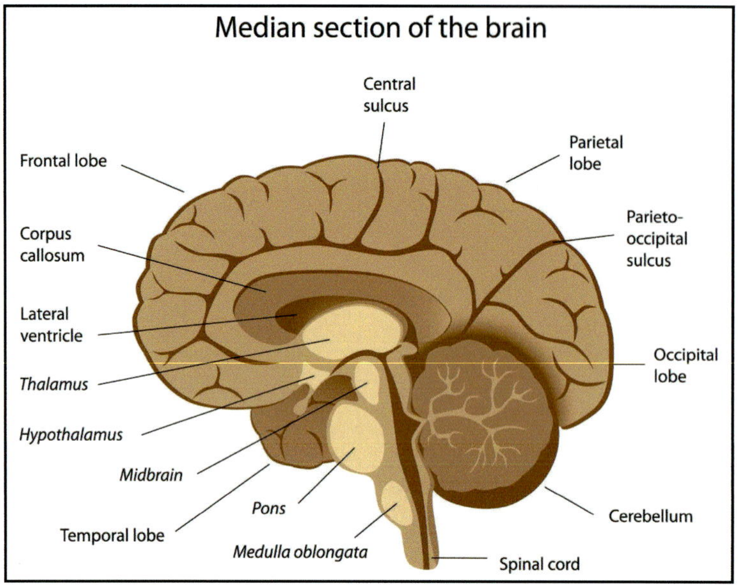

Figure 8-2. A cross-section of the brain. (Alila Medical Images/shutterstock.com)

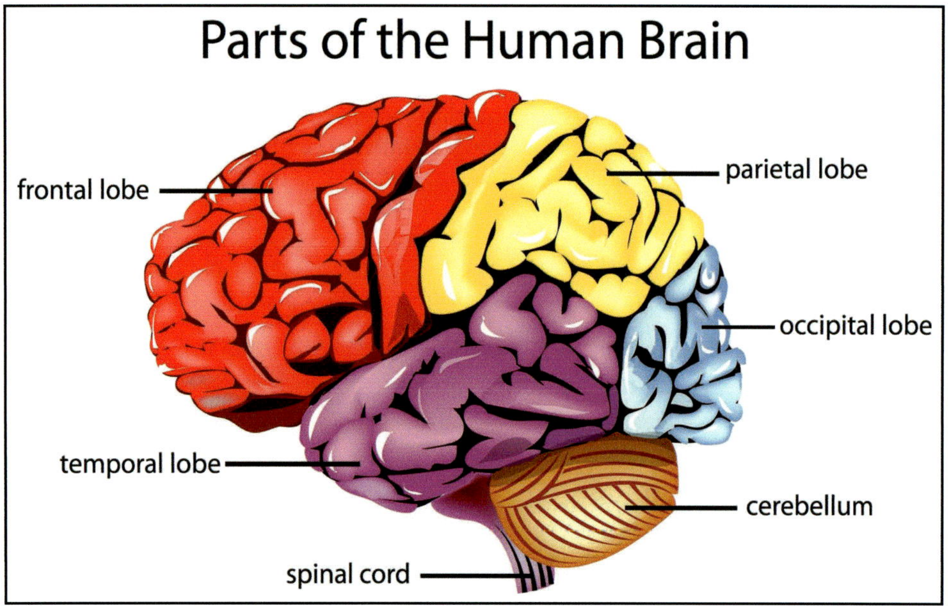

Figure 8-3. Lobes of the brain correspond with the names of the skull bones. (Matthew Cole/shutterstock.com)

Functions of these lobes can be found in Table 8-1 and in Figure 8-4. The cerebrum has a right and left hemisphere and each lobe is represented in both hemispheres. Typically, the right side of the brain controls the left side of the body, and vice versa. On a different note, people are often referred to as "right-brained" or "left-brained," due to the fact that each side of the brain is also responsible for specific nonmotor traits, such as language acquisition or problem solving (Figure 8-5).

The **cerebellum** ("little brain") coordinates muscular movement and balance. The cerebellum is responsible for coordination and equilibrium, so when someone is evaluated for a stroke, athletes are assessed for traumatic brain injury (TBI; concussions), or police perform field sobriety tests for suspicion of driving while intoxicated, the cerebellum is one aspect of the brain being tested.

In the middle of the brain, surrounded by the cerebrum and anterior to the cerebellum, is the **diencephalon** (**di-**—two; **encephal/o**—brain). This structure contains the thalamus and hypothalamus (**hypo-**—below, decreased, deficient, insufficient, low, under). The **thalamus** is often called the relay station of the brain, as it receives and redirects impulses to and from the cerebrum. The **hypothalamus** is in charge of all involuntary actions: regulating blood pressure, heartbeat, glandular functions, and so on.

TABLE 8-1 FUNCTIONS OF THE LOBES OF THE CEREBRUM (FIGURE 8-5)	
LOBE	**FUNCTION**
frontal	• Personality • Speech • Movement
parietal	• Sensation • Language
occipital	• Vision
temporal	• Balance • Coordination • Hearing • Smell

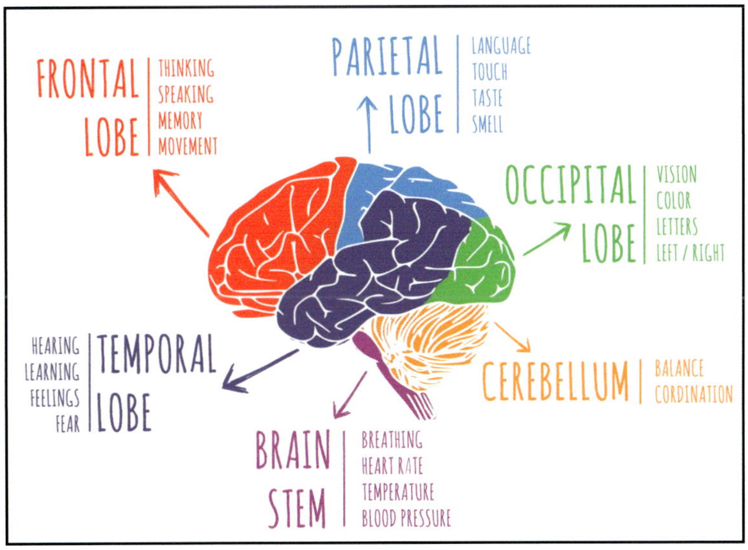

Figure 8-4. Responsibilities of the lobes of the brain. (Noiel/shutterstock.com)

The brainstem is the structure through which all incoming and outgoing information passes. Parts of the brainstem include the **medulla oblongata**, **pons**, and **midbrain** (Figure 8-6). The medulla oblongata (also called the *medulla*), is the main transmitter between the spinal cord and brain. Its primary function is to regulate breathing rhythms. The pons (meaning "bridge") is the connection between the medulla and cerebellum. Finally, the midbrain is another relay center and is the most superior aspect of the brainstem.

Within the brain are small open areas termed ventricles. These ventricles are filled with cerebrospinal fluid (CSF; **cerebr/o**—cerebrum; **spin/o**—spine; **-al**—pertaining to) which circulates through the brain and spinal cord via channels and the subarachnoid space. Ventricles are the structures that are important in certain medical conditions, such as hydrocephalus (**hydro-**—water; **cephal/o**—head), or when using a lumbar puncture to assess for meningitis (**mening/**—membrane, meninges; **-itis**—inflammation). CSF is a slightly yellow fluid that transports nutrients, provides a bit of shock absorption from trauma, and removes waste from the CNS.

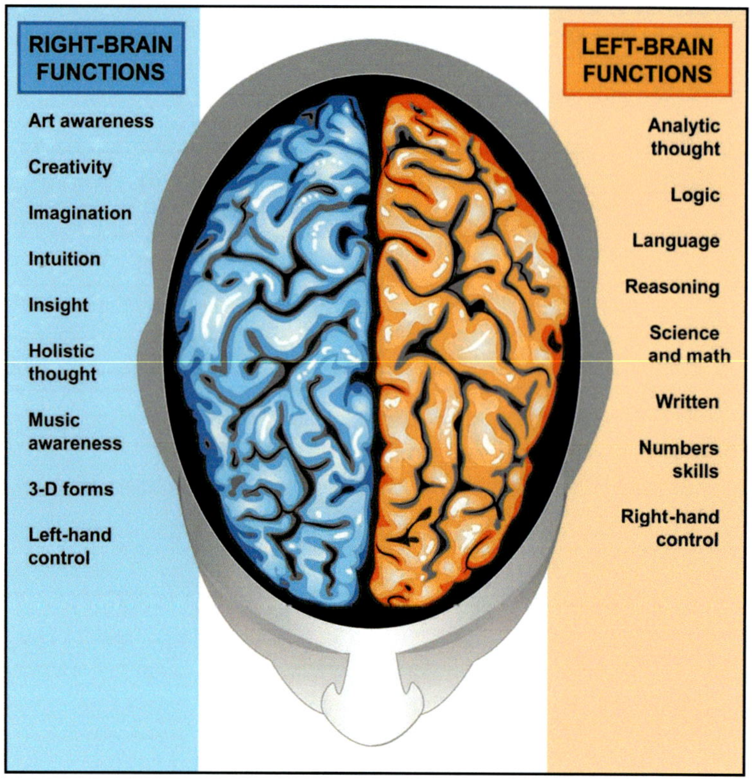

Figure 8-5. Right and left brain functions. (MedusArt/shutterstock.com)

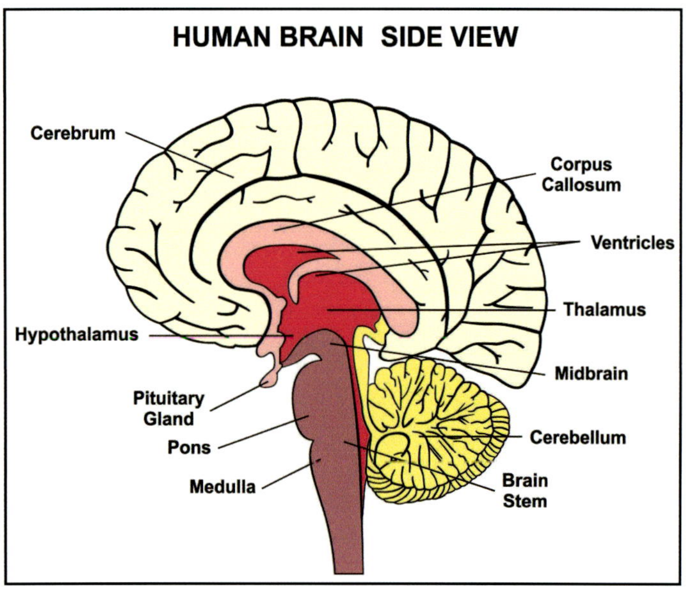

Figure 8-6. Lateral view of the brain. (udaix/shutterstock.com)

The Spinal Cord

The spinal cord runs the length of the spine from the medulla oblongata to the upper lumbar vertebrae (Figure 8-7). As nerves exit the protection of the bony spinal column, they are named for the region of the spine from which they depart (cervical, thoracic, lumbar, and sacral). The spinal cord terminates in a structure called the **cauda equina** (meaning "horse's tail," as this is what it resembles). The cord is made up of cell bodies of motor neurons called **gray matter** and myelin-covered axons extending from the cell bodies. This part of the cord is white, and aptly named **white matter**. As the nerves leave the spinal cord, and exit out of the spinal column they become a part of the PNS (Figure 8-8).

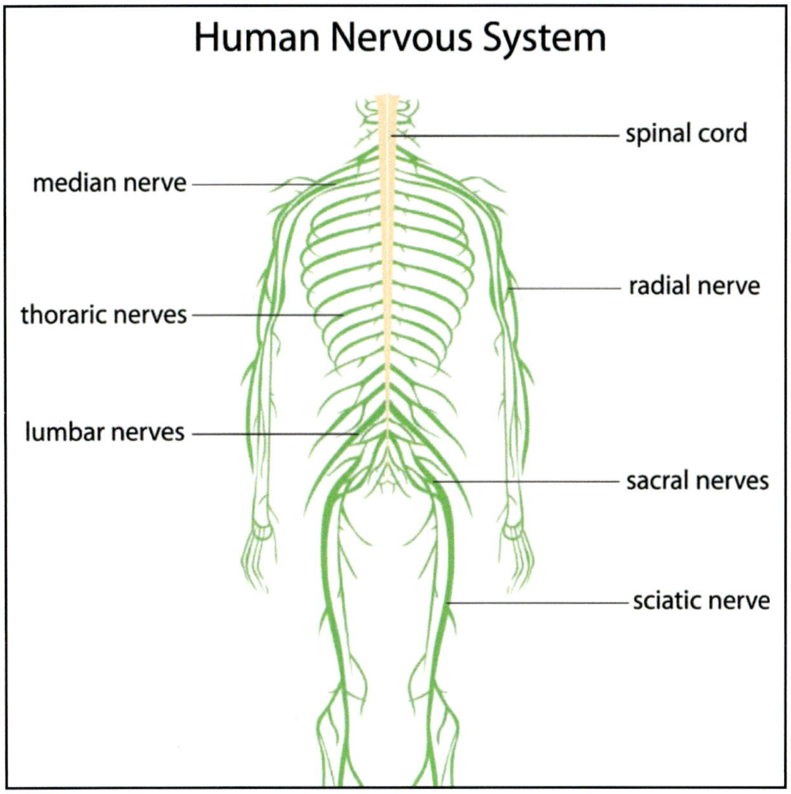

Figure 8-7. The peripheral nervous system. (Alila Medical Images/shutterstock.com)

Figure 8-8. A cross-section of the spinal cord. (Matthew Cole/shutterstock.com)

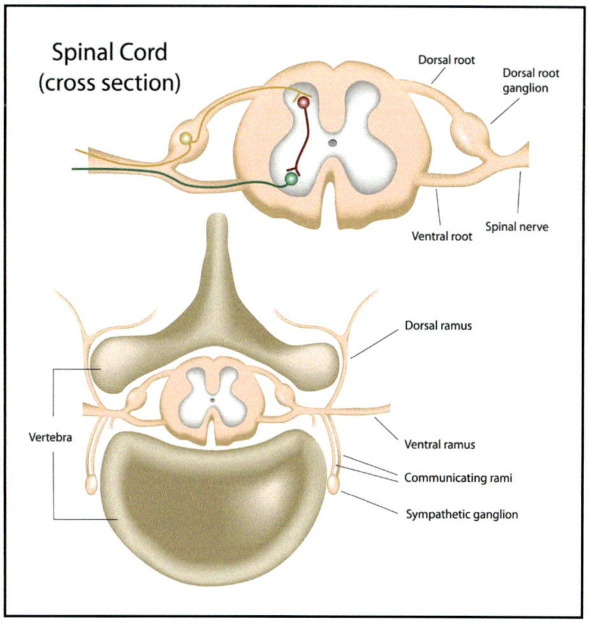

Meninges

As mentioned earlier, the brain is protected by the skull, and the spinal cord is surrounded by the bony spinal column. The spinal column is created by the vertebra and provides a bony tube to shield the spinal cord. There are protective layers of membranes between the skull or spinal column and their bony protectors. These membranes are termed *meninges* and they supply spaces for blood vessels and CSF to provide nutrients to the brain and spinal cord. From the skull (or spinal column) inward toward the brain (or spinal cord), the layer of meninges are (Figure 8-9):

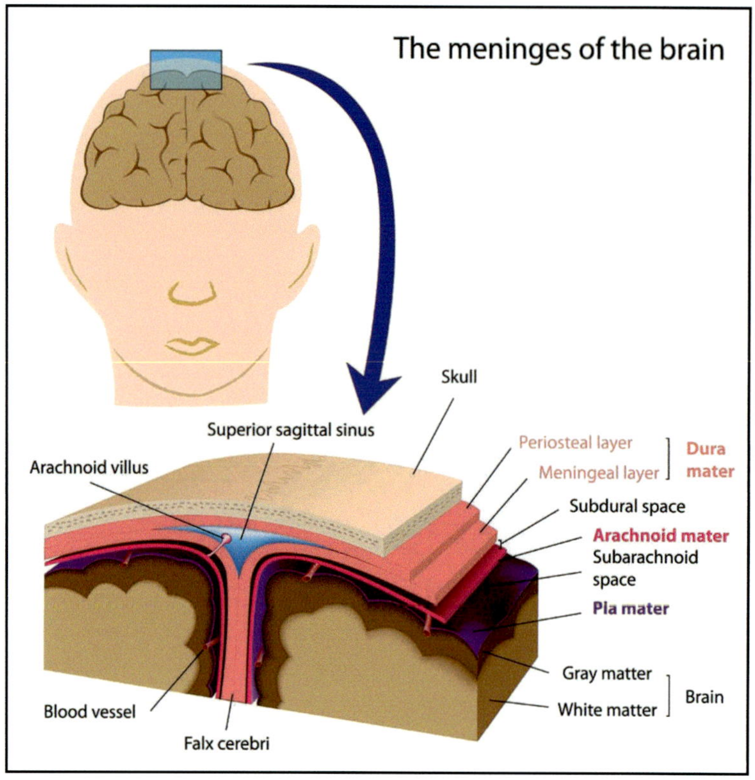

Figure 8-9. The meninges of the brain and spinal cord. (Alila Medical Images/shutterstock.com)

- **Dura mater** ("tough mother")
- **Arachnoid** ("spider-like")
- **Pia mater** ("soft mother")

Above the dura mater is the epidural space (**epi-**—above), and the subdural space (**sub-**—below) lies below it. The dura mater is a tough, fibrous protective layer, whereas the spider-like covering, the arachnoid, adheres more closely to the brain and spinal cord and their curvatures. Underneath the arachnoid is the subarachnoid space. Adhering directly to the brain and spinal cord is the pia mater. It is very difficult to distinguish this layer from the actual brain or spinal cord as it is very closely associated with the neurological tissues. Think of an orange with its tough rind: The layer inside the rind is a thick white membrane akin to the dura mater. The layer holding the sections of orange together is more like the arachnoid, and the innermost membrane that is so closely adhered to the tiny sections of orange is the pia mater.

Cranial Nerves

Cranial (**crani/**—skull; **-al**—pertaining to) nerves are exactly what the name suggests: nerves that arise from the cranium (**-um**—structure, thing). There are 12 pairs of nerves, listed in Roman numbers (I to XII), and each has specific motor (movement) and/or sensory functions. These nerves can be damaged in head injuries, strokes, and certain medical conditions. Table 8-2 and Figure 8-10 provide a list of the cranial nerves and their functions. Look carefully at the names of the nerves, for most can be figured out by understanding their word parts. (Hint: **opt/o** is the word root for vision, **ocul/o** for eye, and **gloss/o** for tongue.)

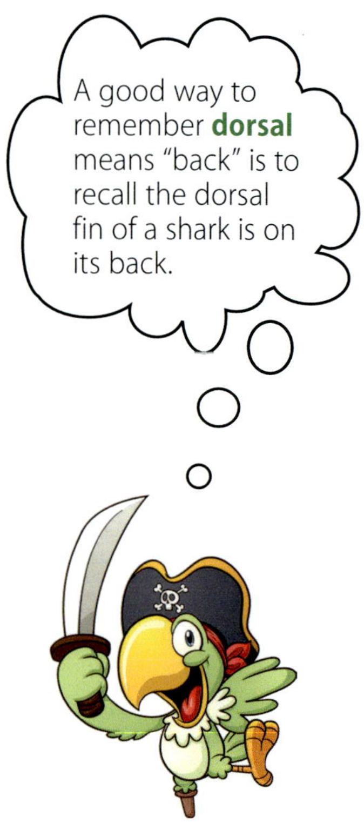
A good way to remember **dorsal** means "back" is to recall the dorsal fin of a shark is on its back.

The Peripheral Nervous System

The PNS begins as nerves leave the protection of the spinal column. Recall from Chapter 5 that the spinal column has several sections (cervical, thoracic, lumbar, sacral, coccygeal). Peripheral nerves, unlike the CNS, can often regenerate if damaged. This is why one may

TABLE 8-2 CRANIAL NERVES (FIGURE 8-10)		
CRANIAL NERVE NUMBER	**NAME**	**FUNCTION**
I	olfactory	Smell
II	optic	Vision (opt/o—vision)
III	oculomotor	Muscular movement of the eyes (ocul/o—eye)
IV	trochlear	Upward movement of the eyes
V	trigeminal	Muscles for chewing
VI	abducens	*Abd*uction of the eyes (looking to the side)
VII	facial	Muscles of the face; sensation of the face
VIII	vestibulocochlear	Hearing and balance (cochlea—balance organ in ear)
IX	glossopharyngeal	Muscles for swallowing (gloss/o—tongue; pharyng/—throat)
X	vagus	Parasympathetic control over the heart, stomach, liver, and other organs
XI	spinal accessory	Movement of shoulder muscles (specifically, the trapezius)
XII	hypoglossal	Movement of the tongue (**hypo-**—below; decreased; deficient; insufficient; low; under; gloss/o—tongue)
Can you tell by the word parts what their functions may be?		

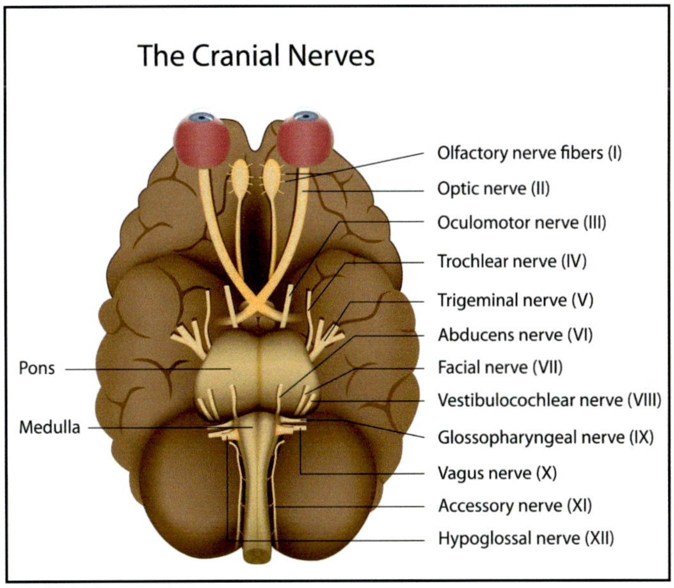

Figure 8-10. Cranial nerves looking from beneath the brain. (Alila Medical Images/shutterstock.com)

sustain a very deep cut or fracture that cuts into the nerves and may slowly regain motor (movement) and sensation to the damaged area. Conversely, when one has a spinal fracture, with intravertebral (**intra-**—inside, within; **vertebr/**—vertebra [spine]) bleeding or pressure where there is damage to the actual spinal cord (of the CNS), the injury to the nerves is likely permanent (paralysis), and both voluntary movement and sensation along the damaged nerves are lost.

The PNS begins as nerves leave the spinal cord (which is a part of the CNS) and travel to specific areas of the body. There are 31 pairs of **spinal nerves**. **Ventral** nerves are nerves that depart the spinal cord on the ventral (front) aspect of the body, and **dorsal** (back) nerves arise from the spinal column on the posterior (dorsal) part of the body. The PNS is divided into two types of nerves: **afferent** and **efferent**. Simply put, afferent nerves are sensory in nature and carry impulses to the brain and spinal cord. Opposite of these nerves are efferent nerves, which carry out motor functions and carry impulses from the brain and spinal cord to the muscles. Both voluntary (skeletal) and involuntary (cardiac and smooth) muscles

Table 8-3

Types of Nerves Assessed When Performing Evaluation for Peripheral Nerve or Intervertebral Disc Injury

TYPE	WHAT IT DOES
dermatome (derm/—skin) (Figure 8-13)	Afferent nerve that carries sensory impulses from the skin to the spinal cord and brain. Sensations such as touch, pressure, and perceptions of temperature all travel on dermatomes. Dermatomes are in specific areas and wrap around the body.
myotome (my/o—muscle)	Muscle or group of muscles innervated by a single motor nerve. Spinal nerve C6 (from the cervical vertebra) typically causes elbow flexion (contracts the biceps brachii muscle).

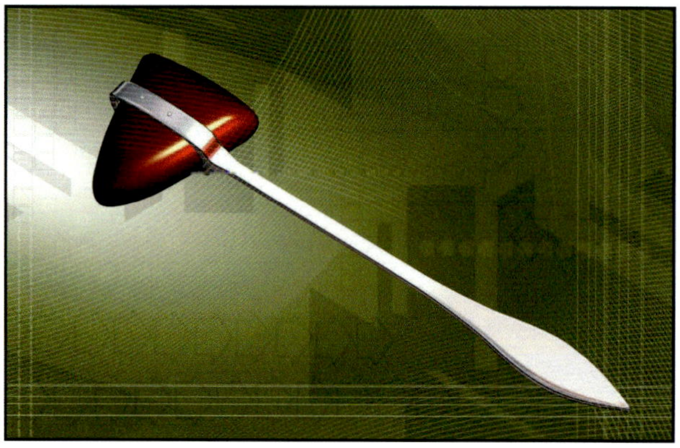

Figure 8-11. A neurological hammer is used to strike a stretched tendon to elicit a response. (Creations/shutterstock.com)

respond to propulsions from the efferent nerves. Health care providers often assess specific nerves or reflexes to determine if the nerve or properties of the nerve are intact (Table 8-3). Reflexes are an involuntary reaction to a stimulus and help determine the integrity of spinal nerves. When a **neurological** (or reflex) hammer (Figure 8-11) is struck on a stretched tendon (biceps, brachioradialis, triceps, patella, or Achilles), an involuntary reflex arc is created from the point of impact to the spinal cord and back to stimulate the tendon to contract. If the nerve is damaged (squeezed by an intervertebral disc, damaged by disease, or blocked) the reflex on that side of the body will be diminished compared to the other side (Figure 8-12).

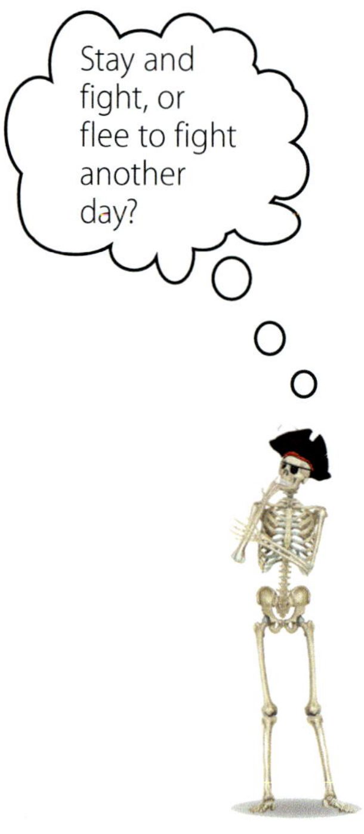

Another aspect of the PNS is the **autonomic nervous system** (ANS), which primarily regulates involuntary responses. It is further subdivided into the **sympathetic** and **parasympathetic nervous systems** (Figures 8-14 and 8-15). The sympathetic nervous system is responsible the "fight-or-flight" response to stress. It addresses blood pressure, heart rate, sweat, and digestive processes as the body prepares to fight (eg, a bicycle pulling out in front of your moving car) or flee (eg, gunfire in a public place) a threat. The parasympathetic nervous system does the opposite of the sympathetic nervous system. It is responsible for the "chill" response and slows down heart rate, breathing, digestion, sweat, and so on.

In addition to nerves, the PNS is composed of receptors and ganglia. Sensory receptors respond to changes in the environment and react to touch, temperature, pain, and pressure. **Ganglia** (singular: ganglion) are clusters of nervous tissue (cells) in the PNS. They resemble swelling along a nerve, but are in fact the areas where impulses leap from nerve to nerve via synapses.

Two different cell types are found in the PNS: parenchymal cells (**neurons**) and stromal cells (**glia**). Neurons are the cells that actually carry out the roles of the nervous system. Glia cells support the role of the neurons. Neurons are not all identical, but they do have similar properties.

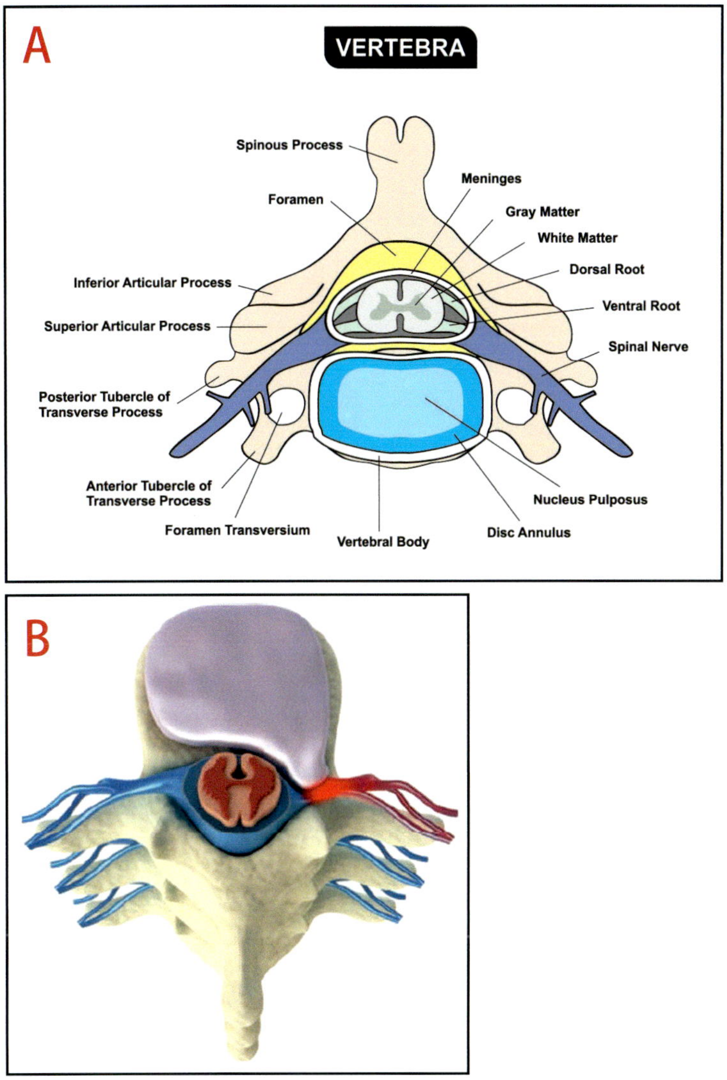

Figure 8-12. (A) Normal anatomy of the relationship between the spinal cord, intervertebral disc, and spinal nerve. (udaix/shutterstock.com) (B) A herniated disc can put pressure on a spinal nerve and block the impulses from fully getting to a muscle, organ, or skin. (Creations/shutterstock.com)

Figure 8-13. Dermatomes. Notice how they appear to wrap around the body. The different colors represent the cervical, thoracic lumbar, and sacral spinal nerves. (Alila Medical Images/shutterstock.com)

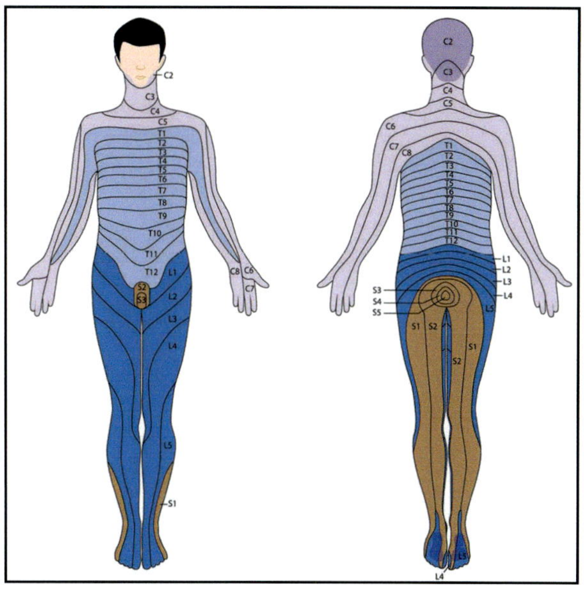

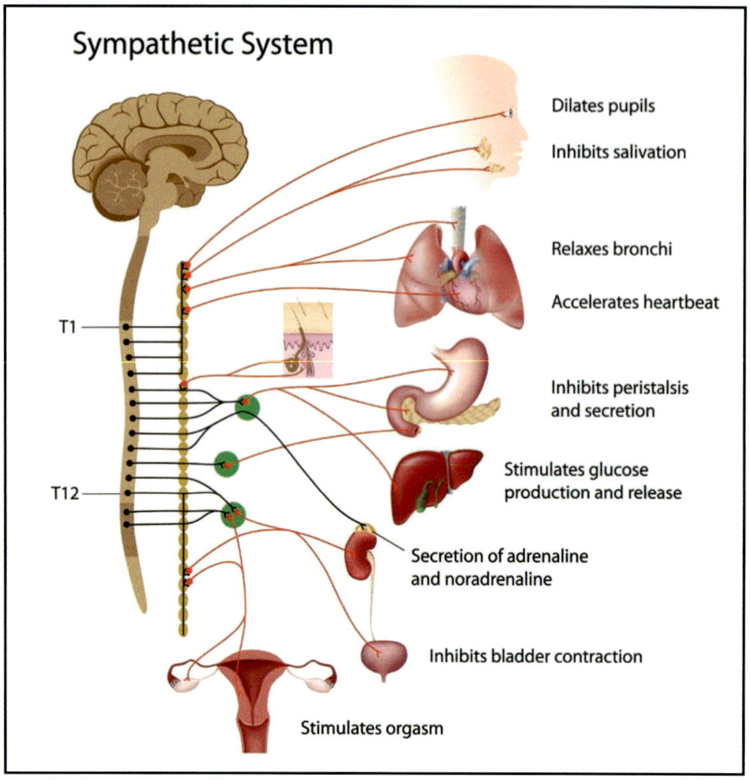

Figure 8-14. The sympathetic nervous system. (Alila Medical Images/shutterstock.com)

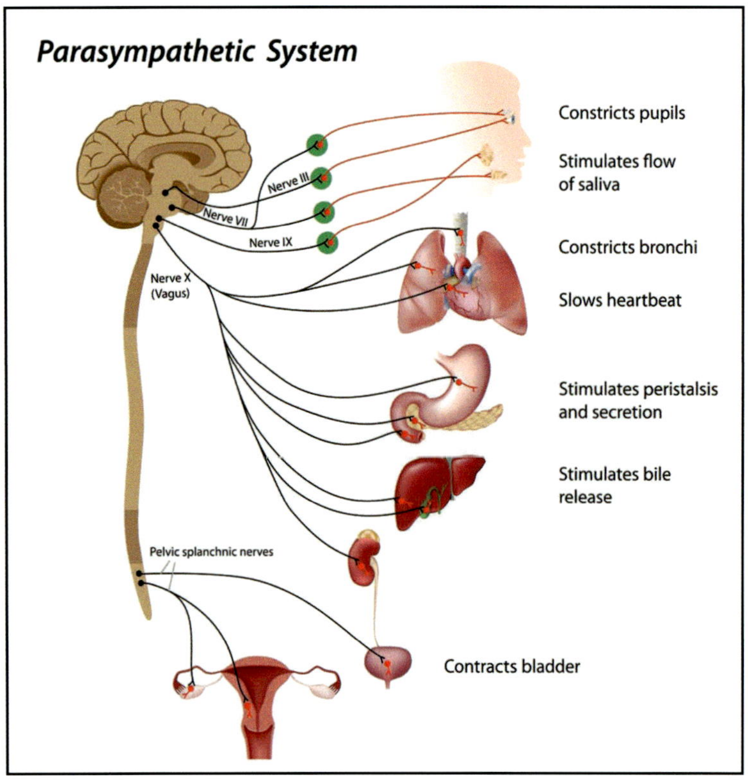

Figure 8-15. The parasympathetic nervous system. (Alila Medical Images/shutterstock.com)

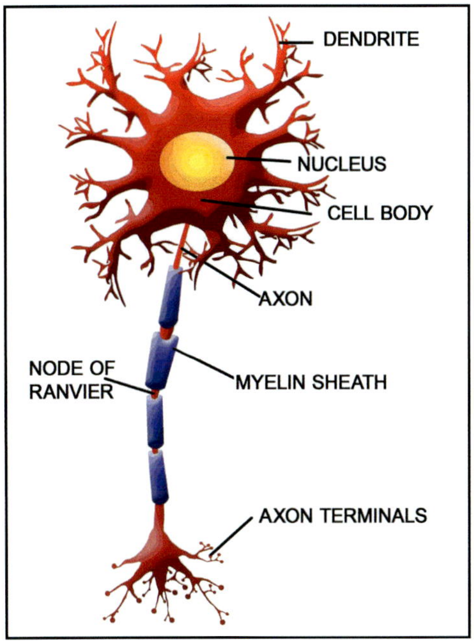

Figure 8-16. Anatomy of a motor neuron. (ducu59us/shutterstock.com)

Figure 8-17. The brachial plexus. (Alila Medical Images/shutterstock.com)

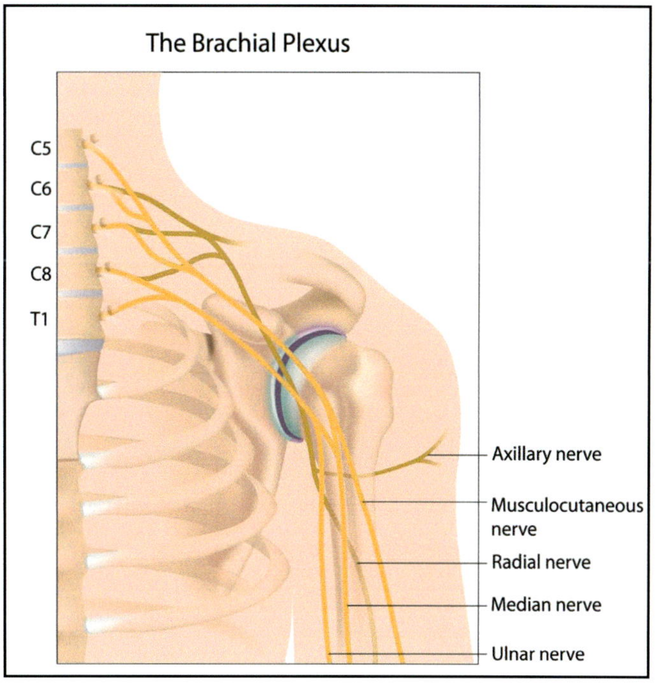

Expanding from the neuron cell bodies are projections called **dendrites** (Figure 8-16). Moving away from the neuron cell body is the **axon**, which is a tube through which the nerve impulse travels away from the cell body toward the target. PNS nerves have a covering, called the **myelin sheath**, protecting and insulating the axon. It is the myelin sheath that allows PNS nerves to regenerate if damaged, as most nerves in the CNS do not have this covering. At the end of the axon is an area called the **axon terminal**. There is a slight space between the axon terminal of one neuron and the dendrite of the cell of the next neuron. Nerve impulses jump this space and continue their path to their target.

Like ligaments, nerves are typically named after the bones or areas of the anatomy in which they reside. Often nerves group into a plexus that travel to a specific region. An example is in Figure 8-17, where the brachial (**brachi/o**—arm) plexus has nerves that describe their location (axillary nerve—near the armpit) or the bones against which they lie (radial and ulnar nerves). The median nerve is in the middle of the arm.

WORD BUILDING

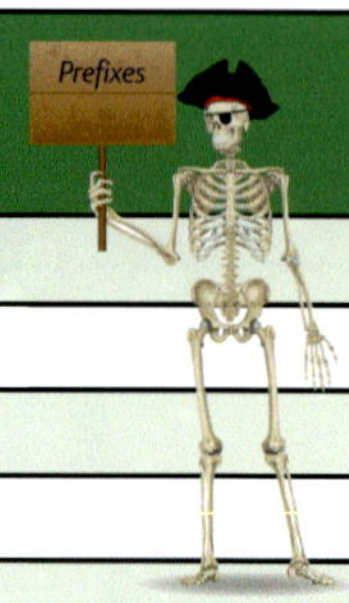

TABLE 8-4
PREFIXES

PREFIX	DEFINITION
a-; an-	not; without
de-	down; take away; without
di-	double
dys-	abnormal; bad; difficult; painful
epi-	above; upon
hemi-	one half
hydro-	water
hyper-	above; excessive; high; increased
hypo-	below; decreased; deficient; insufficient; low; under
intra-	inside; within
mono-	one
pan-	all
par-; para-	beside; near; abnormal
poly-	excessive; many; much; over
pre-	before
sub-	below
tetra-	four

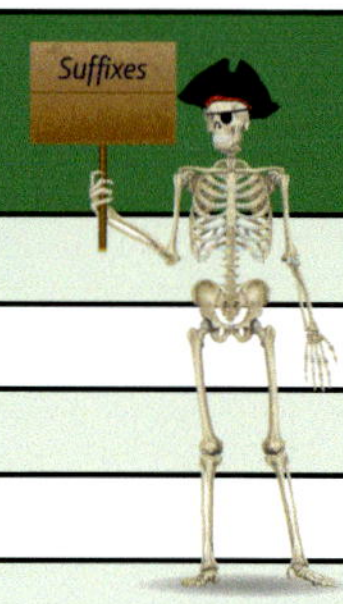

TABLE 8-5
SUFFIXES

SUFFIX	DEFINITION
-al; -ar	pertaining to
-algia	pain
-asthenla	weakness
-cele	hernia; protrusion; swelling
-ectomy	excision; surgical removal
-emic	pertaining to blood
-esthesia	sensation; perception
-gram	record of
-graph	instrument to record
-graphy	process of recording; the act of recording information
-ia	condition
-ic	pertaining to
-ion	process; the act of

(continued)

TABLE 8-5 (CONTINUED)

SUFFIXES

SUFFIX	DEFINITION
-itis	inflammation
-lepsy	seizure
-lysis	breaking down; destruction; loosening; separating; to loosen or break
-malacia	softening
-ology	study of
-oma	mass; tumor
-osis	condition of
-otomy; -tomy	incision; cutting into
-paresis	partial paralysis
-pathy	disease
-phagia	eating or swallowing
-phasia	speaking
-plegia	paralysis
-rrhaphy	surgical repair; suturing
-stomy	surgical opening
-troph	development; growth
-um	structure; thing
-us	pertaining to; condition; structure

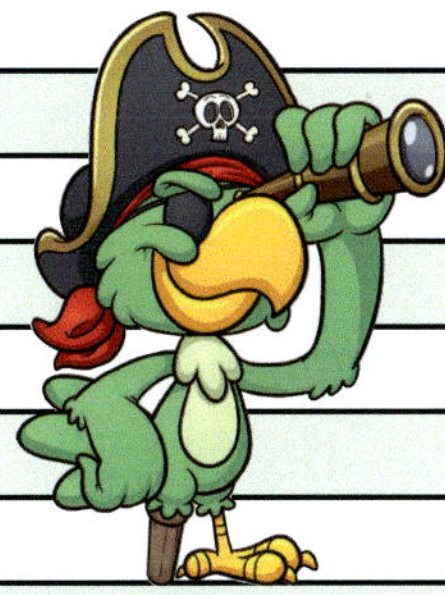

TABLE 8-6

COMBINING FORMS

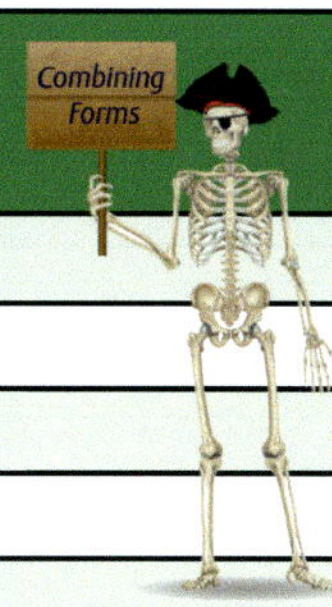

COMBINING FORM	DEFINITION
alges/o	pain
angi/o	vessel
arachn/o	spider
arteri/o	artery
arthr/o	joint
astr/o	star
ather/o	fatty material
blast/o	developing or embryonic cell
brachi/o	arm
cephal/o	head
cerebell/o	cerebellum; little brain
cerebr/o	cerebrum; brain
cortic/o	cortex; outer portion
cran/o; crani/o	cranium; skull
cyt/o	cell

(continued)

Table 8-6 (continued)

Combining Forms

COMBINING FORM	DEFINITION
derm/o	skin
dur/o	hard
electr/o	electricity
embol/o	plug
encephal/o	brain
fibr/o	fiber
gangli/o; ganglion/o	knot; swelling
gli/o	glue
gloss/o	tongue
kinesi/o	movement
lumb/o	low back
lys/o	to break apart
mening/i; mening/o	membrane; meninges
ment/o	mind
my/o	muscle
myel/o	bone marrow; medulla; myelin; spinal cord
narc/o	numbness; stupor; sleep
neur/o	nerve; cord; sinew
ocul/o	eye
opt/o	vision
peritone/o	peritoneum; membrane; to stretch; to stretch over
phas/o; phasi/o	speech
plegi/o	paralysis
poli/o	gray
praxia	to achieve; doing
psych/o	mind
quadr/i; quadr/o	four
radic/o; radicul/o	nerve root
scler/o	hard; hardening; thick; sclera
somat/o	body
somn/o	sleep
spin/o	spine; thorn
taxi/o	response to a stimulus
thalam/o	inner chamber; thalamus
thromb/o	clot
vascul/o	blood vessel
ventricul/o	ventricle; cavity
vertebr/o	vertebra; spine

Signs and Symptoms

Table 8-7 Signs and Symptoms Related to a Neurological Condition		
Recall that a sign is something that is objective and can be measured, whereas a symptom is something a person feels.		
SIGN/SYMPTOM	**WORD PARTS**	**DEFINITION**
amnesia		Loss of memory caused by injury or emotional distress
anesthesia (Table 8-8)	**an-** (without) **-esthesia** (sensation)	Absence of all feeling, especially pain
aphasia	**a-** (without) **-phasia** (speaking)	Inability to speak
ataxia	**a-** (without) taxi/ (reaction to a stimulus)	Impaired ability to perform coordinated movements
athetosis	**-osis** (condition)	Consistent, slow, involuntary writhing movement of the extremities
aura		Precursor to a seizure or headache; premonition of light that precedes a seizure
cephalalgia (Figure 8-18)	cephal/ (head) **-algia** (pain)	Headache
coma		State of decreased consciousness
convulsion		Involuntary muscular spasms
decerebrate posturing	**de-** (down) cerebr/ (cerebrum)	Position of an unconscious person where the upper extremities and lower extremities are extended and the wrists are flexed
decorticate posturing	**de-** (down) cortic/ (cortex; outer portion)	Position of an unconscious person where the upper extremities are flexed and the lower extremities are rigid
dysphasia	**dys-** (difficult) **-phasia** (speaking)	Difficulty speaking
dyssomnia	**dys-** (difficult) somn/ (sleep) **-ia** (condition)	Sleep disorder; difficulty sleeping or staying asleep
fasciculation	**-ion** (the act of)	Involuntary twitching of small muscles
hyperalgesia	**hyper-** (increased) alges/ (pain) **-ia** (condition)	Exceptionally sensitive to painful stimulus
hyperesthesia	**hyper-** (increased) **-esthesia** (sensation)	Increased sensitivity to touch or pain

(continued)

8

Table 8-7 (continued)
Signs and Symptoms Related to a Neurological Condition

SIGN/SYMPTOM	WORD PARTS	DEFINITION
hypokinesia	**hypo-** (decreased) kinesi/ (movement) **-ia** (condition)	Decrease in normal movement; slow movement
monoparesis	**mono-** (one) **-paresis** (partial paralysis)	Partial paralysis of one limb
neuralgia	neur/ (nerve) **-algia** (pain)	Pain in a nerve
paresthesia	**par-** (alongside; around; beside; near) **-esthesia** (sensation)	Abnormal condition where one feels numbness or tingling without a specific cause
radiculopathy	radicul/o (nerve root) **-pathy** (disease)	Disease of a nerve root; also means pain away (more distal) from the injury
sciatica (Figure 8-19)		Inflammation of the sciatic nerve, causing pain/numbness down the back of one leg
seizure		Sudden attack of muscular convulsions or spasms
syncope		Fainting; often due to a lack of blood to the brain
vertigo		Dizziness; sensation or movement when there is no movement

Table 8-8
Types of Anesthesia

TYPE	DEFINITION
general anesthesia	Whole body is without feeling, induced by inhaled or intravenous injection
local anesthesia	Specific area is without feeling, often by an injection
regional anesthesia	Region (eg, arm or leg) is without feeling, usually by a nerve block or **epidural** (**epi-**—above; upon) injection in the back
topical anesthesia	Surface of a tissue is without feeling, usually by a gel, solution, or ointment

Seizure activity varies from a **grand mal seizure** where all muscles contract to a **petit mal seizure** where there is little outward appearance of a seizure and the person appears to have momentarily lost focus.

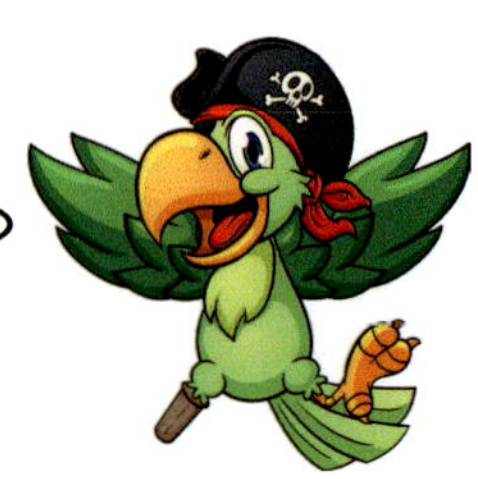

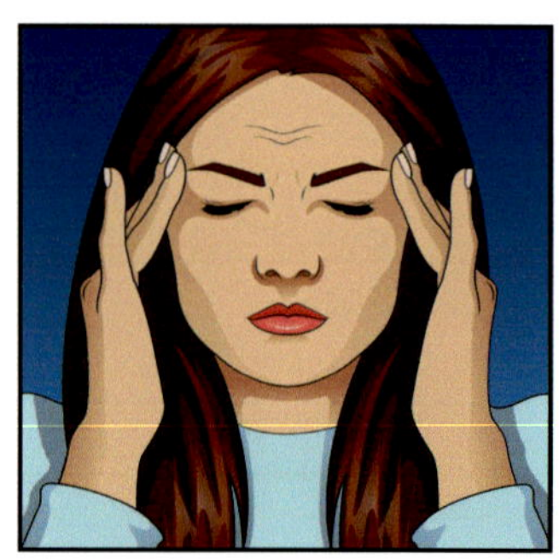

Figure 8-18. Cephalalgia, commonly known as *headache*. (Ed Meden/shutterstock.com)

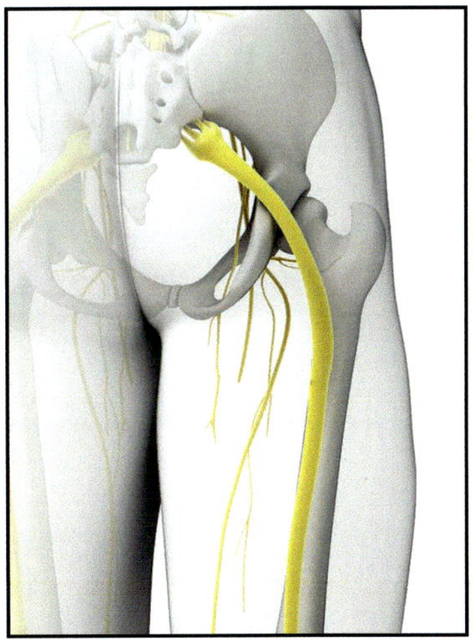

Figure 8-19. The sciatic nerve runs down the posterior aspect of the leg. Sciatica is when there is pain along this nerve. (Sebastian Kaulitzki/shutterstock.com)

MEDICAL CONDITIONS

8

Table 8-9 Medical Conditions Related to the Neurological System		
NAME	**WORD PARTS**	**DEFINITION**
amyotrophic lateral sclerosis (ALS)	**a-** (without) my/o (muscle) **-troph** (development) **-ic** (pertaining to) scler/ (hard) **-osis** (condition)	When the lateral aspects of the spinal column harden, there is progressive atrophy and paralysis; fatal condition; also known as *Lou Gehrig's disease*
astrocytoma	astr/o (star) cyt/ (cell) **-oma** (tumor)	Tumor made of the star-shaped glial cells, which can be malignant
cerebral palsy (CP)	cerebr/ (cerebrum) **-al** (pertaining to)	Partial muscle paralysis occurring since birth
cerebrovascular accident (CVA) (Figure 8-20)	cerebr/o (cerebrum) vascul/ (vessel) **-ar** (pertaining to)	Arrested blood supply in the brain; also known as a *stroke*
dementia	**de-** (down; take away; without) ment/ (mind) **-ia** (condition)	Declining mental function; not associated with age-related memory loss
demyelinating	**de-** (take away) myel/ (myelin)	Removal or destruction of the myelin sheath
duritis	dur/ (hard) **-itis** (inflammation)	Inflammation of the dura mater
encephalitis	encephal/ (brain) **-itis** (inflammation)	Inflammation of the brain; typically transmitted via a mosquito

(continued)

Table 8-9 (continued)

Medical Conditions Related to the Neurological System

NAME	WORD PARTS	DEFINITION
epilepsy	**epi-** (above; upon) **-lepsy** (seizure)	Brain disorder characterized by recurrent seizures
gangliitis	gangli/ (knot; swelling) **-itis** (inflammation)	Inflammation of a ganglion
glioma	gli/ (glue) **-oma** (tumor)	Tumor in neuroglia cells
hydrocephalus	**hydro-** (water) cephal/ (head) **-us** (pertaining to)	Abnormal accumulation of CSF, resulting in an enlarged head
meningitis	mening/ (meninges) **-itis** (inflammation)	Inflammation of the meninges; caused by viral or bacterial infection
meningocele	mening/o (meninges) **-cele** (hernia; protrusion; swelling)	Protrusion or hernia of the meninges through a defect in the spinal column or cranium
multiple sclerosis (MS) (Figure 8-21)	scler/ (hard; hardening; thick) **-osis** (condition)	Progressive disease marked by demyelination of nerve fibers in the brain and spinal cord; characterized by muscle weakness, paresthesia, and visual disturbances
myelitis	myel/ (spinal cord) **-itis** (inflammation)	Inflammation of the spinal cord
narcolepsy (Figure 8-22)	narc/o (sleep) **-lepsy** (seizure)	Disorder characterized by sudden, uncontrollable attacks of sleep and visual/auditory hallucinations
neurapraxia	neur/ (nerve) praxia (to achieve; doing)	Following an injury, the injured nerve is intact but no longer transmits impulses
neuritis	neur/ (nerve) **-itis** (inflammation)	Inflammation of a nerve
neuroblastoma	neur/o (nerve) blast/ (embryonic cell) **-oma** (mass; tumor)	Malignant tumor of the ANS usually found in children under the age of 10
neurofibroma	neur/o (nerve) fibr/ (fiber) **-oma** (tumor)	Benign fibrous tumor made of nervous tissue
neuropathy	neur/o (nerve) **-pathy** (disease)	Disease of the nerves, marked by inflammation or degeneration
poliomyelitis	poli/o (gray) myel/ (spinal cord) **-itis** (inflammation)	Inflammation of the gray matter of the spinal cord caused by a virus; can lead to paralysis; also called *polio*

(continued)

TABLE 8-9 (CONTINUED) MEDICAL CONDITIONS RELATED TO THE NEUROLOGICAL SYSTEM		
NAME	**WORD PARTS**	**DEFINITION**
polyneuritis	**poly-** (many) neur/ (nerve) **-itis** (inflammation)	Inflammation of several nerves
radiculitis	radicul/ (nerve root) **-itis** (inflammation)	Inflammation of a nerve root
transient ischemic attack (TIA)	**-emic** (pertaining to blood)	Brief loss of blood flow to the brain, resulting in temporary neurological dysfunction

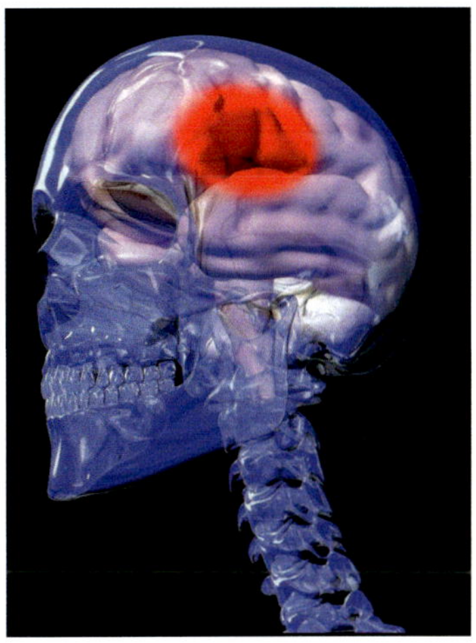

Figure 8-20. A stroke (also known as a *cerebrovascular accident*) is when the blood supply to the brain is interrupted, either by bleeding or occlusion. (BioMedical/shutterstock.com)

8

Figure 8-21. In multiple sclerosis, the normal myelin of the nerves is disrupted. (Blamb/shutterstock.com)

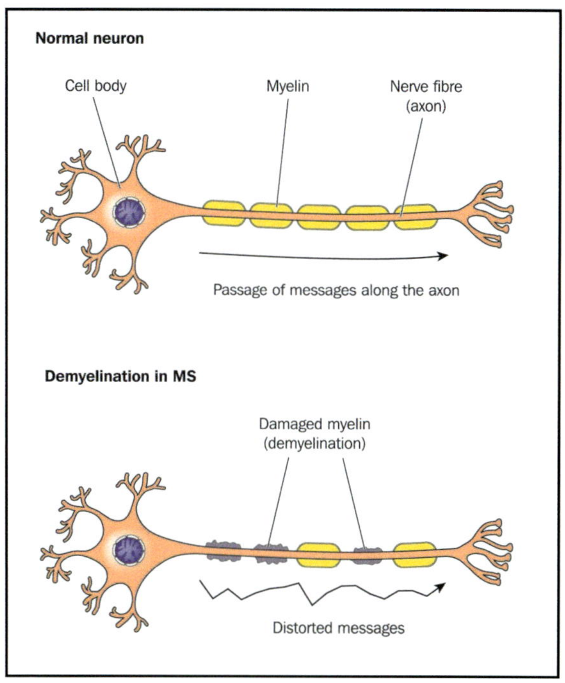

Table 8-10
Neurological Conditions With Specific Names

NAME	DEFINITION
Alzheimer's disease	Progressive neurodegenerative disease of unknown origin
autism	Development disorder that varies greatly with each patient; characterized by withdrawal from reality and impaired social interaction
Bell's palsy (Figure 8-23)	Paralysis of the facial nerve (CN VII) with rapid onset and slow resolution; one side of the face appears distorted
complex regional pain syndrome (CRPS)	Characterized by an overactive sympathetic nervous system; typically follows an insult (no matter how minor) to a nerve
Guillain-Barré syndrome (GBS)	Acute disorder of the peripheral nerves marked by demyelination and rapid degeneration to the point where most patients require hospitalization and breathing assistance; there is no cure, although most patients get better
Huntington's chorea	Genetic disorder that becomes apparent in adulthood; characterized by a progressive deterioration of neuromuscular control and dementia
migraine	Severe headache with side effects; often due to vascular issues
Parkinson's disease	Chronic, degenerative, neurological disease; characterized by tremors and challenges speaking and swallowing
rabies (Figure 8-24)	Infection of the brain due to viral encephalitis caused by the saliva of infected mammals
shingles (Figure 8-25)	Herpes zoster infection that involves peripheral nerves; characterized by pain and blisters along dermatomes
stroke	Lack of oxygen (via blood) in the brain; may lead to permanent paralysis and dysfunction; also called *cerebrovascular accident* (CVA)
Tay-Sachs disease	Genetic disorder resulting in CNS deterioration
Tourette syndrome	Involuntary condition characterized by tics, facial movements, and/or vocal expressions

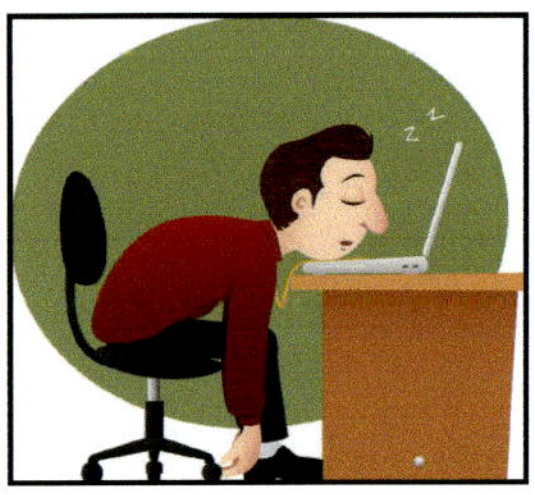

Figure 8-22. Narcolepsy is uncontrollable attacks of sleep. (weniworks/shutterstock.com)

Figure 8-23. Bell's palsy affects cranial nerve VII. (hkannn/shutterstock.com)

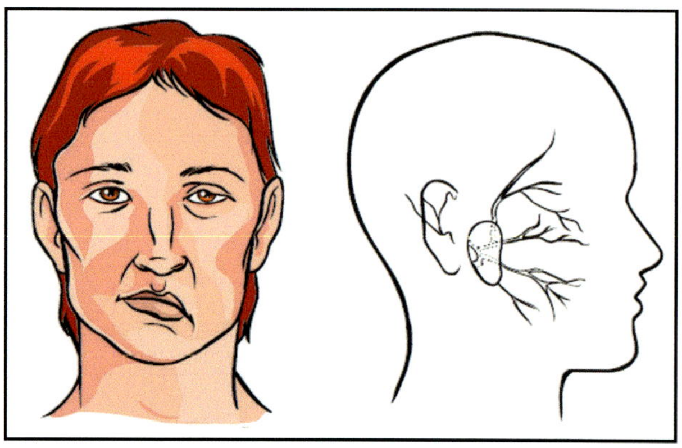

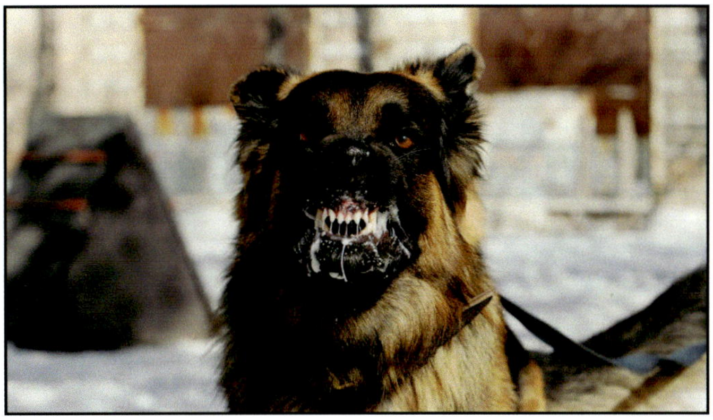

Figure 8-24. Rabies is transmitted through the saliva of infected mammals. (Victoria Antonova/shutterstock.com)

Figure 8-25. Shingles appears along dermatomes and is caused by the herpes (varicella) virus. (Alila Medical Images/shutterstock.com)

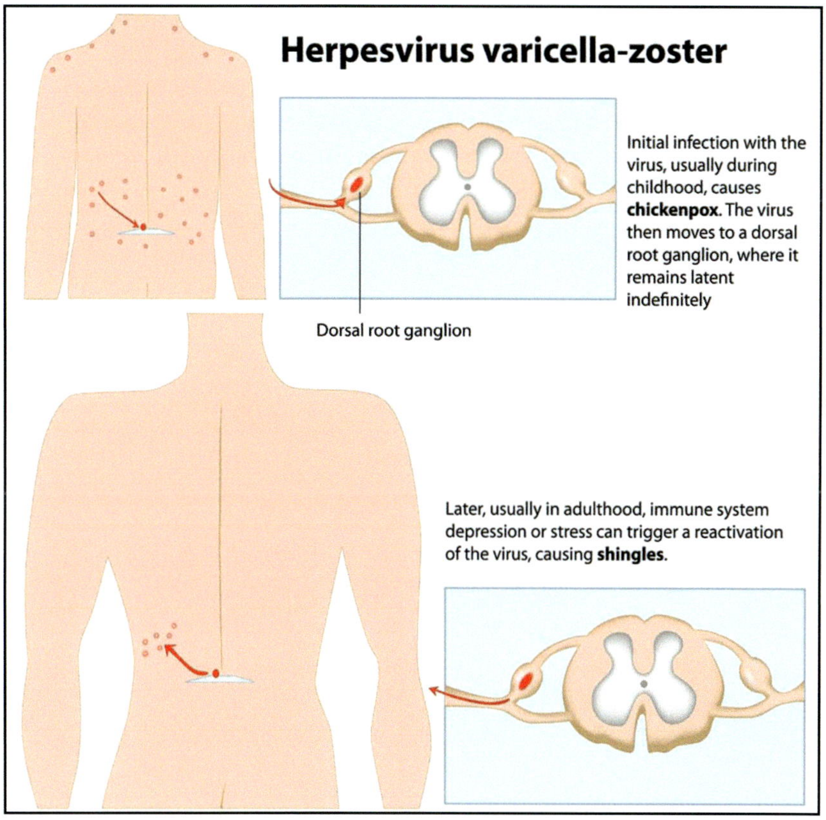

A WORD ABOUT MENINGITIS

If you are entering college, especially if you are planning on living in close quarters with others (such as in a dorm), consider a vaccination against **bacterial meningitis** (also known as *meningococcal meningitis*). Because there are over 100 cases per year on college campuses, and up to 15 college students die annually from it, many colleges require the meningococcal vaccine prior to entrance to college to prevent an outbreak.

A WORD ABOUT CONCUSSIONS

In the world of sports, concussions are a hot topic. A concussion (also called a ***traumatic brain injury*** [TBI]) is any alteration in brain activity, typically following some sort of blow, rapid deceleration, twist, or shake that affects the brain. Signs and symptoms of a concussion can include headache, nausea, vomiting, dizziness, ringing in the ears (tinnitus), mood changes, difficulty sleeping, and difficulty concentrating. Any one of these signs or symptoms following a head injury leads to a diagnosis of a concussion, and the injured person should be referred to qualified medical care.

Note that a person does *not* need to be unconscious to have suffered a concussion. Anyone suspected of a concussion should be referred to a qualified concussion specialist (typically not a regular physician). Athletic trainers are one group of Board-certified, licensed health care providers who have training in concussion management. With specialized training, many other health care providers also become qualified to manage concussions and make return-to-activity, and return-to-learn decisions.

Tests and Procedures

Table 8-11

Tests Related to the Neurological System

NAME	WORD PARTS	PURPOSE
cerebral angiogram	cerebr/ (cerebrum) **-al** (pertaining to) angi/o (vessel) **-gram** (a record of)	Record of the cerebral arteries done via x-ray following the injection of a contrast dye
deep tendon reflex (DTR) testing		Series of tests using a neurological hammer to stimulate tendons to determine if spinal nerves are functioning within normal limits
electroencephalography (EEG) (Figure 8-26)	electr/o (electricity) encephal/o (brain) **-graphy** (process of recording)	Process of recording electrical brain activity
electromyogram (EMG)	electr/o (electricity) my/o (muscle) **-gram** (a record of)	Measures the electrical nerve activity in skeletal muscles via small electrodes (needles) placed in muscles
encephalograph	encephal/o (brain) **-graph** (an instrument to record information)	Instrument for recording brain activity
evoked potential (EP) studies		Group of tests used to diagnose changes in brain waves

(continued)

TABLE 8-11 (CONTINUED) TESTS RELATED TO THE NEUROLOGICAL SYSTEM		
NAME	**WORD PARTS**	**PURPOSE**
lumbar puncture (Figure 8-27)	lumb/ (low back) **-ar** (pertaining to)	Withdrawal of CSF from the subarachnoid space in the lumbar area of the spinal cord; used to determine if one has meningitis, among other things
myelogram	myel/o (spinal cord) **-gram** (a record of)	Record of the spinal cord via x-ray following injection of a contrast dye
nerve conduction study (NCS)		Test of the speed of peripheral nerve impulses
polysomnography (Figure 8-28)	**poly-** (excessive; many; much; over) somn/o (sleep) **-graphy** (process of recording)	Series of tests performed on a sleeping patient; most commonly used to determine sleep apnea (periodic cessation of breathing)

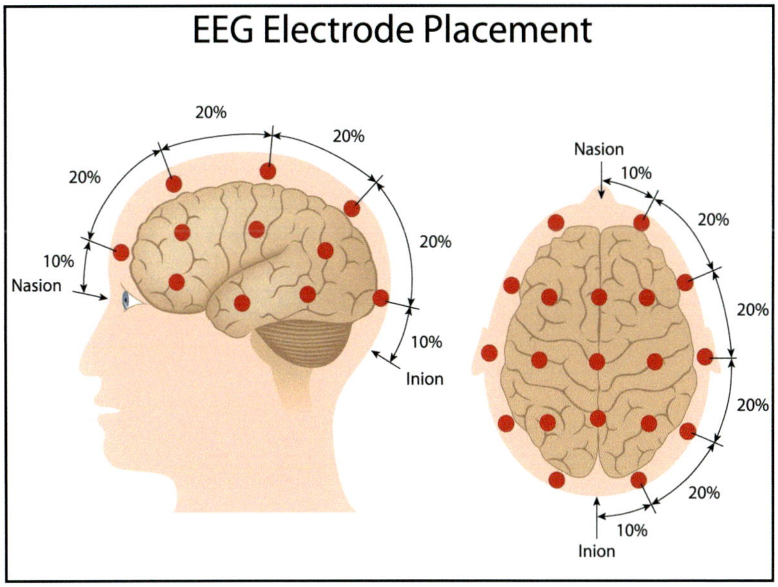

Figure 8-26. During an electroencephalogram, electrodes are placed on the skull to measure brain activity. (Alila Medical Images/shutterstock.com)

Figure 8-27. Lumbar puncture involves taking a sample of the cerebrospinal fluid in the subarachnoid space of the spine. (Grei/shutterstock.com)

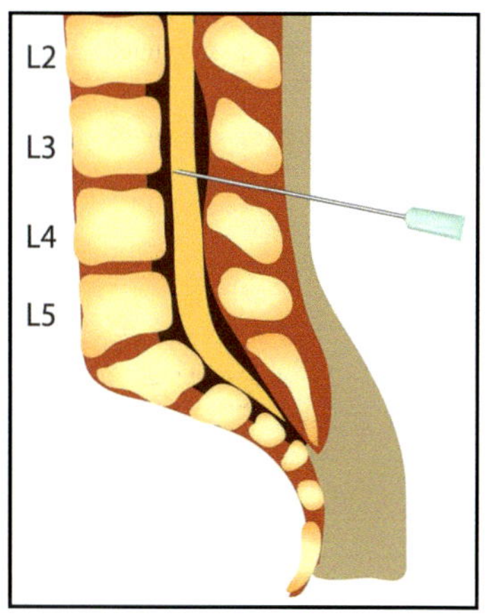

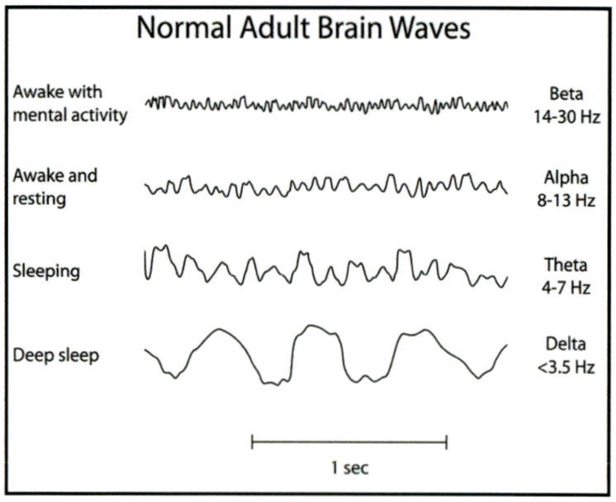

Figure 8-28. Brain wave activity wide awake and working vs in a deep sleep. (Alila Medical Images/shutterstock.com)

Table 8-12

Procedures Related to the Neurological System

NAME	WORD PARTS	PURPOSE
craniectomy	crani/ (skull) **-ectomy** (surgical excision)	Surgical removal of a part of the cranium
craniotomy	crani/ (skull) **-otomy** (incision)	Incision into the cranium
neurectomy	neur/ (nerve) **-ectomy** (surgical excision; removal)	Surgical removal of a nerve
neurolysis	neur/o (nerve) **-lysis** (separating)	Separating lesions (scar tissue) from a nerve; destruction of a nerve
neurorrhaphy	neur/o (nerve) **-rrhaphy** (suturing)	Suturing a nerve
neurotomy	neur/ (nerve) **-otomy** (to cut into)	Cutting into a nerve
radicotomy	radic/ (nerve root) **-otomy** (to cut into)	Incision into a nerve root
vagotomy	**-otomy** (to cut into)	Cutting a part of the vagus nerve, often to reduce secretion of gastric acid into the stomach
ventriculoperitoneostomy	ventricul/o (ventricle) peritone/o (peritoneum; membrane; to stretch; to stretch over) **-stomy** (surgical opening)	Procedure where a shunt is introduced into the brain ventricles with a drain into the abdominal cavity

Mental Health and Behavioral Disorders

Most of the neurological conditions presented so far have measurable signs of physiological changes that cause the condition or disease. Mental health and behavioral disorders are also illnesses that effect the brain, only these conditions are not usually caused by a physical injury or illness (Table 8-13). They are, nonetheless, true neurological conditions and are best treated by psychiatrists (medical doctors who treat mental disorders) in conjunction with licensed psychologists or mental health care providers. As with other pathological conditions, recognition of a mental health problem can lead to diagnosis and treatment. Most who follow their prescribed treatment plan will be able to manage their conditions quite well.

Table 8-13

Mental Health and Behavioral Disorders

NAME	DEFINITION
anorexia nervosa	Eating disorder resulting from low self-image, fear of gaining weight; extreme measures to prevent weight gain
anxiety disorder	Emotional instability brought about due to apprehension of real or imagined events
attention-deficit/hyperactivity disorder (ADHD)	Inability to focus for a period of time due to high energy; similar to attention-deficit disorder (ADD), but with the hyperactivity component
bipolar disorder	Cyclic condition of extreme mania and elevated moods to depression and lethargy
bulimia nervosa	Eating disorder involving uncontrollable eating, followed by purging (eg, vomiting, laxative use)
dementia	Memory loss, confusion, and disorientation
depression (clinical)	Overwhelming feelings of sadness, worthlessness, and despair
mania	Emotional disorder in which a patient is frenzied and has abnormally high psychomotor activity or excitement
neurosis	Emotional disorder characterized by a counterproductive means of coping with stress
obsessive-compulsive disorder (OCD)	Uncontrollable need to act (perform specific motor skills); repetitive behaviors or rituals
paranoia	Condition where the person is convinced they are being persecuted; characterized by mistrust, combativeness
phobia	Intense, irrational fear of something that causes a strong emotional response
posttraumatic stress disorder (PTSD)	Extreme fear/anxiety resulting from a traumatic experience
psychosis	Inability to determine reality from fiction
psychosomatic	Condition where the person imagines symptoms that are not present or who becomes ill (eg, ulcer) due to anxiety
schizophrenia	Group of disorders encompassing an inability to determine reality from nonreality

Bibliography

Broglio SP, Cantu RC, Gioia GA, et al, National Athletic Trainers' Association Position Statement: Management of Sport Concussion. *J Athl Train.* 2014;49(2):245-265.

Casa DJ, Guskiewicz KM, Anderson SA, et al. National Athletic Trainers' Association Position Statement: Preventing Sudden Death in Sports. *J Athl Train.* 2012;47(1):79-101.

Cohen BJ, Jones SA. *Medical Terminology: An Illustrated Guide.* 9th ed. Jones & Bartlett; 2021.

Flanagan KW, Cuppett M. *Neurological Conditions. In Medical Conditions in the Athlete.* 3rd ed. Human Kinetics; 2017.

Mosby's Dictionary of Medicine, Nursing & Health Professions. 10th ed. Elsevier; 2017.

Rice J. *Medical Terminology for Health Care Professionals.* 9th ed. Pearson; 2018.

Venes D, ed. *Taber's Cyclopedic Medical Dictionary.* 24th ed. F. A. Davis; 2021.

Wingerd BD. *Medical Terminology Complete!* Pearson; 2019.

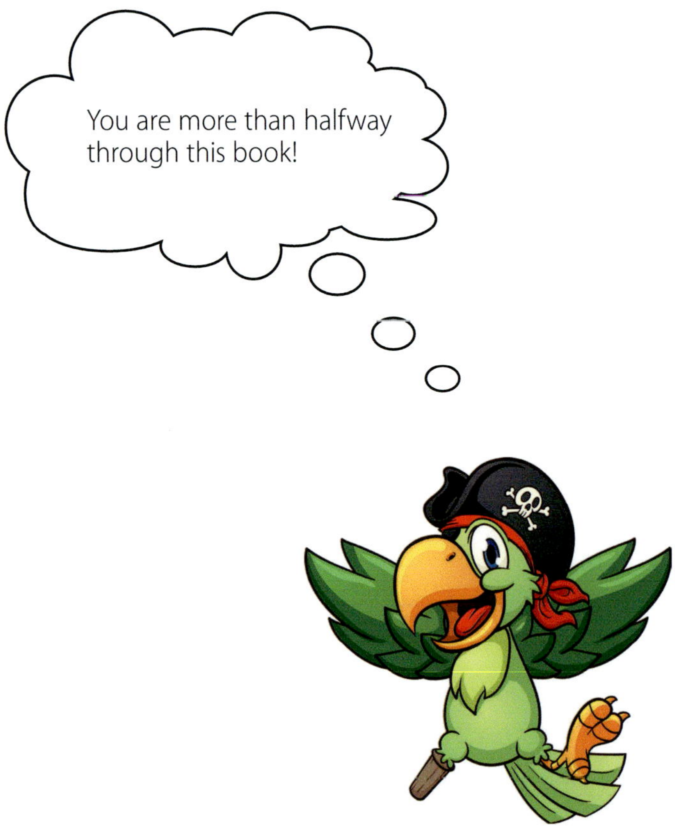

Notes

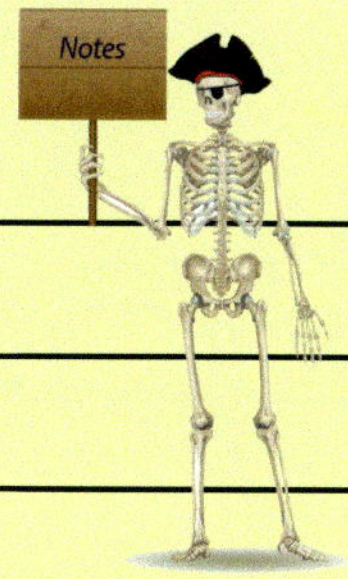

NOTES

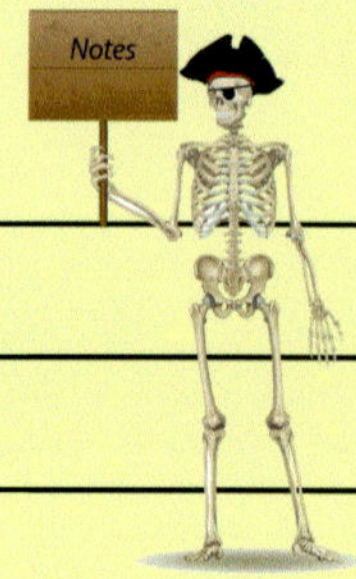

Learning Activities

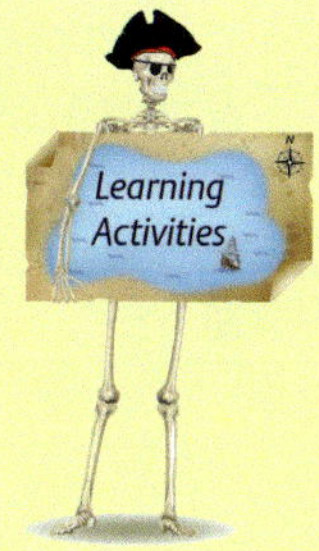

Name:______________________

Neurological System

A. Label the lobes of the brain from the following list.

- frontal__________________
- occipital________________
- cerebellum_______________
- temporal_________________
- parietal_________________

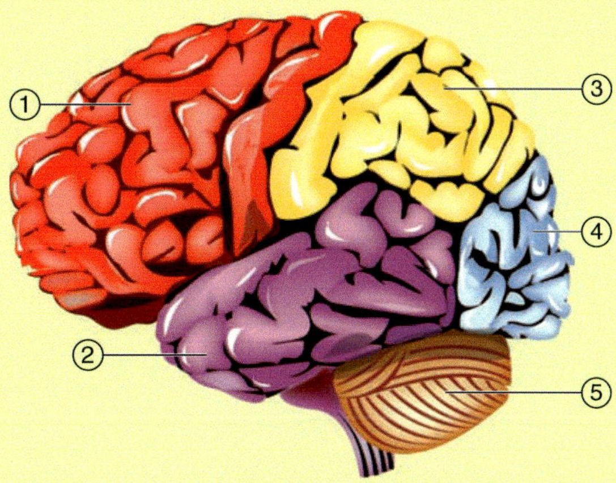

(Matthew Cole/shutterstock.com)

B. Label the bones of the skull from the following list.

- nasal____________
- cervical spine______
- occipital__________
- mandible__________
- temporal__________
- parietal__________
- frontal___________
- maxilla___________
- zygoma___________

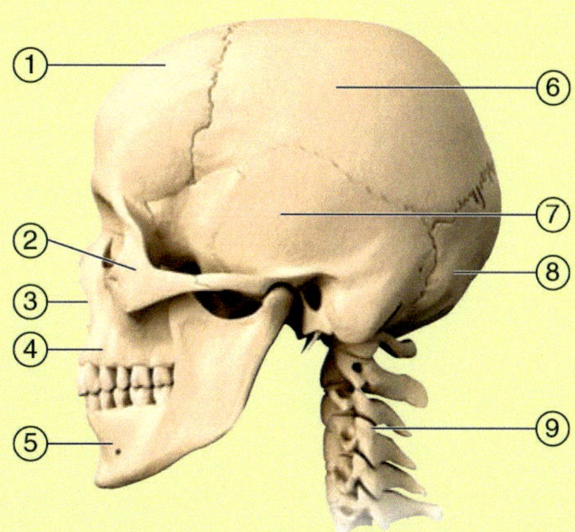

C. Using this chart, indicate whether each is a sign or a symptom. One has been done for you.

TERM	SIGN	SYMPTOM
cephalalgia		*X*
fasciculation		
neuralgia		
syncope		
ataxia		
seizure		

D. Using your knowledge from previous chapters, separate the word elements and define the following words.

1. cerebral arteriosclerosis____________________
2. cerebral thrombosis____________________
3. cerebral aneurysm____________________
4. neurology____________________
5. arachnophobia____________________

E. Matching.

Match the word element with its best meaning.

1. **dys-** ________	a. all
2. **-paresis**______	b. sensation, perception
3. myel/o ______	c. paralysis
4. **pan-**________	d. bad, painful, difficult
5. **-plegia**______	e. response to a stimulus
6. **-al** _________	f. within
7. praxia_______	g. pertaining to
8. **infra-**_______	h. to achieve, doing
9. taxi/o_______	i. partial paralysis
10. **-esthesia**_____	j. spinal cord

F. Build the word.

Using the word root, add the other word element and define the new word created.

1. **hemi-**
   a. **-paresis** ____________________
   b. **-plegia** ____________________
   c. **par-** + **-esthesia** ____________________
   d. **-ataxia** ____________________
   e. **hyper-** + **-trophy** ____________________
2. **para-**
   a. **an-** + **-esthesia** ____________________
   b. **-plegia** ____________________
   c. **-plegic** ____________________
   d. **-lysis** ____________________
   e. **-nasal** ____________________
3. **neur/o**
   a. **-itis** ____________________
   b. **-oma** ____________________
   c. muscul/ + **-ar** ____________________
   d. **-plasty** ____________________
   e. **-genic** ____________________

8

Case Study

Define the numerical terms (1 to 11).

For assistance with medical abbreviations, refer to Appendix A.

History, Chief Complaint

A construction worker was struck on the head with a heavy board that was swinging from a crane. The force knocked her helmet off and she fell to the ground. She experienced no **LOC** (1) and was evaluated by the athletic trainer.

Evaluation

The construction worker has a **HA** (2), eyes were **PERRLA** (3), and she was unsteady on her feet. Her **myotomes** (4) and **dermatomes** (5) were **WNL** (6). All cranial nerve testing was normal with the exception of **CN VIII** (7). She complained of **tinnitus** (8), dizziness, and an upset stomach.

Diagnostic Studies

The worker was sent for a **CT** (9) to **R/O** (10) **intracranial hemorrhaging** (11). The test was normal and she was diagnosed with a concussion. She was referred to her primary physician for post-concussion evaluation and return-to-work progression training.

Terms

1. ______________________________
2. ______________________________
3. ______________________________
4. ______________________________
5. ______________________________
6. ______________________________
7. ______________________________
8. ______________________________
9. ______________________________
10. ______________________________
11. ______________________________

9

Gastrointestinal System

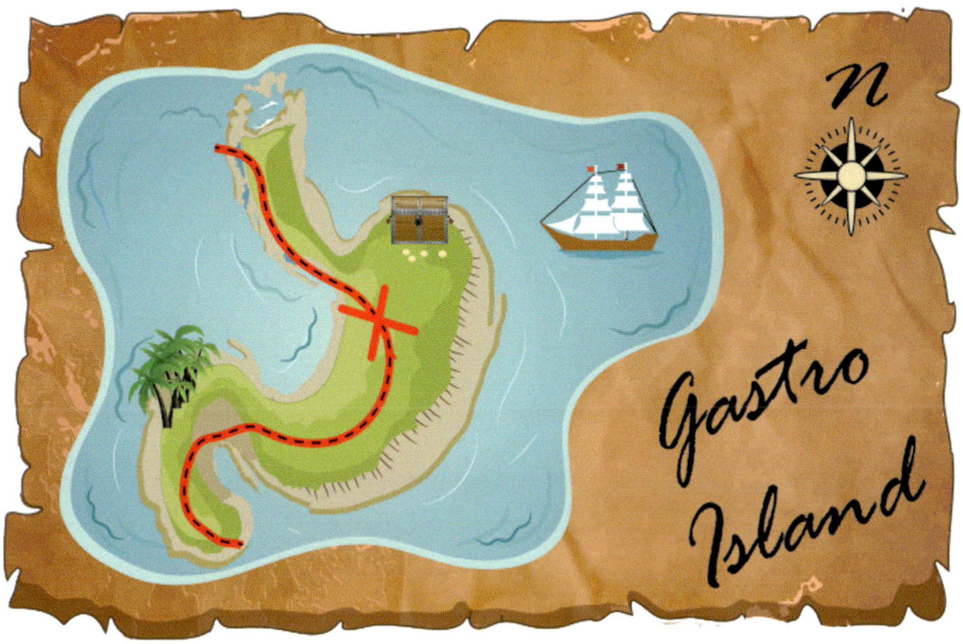

Objectives

After studying this chapter, you will be able to:

1. Identify the major components of the gastrointestinal (GI) system.
2. Describe the relationship between the various aspects of the GI system.
3. Describe the role of the accessory organs and glands play in digestion.
4. Identify and build words relating to the GI system.
5. List signs and symptoms of a condition with the GI system.
6. Describe common medical conditions of the GI system.
7. Identify diagnostic tests and procedures specific to the neurological system.
8. Differentiate between the purposes of classes of medications related to the GI system.

Flanagan KW.
Medical Terminology With Case Studies: A Navigated Guide to Learning for Health Care Professionals, Third Edition (pp 217-253).

Chapter Outline

- Self-assessment
- Checklist for word parts in the chapter
- Checklist of new anatomy
- Introduction
- Anatomy
    - The mouth
    - The intestines
    - Accessory organs and glands
- Word building
    - Prefixes
    - Suffixes
    - Combining forms
- Signs and symptoms
- Medical conditions
- Tests and procedures
- Medication classifications
- Learning activities
- Case study

Self-Assessment

Based on what you have learned so far, can you write the definition of these words?

- gastritis____
- tonsillectomy____
- gastroenterology____
- gastrostomy____
- hemicolectomy____
- hepatitis____

Checklist for Word Parts in the Chapter

Prefixes

- ☐ a-
- ☐ ad-
- ☐ an-
- ☐ anti-
- ☐ bi-
- ☐ dia-
- ☐ dys-
- ☐ eme-
- ☐ endo-
- ☐ epi-
- ☐ extra-
- ☐ hyper-
- ☐ mal-
- ☐ pan-
- ☐ par-
- ☐ peri-
- ☐ re-
- ☐ retro-
- ☐ sub-
- ☐ tri-

Suffixes

- ☐ -ac
- ☐ -al
- ☐ -algia
- ☐ -ary
- ☐ -ase
- ☐ -cele
- ☐ -centesis
- ☐ -dynia
- ☐ -ectomy
- ☐ -emesis
- ☐ -emia
- ☐ -gram
- ☐ -ia
- ☐ -iasis
- ☐ -ic
- ☐ -ion
- ☐ -itis
- ☐ -malacia
- ☐ -megaly
- ☐ -occlus/o
- ☐ -oid
- ☐ -oma
- ☐ -orexia
- ☐ -osis
- ☐ -otomy
- ☐ -pathy
- ☐ -pepsia
- ☐ -plasty
- ☐ -ptosis
- ☐ -rrhaphy
- ☐ -rrhea
- ☐ -scopy
- ☐ -sis
- ☐ -stomy
- ☐ -tomy
- ☐ -tripsy
- ☐ -y

Combining Forms

- ☐ abdomin/o
- ☐ amyl/o
- ☐ an/o
- ☐ append/o
- ☐ bil/i
- ☐ bucc/o
- ☐ cec/o
- ☐ celi/o
- ☐ cheil/o
- ☐ chol/e
- ☐ cholangi/o
- ☐ cholecyst/o
- ☐ choledoch/o
- ☐ cirrh/o
- ☐ col/o
- ☐ colon/o
- ☐ corpor/o
- ☐ cyst/o
- ☐ dent/o
- ☐ diverticul/o
- ☐ duoden/o
- ☐ enter/o
- ☐ esophag/e
- ☐ esophag/o
- ☐ fec/o
- ☐ gastr/o
- ☐ gingiv/o
- ☐ gloss/o
- ☐ halit/o
- ☐ hemat/o
- ☐ hemorrhoid/o
- ☐ hepat/o
- ☐ hern/o
- ☐ herni/o
- ☐ ile/o
- ☐ inguin/o
- ☐ jejun/o
- ☐ labi/o
- ☐ lapar/o
- ☐ leuk/o
- ☐ lingu/o

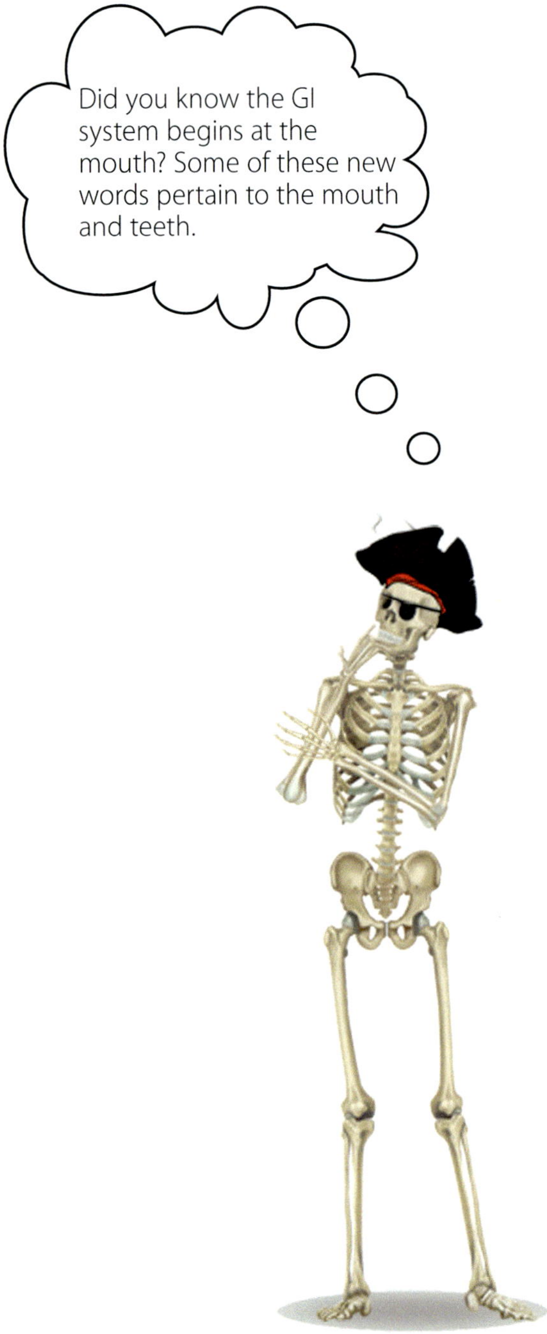

Combining Forms

- ☐ lith/o
- ☐ melan/o
- ☐ my/o
- ☐ nas/o
- ☐ occlus/o
- ☐ occult
- ☐ odont/o
- ☐ or/o
- ☐ ot/o
- ☐ palat/o
- ☐ pancreat/o
- ☐ peps/o
- ☐ pept/o
- ☐ perine/o
- ☐ peritone/o
- ☐ phag/o
- ☐ pharyng/o
- ☐ polyp/o
- ☐ proct/o
- ☐ pub/o
- ☐ py/o
- ☐ pylor/o
- ☐ rect/o
- ☐ rubin/o
- ☐ sial/o
- ☐ sigmoid/o
- ☐ spasm/o
- ☐ steat/o
- ☐ stomat/o
- ☐ uvul/o
- ☐ verm/i

Checklist of New Anatomy

Mouth

- ☐ Buccal cavity
- ☐ Teeth
    - ☐ Gingiva
    - ☐ Crown
    - ☐ Dentin
    - ☐ Pulp
- ☐ Tongue
    - ☐ Lingual frenulum
- ☐ Palate
    - ☐ Hard palate
    - ☐ Soft palate
- ☐ Uvula
- ☐ Salivary glands
    - ☐ Parotid
    - ☐ Sublingual
    - ☐ Submandibular

Throat

- ☐ Epiglottis
- ☐ Trachea
- ☐ Esophagus
- ☐ Lower esophageal sphincter

Stomach

- ☐ Fundus
- ☐ Antrum
- ☐ Pyloric sphincter

Intestines

- ☐ Small intestine
    - ☐ Duodenum
    - ☐ Jejunum
    - ☐ Ileum
    - ☐ Ileocecal valve
- ☐ Large intestine
    - ☐ Cecum
    - ☐ Appendix
    - ☐ Ascending colon
    - ☐ Transverse colon
    - ☐ Descending colon
    - ☐ Sigmoid colon
    - ☐ Rectum
    - ☐ Anus

Accessory Organs

- ☐ Liver
- ☐ Gallbladder
    - ☐ Cystic duct
    - ☐ Common bile duct
- ☐ Pancreas
    - ☐ Pancreatic duct

Introduction

Gastro Island is home to combining forms distinctive to the GI system. As you may have noted in your travel to other islands, several prefixes and suffixes are utilized in conjunction with word roots related to the GI system. The gold and silver coins (prefixes and suffixes) of word parts travel easily from body system to body system, and alter the word root or combining form to make it identifiable in relation to the system. Gastro Island contains words and word parts related to the teeth, mouth, stomach, and digestive tract, as well as the liver and pancreas.

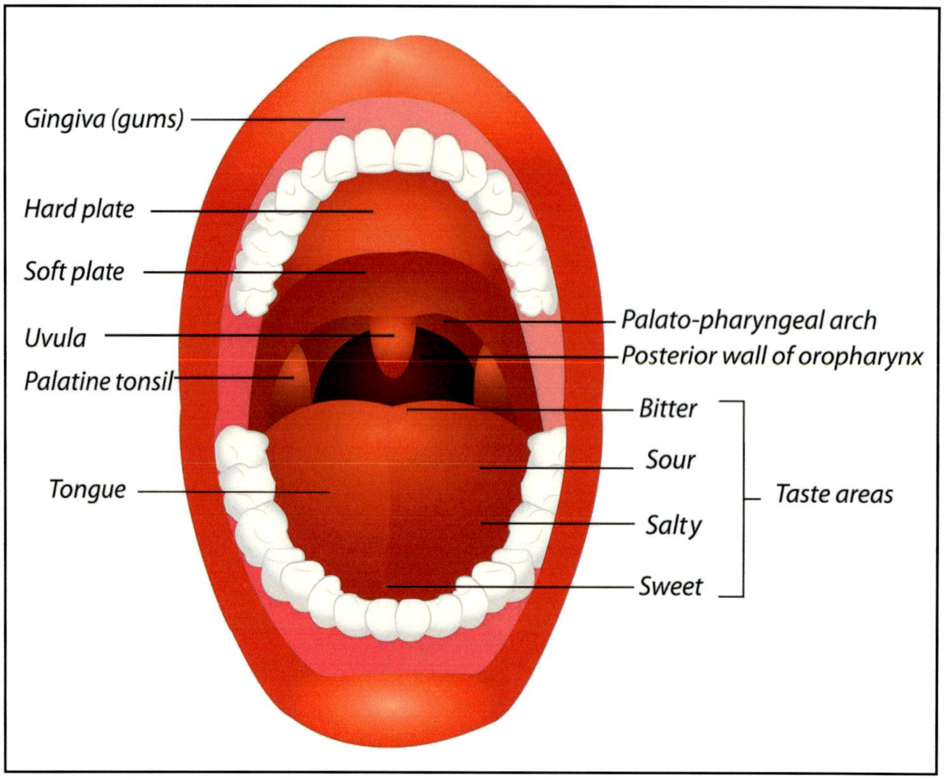

Figure 9-1. Digestion begins at the mouth with the teeth and tongue. (GRei/shutterstock.com)

Anatomy

The Mouth

The GI system is also referred to as the **alimentary tract** or **digestive system**. Digestion begins at the mouth, or the **buccal** (oral) cavity, where food is broken into smaller pieces by the teeth (Figure 9-1). The adult human has 32 permanent **teeth**, which are formed in 16 pairs that have special functions (Table 9-1 and Figure 9-2). **Deciduous teeth** are also referred to as **primary** or **baby teeth**, and appear shortly after birth until they are eventually replaced (6 to 21 years of age). Teeth are housed in the **gingiva** (gum), which is the top layer above the bones (the mandible and maxilla) holding them in place. The visible aspect of each tooth is covered in enamel and is called the **crown** when observable above the gingiva. Under the hard crown is the softer, spongy **dentin** layer, followed by the **pulp**. Each tooth root has its own blood and nerve supply within the pulp (Figure 9-3).

The roof of the mouth is actually termed the **palate** and is formed by bone in the anterior aspect of the mouth. As the palate moves posteriorly, it becomes the **soft palate**, made of soft tissue. From the soft palate hangs the **uvula**, which is a fleshy tissue used primarily in speech. As food is passed through the mouth by the muscular actions of the **tongue** and chewing (**mastication**), it is lubricated with **saliva**, which contains certain enzymes (**amylase**) that facilitate the breakdown of food. This partially chewed and moistened food is termed **bolus**. The tongue itself is a large muscle that has specific taste buds that primarily identify sweet, salty, sour, or bitter in different regions of the tongue. One cannot "swallow" their tongue, as it is firmly attached to the hyoid bone, epiglottis, and pharynx. Anteriorly, it is attached under the tongue by a thin membrane called the **lingual frenulum**.

Table 9-1

Names and Functions of Adult Teeth

NAME	AMOUNT (TOP/BOTTOM)	FUNCTION	LOCATION
incisors	4/4	Biting	Front of the mouth
cuspid (canine)	2/2	Tearing food into smaller pieces	Lateral and behind the incisors
bicuspid (premolars) **bi-** (two)	4/4	Tearing and grinding	Posterior to the cuspids (**bi-**—two; they have two surface points)
tricuspid (molars) **tri-** (three)	6/6	Grinding	Rear of the mouth (**tri-**—three; they have three surface points)

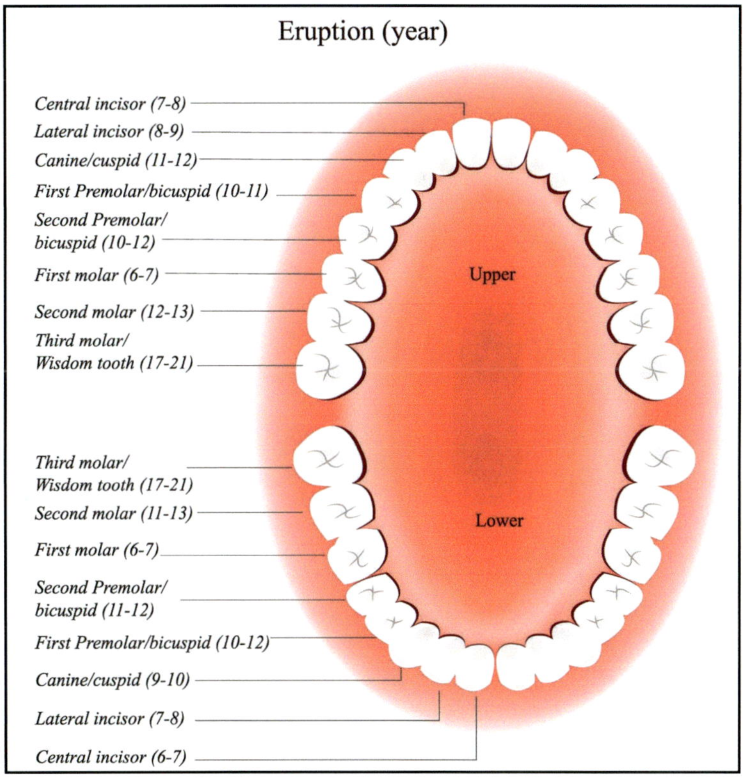

Figure 9-2. Teeth of the adult mouth. (GRei/shutterstock.com)

9

There are three main salivary glands, and they are named for the anatomical location in which they lie (Figure 9-4):

1. **Parotid salivary gland** (**par-**—near; **ot/**—ear; **nas/o**—nose; **pharyng/**—throat) the largest of the salivary glands
2. **Sublingual salivary gland** (**sub-**—under; **lingu/**—tongue) under the tongue
3. **Submandibular salivary gland** (**sub-**—under) under the mandible (jaw) bone

As moistened food passes the soft palate enroute to the pharynx (throat), swallowing reflexes pass the bolus into the esophagus.

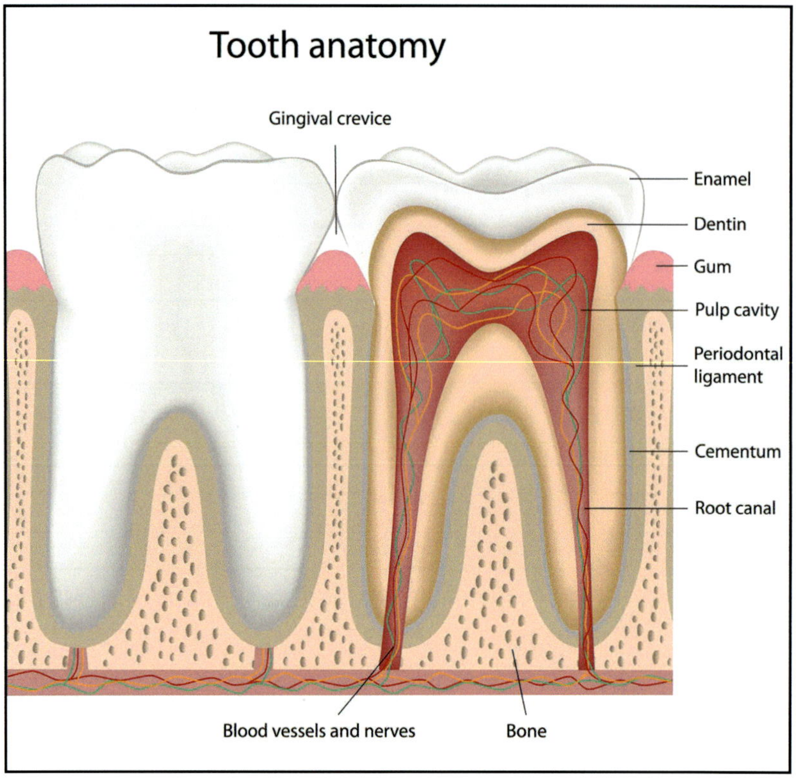

Figure 9-3. Anatomy of a tooth. (Alila Medical Images/shutterstock.com)

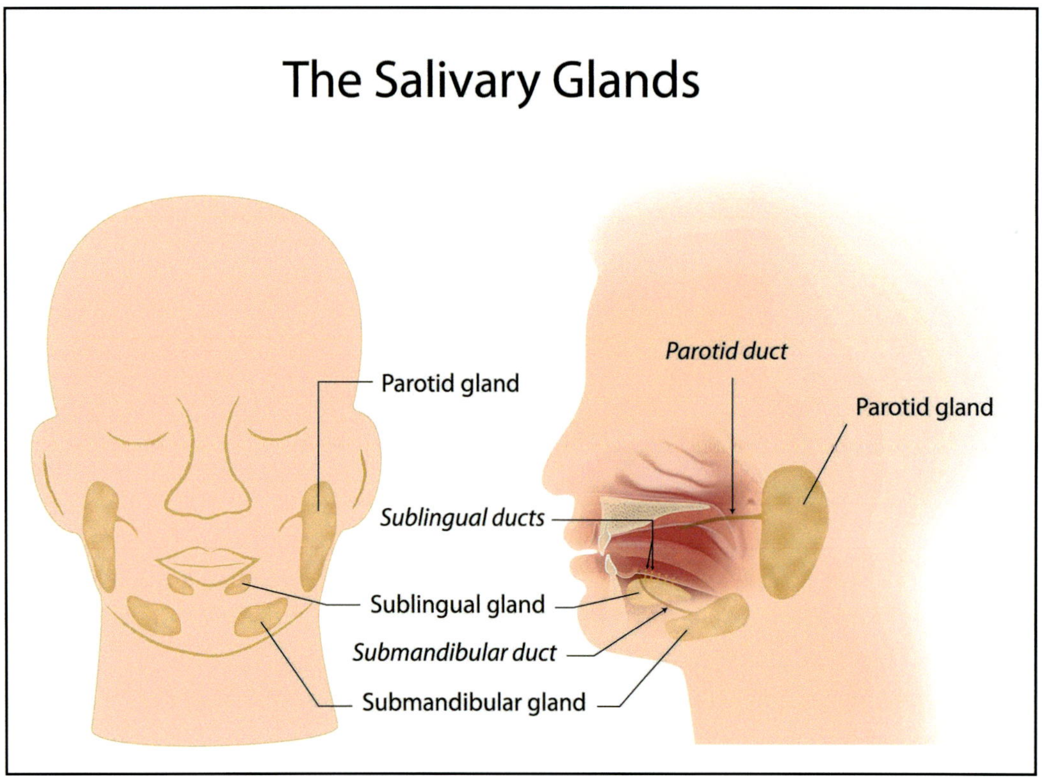

Figure 9-4. The salivary glands and ducts. (Alila Medical Images/shutterstock.com)

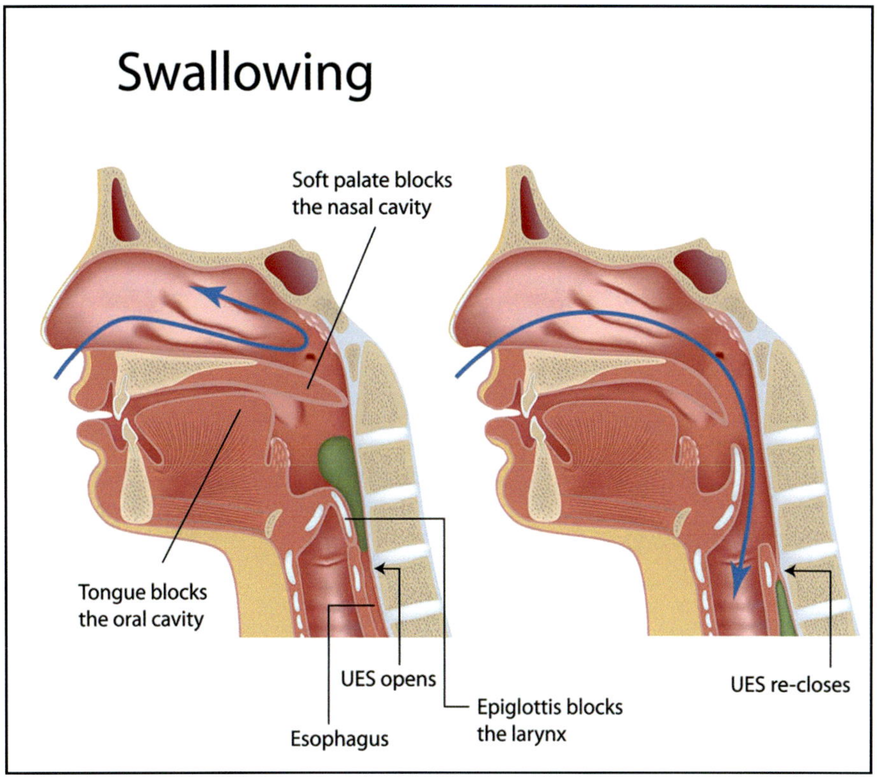

Figure 9-5. The epiglottis closes over the trachea to prevent food from entering it. (UES = upper esophageal spinchter.) (Alila Medical Images/shutterstock.com)

9

The **epiglottis** (**epi-**—above) prevents food from entering the **trachea** and **bronchi** by closing over the **larynx** each time a person swallows (Figure 9-5). An involuntary muscular action, **peristalsis**, moves food along the esophagus past the lower esophageal sphincter (**LES**), which opens into the stomach (Figure 9-6). The LES is also termed the **cardiac sphincter** and it keeps food from moving back up the esophagus after it enters the kidney-shaped stomach. In the stomach (word root: **gastr/o**) food is further broken down mainly due to hydrochloric acid (HCL). The upper aspect of the stomach is called the **fundus**, the middle portion is the **body**, and the lower end is the **antrum**. There are folds in the stomach (rugae) that stretch and expand to accommodate food and liquid (think: Thanksgiving dinner). In the stomach, the bolus is further decomposed with the help of HCL and enzymes into a semiliquid **chyme** (Figure 9-7).

The Intestines

Recall from Chapter 3 ("Body Organization and Anatomical Directions") that there are imaginary lines dividing the abdomen into quadrants. The umbilicus serves as the horizontal divider, and the *linea alba* (the fibrous tissue separating the vertical "six-pack" of the rectus abdominis muscle) acts as the vertical divider. These areas are most often abbreviated; for example, URQ is upper right quadrant, which is divided into the right and left sides by the umbilicus (navel).

The intestines and many organs of the abdomen are encased within a tough membrane, the **peritoneum**. Contents within the peritoneal cavity often do not have the same response to pain as do other structures outside of the peritoneum (eg, the kidneys, which lie in the retroperitoneal area [**retro-**—back, backward, behind]). Injuries or conditions arising within the peritoneum are often perceived as nonspecific pain, or as pressure instead of sharp pain. This is why some acute infections, such as appendicitis, often present as vague pain and pressure at first, and have pain away from the site of injury/infection. Both the appendix (**McBurney's point**: pain midway between the umbilicus [naval] and anterior superior iliac spine of the right ileum) and spleen (**Kerh's sign**: referred pain to left shoulder) can have pain away from the actual organ when injured.

The intestines begin at the distal end of the stomach where the chyme leaves and passes through the **pyloric sphincter.** There are two divisions of the **alimentary tract**: the small and large intestines (Figure 9-8). The small intestine is about 21 feet long and winds through the abdominal cavity where it has three distinct sections: the **duodenum**, **jejunum**, and **ileum**. The duodenum is merely an extension of the stomach and is less than 1 foot long, whereas the jejunum is about 8 feet in length, followed by the longest section of the intestine, the 12 feet of ileum. In the small intestine, bile from the liver and gallbladder and enzymes from the pancreas assist with breakdown and absorption of food nutrients as well as absorption and distribution of vitamins, minerals, and water. Small projections in the lining of the intestines (called **villi**) assist with removing essential nutriments and passing them along through capillaries and lymph to be distributed via the heart throughout the body.

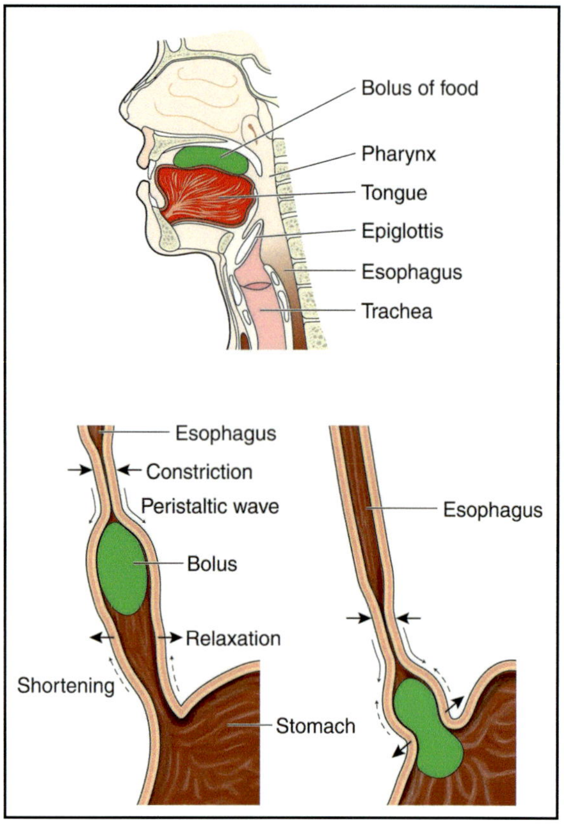

Figure 9-6. Swallowing occurs via peristalsis. (Blamb/shutterstock.com)

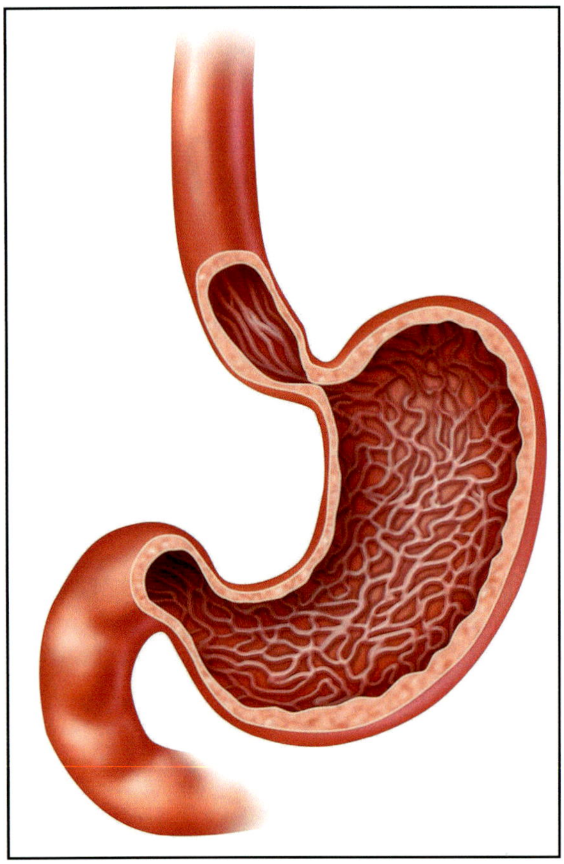

Figure 9-7. The stomach. (Lightspring/shutterstock.com)

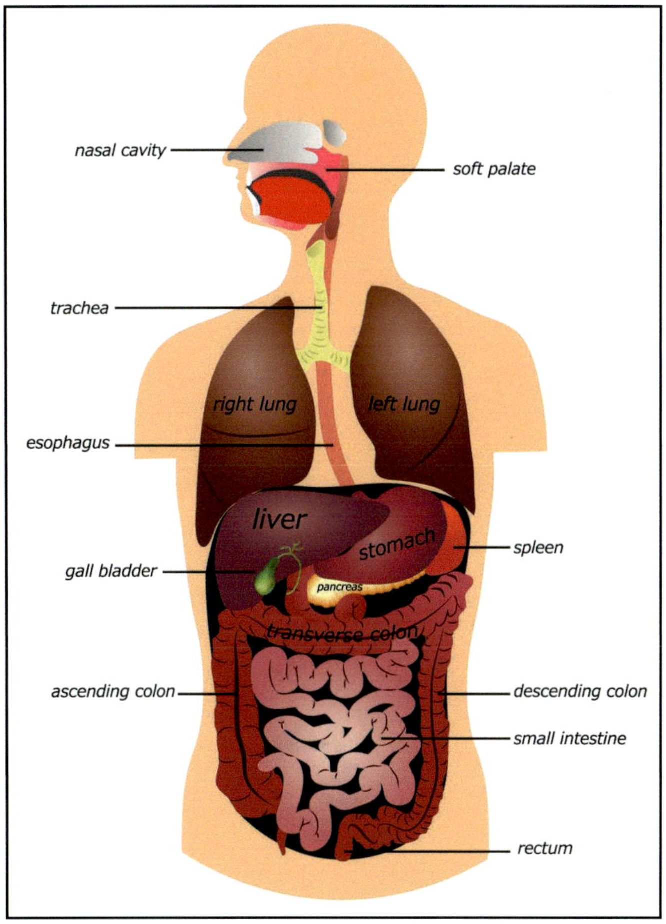

Figure 9-8. Overview of the organs of the GI system. (GRei/shutterstock.com)

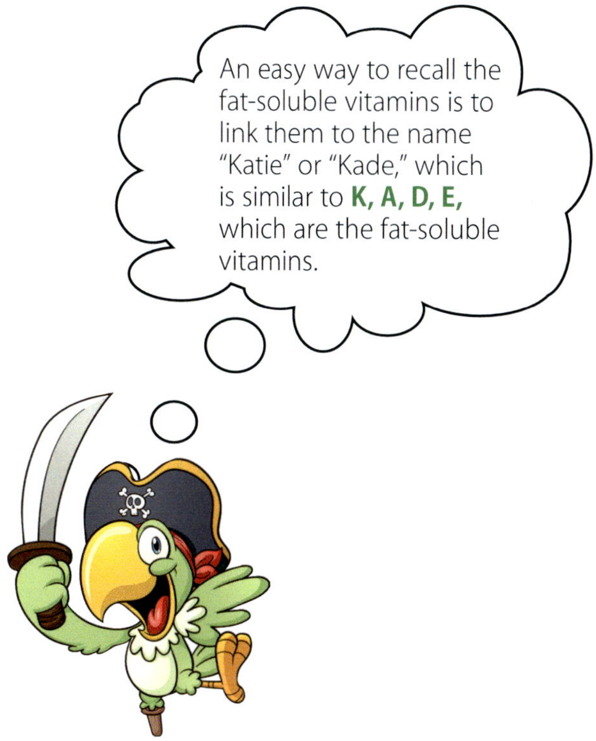
An easy way to recall the fat-soluble vitamins is to link them to the name "Katie" or "Kade," which is similar to **K, A, D, E,** which are the fat-soluble vitamins.

The 5-foot long large intestine begins with the **ileocecal valve** that joins the small intestine to the **cecum**, a small pouch that joins the two intestines. The **vermiform appendix** (called simply, *the appendix*) is a small sack with little known function that attaches to the cecum (vermiform comes from a word meaning "worm-like"). The large intestine, often referred to as the **colon**, begins in the lower right quadrant (LRQ) of the abdomen and moves superiorly as the **ascending colon** to the upper right quadrant (URQ), then across to the upper left quadrant (ULQ; **transverse colon**), then inferiorly as the **descending colon**, ending at the S-shaped **sigmoid colon** in the lower left quadrant (LLQ). The large intestine ends with the **rectum**, where waste is stored until eliminated voluntarily via the **anus**.

Accessory Organs and Glands

Digestion occurs with the aid of several accessory organs and glands. It begins in the mouth with salivary **amylase**, an enzyme secreted from the salivary glands into saliva that helps break down carbohydrates. The **liver**, the largest organ within the body, is said to have over 500 functions, and is located in the upper right quadrant of the abdomen. In the GI system, the liver manages metabolism of carbohydrates, proteins, and fats. It also changes glucose (sugar) to glycogen to stockpile it for later use and stores fat-soluble vitamins (K, A, D, E) and iron. The liver secretes **bile**, which is a compound that emulsifies (breaks down) fats into smaller units, into the duodenum and stores the bile in the **gallbladder** housed under the liver. Another critical aspect of digestion comes from the **pancreas**. This gland secretes digestive enzymes as well as bicarbonate to neutralize the HCL in the stomach. The pancreas is discussed in more detail in Chapter 11 ("Endocrine System"). Both the gallbladder and pancreas have ducts that provide a means to transport necessary digestive components to the small intestine. The gallbladder has a **cystic duct** and **common bile duct**, and the pancreas has the **pancreatic duct** emptying into the small intestine to facilitate digestion (Figure 9-9). These pathways are often used in describing locations for medical conditions or procedures. It can take 4 to 12 hours to complete a digestive process, from ingestion to voluntary elimination, depending on the person and food consumed.

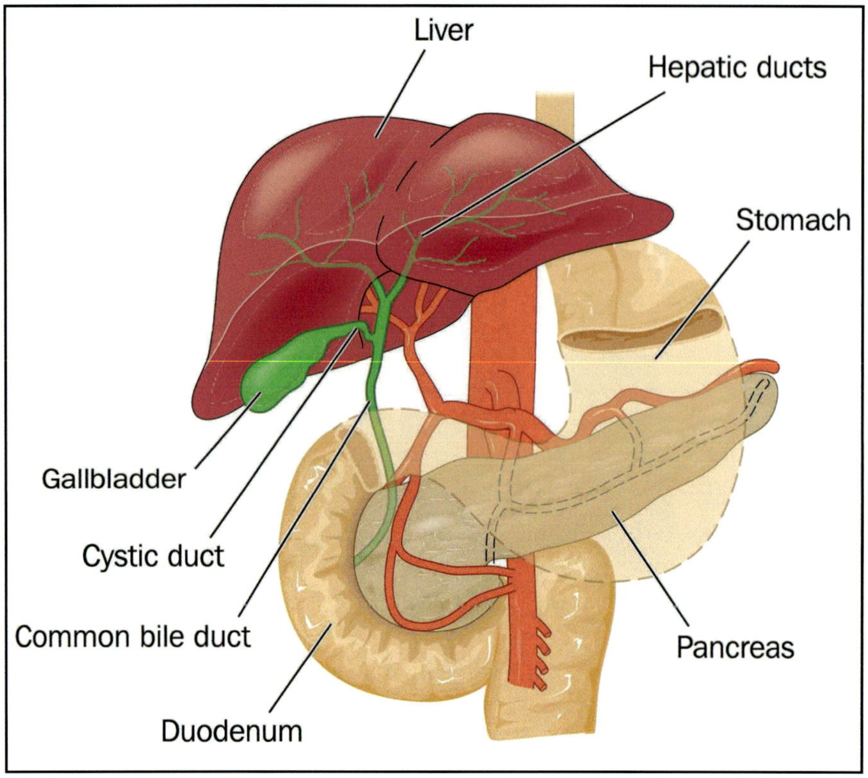

Figure 9-9. The ducts of the gallbladder. (Blamb/shutterstock.com)

Word Building

Table 9-2
Prefixes

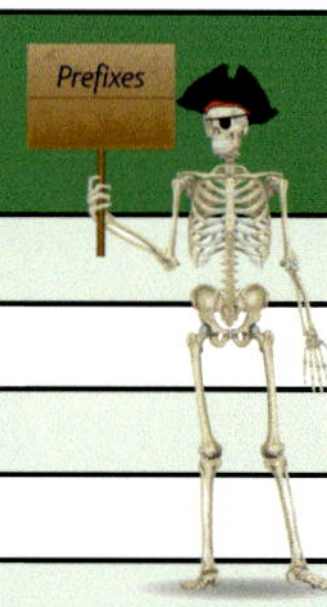

PREFIX	DEFINITION
a-; an-	not; without
ad-	toward; near
anti-	against
bi-	two
dia-	across; through
dys-	painful; difficult; abnormal; bad
eme-	to vomit
endo-	in; within
extra-	outside
hyper-	above; excessive; high; increased
mal-	bad
pan-	all
par-	alongside; around; beside; near
peri-	around
re-; retro-	back; backward; behind
sub-	under; below
tri-	three

TABLE 9-3
SUFFIXES

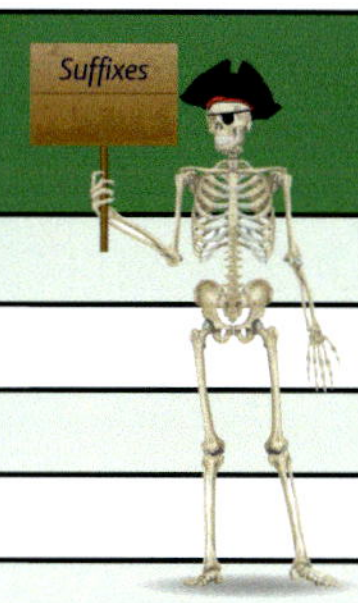

SUFFIX	DEFINITION
-ac; -al	pertaining to
-algia	pain
-ary	pertaining to
-ase	enzyme
-cele	hernia; protrusion; swelling
-centesis	puncture; surgical puncture
-dynia	pain
-ectomy	excision; surgical removal
-emesis	vomiting
-emia	blood condition
-gram	a record of
-ia	condition
-iasis	condition
-ic	pertaining to
-ion	process; the act of
-itis	inflammation
-malacia	softening
-megaly	abnormally large; enlargement
-occlus/o	to close
-oid	resembling
-oma	mass; tumor
-orexia	appetite
-osis	condition
-otomy	incision; cutting into
-pathy	disease
-pepsia	digestion
-plasty	reconstruction; repair; plastic surgery
-ptosis	drooping; falling; prolapse
-rrhaphy	suture; surgical repair
-rrhea	excessive flow; discharge
-scopy	examination of
-sis	condition; state of
-stomy	surgical opening
-tomy	incision; to cut into
-tripsy	crushing
-y	process of

Table 9-4
Combining Forms

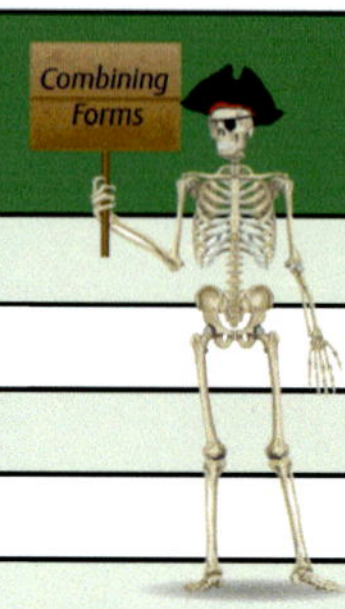

COMBINING FORM	DEFINITION
abdomin/o	abdomen
amyl/o	starch
an/o	anus
append/o	appendix
bil/i	bile
bucc/o	cheek
cec/o	cecum; intestine
celi/o	abdomen
cheil/o	lip
chol/e	bile; gall
cholangi/o	bile vessel
cholecyst/o	gallbladder (cyst = bladder)
choledoch/o	bile duct
cirrh/o	orange
col/o; colon/o	colon
corpor/o	body
cyst/o	bladder; sac
dent/o	teeth; dental
diverticul/o	small pouch
duoden/o	duodenum
esophag/e; esophag/o	esophagus
fec/o	feces; stool
gastr/o	stomach; abdomen
gingiv/o	gum
gloss/o	tongue
halit/o	breath
hemat/o	blood
hemorrhoid/o	vascular protrusion through a weakened wall or membrane of the anus
hepat/o	liver
hern/o; herni/o	hernia, rupture, or weakened wall/membrane
ile/o	ileum
inguin/o	groin
jejun/o	jejunum; empty
labi/o	lip
lapar/o	abdomen
leuk/o	white
lingu/o	tongue

(continued)

Table 9-4 (continued)
Combining Forms

COMBINING FORM	DEFINITION
lith/o	stone
melan/o	black
my/o	muscle
occlus/o	to close
occult	hidden
odont/o	tooth
or/o	mouth
ot/o	ear
palat/o	palate; roof of mouth
pancreat/o	pancreas; sweetbread
peps/o; pept/o	digestion
perine/o	perineum
peritone/o	peritoneum; membrane; to stretch; to stretch over
phag/o	eating; swallowing
pharyng/o	throat; pharynx
polyp/o	polyp; a small growth
proct/o	rectum; anus
py/o	pus
pylor/o	pylorus; gatekeeper
rect/o	rectum; erect; straight
rubin/o	red pigment
sial/o	saliva
sigmoid/o	the letter S
spasm/o	spasm; sudden involuntary contraction
steat/o	fat
stomat/o	mouth
uvul/o	grape; mouth
verm/i	worm

Signs and Symptoms

Table 9-5

Signs and Symptoms Related to the Gastrointestinal System

SIGN/SYMPTOM	WORD PARTS	DEFINITION
anorexia	**an-** (without) **-orexia** (appetite)	Lack of appetite (not like anorexia nervosa, a separate condition with behavioral issues)
aphagia	**a-** (without) phag/ (swallowing) **-ia** (condition)	Inability to swallow
dentalgia	dent/ (tooth) **-algia** (pain)	Toothache
diarrhea	**dia-** (across; through) **-rrhea** (excessive flow)	Excessive watery discharge of feces
dyspepsia	**dys-** (difficult) **-pepsia** (digestion)	Indigestion, difficult digestion
dysphagia	**dys-** (difficult) phag/ (swallowing) **-ia** (condition)	Difficulty swallowing
eructation		Producing gas from the stomach through the mouth (belching)
gastrodynia	gastr/o (stomach) **-dynia** (pain)	Stomachache
halitosis	halit/ (breath) **-osis** (condition)	Bad breath
hematemesis	hemat/ (blood) **-emesis** (vomiting)	Vomiting blood
hepatomegaly	hepat/o (liver) **-megaly** (enlargement)	Enlarged liver
hyperbilirubinemia	**hyper-** (excessive) bil/i (bile) rubin/ (red pigment) **-emia** (blood condition)	Excessive levels of red bile pigment in the blood
jaundice		Yellowing of the skin, mucous membranes, and eyes due to the liver's inability to remove bilirubin
malocclusion	**mal-** (bad) occlus/ (to close) **-ion** (the act of)	Situation where the jaw does not close properly, creating malalignment of teeth; may be caused by mandible deformity
melena	melan/ (black)	Black, tarry stools; usually caused by the presence of partially digested blood in the feces

(continued)

TABLE 9-5 (CONTINUED) SIGNS AND SYMPTOMS RELATED TO THE GASTROINTESTINAL SYSTEM		
SIGN/SYMPTOM	**WORD PARTS**	**DEFINITION**
pyorrhea	py/o (pus) **-rrhea** (discharge)	Discharge of pus; in this situation it is the inflammation of the gums in the mouth distinguished by purulent material and eventual loosening of the teeth
reflux (Figure 9-10)	**re-** (back)	To flow backward; regurgitation into esophagus
steatorrhea	steat/o (fat) **-rrhea** (excessive flow)	Abnormal levels of fat in the feces

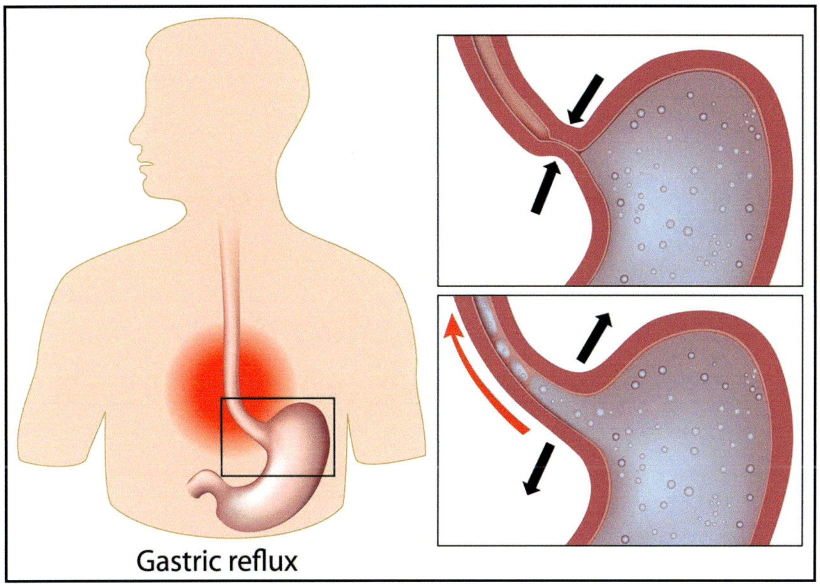

Figure 9-10. The mechanism of reflux is when stomach contents are able to pass back up past the lower esophageal sphincter. (Alila Medical Images/shutterstock.com)

MEDICAL CONDITIONS

TABLE 9-6 MEDICAL CONDITIONS RELATED TO THE GASTROINTESTINAL SYSTEM		
NAME	**WORD PARTS**	**DEFINITION**
appendicitis (Figure 9-11)	append/ (appendix) **-ic** (pertaining to) **-itis** (inflammation)	Inflammation of the appendix
cholangioma	cholangi/ (bile vessel) **-oma** (tumor)	Tumor originating from the bile duct
cholecystitis	chol/e (gall) cyst/ (bladder) **-itis** (inflammation)	Inflammation of the gallbladder
		(continued)

9

Table 9-6 (continued)
Medical Conditions Related to the Gastrointestinal System

NAME	WORD PARTS	DEFINITION
choledocholithiasis	choledoch/o (bile duct) lith/ (stone) **-iasis** (condition)	Gallstones in the bile duct
cholelithiasis (Figure 9-13)	chol/e (gall) lith/ (stone) **-iasis** (condition)	Gallstones
cirrhosis (Figure 9-14)	cirrh/ (orange) **-osis** (condition)	Chronic degenerative liver disorder resulting in the organ being infiltrated with fat
diverticulitis (Figure 9-15)	diverticul/ (small pouch) **-itis** (inflammation)	Inflammation of the diverticula (small pouches) within the colon
diverticulosis	diverticul/ (small pouch) **-osis** (condition)	Abnormal small pouches in the colon
dysentery	**dys-** (difficult; bad; painful) enter/ (intestines) **-y** (process of)	Severe inflammation of the small intestine; often caused by an infection
enteritis	enter/ (intestines) **-itis** (inflammation)	Inflammation of the small intestine
gastritis	gastr/ (stomach) **-itis** (inflammation)	Inflammation of the stomach
gastroenterocolitis	gastr/o (stomach) enter/o (intestines) col/ (colon) **-itis** (inflammation)	Inflammation of the stomach, small intestine, and colon
gastroenteritis	gastr/o (stomach) enter/ (intestines) **-itis** (inflammation)	Inflammation of the stomach and small intestine
gastroesophageal reflux disease (GERD)	gastr/o (stomach) esophag/ (esophagus) **-al** (pertaining to) **re-** (back)	Condition when stomach contents back up the esophagus out of the stomach due to a weak or ineffective esophageal sphincter
gastromalacia	gastr/o (stomach) **-malacia** (softening)	Softening of the lining of the stomach
gingivitis (Figure 9-16)	gingiv/ (gums) **-itis** (inflammation)	Inflammation of the gums
glossopathy	gloss/o (tongue) **-pathy** (disease)	Disease of the tongue
hemorrhoid (Figure 9-17)	hemorrh/ (likely to bleed) **-oid** (resembling)	Varicose vein near the anus that may cause bleeding

(continued)

Table 9-6 (continued)

Medical Conditions Related to the Gastrointestinal System

NAME	WORD PARTS	DEFINITION
hepatitis	hepat/ (liver) **-itis** (inflammation)	Inflammation of the liver; it has several varieties (A to D) caused by contact with contaminated blood, food, or sexual contact
hepatoma	hepat/ (liver) **-oma** (tumor)	Tumor of the liver
hepatomegaly	hepat/o (liver) **-megaly** (enlargement)	Enlargement of the liver
leukoplakia	leuk/o (white)	Abnormal thickening of the mucous membranes of the mouth and tongue; appears white and may be a precursor of oral cancers
palatitis	palat/ (roof of mouth) **-itis** (inflammation)	Inflammation of the roof of the mouth
pancreatitis (Figure 9-18)	pancreat/ (pancreas) **-itis** (inflammation)	Inflammation of the pancreas
parotitis	**par-** (near) ot/ (ear) **-itis** (inflammation)	Inflammation of the parotid (saliva) gland; also called *mumps*
periodontal disease (Figure 9-19)	**peri-** (around) odont/ (tooth)	Group of conditions that lead to inflammation around the tooth, including gingivitis
peritonitis	perit/ (peritoneum) **-itis** (inflammation)	Inflammation of the peritoneum
polyposis	polyp/ (polyp) **-osis** (condition)	Condition of many polyps in the colon
proctoptosis	proct/o (rectum/anus) **-ptosis** (falling; prolapse)	Prolapse or falling of the rectum through the anus
rectocele	rect/o (rectum) **-cele** (hernia)	A hernia of part of the rectum
sialoadenitis	sial/o (saliva) aden/ (gland) **-itis** (inflammation)	Inflammation of the salivary gland
sialolith	sial/o (saliva) lith/ (stone)	Calcified or mineralized object, or stone, in the saliva gland
stomatitis	stomat/ (mouth) **-itis** (inflammation)	Inflammation in the mouth, often called *canker sores*

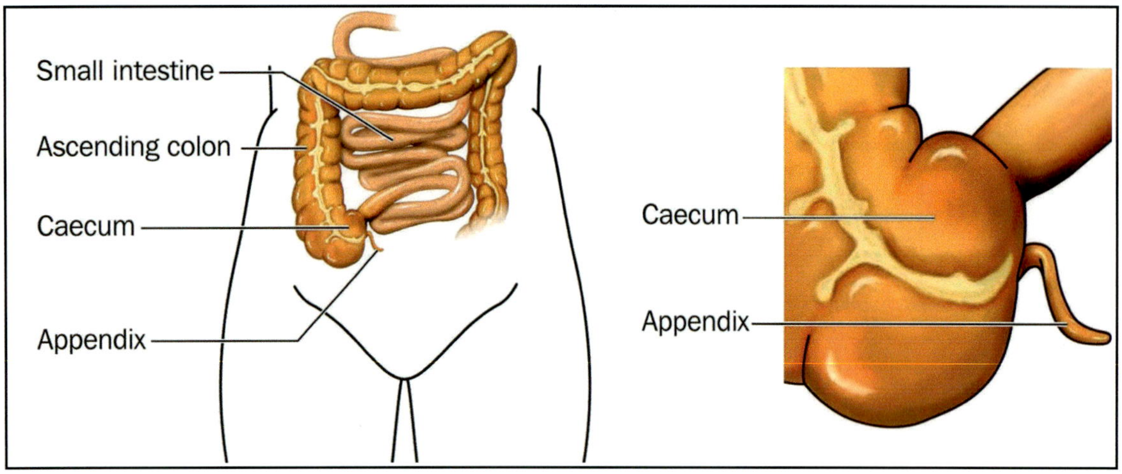

Figure 9-11. Appendicitis is an inflammation of the vermiform appendix. (Blamb/shutterstock.com)

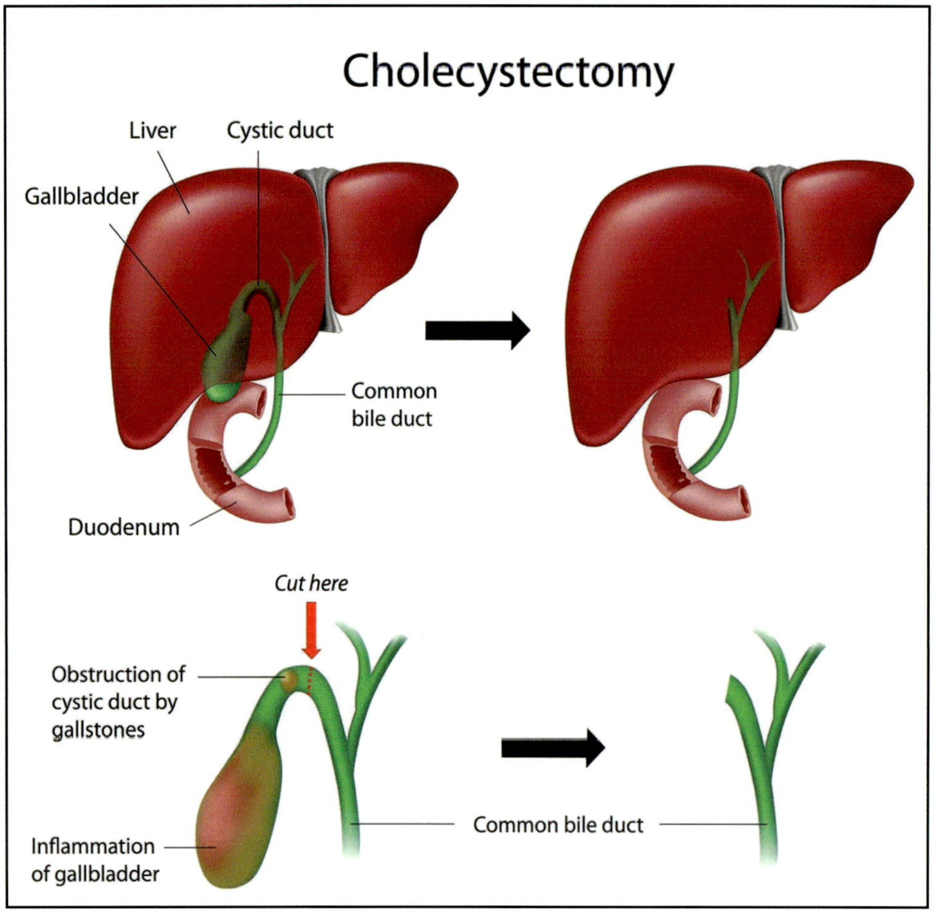

Figure 9-12. Cholecystectomy. (Alila Medical Images/shutterstock.com)

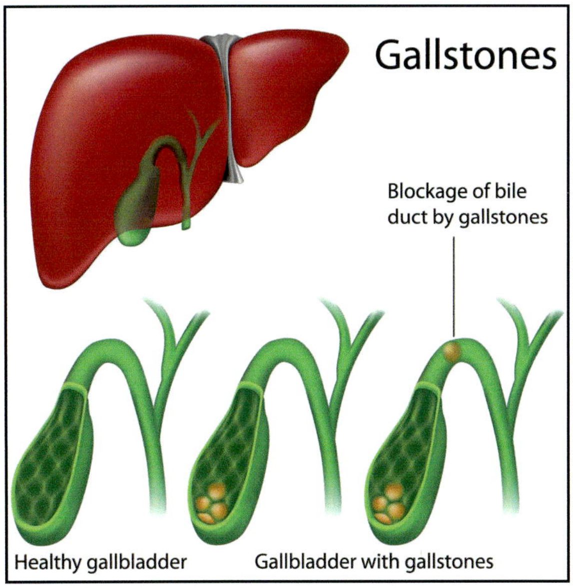

Figure 9-13. Choledocholithiasis, or gallstones, in the common bile duct. (Alila Medical Images/shutterstock.com)

Figure 9-14. Comparison of a normal liver (bottom) and one with cirrhosis (top). (ANATOMIA3D/shutterstock.com)

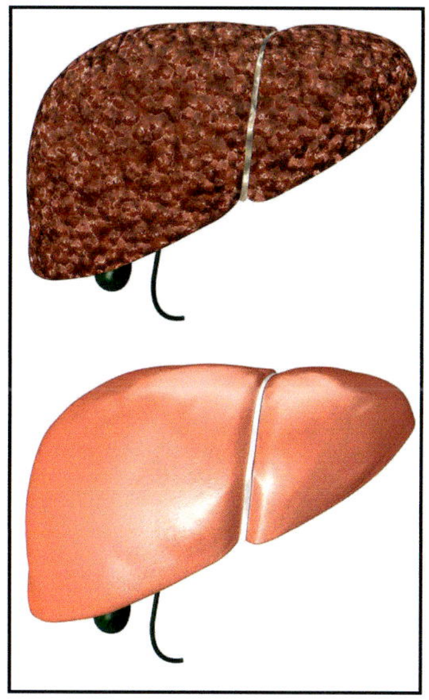

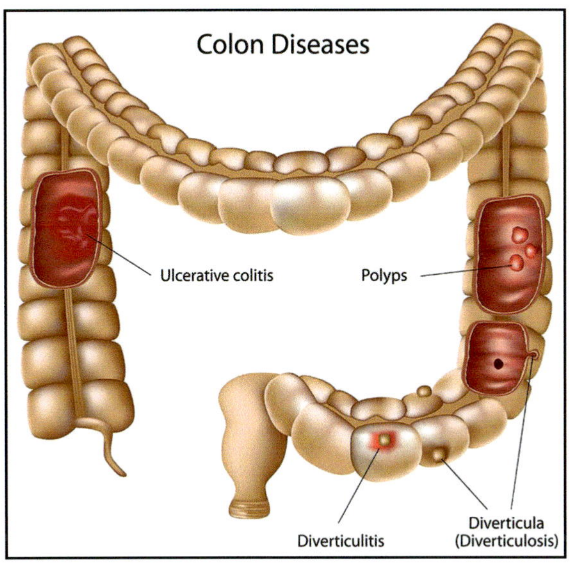

Figure 9-15. Diverticulitis and polyps in a colon. (Alila Medical Images/shutterstock.com)

Figure 9-16. Gingivitis, or inflammation of the gums. (miucci/shutterstock.com)

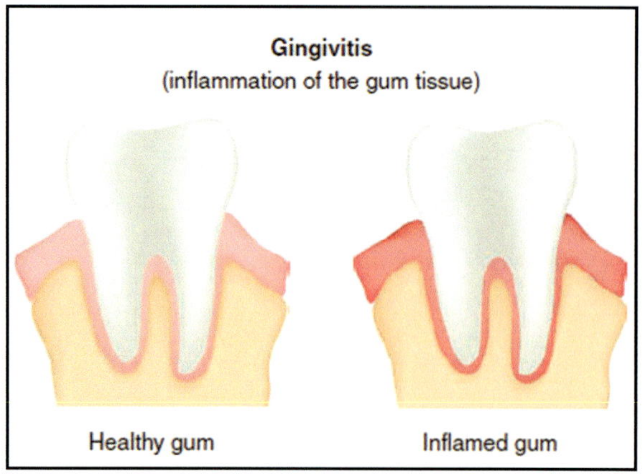

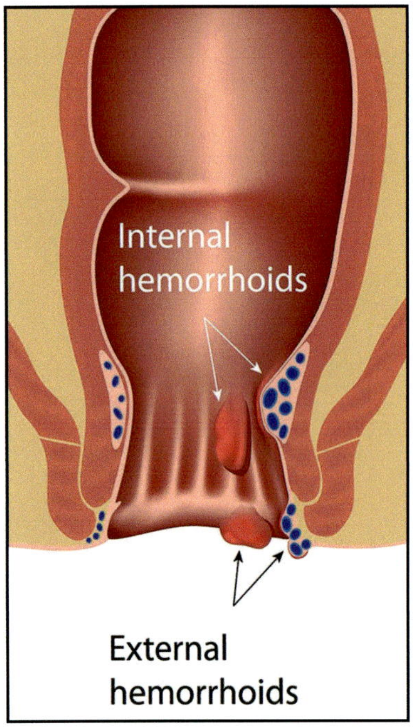

Figure 9-17. Hemorrhoids are found both internal and external to the anus. (Alila Medical Images/shutterstock.com)

Figure 9-18. Acute pancreatitis may have several causes, including a blocked pancreatic duct. (Alila Medical Images/shutterstock.com)

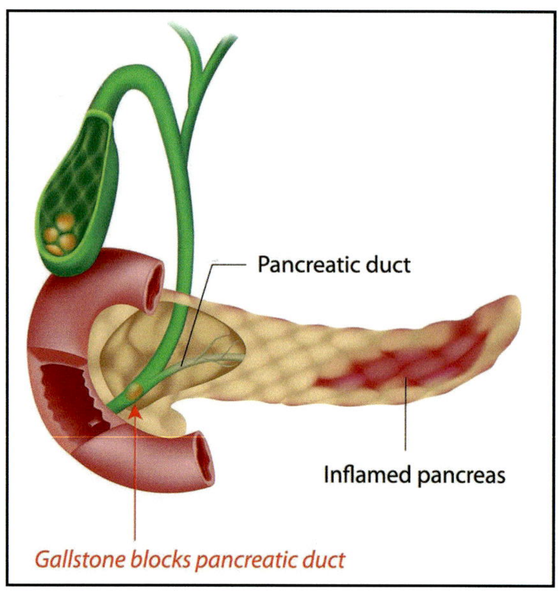

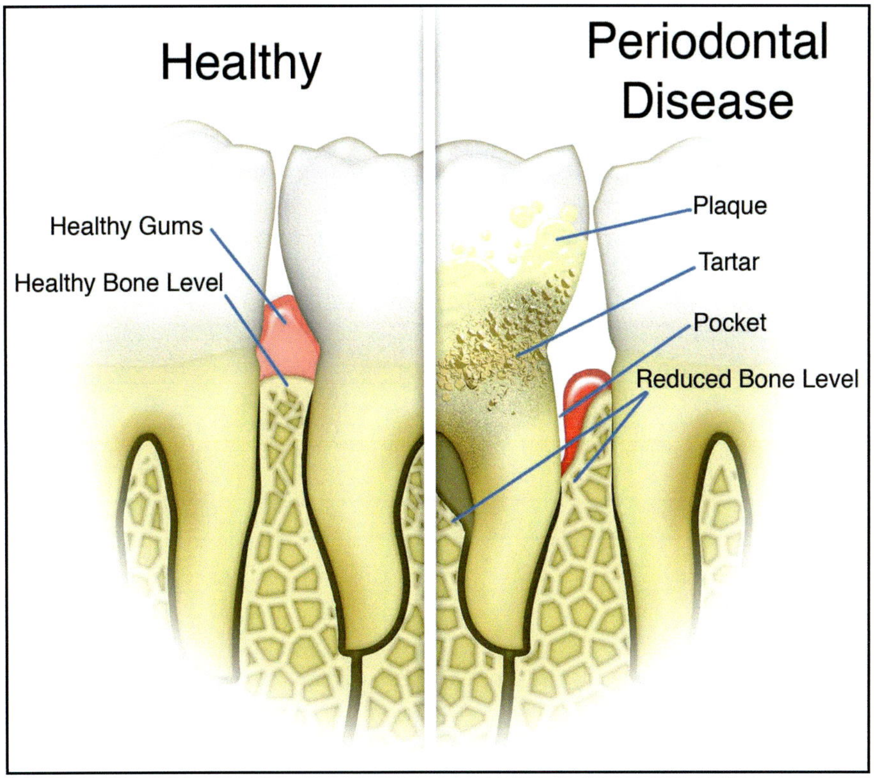

Figure 9-19. Comparison of healthy teeth and gums and periodontal disease. (Highforge Solutions/shutterstock.com)

Table 9-7
Gastrointestinal Terms Without Common Word Parts

TERM	DEFINITION
ascites	Accumulation of serous fluid in the abdominal (peritoneal) cavity
borborygmus	Audible noise of digestion caused by gases moving through the digestive tract
cleft palate	Birth defect where an infant's palate and/or lip do not join as normal
Crohn's disease	chronic inflammation of the GI tract; most often in the ileum
gavage	To provide liquid or semisolid material via a feeding tube
giardiasis	Infection caused by a protozoa, causing vomiting, cramping, and diarrhea
inflammatory bowel disease (IBD)	Group of conditions causing inflammation in the GI tract
irritable bowel syndrome (IBS)	Chronic GI condition that vacillates between diarrhea and constipation
lavage	Process of washing a cavity (eg, stomach, abdominal cavity) with saline solution, typically prior to or following endoscopy or surgery
mumps	Acute viral disease (usually in children) characterized by swelling of the parotid glands
temporomandibular joint (TMJ) dysfunction	Pain at the joint where the mandible (jaw) and temporal (skull) bones join; often due to grinding teeth while sleeping
volvulus	Obstructed intestine due to its twisting on itself

Table 9-8
Types of Hernias

TYPE	LOCATION/DEFINITION
hiatal hernia (Figure 9-20)	Hernia that protrudes upward into the aspect of the diaphragm where the esophagus usually passes; also termed *esophageal hiatus*
inguinal hernia	When an aspect of the small intestine protrudes through the abdominal wall into the inguinal (groin) area
sports hernia (athletic pubalgia)	Unlike a hernia, this is a soft tissue (muscle, tendon) strain in the region of the groin and is a musculoskeletal injury, not a GI condition (pub/o—pubic bone; **-algia**—pain)
strangulated hernia	When a hernia is constricted, reducing blood flow to nearby organs
umbilical hernia	When a portion of the small intestine protrudes through the abdominal wall near the naval (umbilicus)
Hernias are named after their anatomical location or condition.	

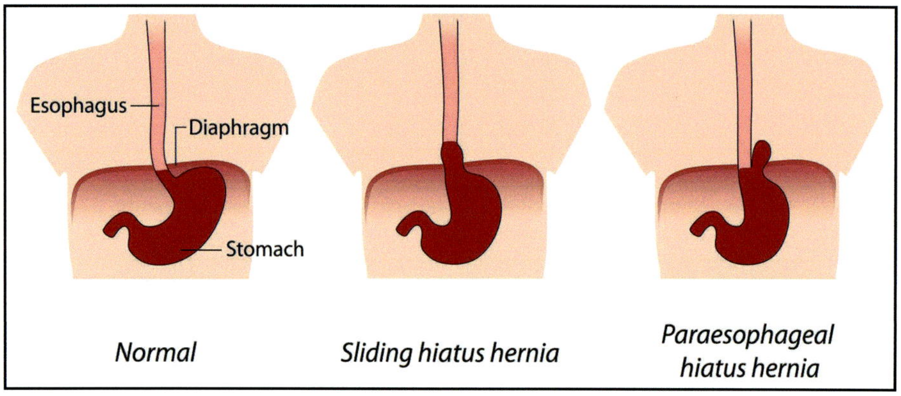

Figure 9-20. Hiatal hernia is when part of the stomach protrudes into and above the diaphragm. (Alila Medical Images/shutterstock.com)

Tests and Procedures

Table 9-9
Tests and Procedures Related to the Gastrointestinal System

NAME	WORD PARTS	PURPOSE
abdominocentesis	abdomin/o (abdomen) **-centesis** (surgical puncture)	Surgical puncture into the abdominal cavity to remove excess fluid; also termed *paracentesis*
abdominoplasty	abdomin/o (abdomen) **-plasty** (repair)	Surgical repair of the abdomen
anoplasty	an/o (anus) **-plasty** (repair)	Surgical repair of the anus
appendectomy	append/ (appendix) **-ectomy** (surgical removal)	Surgical removal of the appendix

(*continued*)

TABLE 9-9 (CONTINUED) TESTS AND PROCEDURES RELATED TO THE GASTROINTESTINAL SYSTEM		
NAME	**WORD PARTS**	**PURPOSE**
celiotomy	celi/ (abdomen) **-otomy** (incision)	Surgical incision into the abdominal cavity
cheilorrhaphy	cheil/o (lip) **-rrhaphy** (suturing)	Suturing of the lip
cholangiogram	cholangi/o (bile vessel) **-gram** (a record of)	X-ray image using contrast medium injected in the vessels that provides an image of the bile ducts
cholecystectomy	chol/e (gall) cyst/ (bladder) **-ectomy** (surgical removal)	Surgical removal of the gallbladder
choledocholithotomy	choledoch/ (bile duct) lith/ (stone) **-otomy** (incision)	Cutting into the common bile duct (usually to remove stones)
colectomy (Figure 9-21)	col/ (colon) **-ectomy** (surgical removal)	Surgical removal of all or part of the colon
colonoscopy (Figure 9-22)	colon/o (colon) **-scopy** (examination of)	Visual examination of the colon using a colonoscope
endoscopic examination	**endo-** (within) **-scopic** (pertaining to visual examination)	Use of an endoscope to view within the body cavities, usually within the GI system
esophagogastro-duodenoscopy (EGD)	esophag/o (esophagus) gastr/o (stomach) duoden/o (duodenum) **-scopy** (examination of)	Visual examination of the esophagus, stomach, and duodenum using an endoscope
extracorporeal shock wave	**extra-** (outside) corpor/ (body) **-al** (pertaining to)	Noninvasive procedure using ultrasonic sound waves to crush gallbladder or kidney stones
fecal occult blood test	fec/ (feces; stool) **-al** (pertaining to) occult/ (hidden)	Fecal smear test examining for hidden blood in the stool (feces)
hemorrhoidectomy	hemorrhoid/ (vascular protrusion through a weakened wall or membrane of the anus) **-ectomy** (surgical removal)	Surgical removal of hemorrhoids
herniorrhaphy	herni/o (hernia) **-rrhaphy** (surgical repair)	Surgical repair of a hernia

(continued)

Table 9-9 (continued)
Tests and Procedures Related to the Gastrointestinal System

NAME	WORD PARTS	PURPOSE
laparotomy	lapar/ (abdomen) **-otomy** (incision)	Minimally invasive procedure to perform abdominal surgeries
lithotripsy (Figure 9-23)	lith/o (stone) **-tripsy** (crushing)	Procedure for crushing stones in the gallbladder or kidney so they may be small enough to be eliminated
nasal cannula	nas/ (nose)	Tubes inserted at the tip of the nares to provide oxygen
nasogastric intubation	nas/o (nose) gastr/ (stomach) **-ic** (pertaining to)	Tube inserted through the nostril to the stomach to remove gases or food, or introduce medications or food
odontectomy	odont/ (tooth) **-ectomy** (surgical removal)	Surgical extraction of a tooth
palatoplasty	palat/o (palate) **-plasty** (repair)	Surgical repair of the palate
pyloromyotomy	pylor/o (pylorus) my/o (muscle) **-tomy** (incision)	Incision into the pyloric sphincter to broaden the opening

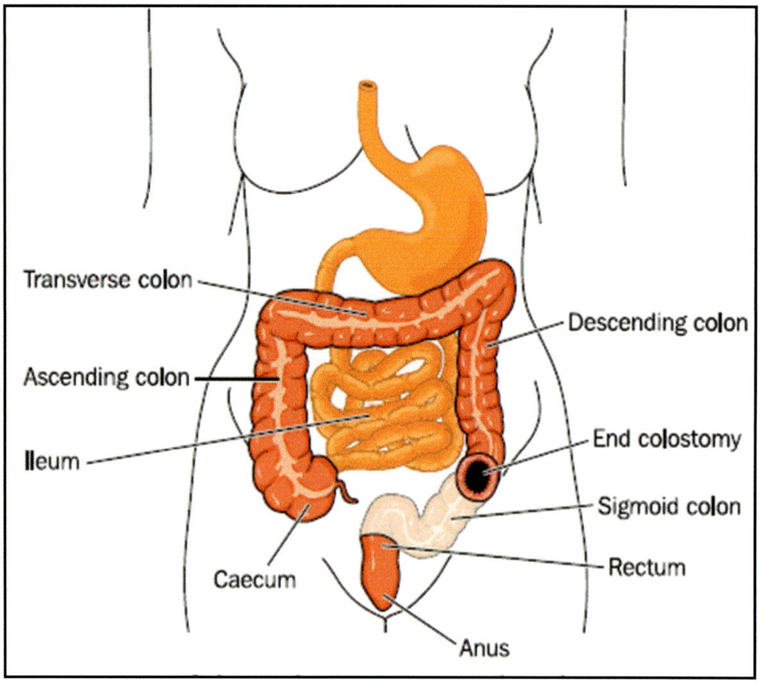

Figure 9-21. When a portion of the colon is removed (colectomy), an artificial opening (stoma) is created to eliminate waste. (Alila Medical Images/shutterstock.com)

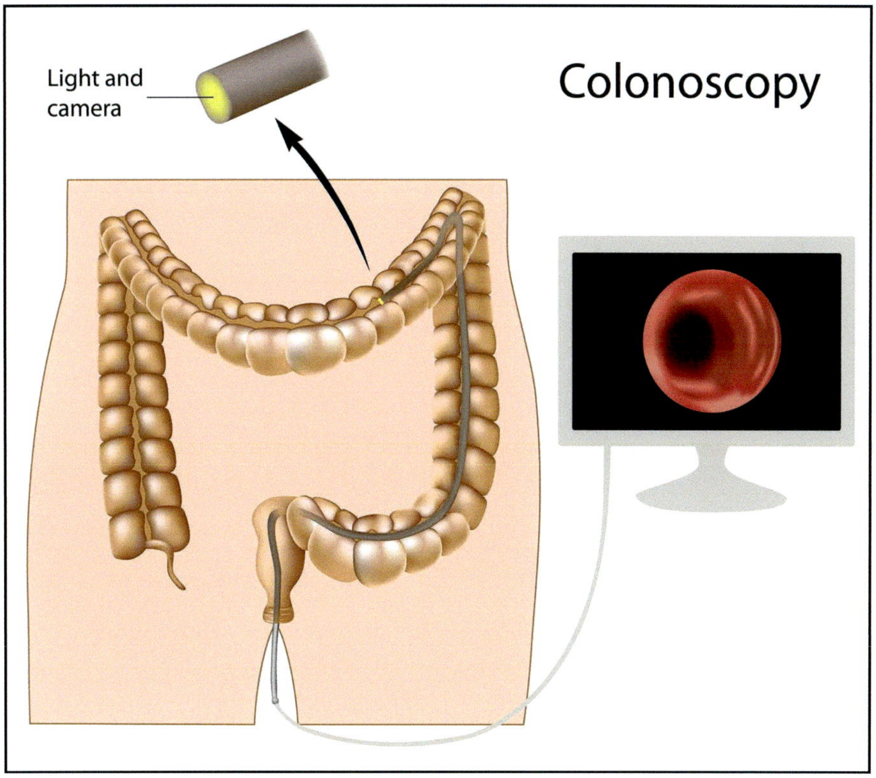

Figure 9-22. Colonoscopy. (Alila Medical Images/shutterstock.com)

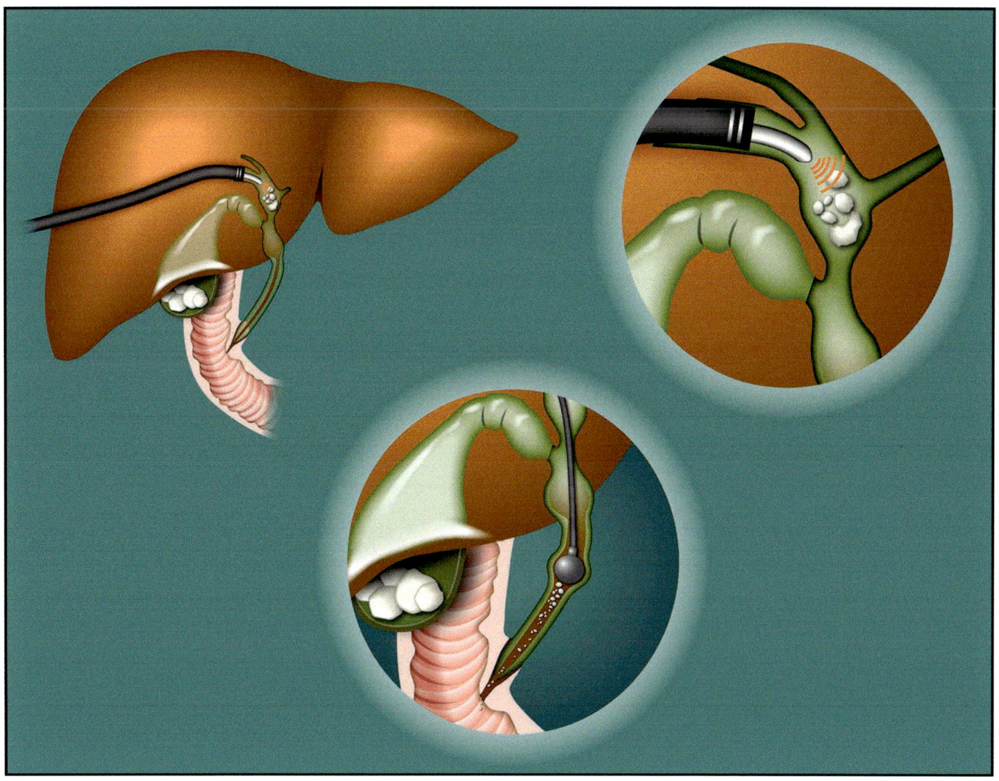

Figure 9-23. Lithotripsy of gallstones. (Alexonline/shutterstock.com)

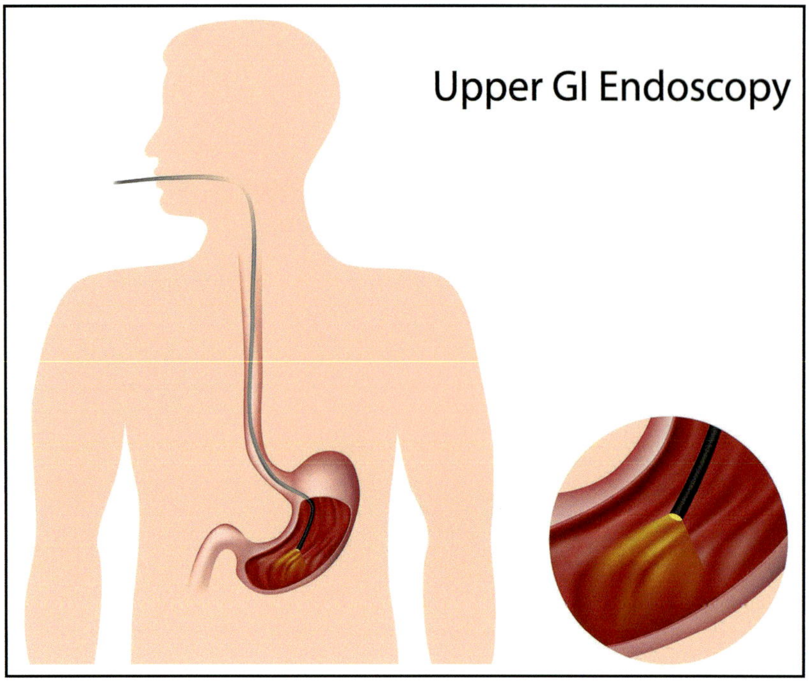

Figure 9-24. Upper GI endoscopy. (Alila Medical Images/shutterstock.com)

Endoscopy is a visual examination of a cavity. In the GI system it can mean:

Upper GI endoscopy (Figure 9-24)	• Esophagoscopy • Gastroscopy • Duodenoscopy
Lower GI endoscopy	• Colonoscopy • Sigmoidoscopy • Proctoscopy

The following are terms relating to creating an artificial opening that acts as a means to remove fecal matter (Figure 9-25):

Word root + **-ostomy**	Defined as a new surgical opening into:
col**ostomy**	the colon
gastr**ostomy**	the stomach
ile**ostomy**	the ileum

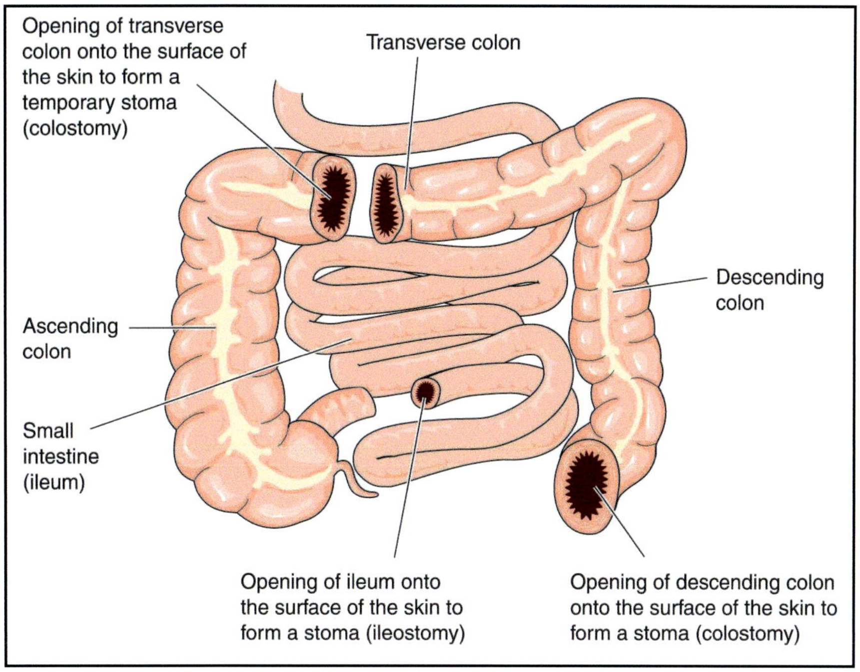

Figure 9-25. Various colostomy and ileostomy sites. (Blamb/shutterstock.com)

9

Medication Classifications

Table 9-10

Medication Classifications Used in Treatment of Gastrointestinal Conditions

CATEGORY	WHAT IT DOES
antacid	Prevents acid production; neutralizes acid in the stomach
antiemetic **anti-** (against) **eme-** (to vomit) **-ic** (pertaining to)	Stops vomiting
antispasmodic **anti-** (against) spasm/ (spasm) **-ic** (pertaining to)	Slows normal peristalsis to alleviate diarrhea
emetics **eme-** (to vomit) **-ic** (pertaining to)	Induce vomiting; used in certain situations of overdoses with noncorrosive agents
laxatives	Increase peristaltic activity to assist with defecation
proton pump inhibitor (PPI)	Inhibits gastric acid secreting into the stomach

Bibliography

Basco R, Allan B. *Medical Language for Modern Health Care.* 5th ed. McGraw-Hill; 2023.
Fremgen BF, Frucht SS. *Medical Terminology: A Living Language.* 7th ed. Pearson; 2019.
Hutton A. *Medical Terminology for Health Care.* 5th ed. Churchill Livingstone; 2017.
Kotzwinkle W, Murray G, Colman A, Morrison P. *Walter, the Farting Dog.* Frog, Ltd; 2001.
Mosby's Dictionary of Medicine, Nursing & Health Professions. 10th ed. Elsevier; 2017.
Rice J. *Medical Terminology for Health Care Professionals.* 9th ed. Pearson; 2018.
Venes D, ed. *Taber's Cyclopedic Medical Dictionary.* 24th ed. F. A. Davis; 2021.

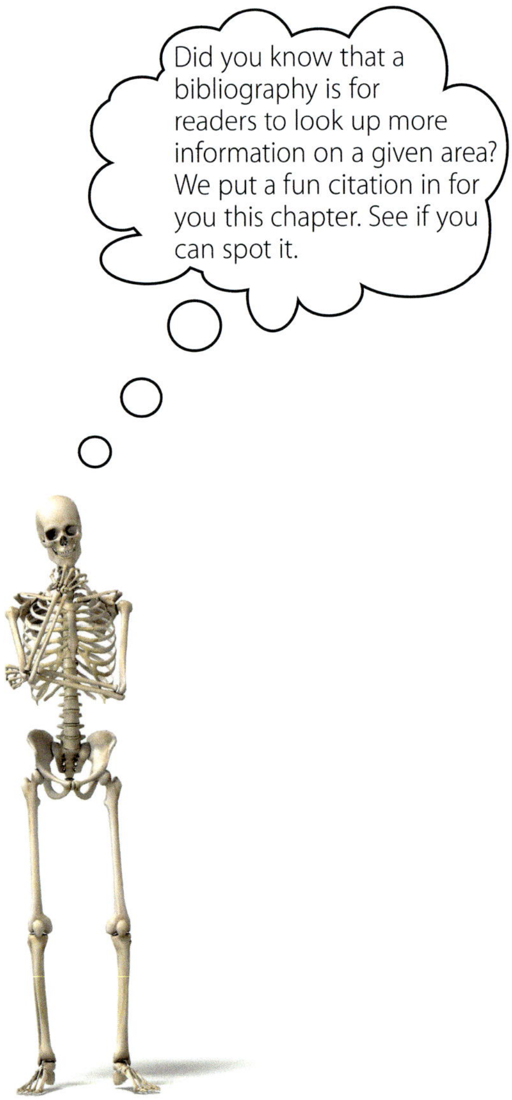

NOTES

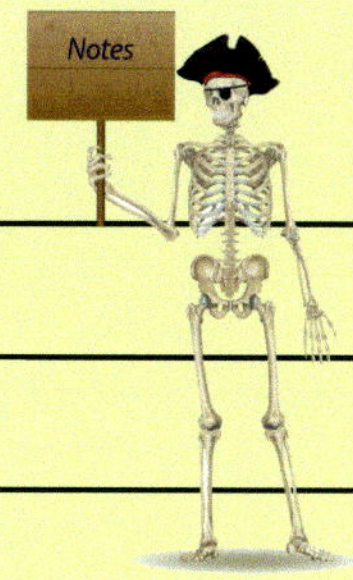

NOTES

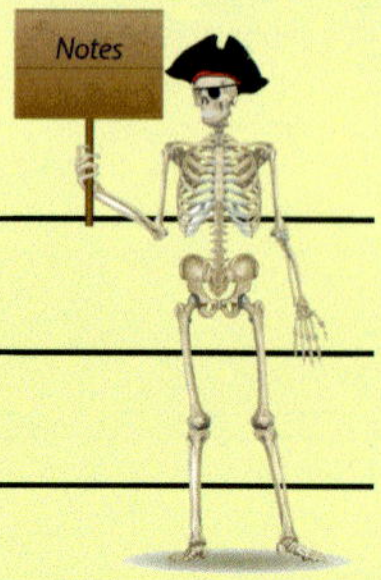

Learning Activities

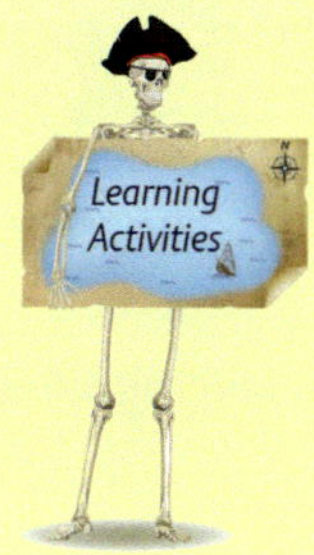

Name:____________________

Gastrointestinal System

A. Using the bulleted list of anatomy, list the number on the drawing that corresponds with the anatomical part.

- transverse colon__________
- stomach__________
- pancreas__________
- descending colon__________
- appendix__________
- sigmoid colon__________
- antrum__________
- small intestine__________
- ascending colon__________
- duodenum__________
- gallbladder__________
- esophagus__________
- fundus__________

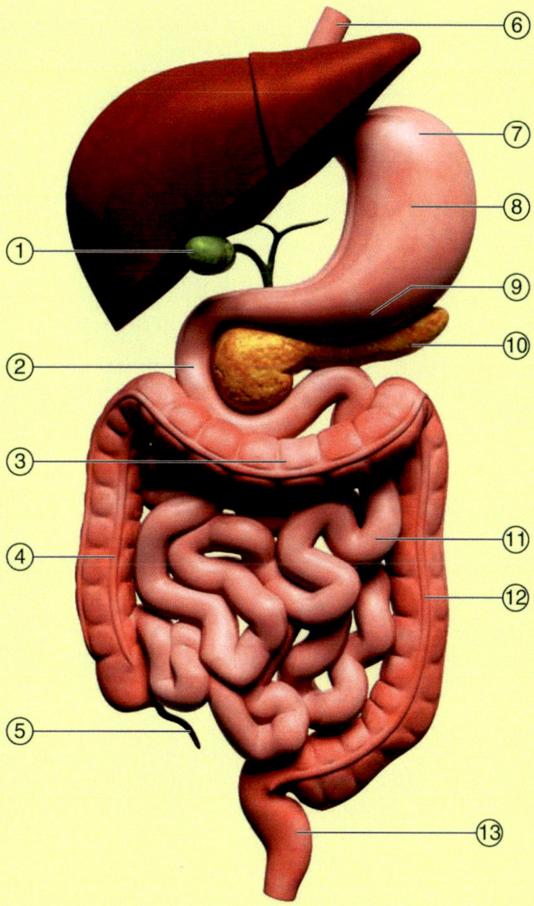

B. Label the salivary glands from the following list of words.

- submandibular gland _______
- parotid gland______________
- sublingual gland___________

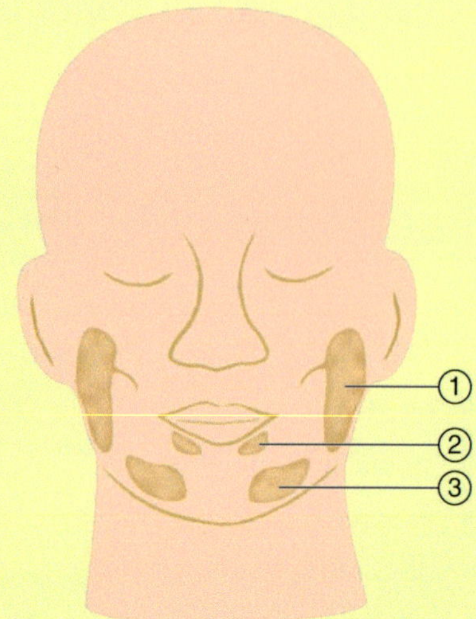

(Alila Medical Images/shutterstock.com)

C. Matching.

Match the word with its best meaning.

1. aphagia___________________	a. difficulty swallowing
2. hematemesis________________	b. pus around the gums
3. steatorrhea________________	c. stomachache
4. cholelithiasis______________	d. enlargement of the liver
5. pyorrhea__________________	e. inflammation of the small intestine
6. dysphagia_________________	f. inability to swallow
7. hepatomegaly______________	g. vomiting blood
8. gingivitis_________________	h. fat in the feces
9. enteritis__________________	i. inflammation of the gums
10.gastrodynia________________	j. having gallstones

D. Build the word.

Using the suffix that follows, add the other word element and define the new word created.

1. **-itis**
   a. cheil/______________________________
   b. esophag/____________________________
   c. enter/______________________________
   d. col/________________________________
   e. cholecyst/___________________________
   f. ile/________________________________
   g. hepat/______________________________
   h. gloss/______________________________
   i. proct/______________________________
2. **-scopy**
   a. proct/o_____________________________
   b. lapar/o_____________________________
   c. sigmoid/o___________________________
   d. **endo-**_____________________________
   e. gastr/o_____________________________
   f. esophag/o___________________________

3. **-ectomy**
   a. diverticul ____________________
   b. polyp ____________________
   c. uvul ____________________
   d. gastr ____________________
   e. gingiv____________________

E. Separate the word elements of the following terms and define them.

1. gastroenterocolitis ____
2. cholangiogram ____
3. cholecystectomy ____

F. From the following list, choose the two word elements that match the meaning of the words.

- odont/o
- an/o
- or/o
- labi/o
- dent/o
- gloss/o
- proct/o
- stomat/o
- lingu/o
- cheil/o

1. mouth____
2. lip____
3. anus____
4. tongue____
5. teeth ____

G. Fill in the blanks.

1. the place where pain is felt in appendicitis____
2. to have no appetite____
3. the involuntary muscular action that moves food along the esophagus and alimentary tract____________________
4. chewing____
5. the enzyme in saliva that begins the breakdown of carbohydrates____
6. when the jaw does not close properly____

9

Case Study

Define the numerical terms (1 to 18) and draw the alphabetical terms (A to C) on the anatomy figure.
For assistance with medical abbreviations, refer to Appendix A.

History, Chief Complaint

A high school gymnast complained of **dyspepsia** (1) and **epigastric** (2) pain in this afternoon's practice. He ate yogurt, nuts, and a banana for breakfast and a Lean Cuisine (Nestlé S.A.) for lunch. He just started feeling bad about 1 hour ago. He denied **diarrhea** (3), constipation, **anorexia** (4), and **emesis** (5).

Evaluation

He did not appear to have **jaundice** (6), and his oral temperature was 101°F. On palpation, he did not have **hepatomegaly** (7, A) or **splenomegaly** (8, B), but did have pain upon palpation in the **LRQ** (9, C). Specifically, he had pain at **McBurney's point** (10).

Treatment

The gymnast had both a **UA** (11) and **CBC** (12). The UA was **WNL** (13), but the CBC revealed **leukocytosis** (14). **Ultrasonography** (15) revealed **acute** (16) **appendicitis** (17), and an **appendectomy** (18) was scheduled.

Terms

1. ____________________
2. ____________________
3. ____________________
4. ____________________
5. ____________________
6. ____________________
7. ____________________
8. ____________________
9. ____________________
10. ____________________
11. ____________________
12. ____________________
13. ____________________
14. ____________________
15. ____________________
16. ____________________
17. ____________________
18. ____________________

Anatomy

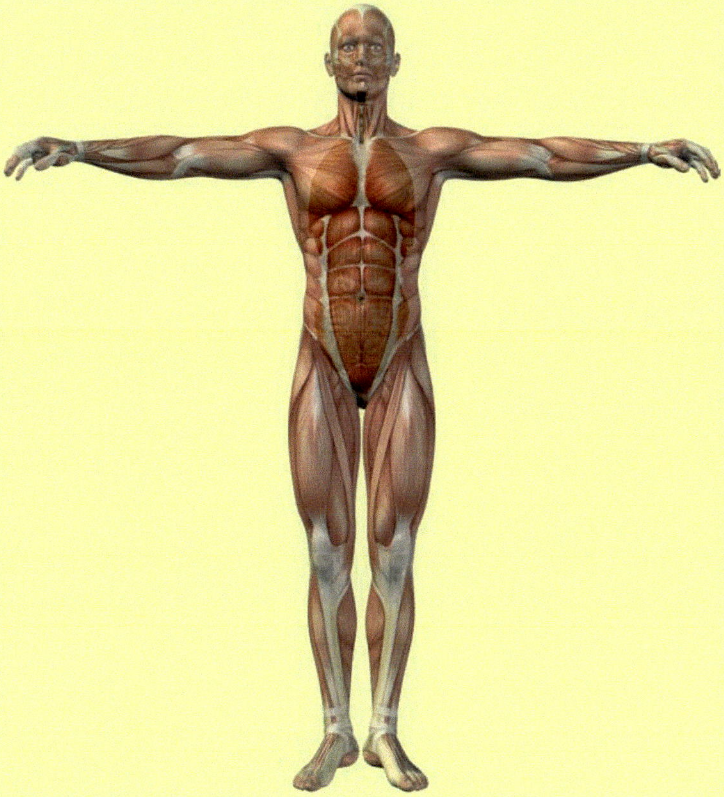

Flanagan KW. *Medical Terminology With Case Studies: A Navigated Guide to Learning for Health Care Professionals, Third Edition*. © 2023 Taylor & Francis Group.

10

Integumentary System

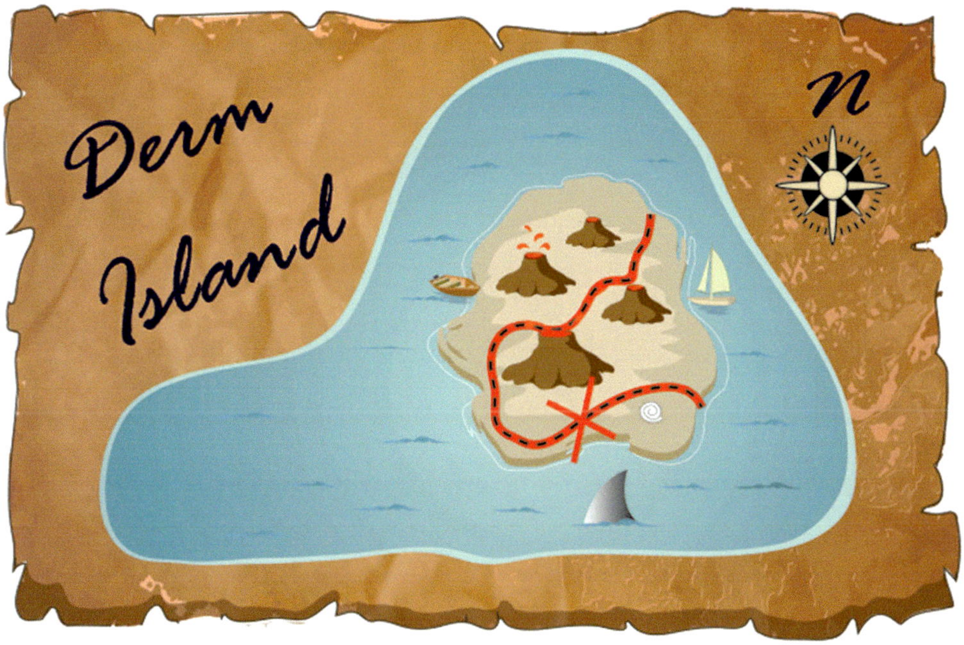

OBJECTIVES

After studying this chapter, you will be able to:

1. Identify the major components of the integumentary system.
2. Build words relating to the integumentary system.
3. List signs and symptoms of dermatological issues.
4. Identify and describe lesions.
5. Explain the ABCDE system as it pertains to skin cancers.
6. Describe basic abnormalities or conditions of the dermatological system.
7. Explain diagnostic tests and procedures specific to the integumentary system.
8. Identify classifications of medications used to treat pathological conditions related to the skin and its structures.

Flanagan KW.
Medical Terminology With Case Studies: A Navigated Guide to Learning for Health Care Professionals, Third Edition (pp 255-290).

Chapter Outline

- Self-assessment
- Checklist for word parts in the chapter
- Checklist of new anatomy
- Introduction
- Anatomy
  - The skin
  - Accessory glands
  - Hair and nails
- Word building
  - Prefixes
  - Suffixes
  - Combining forms
- Signs and symptoms
- Medical conditions
- Tests and procedures
- Medication classifications
- Learning activities
- Case study

Self-Assessment

Based on what you have learned so far, can you write the definition of these words?

- dermatitis________________________________
- melanoma________________________________
- hidrosis________________________________
- scleroderma________________________________
- percutaneous________________________________
- transdermal________________________________
- hyperplasia________________________________
- dorsum________________________________

Checklist for Word Parts in the Chapter

Prefixes

- ☐ a-
- ☐ actin-
- ☐ allo-
- ☐ an-
- ☐ anti-
- ☐ auto-
- ☐ caus-
- ☐ caut-
- ☐ de-
- ☐ dia-
- ☐ ec-
- ☐ epi-
- ☐ ex-
- ☐ hyper-
- ☐ hypo-
- ☐ intra-
- ☐ par-
- ☐ per-
- ☐ sub-
- ☐ syn-
- ☐ tel-
- ☐ trans-

Suffixes

- ☐ -al
- ☐ -algia
- ☐ -ar
- ☐ -cyte
- ☐ -ectasia
- ☐ -ectasis
- ☐ -ectomy
- ☐ -esthesia
- ☐ -ferous
- ☐ -ia
- ☐ -ic
- ☐ -in
- ☐ -ion
- ☐ -is
- ☐ -ism
- ☐ -itis
- ☐ -ium
- ☐ -lysis
- ☐ -malacia
- ☐ -oid
- ☐ -oma
- ☐ -osis
- ☐ -ous
- ☐ -plasty
- ☐ -rrhea
- ☐ -um
- ☐ -us

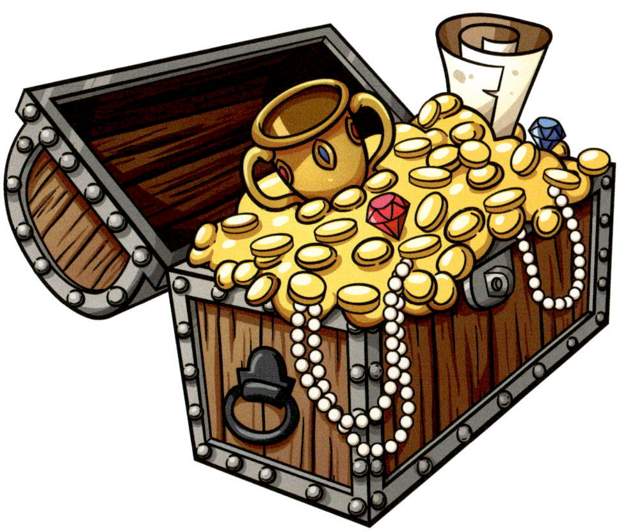

Many of these prefixes and suffixes should look familiar now. How are you doing on learning their meanings?

Combining Forms

- ☐ acr/o
- ☐ aden/o
- ☐ adip/o
- ☐ albin/o
- ☐ ang/i
- ☐ axill/o
- ☐ bas/o
- ☐ capit/o
- ☐ carcin/o
- ☐ cellul/o
- ☐ chord/o
- ☐ chym/o
- ☐ corpor/o
- ☐ crur/o
- ☐ cry/o
- ☐ crypt/o
- ☐ cubit/o
- ☐ cutane/o
- ☐ derm/a
- ☐ derm/o
- ☐ dermat/o
- ☐ electr/o
- ☐ eryth/o
- ☐ erythr/o
- ☐ follicul/o
- ☐ hidr/o
- ☐ kel/o
- ☐ kerat/o
- ☐ leuk/o
- ☐ lip/o
- ☐ lun/o
- ☐ melan/o
- ☐ miliar
- ☐ my/o
- ☐ myc/o
- ☐ onych/o
- ☐ pachy
- ☐ pallor
- ☐ papill/o
- ☐ ped/o
- ☐ pedicul/o
- ☐ pil/o
- ☐ prurit/o
- ☐ rhytid/o
- ☐ rubor
- ☐ scler/o
- ☐ seb/o

10

Combining Forms

- ☐ **sudor/o**
- ☐ **therm/o**
- ☐ **top/o**
- ☐ **trich/o**
- ☐ **ungu/o**
- ☐ **vascul/o**
- ☐ **xanth/o**
- ☐ **xen/o**
- ☐ **xer/o**

Checklist of New Anatomy

Skin

- ☐ Epidermis
  - ☐ Stratum corneum
  - ☐ Stratum lucidum
  - ☐ Stratum granulosum
  - ☐ Stratum spinosum
  - ☐ Stratum basale
- ☐ Dermis
  - ☐ Papillary
  - ☐ Reticular region
- ☐ Subcutaneous

Glands, Hair, and Nails

- ☐ Sudoriferous glands
  - ☐ Pores
- ☐ Sebaceous glands
  - ☐ Pores
  - ☐ Sebum
- ☐ Hair
  - ☐ Shaft
  - ☐ Papilla
- ☐ Nails
  - ☐ Nail plate
  - ☐ Nail matrix
  - ☐ Nail bed
  - ☐ Lunula
  - ☐ Cuticle
  - ☐ Paronychium

Introduction

Derm Island is full of volcanic eruptions, as it represents the integumentary (also known as the *dermatological*) system, and these eruptions resemble outbreaks on skin. The island contains combining forms distinctive to the integumentary system, which involves the skin, nails, hair follicles, and sweat and oil glands.

Anatomy

The word *integument* means "covering," which is the purpose of the skin and the rest of the **integumentary system**. The skin is actually the largest organ of the body (the liver is the largest organ inside the body), as it is first in line to protect it from harm. It is an external barrier that offers a shielding layer between the environment and muscle, bone, tissues, and other organs. The skin assists in temperature regulation and provides awareness to the brain of surface pressure, temperature, proprioception, and sensation. It also provides a layer of protection against ultraviolet radiation, fluid loss, and trauma. As a system, the integument works together with accessory structures, **hair** and **nails**, and **sebaceous** (oil) and **sudoriferous** (sweat) glands. It exchanges gases, synthesizes vitamin D, and provides information in some medical diagnoses though skin condition, color, and texture.

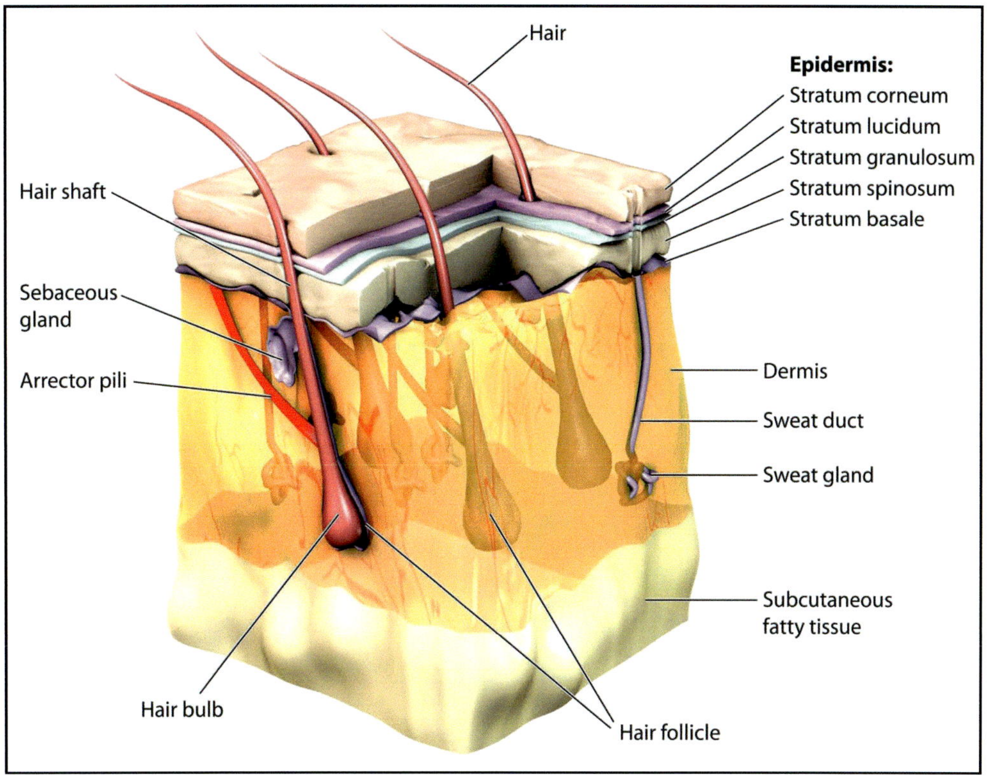

Figure 10-1. Layers of the skin. (Blamb/shutterstock.com)

10

The Skin

The two layers of the skin consist of the **epidermis** (**epi-**—above; **derm/**—skin), and **dermis**, also referred to as the *corium* (Figure 10-1). Beneath the dermis is a layer of fat (**adipose**) and connective tissue called the **subcutaneous** (**sub-**—under; **cutane/**—skin). The subcutaneous is also called the **hypodermis** (**hypo-**—below; **derm/**—skin). Within each layer are divisions of different cell types that are arranged in layers (**strata**) of epithelial tissue. The epidermis is largely composed of layers of dead cells, and it is constantly sloughing off old cells and moving these cells up toward the surface. It takes about 30 days for a cell to move from the bottom (basal) layer to the top (**stratum corneum**) layer. The dead cells are called **keratinocytes** (**-cyte**—cell) and are filled with **keratin** (**kerat/o**—hard), which is a hard protein that assists with maintaining homeostasis (Figure 10-2). Due to its waterproofing attribute, keratin prevents water loss due to evaporation and also prevents moisture from entering the body. The deepest layer of the epidermis, the **stratum basale**—or simply, *basal layer*—houses specialized cells called **melanocytes** (**melan/o**—black; **-cyte**—cell). Melanocytes produce **melanin**, which is a black pigment. The amount of melanin one has is genetically determined. Darker-skinned individuals produce larger quantities of melanin than do those with a lighter complexion, and are less prone to wrinkles. People with freckles and moles have a dense local collection of melanin at that site.

The layers of the epidermis are, from the surface inward:

- **Stratum corneum**: Primarily keratinized, dead cells
- **Stratum lucidum**: A thin, clear layer found only in the palms of the hands and soles of the feet
- **Stratum granulosum**: Layers of granular cells
- **Stratum spinosum**: Several layers of cells that have spine-like projections
- **Stratum basale**: A single layer of cells that contain melanocytes, the cell that produces pigment.

Skin cancers are typically named after the layer or cell from which they arise. For example, **basal cell carcinomas (BCC)** (**carcin/o**—cancer, **-oma**—mass; tumor) arise from the stratum basale, and **melanomas** develop from abnormal melanocytes.

The dermis lies beneath the epidermis and contains blood and lymph vessels, nerves, muscles that erect hair shafts, hair follicles, and glands. This layer is further subdivided into the upper area, the papillary region, and the lower layer of the reticular region. Under the dermal layer is the subcutaneous layer of fat and connective tissue that provides a joining between this sheet and underlying tissues (muscles, bones, organs). The subcutaneous layer is also a protective and insulating barrier to the body.

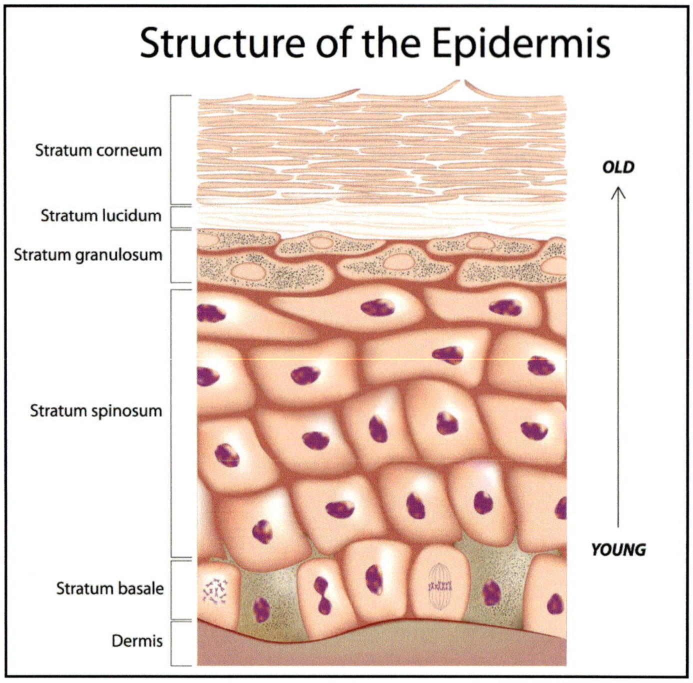

Figure 10-2. Movement of keratinocytes to the surface where they flake off. (Alila Medical Images/shutterstock.com)

Accessory Glands

Sweat glands, called **sudoriferous glands** (**sudor/o**—sweat), originate from the dermis layer of the skin and assist with thermoregulation of the skin and body. When the body gets too hot, the glands secrete perspiration through tiny openings in the epidermis called **pores** (see Figure 10-1). Certain areas of the body—the soles of the feet, axilla, palms, groin, upper lip, and forehead—have large numbers of sweat glands, but they can be found everywhere on the body. The other gland associated with skin is the **sebaceous gland**. This gland is responsible for secreting an oily, acidic material called **sebum** (**seb/o**—oil). The purpose of sebum is to provide lubrication to the skin surface and hair. Because of the acidic properties, sebum also contributes to inhibiting the growth of bacteria on the skin's surface. **Acne** occurs when these external pores become blocked. As with hair, sebaceous glands can be found most anywhere on the body, but are more frequent on the scalp and face and around the openings to internal body cavities. The amount of sebum secreted is largely dependent on hormones and decreases with age.

Hair and Nails

It is possible to have hair on almost every surface of skin, except the palms of the hands, soles of the feet, lips, nipples, and some external genitalia. The type and texture of hair is different on various aspects of the body and is distinguishable under microscopic examination (cue *CSI*). Hair roots are embedded in the dermis, with the visible **hair shaft** apparent above the surface. At the base of each hair follicle are capillaries within a covering called the **papilla**. As long as the papilla is intact, DNA can be analyzed, which is why scientists want complete hair follicles when investigating a crime scene. Also at the base of the hair follicles are melanocytes that dictate each strand's hair color. The amount of melanin determines whether a given shaft is yellow, red, brown, or black. Both age and genetics determine hair color. The main function of hair is to protect and thermoregulate the body. When a person is cold, the **arrector pili**, the muscle associated with each shaft, constricts and reacts causing hair to stand erect (**piloerection**; **pil/o**—hair), what we commonly refer to as *goose bumps*. This action provides a layer of insulation to the skin to keep it warmer.

Fingernails and toenails are keratin coverings found on the dorsal and distal aspects of all fingers and toes. There are two main aspects of nails; the visible and hard **nail plate** and the hidden **nail matrix** that lies on the proximal aspect of each nail, under the skin (Figure 10-3). Under the nail plate is the highly vascular **nail bed**. This blood supply is the reason nails appear pinkish when healthy, and bluish when deficient in blood or oxygen. Near the base of each nail is a moon-shaped area called the **lunula** (**lun/o**—moon). Nail growth occurs proximal to the lunula. The tiny layer of skin on the most proximal nail near the matrix is termed the **cuticle**, and the skin fold along the edges of the nail is the **paronychium** (**par-**—alongside; **onych/**—nail; **-ium**—membrane).

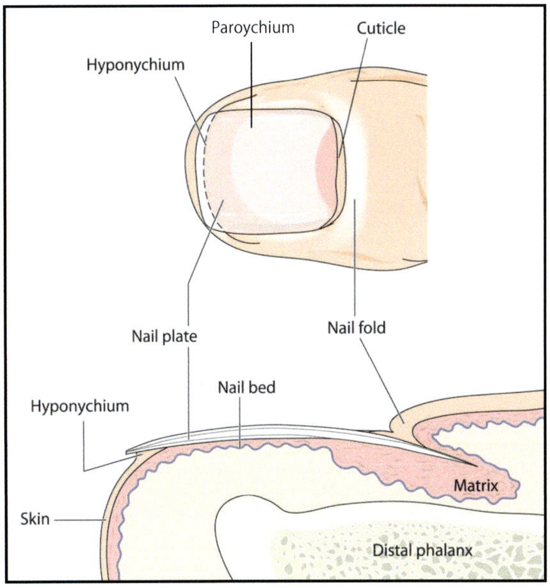

Figure 10-3. Anatomy of the nail. (Blamb/shutterstock.com)

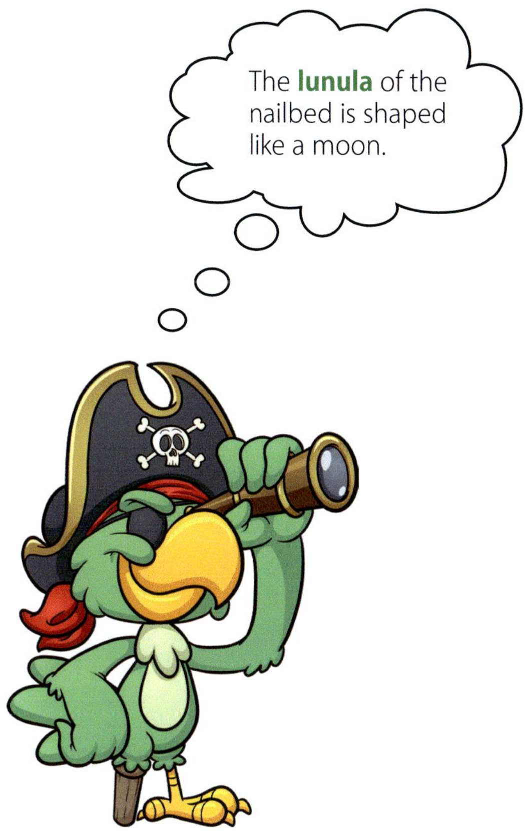

Word Building

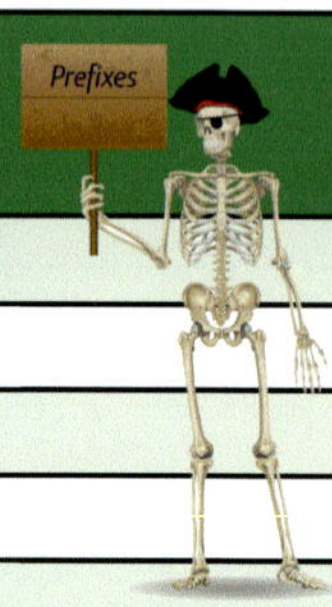

Table 10-1

Prefixes

PREFIX	DEFINITION
a-	without
actin-	ray; radiation
allo-	other; different
an-	not; without
anti-	against
auto-	self; own
caus-; caut-	burn; heat
de-	down; take away; without
dia-	across; through
ec-	out; outside
epi-	above; upon
ex-	away; away from; out; outside
hyper-	above; excessive; high; increased
hypo-	below; decreased; deficient; insufficient; low; under
intra-	inside; within
par-	alongside; around; beside; near
per-	through
sub-	under; below
syn-	union; together
tel-	end
trans-	across; through

Table 10-2
Suffixes

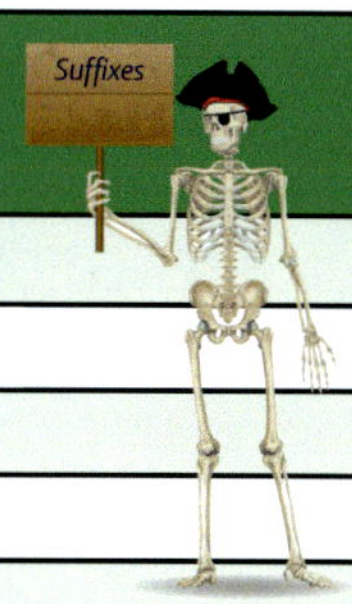

SUFFIX	DEFINITION
-al	pertaining to
-algia	pain
-ar	pertaining to
-cyte	cell
-ectasia; -ectasis	dilation; expansion
-ectomy	surgical removal; excision
-esthesia	perception; sensation
-ferous	pertaining to; carrying
-ia	condition
-ic	pertaining to
-in	substance
-ion	process; the act of
-is	pertaining to; structure
-ism	condition
-itis	inflammation
-ium	structure; membrane
-lysis	breaking down; destruction; loosening; separating; to loosen or break
-malacia	softening
-oid	resembling
-oma	mass; tumor
-osis	condition
-ous	pertaining to
-plasty	reconstruction; repair; plastic surgery
-rrhea	discharge; excessive flow
-um	structure; thing
-us	pertaining to; structure

Table 10-3
Combining Forms

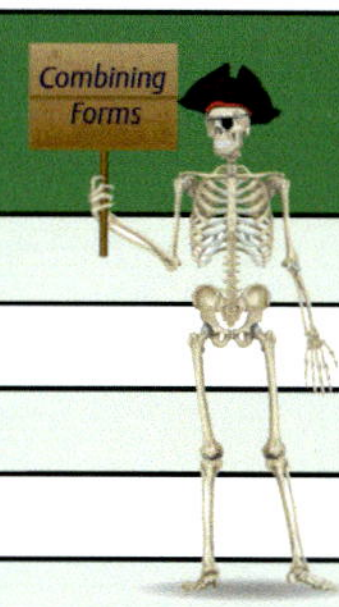

COMBINING FORM	DEFINITION
acr/o	extremity
aden/o	gland
adip/o	fat
albin/o	white
ang/i	vessel
axill/o	armpit

(continued)

Table 10-3 (continued)

Combining Forms

COMBINING FORM	DEFINITION
bas/o	base; bottom
capit/o	head
carcin/o	cancer
cellul/o	cell
chord/o	cord; spinal cord
chym/o	juice
corpor/o	body
crur/o	leg
cry/o	cold
crypt/o	hidden
cubit/o	elbow
cutane/o	skin
derm/a; derm/o; dermat/o	skin
follicul/o	little bag
hidr/o	sweat
kel/o	tumor; fibrous growth
kerat/o	cornea; hard; horn-like
miliar	tiny
myc/o	fungus
onych/o	nail
pachy	thick
papill/o	papilla; nipple
ped/o	foot; child
pedicul/o	lice (singular—louse)
pil/o	hair
prurit/o	itching
rhytid/o	wrinkle
scler/o	hard; hardening; thick; sclera
seb/o	oil; sebum
sudor/o	sweat
therm/o	heat; temperature
top/o	place; location
trich/o	hair
ungu/o	nail
vascul/o	blood vessel
xer/o	dry

Table 10-4

Combining Forms Related to Color

COMBINING FORM	DEFINITION
eryth/o; erythr/o	red
leuk/o	white
melan/o	black
pallor	pale
rubor	red
xanth/o	yellow

Table 10-5

Terms Related to Skin

TERM	WORD PARTS	DEFINITION
cutaneous	cutane/ (skin) **-ous** (pertaining to)	Pertaining to the skin
hypodermic	**hypo-** (under) derm/ (skin) **-ic** (pertaining to)	Pertaining to under the skin
intradermal	**intra-** (within) derm/ (skin) **-al** (pertaining to)	Pertaining to within the skin
percutaneous	**per-** (through) cutane/ (skin) **-ous** (pertaining to)	Pertaining to through the skin
subcutaneous	**sub-** (under) cutane/ (skin) **-ous** (pertaining to)	Pertaining to under the skin; also referred to as *sub-Q*
transcutaneous; transdermal	**trans-** (across; through) cutane/; derm/ (skin) **-ous; -al** (pertaining to)	Across or through the skin, as in a transdermal patch to deliver medication

Signs and Symptoms

Table 10-6

Signs and Symptoms of Dermatological Conditions

SIGN/SYMPTOM	WORD PARTS	DEFINITION
causalgia	**caus-** (heat) **-algia** (pain)	Sensation of burning
cellulitis	cellul/ (cell) **-itis** (inflammation)	Acute inflammation of the skin in response to an infection; characterized by red, hot, painful, and swollen skin
dermatitis	dermat/ (skin) **-itis** (inflammation)	Inflammation of the skin
ecchymosis (Figure 10-4)	**ec-** (out; outside) chym/ (juice) **-osis** (condition)	Bruise; discoloration caused by blood seeping under the skin
erythema	eryth/ (red)	Redness of the skin caused by any number of things; examples are exposure to hot/cold temperatures, inflammation
erythroderma	erythr/o (red) derm/a (skin)	Redness of the skin
keloid	kel/ (tumor; fibrous growth) **-oid** (resembling)	Tissue that resembles a tumor, but is an overreaction to an injury, creating excessive scarring
pruritus	prurit/ (itching) **-us** (pertaining to)	Itching
thermanesthesia	therm/ (heat; temperature) **an-** (without) **-esthesia** (perception)	Unable to determine temperature differences (hot or cold)
xanthoma	xanth/ (yellow) **-oma** (tumor)	Yellow tumor; typically found on the eyelid or near the eye
xanthoderma	xanth/o (yellow) derm/a (skin)	Yellow-colored skin
xeroderma	xer/o (dry) derm/a (skin)	Dry skin
xerosis	xer/ (dry) **-osis** (condition)	Dryness of skin, mucous membranes, and the eye

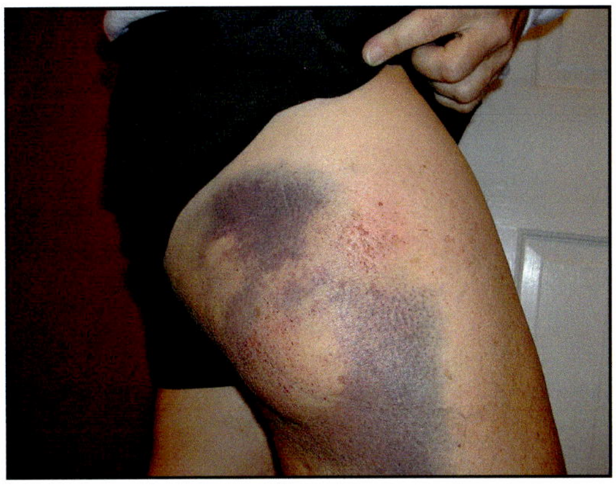

Figure 10-4. Ecchymosis, otherwise known as a bruise, can take on many colors.

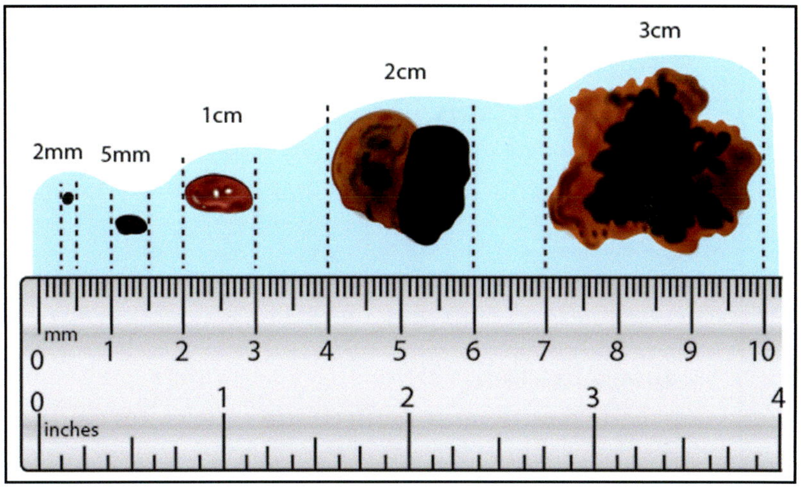

Figure 10-5. Size of lesions.

Medical Conditions

In dermatology, the term lesion is used for any situation where the skin has been altered due to trauma or infection. Lesions are either **primary** (initial reaction to injury or infection) or **secondary** (alterations to the original lesion due to infection, disease, scratching, etc). It is important to describe lesions in terms of size (Figure 10-5) and type (Figure 10-6).

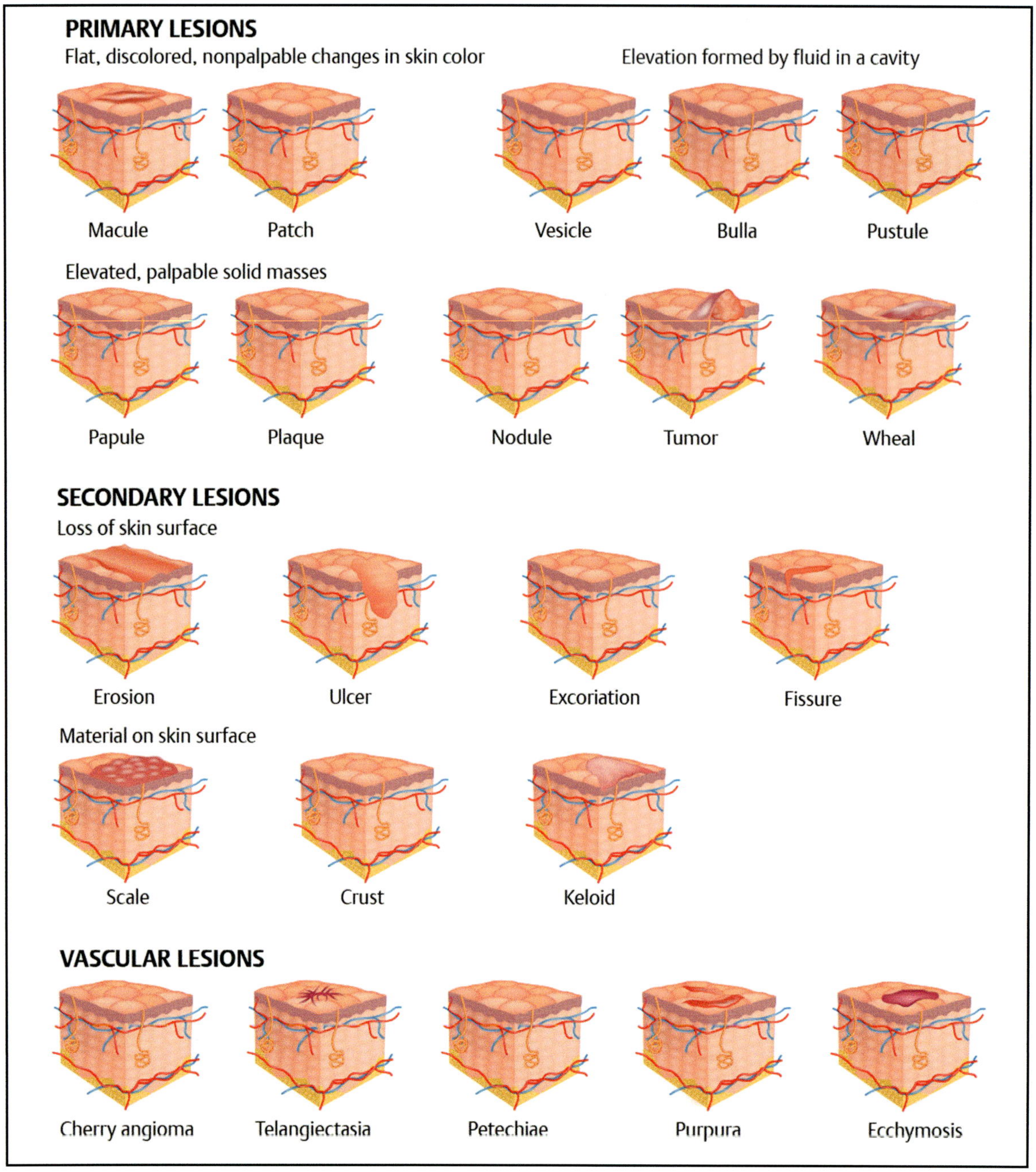

Figure 10-6. Primary and secondary lesions.

Table 10-7

Medical Conditions Related to the Skin

NAME	WORD PARTS	DEFINITION
acrochordon (Figure 10-7)	acr/o (extremity) chord/ (spinal cord)	Tiny benign outgrowths of skin; also called *skin tags*
actinic dermatitis (Figure 10-8)	**actin-** (radiation) **-ic** (pertaining to) dermat/ (skin) **-itis** (inflammation)	Red inflamed skin due to overexposure to radiant energy (eg, sun, x-rays, ultraviolet light)
actinic keratosis (AK)	**actin-** (radiation) **-ic** (pertaining to) kerat/ (hard) **-osis** (condition)	Premalignant lesion that has a slow-developing thickening and scaling due to chronic sun exposure
albinism	albin/ (white) **-ism** (condition)	Genetic condition of complete or partial absence of pigment in skin, eyes, and hair
atopic dermatitis	**a-** (without) top/ (location) **-ic** (pertaining to) dermat/ (skin) **-itis** (inflammation)	Inflammatory, itchy condition found typically on the face, antecubital (bend in elbow) and popliteal (behind the knee) areas
basal cell carcinoma (BCC)	bas/ (base) **-al** (pertaining to) carcin/ (cancer) **-oma** (mass; tumor)	Epithelial tumor that is malignant, but rarely metastasizes to other areas
decubitus ulcer (Figure 10-9)	**de-** (down) cubit/ (elbow) **-us** (structure)	Area of skin (often the buttocks) that becomes broken down due to pressure; also known as a *pressure ulcer* or *bedsore*
dermatomyositis	dermat/o (skin) my/o (muscle) **-itis** (inflammation)	Connective tissue disease involving destruction of the muscle tissue
dermatomycosis	dermat/o (skin) myc/ (fungus) **-osis** (condition)	Skin condition caused by fungus
keratosis	kerat/ (horn) **-osis** (condition)	Localized dry, hard skin that can arise in several forms (AK, keratosis senilis [in older adults], or seborrheic keratosis)
melanocarcinoma	melan/o (black) carcin/ (cancer) **-oma** (mass; tumor)	Malignant carcinoma
miliaria	miliar (tiny) **-ia** (condition)	Red skin with tiny vesicles and papules caused by blocked sweat ducts; typically found in hot, humid conditions; also called *prickly heat*

(continued)

Table 10-7 (continued)
Medical Conditions Related to the Skin

NAME	WORD PARTS	DEFINITION
pachyderma	pachy/ (thick) derm/a (skin)	Overgrowth or thickening of the skin and subcutaneous tissues
pediculosis	pedicul/ (lice) **-osis** (condition)	Infestation of body lice
scleroderma	scler/o (hardening) derm/a (skin)	Chronic condition consisting of hardening of the skin and connective tissue
telangiectasia (Figure 10-10)	**tel-** (end) ang/i (vessel) **-ectasia** (dilation)	Permanent dilation of superficial blood vessels that form a vascular lesion; one form of this is also known as *spider veins*

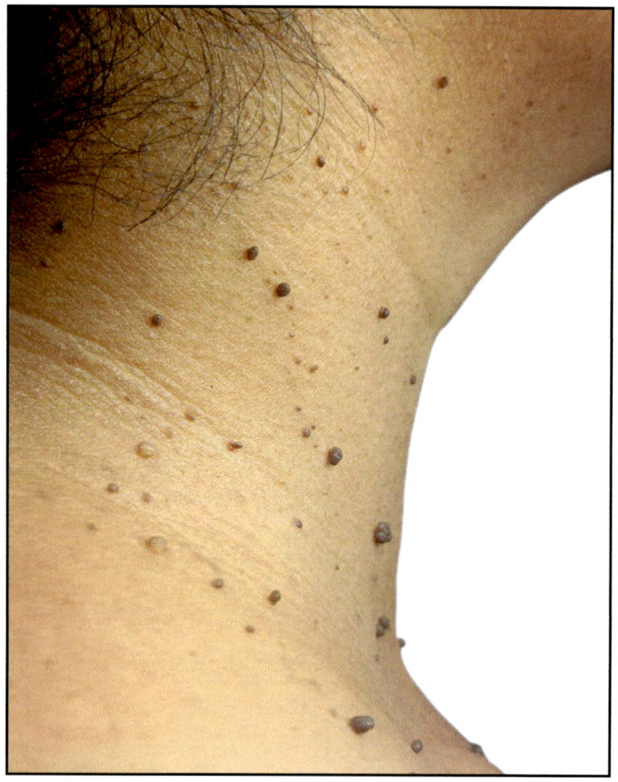

Figure 10-7. Acrochordon, also known as a *skin tag*. (Dhujmontra/shutterstock.com)

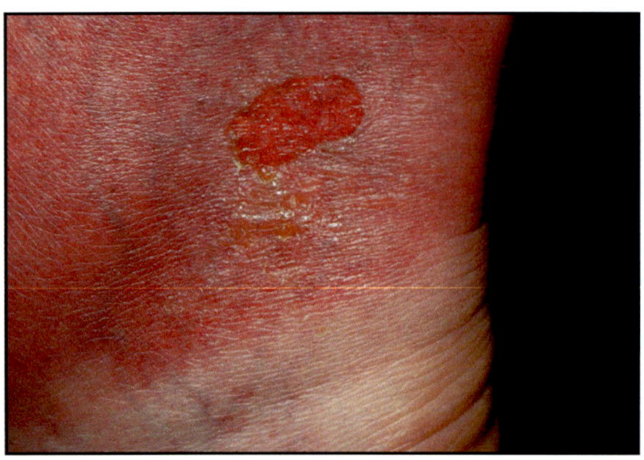

Figure 10-8. Actinic dermatitis from overexposure to the sun. (falk/shutterstock.com)

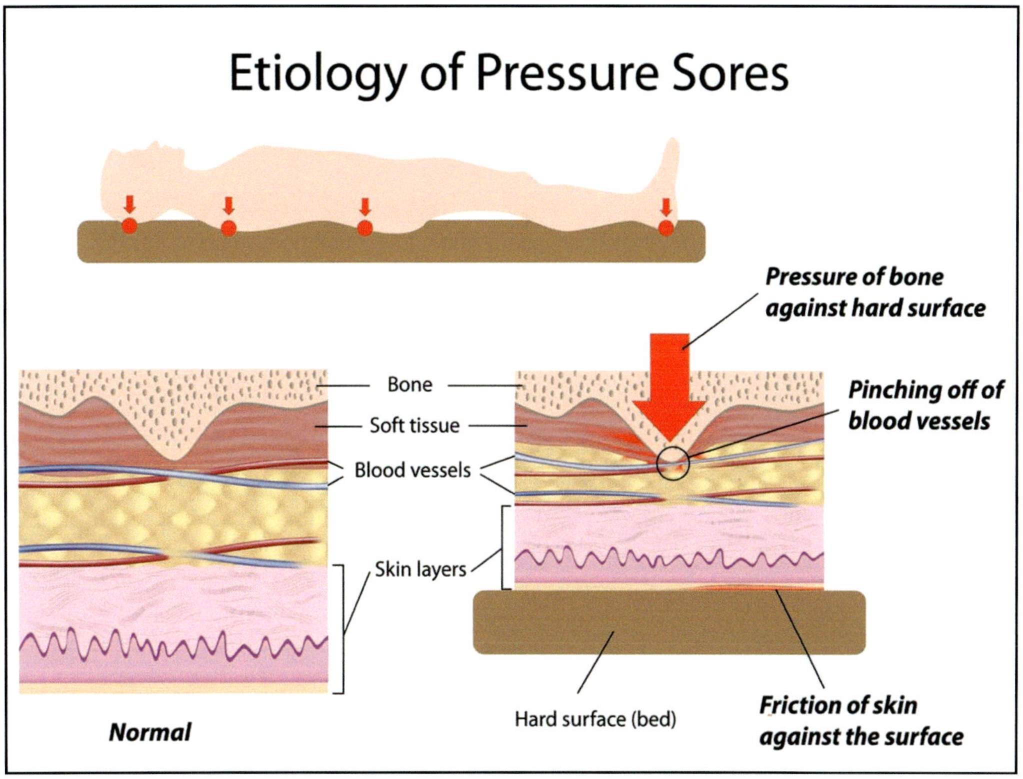

Figure 10-9. A decubitus ulcer caused by pressure; also known as a *bedsore*. (Alila Medical Images/shutterstock.com)

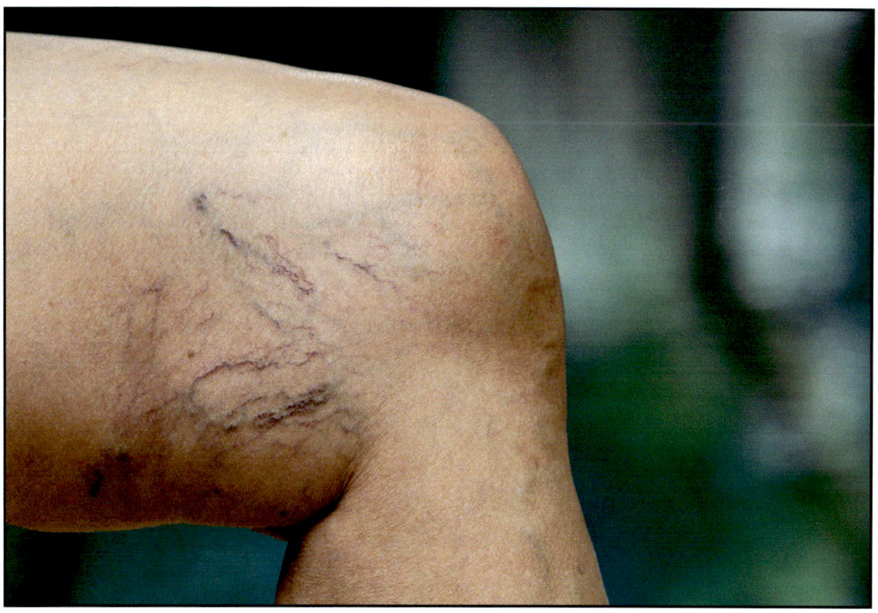

Figure 10-10. A form of telangiectasia known as *spider veins*. (eyepark/shutterstock.com)

Table 10-8

Dermatological Terms Without Common Word Parts

TERM	DEFINITION
acne	Inflamed sebaceous glands; also known as pimples
bedbugs (Figure 10-11)	Blood-sucking arthropod whose bite causes pain, red skin, and severe itching (*Cimex lectularius*)
boil	Localized, small infection in the subcutaneous tissues, hair follicle, or gland
bulla	Fluid-filled sac; another word for a blister (plural—bullae)
callus	Painless hardened thickening of the stratum corneum in areas of pressure or friction; also called *callous* or *keratoma*
candidiasis	Yeast infection of the skin or mucous lining
carbuncle	Infection of the subcutaneous tissues, typically presented as a cluster of boils
cicatrix	Soft, avascular, red scar tissue after an acute healing phase
comedo (Figure 10-12)	Lesion associated with acne; a blackhead is an open comedo; a whitehead is a closed comedo
corn	Hard mass of epithelial cells over a bony prominence; can become soft (macerated) by perspiration; named "corn" due to its shape under the skin
cyst	Normal-occurring closed sac under the skin filled with fluid, semi-solid, or solid material
dehiscence	Splitting of layers of a wound as it heals
eczema	Inflammatory skin disorder; characterized by erythema, papules, vesicles, pustules, scales, crusts, or scabs
eschar (Figure 10-13)	Scab or crust from trauma
exudate	Producing serum or pus
gangrene	Necrosis of tissue, usually due to deficient blood supply
herpes (Figure 10-14)	Inflammatory skin disorder caused by a virus; herpes simplex virus (HSV) when it affects the lips and mouth and is known as a cold sore; in the genitals it is known as *genital herpes* (HSV-2); and herpes zoster is known as *shingles*
hives (Figure 10-15)	Red, itchy, swollen skin in response to an allergen; also called *urticaria*
impetigo	Skin infection characterized by crusty vesicles or bullae
Kaposi's sarcoma	Malignant condition characterized by dark (brown or purple) papules on the feet, spreading to other areas of the skin
lentigo	Flat, brown mark on the skin, often caused by sun exposure; also called a *freckle*
macerated	Breakdown of skin due to prolonged exposure to water or moisture
milia	Superficial cysts caused by clogged oil ducts
mole (Figure 10-16)	Raised, discolored spot on the skin; also known as a *nevus*
nevus flammeus (Figure 10-17)	Vascular birthmark with superficial and deep dilated capillaries present at birth; usually temporary; also called a *stork bite* or *port wine stain*
petechiae	Small, pinpoint, red or blue hemorrhagic area on skin
psoriasis (Figure 10-18)	Chronic skin condition marked by itching and raised patches of white scales on the skin or scalp; can appear and dissipate

(continued)

TABLE 10-8 (CONTINUED) DERMATOLOGICAL TERMS WITHOUT COMMON WORD PARTS	
TERM	**DEFINITION**
purpura	Group of bleeding disorders characterized by hemorrhage into the tissues
roseola	Rose-colored rash on the skin
rubella	Acute, contagious, systemic disease characterized by a red rash and fever; a preventative vaccine, MMR (measles-mumps-rubella vaccine), is available for infants; also known as the *German measles* or *3-day measles*
rubeola	One of the most contagious diseases, marked by a fever and rash; also preventable by the MMR vaccine; known simply as *measles* or *red measles*
scabies	Contagious disease caused by a mite that burrows beneath the skin; characterized by intense itching and rash
sebum	Oily secretions produced by sebaceous glands
striae	Streaks or lines caused by stretched skin to accommodate growth during weight gain/loss or pregnancy; also called *stretch marks*
varicella (Figure 10-19)	Communicable disease marked by headache and a rash that leads to vesicles; the vaccine Varivax is provided to children to prevent this disease; also called *chickenpox*
verruca	Benign lesion marked by a rough papillomatous surface, caused by a contagious virus; also known as a *wart*
vitiligo	Patches of skin without pigment; benign condition with no known cause

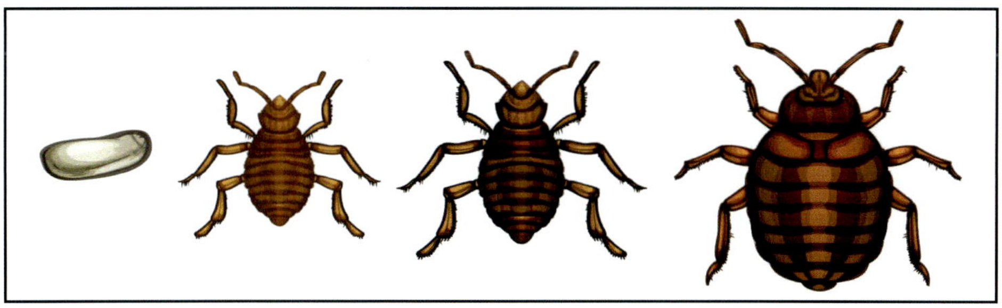

Figure 10-11. The lifecycle of a bedbug (*Cimex lectularius*). (BlueRingMedia/shutterstock.com)

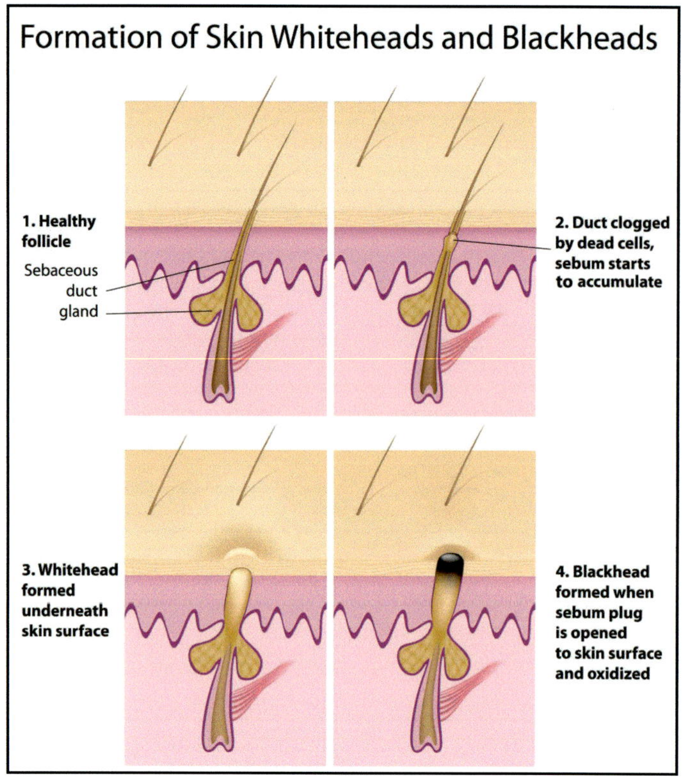

Figure 10-12. Open and closed comedones. (Alila Medical Images/shutterstock.com)

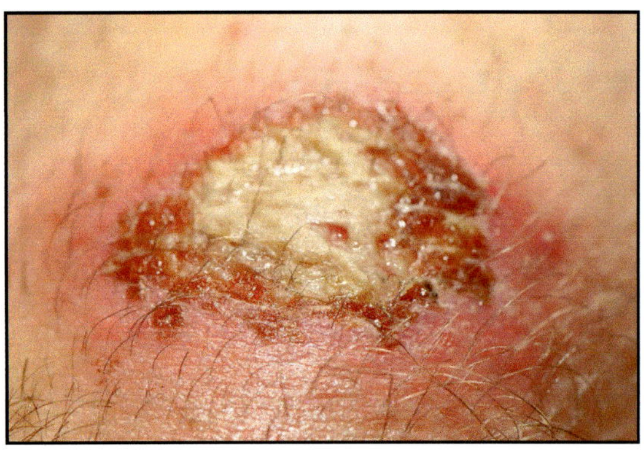

Figure 10-13. A healing abrasion with an eschar forming. (Kondor83/shutterstock.com)

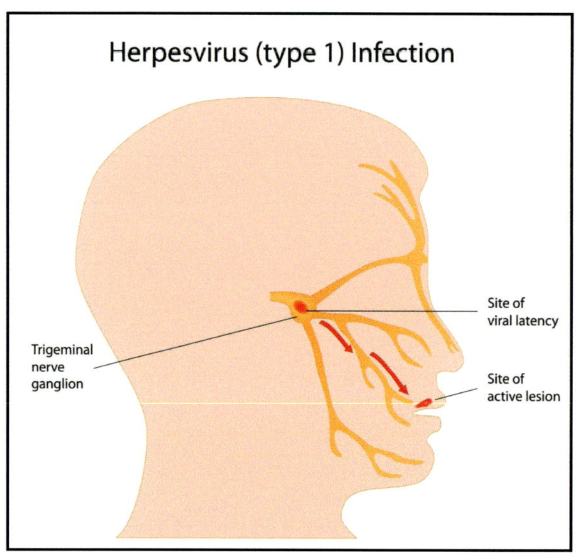

Figure 10-14. Herpes simplex virus 1. (Alila Medical Images/shutterstock.com)

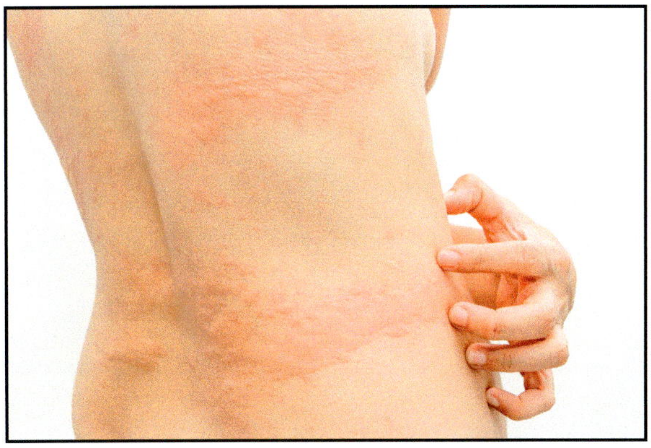

Figure 10-15. Hives, also known as *urticaria.* (namtipStudio/shutterstock.com)

Figure 10-16. A nevus, also known as a *mole.* (Nathalie Speliers Ufermann/shutterstock.com)

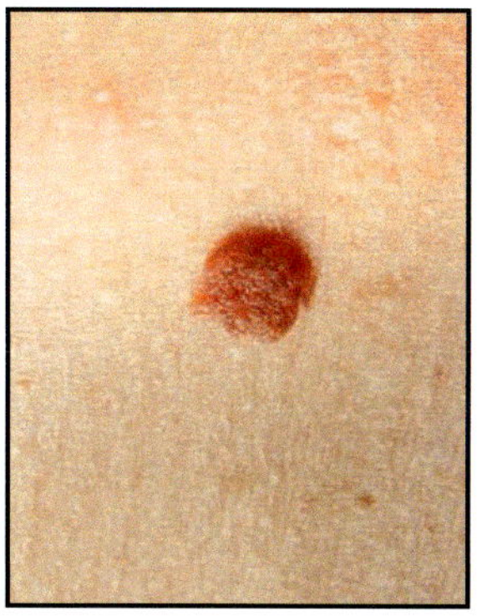

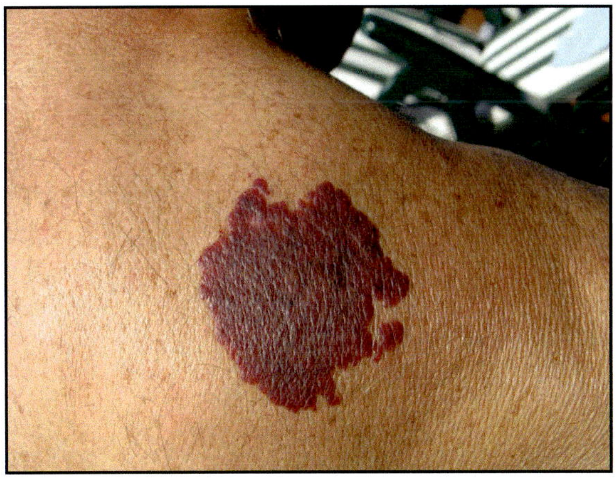

Figure 10-17. A nevus flammeus, also known as a *stork bite* due to its presence at birth, or a *port wine stain*. (guentermanaus/shutterstock.com)

Figure 10-18. Psoriasis. (kenxro/shutterstock.com)

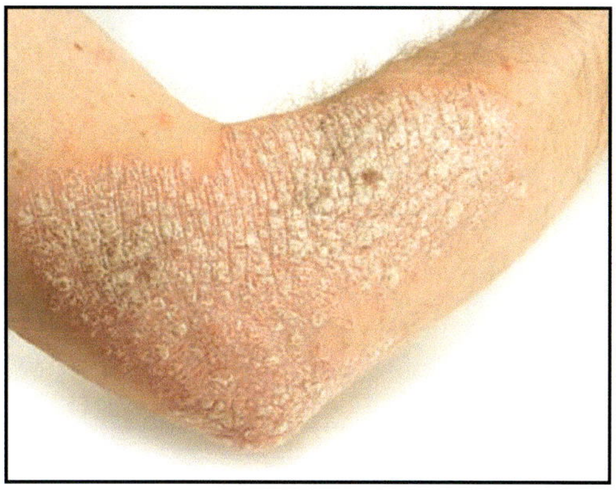

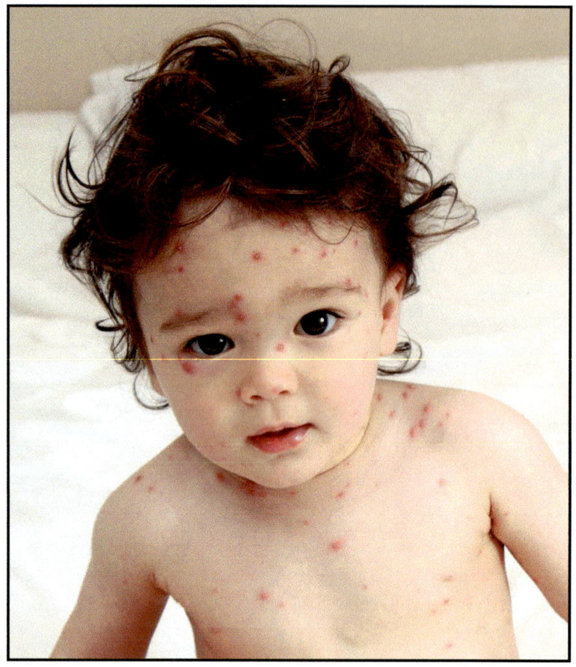

Figure 10-19. Varicella, also known as *chickenpox*. (hartphotography/shutterstock.com)

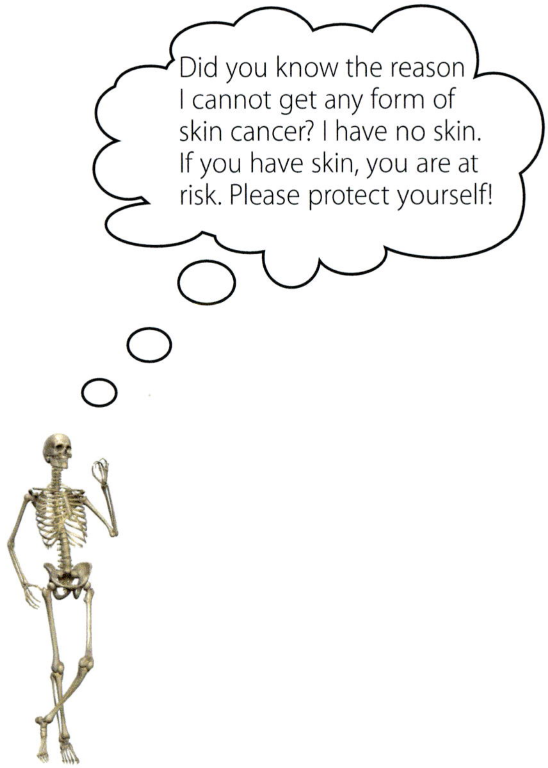
Did you know the reason I cannot get any form of skin cancer? I have no skin. If you have skin, you are at risk. Please protect yourself!

A WORD ABOUT SKIN CANCER

There are two common forms of skin cancer: **nonmelanoma** (rarely metastasize) and **melanoma** (the most malignant of all skin cancers; Table 10-9). Melanoma may be congenital or brought about from sun exposure or from sunburns at a young age. Although skin cancers are not contained to only those with fair skin, those with a lighter complexion are at a higher risk. Skin cancer often is first noted as a difference in the size or shape of marks on the skin. A mark could be a freckle or mole. Dermatologists promote **ABCDE** to reference changes on the surface of the skin in relation to skin cancers:

- **A** **Asymmetry**: If divided in half, each size of a mole should resemble each other
- **B** **Border**: Edges of moles should be smooth and distinct
- **C** **Color**: Freckles and moles should be uniform in color
- **D** **Diameter**: Freckles and moles should be less than 6 mm (the size of a pencil eraser)
- **E** **Evolving**: A skin marking should not change much over time

According to the Centers for Disease Control and Prevention, nearly 66,000 people were diagnosed with melanoma in 2011, and over 9000 died of it. Since the incidence of skin cancer has increased each year, awareness of the danger of sun exposure is important. Some states are voting on laws that ban tanning beds to those under 18 years old in an attempt to prevent skin cancers. Other preventative strategies include:

- Limit outdoor activity to before 10:00 am or after 4:00 pm.
- Apply sunscreen 20 to 30 minutes prior to going outdoors.
- Use sunscreens with a high SPF (sun protection factor), as well as both UVA and UVB protection.
- Apply plenty of sunscreen (at least a shot-glass worth) each application.
- Clothing typically provides an SPF of 5.

Table 10-9 Types of Skin Cancer	
TYPE	**SUBCATEGORY**
melanoma (Figure 10-20)	• Superficial spreading melanoma • Nodular melanoma
nonmelanoma skin cancer	• Basal cell carcinoma (BCC) • Squamous cell carcinoma (SCC)

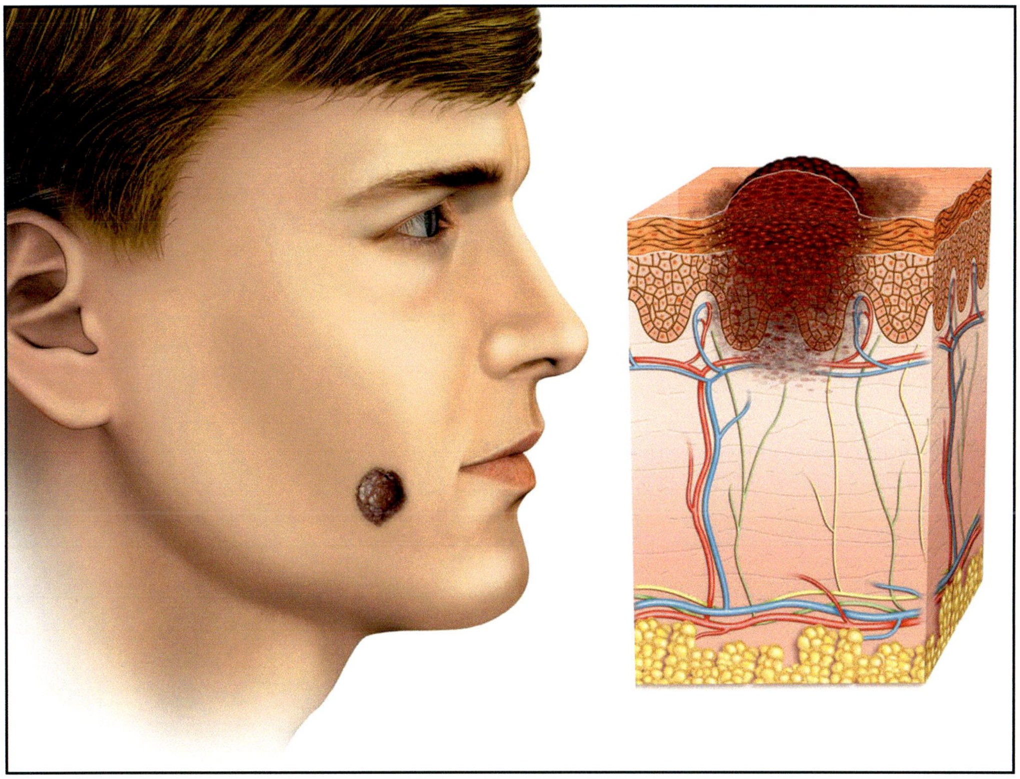

Figure 10-20. Melanoma. (Alex Luengo/shutterstock.com)

Table 10-10
Medical Conditions Related to the Hair Follicle and Sebaceous and Sudoriferous Glands

NAME	WORD PARTS	DEFINITION
alopecia (Figure 10-21)	**a-** (without) **-ia** (condition)	Loss or absence of hair due to the death of the papilla; usually on head (baldness)
anhidrosis	**an-** (without) hidr/ (sweat) **-osis** (condition)	Lack of sweating; could be a temporary sign of an emergency condition, related to a disease, or genetic tendencies
folliculitis	follicul/ (little bag) **-itis** (inflammation)	Inflammation of the hair follicle
hidradenitis	hidr/ (sweat) aden/ (gland) **-itis** (inflammation)	Inflammation to the sweat glands
hyperhidrosis	**hyper-** (excessive) hidr/ (sweat) **-osis** (condition)	Excessive sweating
seborrhea (Figure 10-22)	seb/o (oil) **-rrhea** (excessive flow)	Any one of many dermatological conditions causing an overproduction of oil from the sebaceous glands, causing excessive oiliness or dry scales
trichomycosis	trich/o (hair) myc/ (fungus) **-osis** (condition)	Fungal condition of the hair

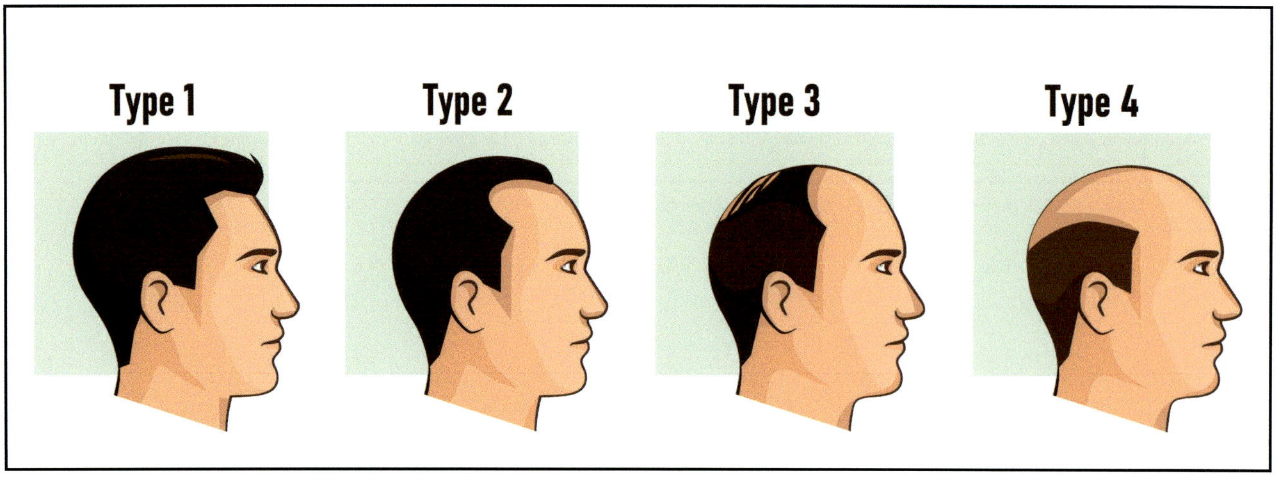

Figure 10-21. Androgenetic alopecia. (logika600/shutterstock.com)

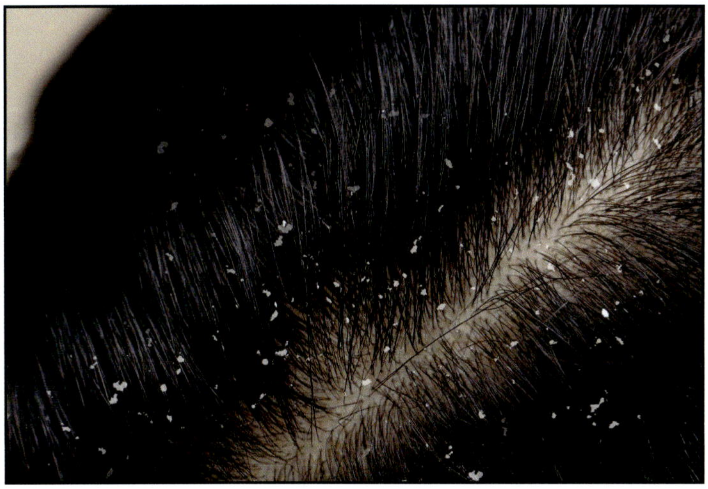

Figure 10-22. One form of seborrheic dermatitis is dandruff. (New Africa/shutterstock.com)

10

Table 10-11

Medical Conditions Related to the Nail and Nail Bed

NAME	WORD PARTS	DEFINITION
leukonychia	leuk/o (white) onych/ (nail) **-ia** (condition)	Small white spots under the nails due to microtrauma
onychitis	onych/ (nail) **-itis** (inflammation)	Inflammation of the nail
onychocryptosis (Figure 10-23)	onchy/o (nail) crypt/ (hidden) **-osis** (condition)	Ingrown nail (one that is hidden)
onycholysis	onych/o (nail) **-lysis** (separating)	Separation of the nail from the nail bed
onychomalacia	onych/o (nail) **-malacia** (softening)	Softening of the nails
onychomycosis (Figure 10-24)	onych/o (nail) myc/ (fungus) **-osis** (condition)	Fungal infection in the nail bed
paronychia	**par-** (around) onych/ (nail) **-ia** (condition)	Bacterial infection around the nail margins
subungual (Figure 10-25)	**sub-** (under) ungu/ (nail) **-al** (pertaining to)	Pertaining to under the nail
xanthoderma	xanth/o (yellow) derm/a (skin)	Yellow-colored skin

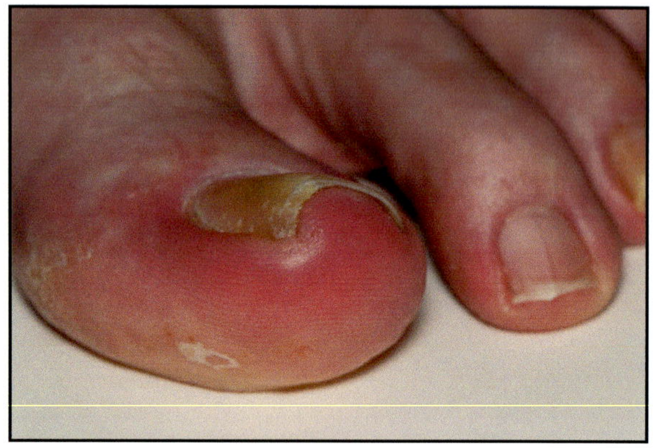

Figure 10-23. An onychocryptosis. (Brett Hondow/shutterstock.com)

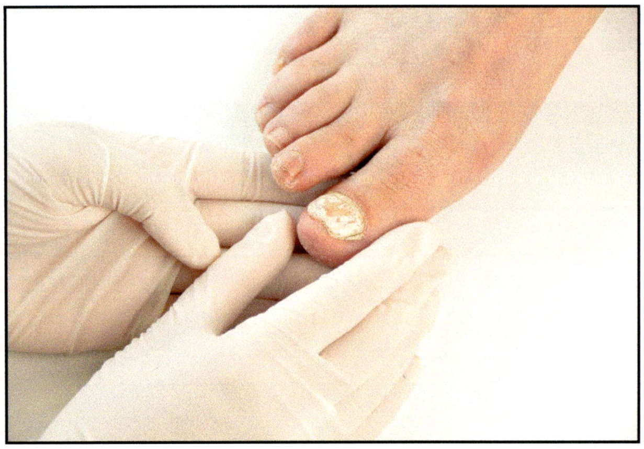

Figure 10-24. Nails with a fungal infection appear thicker and yellow. (cunaplus/shutterstock.com)

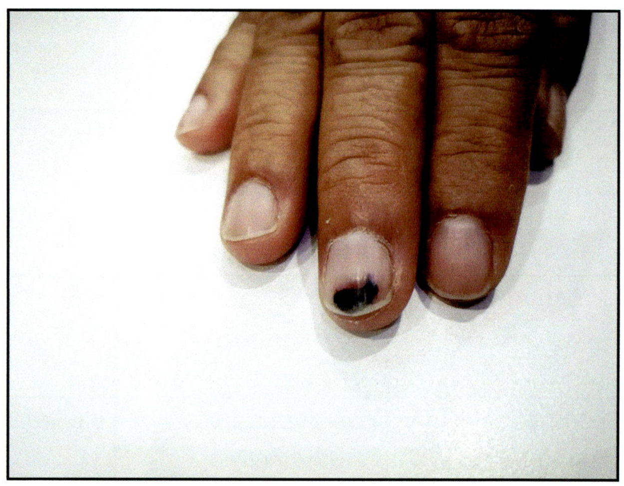

Figure 10-25. A subungual hematoma, or bleeding under the fingernail. (premkamon/shutterstock.com)

Table 10-12

Types of Tinea Infections

TINEA +	DEFINITION
capitis capit/ (head) **-is** (pertaining to)	Ringworm on the scalp
corporis corpor/o (body) **-is** (pertaining to)	Commonly called *ringworm*, tinea corporis can appear on the body, typically in non-hairy areas
cruris crur/ (leg) **-is** (pertaining to)	Occurs in the groin, typically during the summer months; also known as *jock itch*
pedis ped/ (foot) **-is** (pertaining to)	Tinea pedis is found in the foot, between the toes; also known as *athlete's foot* (Figure 10-26)
unguium ungu/ (nail) **-um** (structure)	Thickening of the nails involving the nail beds of the fingers and toes
versicolor	Noncontagious yeast infection that presents in a patchy section of skin with different pigment than the surrounding area; affected areas do not tan

Tinea infections are topical (surface) fungal infections that develop in dark, damp, and humid conditions.

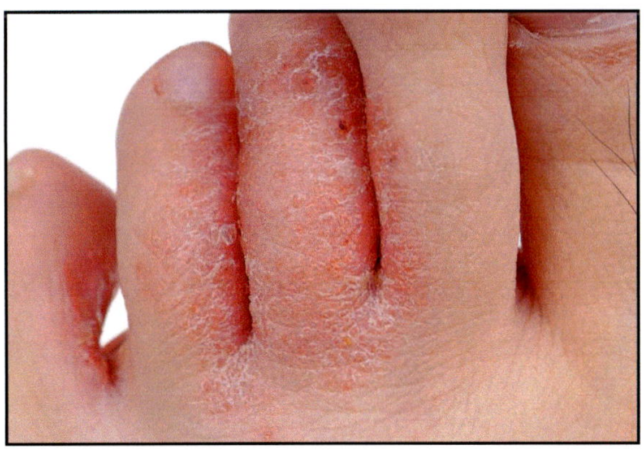

Figure 10-26. Athlete's foot, also known as *tinea pedis*. (carroteater/shutterstock.com)

10

Tests and Procedures

Table 10-13 Tests and Procedures Related to the Integumentary System	
NAME	**PURPOSE**
biopsy	Microscopic examination on a piece of tissue that has been removed; does *not* mean the tissue is cancerous, but only that it is being studied
cauterization **caut-** (heat)	Destruction of tissues through chemicals, freezing, or electric current
chemical peel	Use of chemicals to remove the outer layers of the skin (Figure 10-27)
cryosurgery **cry/o-** (cold)	Use of liquid nitrogen (most often) to freeze and destroy tissues (eg, warts, topical cancers, infections)
debridement	Removal of foreign material or dead tissue using chemical agent or surgical excision
dermabrasion derm/a (skin)	Use of sandpaper or wire brushes to mechanically scrape away the upper layer of skin; most often used in treating scars and wrinkles or removing tattoos
electrocautery electr/o (electricity) **caut-** (burn)	Destruction of tissues via an electrical current
fulguration	Use of a high-frequency electronic current to destroy unwanted tissue
incision and drainage (I&D)	Cutting into a lesion and draining it
laser therapy	Destruction of skin lesions via laser beam
liposuction (lip/o—fat)	Removal of subcutaneous fat through small holes via suction
skin test	Allergen is applied to the skin, either topical of injected; used to determine allergies and reactions; also called a *patch test* (Figure 10-29)
Tzanck test	Microscopic examination of a lesion

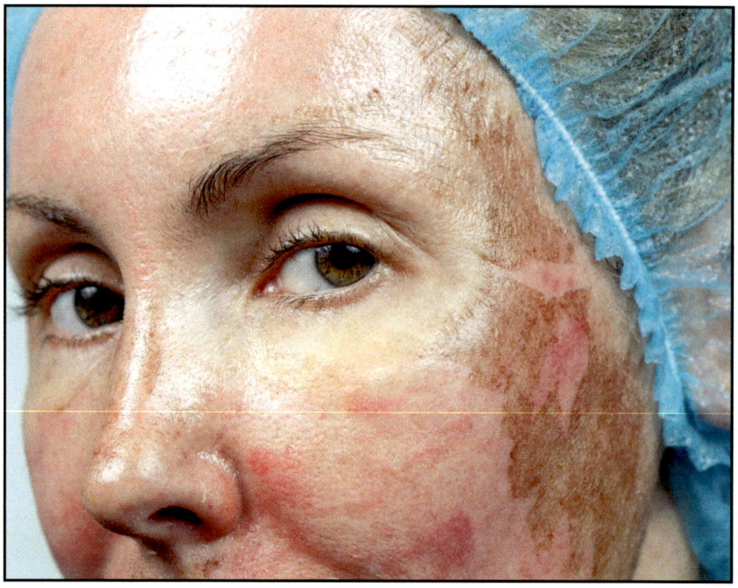

Figure 10-27. A chemical peel causes the superficial layers of the skin to peel off and allows healthy skin to grow. (KKulikov/shutterstock.com)

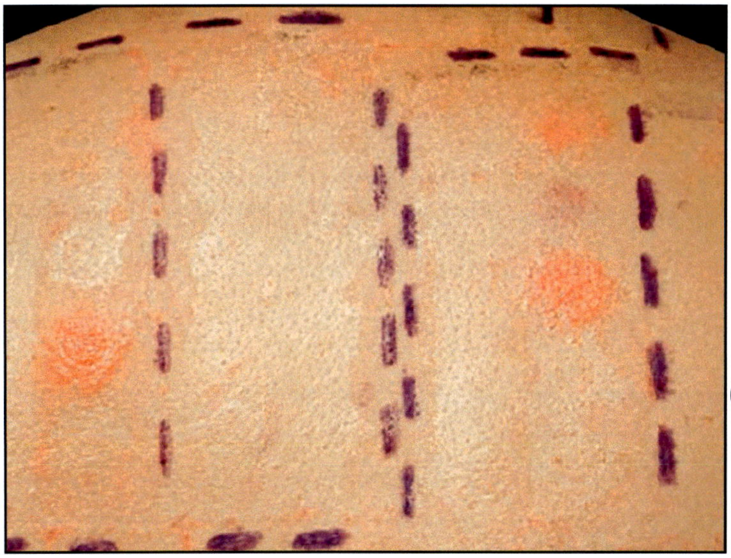

Figure 10-28. An example of a skin test for allergies. (Andy Lidstone/shutterstock.com)

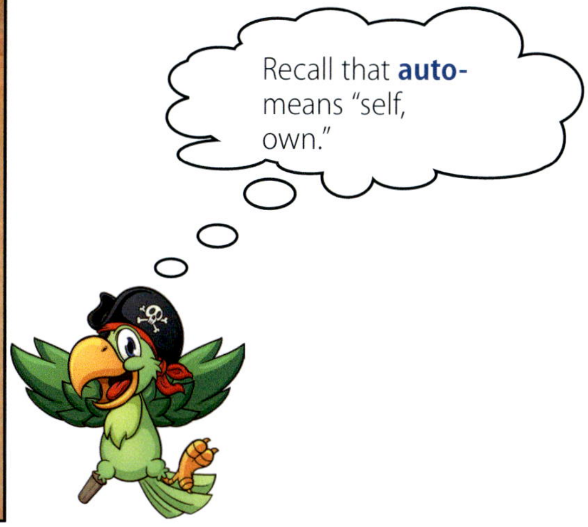

Table 10-14
Terms Related to Tissue Grafting

TERM	WORD PARTS	PURPOSE
allograft	**allo-** (different)	Graft taken from one human and transferred to another part of a different person; typically involves cadaver parts
autograft	**auto-** (self)	Graft taken from one part of a person and transferred to another part of the same person
synthetic	**syn-** (joined)	Artificial material used to create imitation skin
xenograft	xen/o (foreign)	Graft taken from one species and transferred to another species

Table 10-15
Procedures of the Skin and Nails

NAME	WORD PARTS	PURPOSE
dermoplasty	derm/o (skin) **-plasty** (repair)	Surgical repair of the skin
onychectomy	onych/ (nail) **-ectomy** (surgical removal)	Surgical removal of the nail
rhytidectomy	rhytid/o (wrinkle) **-ectomy** (surgical removal)	Cutting away excess skin to remove wrinkles; also known as a *facelift*
rhytidoplasty	rhytid/o (wrinkle) **-plasty** (plastic surgery)	Plastic surgery for the removal of wrinkles
sclerotherapy	scler/o (hard; hardening; thick)	Highly concentrated saline solution is injected into dilated (varicose or spider) veins, or hemorrhoids to destroy (harden) the lumen of the vein

Medication Classifications

Table 10-16

Medication Classifications Used in Treatment of Integumentary Conditions

CATEGORY	WHAT IT DOES
antibiotic	Destroys or interferes with bacterial growth; different subcategories of this medication are used to treat different forms of bacteria
antifungal	Retards fungal growth
antihistamine	Inhibits allergic responses (eg, inflammation, redness, itching) due to histamine
antipruritic	Stops itching
antiseptic	Inhibits bacterial growth; applied topically (on the surface)
antiviral	Destroys or inhibits viruses
corticosteroid	Decreases inflammation
emollient	Softens the skin
keratolytic	Helps loosen and shed the superficial layer of skin
parasiticides	Destroys insect parasites (eg, lice, mites)

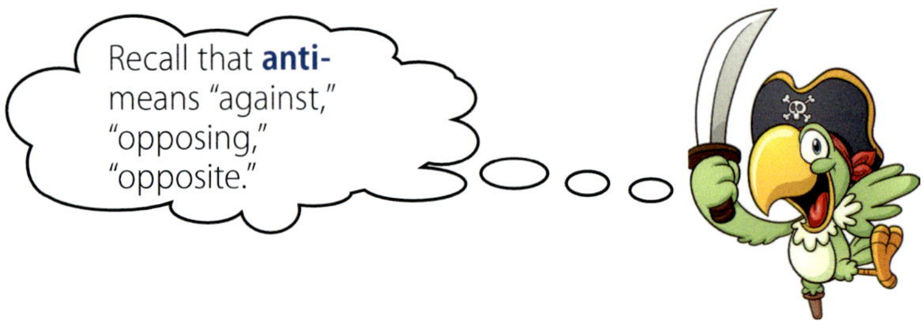

Bibliography

Centers for Disease Control and Prevention. *The Surgeon General's Call to Action to Prevent Skin Cancer.* Published July 2014. Accessed August 31, 20222. https://www.cdc.gov/cancer/skin/pdf/consumer-booklet.pdf

Flanagan KW, Cuppett M. Dermatological conditions. In *Medical Conditions in the Athlete.* 3rd ed. Human Kinetics; 2017.

Guy GP Jr, Thomas CC, Thompson T, Watson M, Massetti GM, Richardson LC. Vital signs: melanoma incidence and mortality trends and projections—United States, 1982–2030. *MMWR.* 2015;64(21):591-596.

Mosby's Dictionary of Medicine, Nursing & Health Professions. 10th ed. Elsevier; 2017.

Skin Cancer Foundation. Skin cancer facts and statistics. Published January 2021. Updated May 2022. Accessed August 30, 2022. https://www.skincancer.org/skin-cancer-information/skin-cancer-facts

US Environmental Protection Agency. Pest control and pesticides safety for consumers. Published October 25, 2021. Updated April 21, 2022. Accessed August 31, 2022. https://www.epa.gov/safepestcontrol

Venes D, ed. *Taber's Cyclopedic Medical Dictionary.* 24th ed. F. A. Davis; 2021.

Weir HK, Thompson TD, Stewart SL, White, MC. Cancer incidence projections in the United States between 2015 and 2050. *Prev Chron Dis.* 2021;18:210006.

Wingerd BD. *Medical Terminology Complete!* Pearson; 2019.

Notes

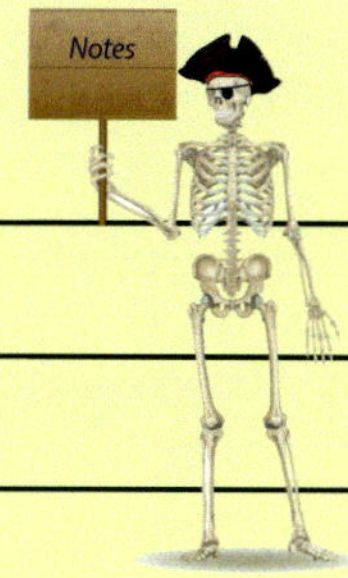

NOTES

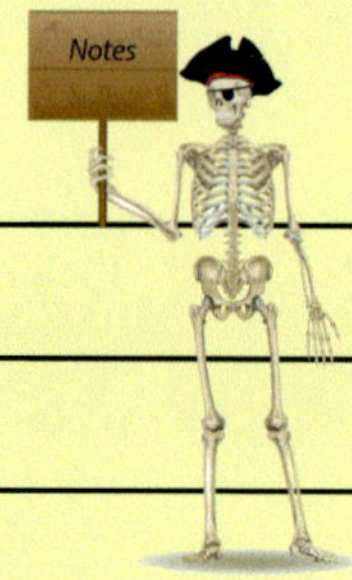

Learning Activities

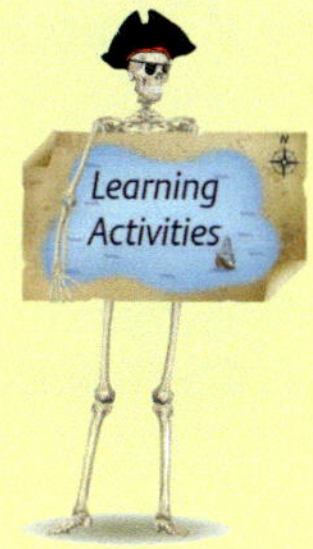

Name:______________________

Integumentary System

A. Label the aspects of the dermis from the following list of words.

- dermis__________________
- hair bulb________________
- sebaceous gland___________
- pore____________________
- sudoriferous gland_________
- arrector pili muscle________
- hair shaft________________
- subcutaneous layer_________

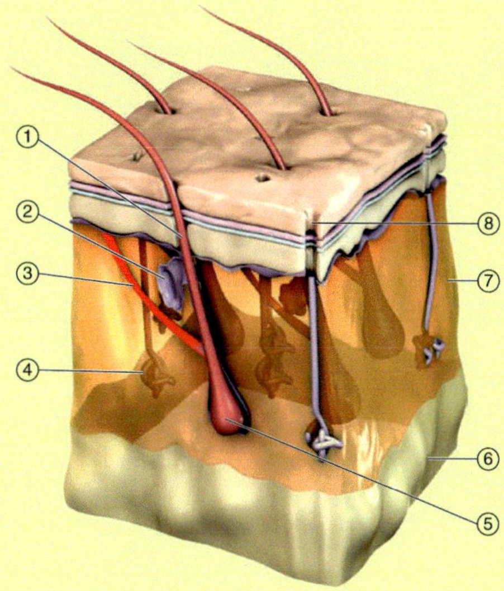

(Blamb/shutterstock.com)

B. Label the aspects of the fingernail from the following list of words.

- nail plate__________
- nail matrix_________
- nail bed___________
- lunula_____________
- cuticle_____________
- paronychium_______

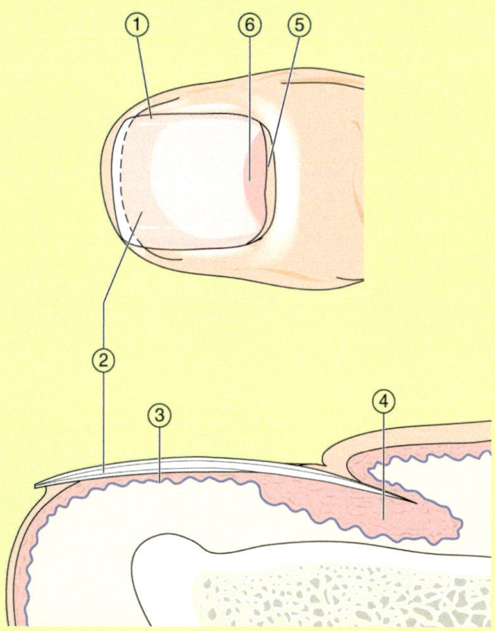

(Blamb/shutterstock.com)

C. Matching.

Match the word element with its best meaning.

1. xanth/o______________	a. hair
2. sudor______________	b. oil
3. ped______________	c. leg
4. rhytid/o______________	d. pale
5. crur/o______________	e. bottom
6. pallor______________	f. foot
7. trich/o______________	g. sweating
8. albin/o______________	h. yellow
9. seb______________	i. wrinkle
10. bas______________	j. white

D. Write the medical word for the following common terms.

1. blister______________________________
2. German measles______________________
3. freckle______________________________
4. skin tag_____________________________
5. stretch marks_______________________
6. pimple______________________________
7. chickenpox__________________________
8. hives_______________________________
9. scar________________________________
10. blackhead__________________________
11. wart_______________________________
12. athlete's foot________________________

E. Indicate if the word listed is a disease/infection, treatment, or parasite.

WORD	DISEASE/INFECTION	TREATMENT	PARASITE
sclerotherapy			
debridement			
varicella			
fulguration			
carbuncle			
dermoplasty			
scabies			
rubella			
xenograft			
Cimex lectularius			

F. Separate the word elements in the following terms and define them.

1. dermatomyositis____________________
2. melanocarcinoma____________________
3. onychoplasty____________________
4. intradermal____________________

G. Write the medical terms that are used to describe these conditions.

1. the layer of skin found only on the soles and palms____________________
2. the bottom-most layer of the dermis____________________
3. inability to distinguish between hot or cold temperatures____________________
4. a layer with cells that have spine-like projections____________________
5. a sensation of burning____________________

H. Describe what the following medications do.

1. emollient ____________________
2. antipruritic ____________________
3. antifungal ____________________
4. antiseptic ____________________
5. keratolytic ____________________

Case Study

Define the numerical terms (1 to 14).

History, Chief Complaint

A wrestler presented with tender, raised **erythroderma** (1) with **bullae** (2) on his knees. He wrestled in a meet 2 days ago, and had not noticed them until just now. He says the lesions are **pruritic** (3). He also noted he was wearing his lucky kneepads, and has not washed them this season (which began 2 months ago). He has a history of **psoriasis** (4).

Evaluation

The lesions do not appear to be **urticaria** (5), **milia** (6), **comedones** (7), **boils** (8), or **folliculitis** (9). The wrestler has had **varicella** (10), so that was ruled out. The athlete was **afebrile** (11) and had no **lymphadenopathy** (12).

Treatment

The wrestler was diagnosed with **impetigo** (13), which is quite contagious. He was prescribed **antibiotics** (14) and is to abstain from contact with others until the lesions are completely cleared. His lucky knee pads were laundered in bleach.

Terms

1. ______________________
2. ______________________
3. ______________________
4. ______________________
5. ______________________
6. ______________________
7. ______________________
8. ______________________
9. ______________________
10. ______________________
11. ______________________
12. ______________________
13. ______________________
14. ______________________

11

Endocrine System

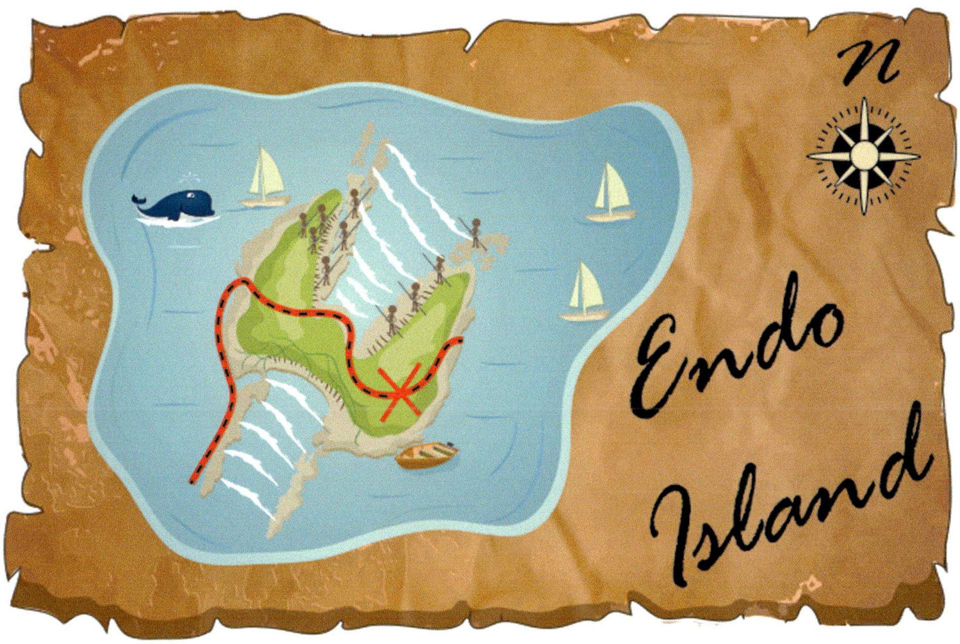

Objectives

After studying this chapter, you will be able to:

1. Identify the major components of the endocrine system.
2. Recall the names of hormones, their gland of origin, and the target organs.
3. List the glands responsible for secreting specific hormones.
4. Explain the role of hormones in ovulation.
5. List signs and symptoms of endocrine disorders.
6. Describe basic abnormalities or conditions of the endocrine system.
7. Describe what roles hormones play in diabetes.
8. Explain diagnostic tests, procedures, and treatments specific to the endocrine system.
9. Identify classifications of medications used to treat pathological conditions related to the endocrine system.

Flanagan KW.
Medical Terminology With Case Studies: A Navigated Guide to Learning for Health Care Professionals, Third Edition (pp 291-327).

Chapter Outline

- Self-assessment
- Checklist for word parts in the chapter
- Checklist of new anatomy
- Checklist of gonad and mammary gland anatomy
- Introduction
- Anatomy
  - Endocrine glands in the head and neck
  - Endocrine glands of the chest and abdomen
  - The gonads
  - Physiology of ovulation
  - The testes
  - The mammary glands
- Word building
  - Prefixes
  - Suffixes
  - Combining forms
- Signs and symptoms
- Medical conditions
- Tests and procedures
- Medication classifications
- Learning activities
- Case study

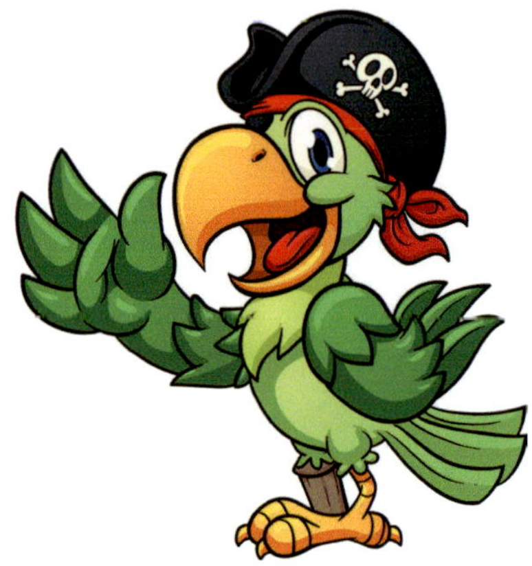

Self-Assessment

Based on what you have learned so far, can you write the definition of these words?

- adenocarcinoma____________________
- mastitis____________________
- oogenesis____________________
- glucometer____________________
- thyroidectomy____________________

Checklist for Word Parts in the Chapter

Prefixes

- ☐ ad-
- ☐ an-
- ☐ anti-
- ☐ crypt-
- ☐ dys-
- ☐ endo-
- ☐ epi-
- ☐ ex-
- ☐ exo-
- ☐ hyper-
- ☐ hypo-
- ☐ pan-
- ☐ para-
- ☐ poly-
- ☐ supra-
- ☐ syn-

There are lots of new terms in the endocrine system, but by now, most of the prefixes and suffixes should be familiar to you. Use them to assist you in understanding the whole word.

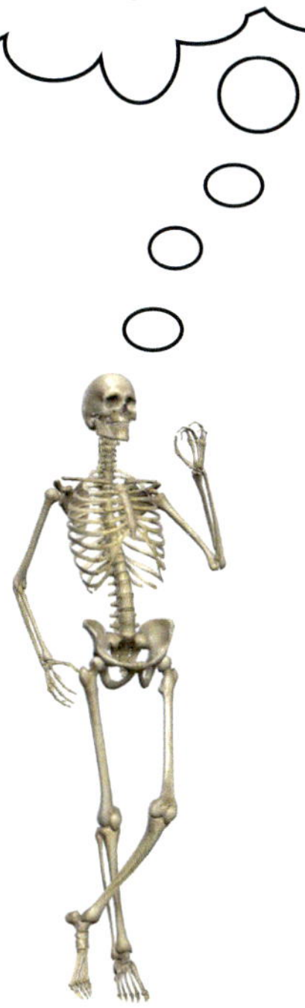

Suffixes

- ☐ -al
- ☐ -arche
- ☐ -ation
- ☐ -cele
- ☐ -crine
- ☐ -drome
- ☐ -ectomy
- ☐ -edema
- ☐ -emia
- ☐ -graphy
- ☐ -ia
- ☐ -ic
- ☐ -ism
- ☐ -itis
- ☐ -megaly
- ☐ -meter
- ☐ -oid
- ☐ -oma
- ☐ -osis
- ☐ -ostomy
- ☐ -otomy
- ☐ -pathy
- ☐ -penia
- ☐ -penic
- ☐ -pexy
- ☐ -physis
- ☐ -plasia
- ☐ -plasty
- ☐ -ptosis
- ☐ -rrhagia
- ☐ -rrhaphy
- ☐ -rrhea
- ☐ -rrhexis
- ☐ -tic
- ☐ -tomy
- ☐ -troph
- ☐ -uria

Combining Forms

- ☐ acid/o
- ☐ aden/o
- ☐ adren/o
- ☐ andr/o
- ☐ calc/i
- ☐ calc/o
- ☐ carcin/o
- ☐ chrom/o
- ☐ cortic/o
- ☐ crin/o
- ☐ cyst/o
- ☐ cyt/o
- ☐ didym/o
- ☐ dips/o
- ☐ galact/o
- ☐ gluc/o
- ☐ glyc/o
- ☐ glycos/o
- ☐ gonad/o
- ☐ gynec/o
- ☐ hormon/o
- ☐ hydr/o
- ☐ hypophys/o
- ☐ idi/o
- ☐ kal/o
- ☐ ket/o
- ☐ keton/o
- ☐ lact/o
- ☐ mamm/o
- ☐ mast/o
- ☐ men/o
- ☐ metr/o
- ☐ myx/o
- ☐ nat/o
- ☐ neur/o
- ☐ oophor/o
- ☐ ophthalm/o
- ☐ orch/o
- ☐ orchi/o
- ☐ orchid/o
- ☐ ov/i
- ☐ ov/o
- ☐ ovari/o
- ☐ ovul/o
- ☐ pancreat/o
- ☐ papill/o

Combining Forms

- ❒ **phe/o**
- ❒ **pituitar/o**
- ❒ **prolactin/o**
- ❒ **pub/o**
- ❒ **ren/o**
- ❒ **scrot/o**
- ❒ **somat/o**
- ❒ **test/o**
- ❒ **thel/e**
- ❒ **thym/o**
- ❒ **thyr/o**
- ❒ **troph/o**
- ❒ **ur/o**
- ❒ **varic/o**

Checklist of New Anatomy

- ❒ Hypothalamus
- ❒ Pituitary gland
  - ❒ Anterior lobe (adenohypophysis)
  - ❒ Posterior lobe (neurohypophysis)
- ❒ Pineal gland
- ❒ Thyroid gland
  - ❒ Isthmus
- ❒ Parathyroid gland
- ❒ Thymus gland
- ❒ Pancreas
- ❒ Islets of Langerhans
  - ❒ Alpha cells
  - ❒ Beta cells
  - ❒ Delta cells
- ❒ Adrenal glands (suprarenal glands)
  - ❒ Adrenal cortex
  - ❒ Adrenal medulla

Checklist of Gonad and Mammary Gland Anatomy

- ❒ Ovaries
  - ❒ Broad ligament
  - ❒ Suspensory ligament
  - ❒ Cortex
  - ❒ Follicles
- ❒ Medulla
- ❒ Ovum
- ❒ Testicles
  - ❒ Seminiferous tubules
  - ❒ Spermatozoa
  - ❒ Epididymis
  - ❒ Vas deferens
  - ❒ Spermatic cord
  - ❒ Scrotum
- ❒ Mammary glands
  - ❒ Lactiferous glands
  - ❒ Lactiferous ducts
  - ❒ Nipple
  - ❒ Areola

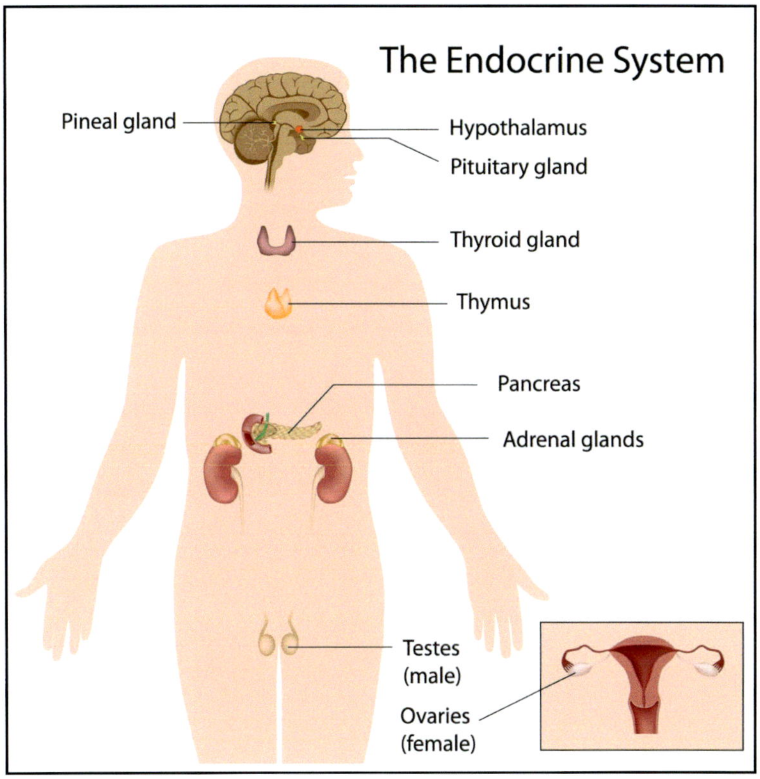

Figure 11-1. Glands of the endocrine system. (Alila Medical Images/shutterstock.com)

11

Introduction

Welcome to Endo Island, home of the **endocrine** (**endo**-—within; **-crine**—to secrete) system, which is composed of glands that secrete hormones directly into the bloodstream and whose functions are to regulate the body. Different from endocrine glands are **exocrine** (**exo**-—away, away from, out, outside) glands that secrete directly to the skin's surface via a duct. Sudoriferous (sweat) and sebaceous (oil) glands are examples of exocrine glands.

Endo Island contains words and combining forms distinctive to the endocrine system. Because the ovaries and testes also function as endocrine glands, terms related to them are found in this chapter, but other terms associated with reproduction are found in Chapter 13 ("Reproductive System"). By now, most of the suffixes and prefixes listed in this chapter should be familiar, as they have traveled with you from previously visited islands. Endo Island resembles the thyroid gland with its channels acting as the trachea. It contains words and word parts related to the hypothalamus, pituitary, pineal, thyroid, parathyroid, thymus, adrenal, pancreas, and sex (ovaries and testes) glands (Figure 11-1).

Anatomy

As a system, endocrine glands secrete hormones directly into the bloodstream that are carried by the blood vessels to specific target organs or tissues. The word *hormone* is Greek for "to set in motion," as each hormone has a specific target cell upon which it acts. Generally, a gland's primary function is to secrete hormones and other substances. The purposes of some hormones are to initiate or inhibit the release of other hormones. Once a given hormone reaches its **target cell**, chemical changes occur that alter the target cell roles. Each target cell has unique properties that can receive the appropriate hormone; likewise, target cells will not respond to hormones from glands that do not target them. For example, insulin secreted by the pancreas will only produce a reaction to its target organ (liver) and not have any effect on another organ (eg, the testes). Overall there are 10 glands that secrete hormones, three of which are paired glands (adrenal gland, ovary, and testis). This section divides review of these glands by anatomical location within the body. Within the head and neck are the hypothalamus, pineal, pituitary, thyroid, and parathyroid glands; the thymus, pancreas, and adrenal glands are found in the body proper; and the gonads, the collective term for sex glands (ovary and testis), are discussed last. Keep in mind that the chief purpose of this textbook is to learn medical words, not be a primary source for anatomy or physiology. There will be enough information provided to understand why terms are named what they are, but do not go into the minute science of the endocrine system.

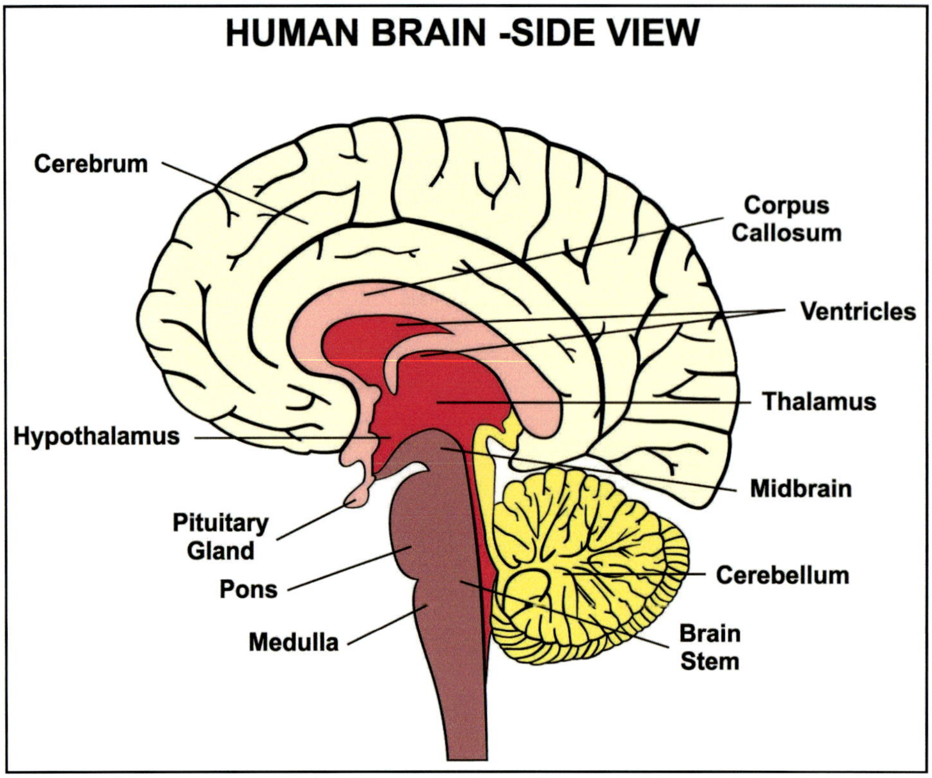

Figure 11-2. Location of the hypothalamus and pituitary glands. (udaix/shutterstock.com)

Endocrine Glands in the Head and Neck

The three endocrine glands in the head are the hypothalamus, pituitary, and pineal glands. Figure 11-2 provides a reminder of their relationship in the brain. The endocrine glands in the neck are the thyroid and parathyroid.

The **hypothalamus** is the connector between the nervous and endocrine systems. Hormones released by the posterior lobe of the pituitary gland (the neurohypophysis) actually originate from nerve cell bodies in the hypothalamus and travel via neurons to the pituitary gland (Figure 11-3). There is much discussion over whether it is the hypothalamus or the pituitary gland that has the nickname the *master gland*, as both control homeostasis as well as regulate other glands.

The **pituitary** gland (combining forms are: **pituitar/o**; **hypophys/o**) has regulatory control over the body and all other glands. Also termed the **hypophysis** (**hypo**-—below; -**physis**—growth), it is the size of a small pea and is located under the brain and connected to the hypothalamus. There are two very distinct lobes of this gland, the anterior and posterior lobes. Each has very specific functions. The **anterior lobe** (also called the **adenohypophysis**) regulates activity of other endocrine glands, whereas the **posterior lobe** (also called the **neurohypophysis**) is controlled by the hypothalamus and receives hormones from neurons from the hypothalamus. From a medical terminology view they are easy to remember: the anterior lobe controls other glands (**adenohypophysis**: **aden/o**—gland); and the posterior lobe houses neurons (**neurohypophysis**; **neur/o**—nerve). Table 11-1 displays some of the major hormones secreted by the lobes of the pituitary gland.

The **pineal gland** is so named because it resembles a pinecone. Its primary function is to secrete **melatonin**, the hormone responsible for regulating sleep and for controlling female reproductive hormones. Melatonin is an interesting hormone as it is produced more when it is dark and less in the light. People often use the hormone to counteract jet lag or shiftwork, when exposure to constant light disrupts the normal circadian rhythm. In people who menstruate, melatonin determines when they begin menstruation, the frequency and duration of their cycles, and onset of menopause (the cessation of menstruation; Table 11-2).

The **thyroid** (**thyr/o**) is the largest gland of the system, and is represented as Endo Island in the opening of this chapter. It is an H-shaped gland that lies anterior to the trachea, inferior to the larynx (voice box; Figure 11-4). Joining the two halves (lobes) of the thyroid is a piece of tissue called the **isthmus** (Figure 11-5). Hormones secreted to the bloodstream from the thyroid have an impact on almost every function in the body (Table 11-3).

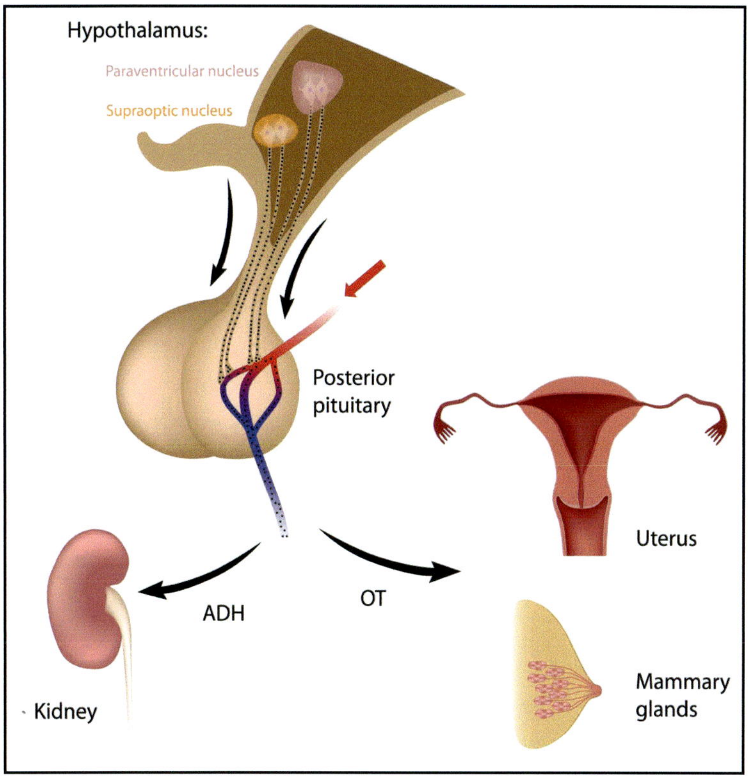

Figure 11-3. The relationship of the hypothalamus and the posterior lobe of the pituitary gland. (Alila Medical Images/ shutterstock.com)

11

Table 11-1
Hormones Secreted by the Anterior Lobe of the Pituitary Gland

ANTERIOR LOBE HORMONES	TARGET ORGANS/ TISSUES	PURPOSE
adrenocorticotropic hormone (ACTH)	adrenal cortex	Affects adrenal cortex; releases are increased during stressful periods (final exams, anyone?)
follicle-stimulating hormone (FSH)	ovaries/testes	Stimulates development of ova (egg) and sperm
growth hormone (GH) or somatotropin	bone, cartilage, muscles, liver	Stimulates growth, cellular division, and protein synthesis
luteinizing hormone (LH)	ovaries/testes	Stimulates gonads to secrete hormones
melanocyte-stimulating hormone (MSH)	skin	Stimulates melanocytes to increase skin pigmentation
prolactin (PRL)	mammary glands (breasts)	Stimulates mammary glands to produce milk
thyroid-stimulating hormone (TSH)	thyroid gland	Stimulates the thyroid gland
antidiuretic hormone (ADH) also called *vasopressin*	kidneys	Maintains homeostasis by maintaining the proper amount of water in the blood
oxytocin	uterus, breasts	Stimulates uterine contractions to initiate labor; milk production of the mammary glands

TABLE 11-2 HORMONE SECRETED BY THE PINEAL GLAND	
PINEAL GLAND HORMONE	**PURPOSE**
melatonin	Regulates biorhythms (sleep) and sexual development

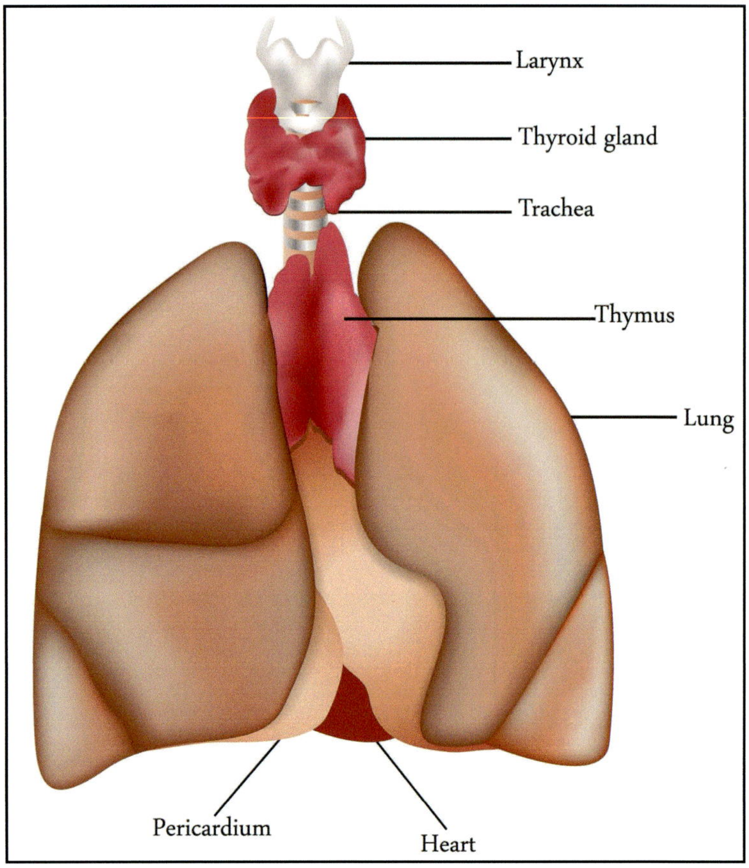

Figure 11-4. Location of the thyroid and thymus glands. (GRei/shutterstock.com)

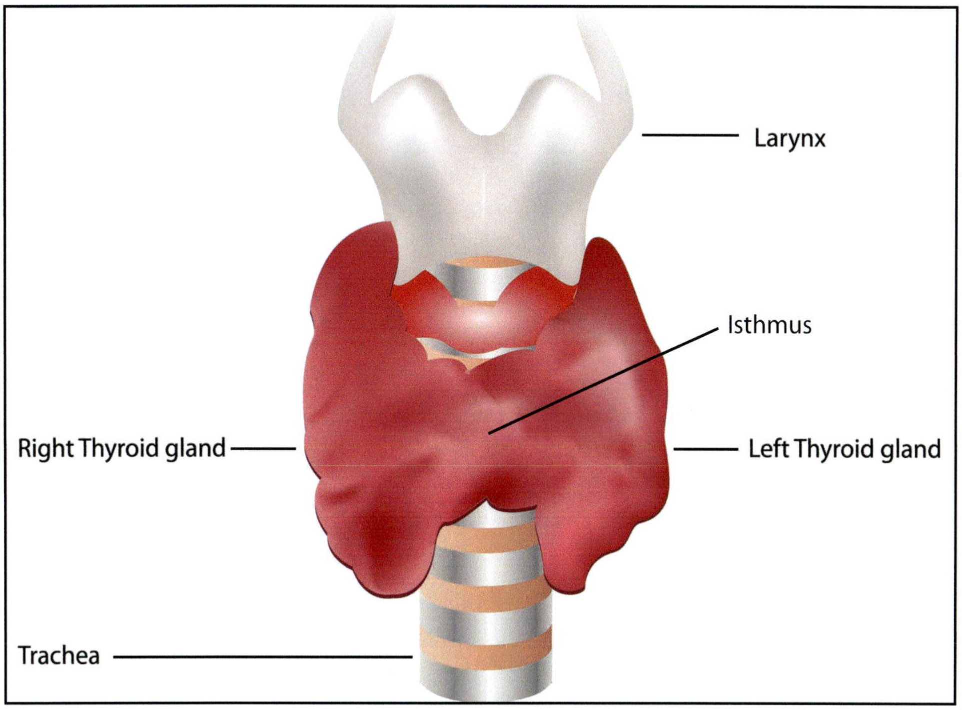

Figure 11-5. The thyroid gland has left and right aspects to it. (GRei/shutterstock.com)

Table 11-3
Hormones Secreted by the Thyroid Gland

THYROID HORMONES	PURPOSE
calcitonin	Regulates calcium levels in the blood
triiodothyronine (T3)	Increases protein synthesis and energy production
thyroxine (T4)	Increases protein synthesis and energy production

Table 11-4
Hormones Secreted by the Parathyroid Gland

PARATHYROID HORMONES	TARGET ORGANS/TISSUES	PURPOSE
parathyroid hormone (PTH)	bone, kidney, small intestine	Regulates calcium levels in the blood

The **parathyroid** glands (**para-**—beside, near, abnormal) are four small, oval-shaped glands adjacent to the thyroid gland in the anterior neck. The parathyroid releases parathyroid hormone (PTH), which controls calcium levels in the body (Table 11-4). PTH performs this function by causing bones to release calcium into the blood and maintaining calcium levels in the kidney (Figure 11-6).

Endocrine Glands of the Chest and Abdomen

The thymus, pancreas, and adrenal glands comprise the endocrine glands of the body proper. The **thymus** (thym/o) is the main component of the **lymph** system, but it also has endocrine properties. It is located behind the sternum in the mediastinum, superior to the heart, and slowly grows in size until about puberty, then diminishes via involution (see Figure 11-4). The hormone **thymosin** is secreted by the thymus and has immunological functions for the whole body (Table 11-5).

Figure 11-6. The parathyroid glands appear to be within the thyroid gland. (O2creationz/shutterstock.com)

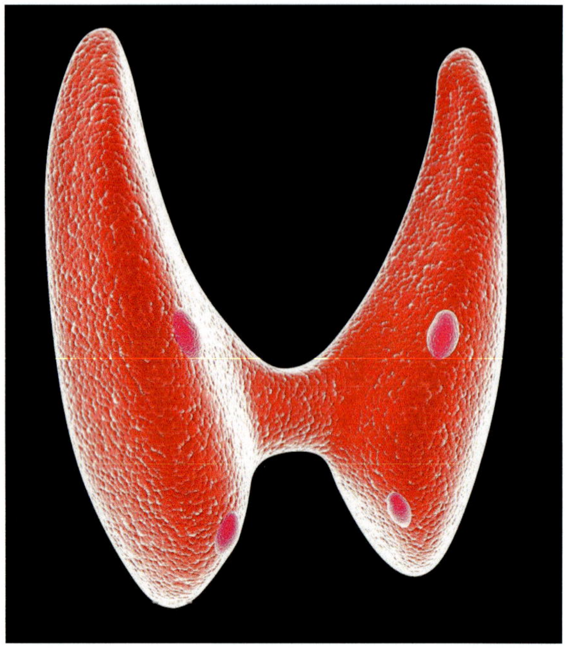

Table 11-5 Hormone Secreted by the Thymus Gland		
THYMUS HORMONE	**TARGET ORGANS/TISSUES**	**PURPOSE**
thymosin	T-cells (lymphocytes)	Maturation and development of the immune system (T lymphocytes)

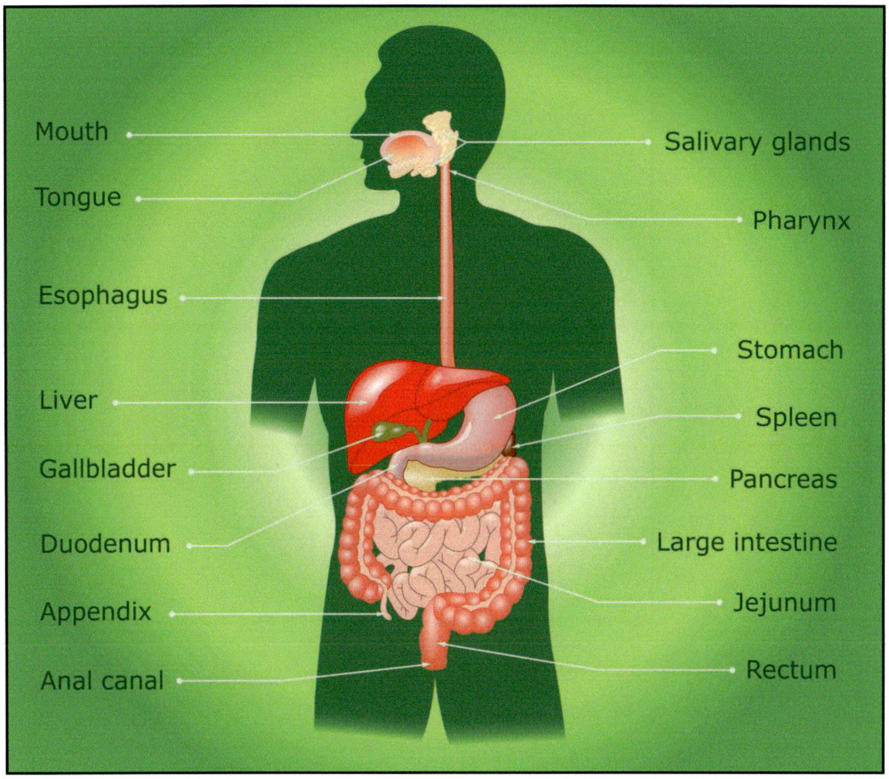

Figure 11-7. The pancreas has a close relationship with the digestive system. (dr OX/shutterstock.com)

11

Table 11-6

Hormones Secreted by the Pancreas

PANCREAS HORMONES	TARGET ORGANS/ TISSUES	PURPOSE
alpha cells (glucagon)	liver, muscles, blood, adipose tissues	Increases blood glucose by accelerating conversion of glycogen from the liver into usable glucose
beta cells (insulin)	liver, muscles, adipose tissues	Accelerates glucose transport into cells; lowers blood glucose
delta cells (somatostatin)	alpha cells, beta cells	Suppresses the release of glucagon and insulin

Playing a huge role in glucose absorption is the **pancreas**. The pancreas has a close relationship with the digestive system (Figure 11-7) and is located in the upper aspect of the abdominal cavity. A specialized cluster of cells in the pancreas called the **islets of Langerhans** secrete hormones that regulate sugar (glucose) levels in the body. Two types of cells within the islets of Langerhans called the **alpha** and **beta cells** secrete the two different hormones (glucagon and insulin, respectively). A third specialized unit is the **delta cells**, which counteracts the alpha and beta cells (Table 11-6). When these cells malfunction, the result is often a medical condition having to do with glucose levels in the blood (eg, diabetes mellitus or hypoglycemia).

Located as pairs just superior to each kidney are the **adrenal** glands (**adren/o**) glands (Figure 11-8). Also known as the **suprarenal** (**supra**-—above; **ren/o**—kidney; **-al**—pertaining to) glands, they have an outer area (**adrenal cortex**) and an inner layer called the **adrenal medulla** (Figure 11-9). These two anatomical areas secrete different hormones to the bloodstream (Table 11-7). The adrenal cortex responds to adrenocorticotropic (**adren/o**—adrenal gland; **cortic/o**—cortex, outer portion; **troph/o**—development, growth, nourishment; **-ic**—pertaining to) hormones secreted from the anterior pituitary gland to release androgens (steroid hormones). Hormones of the medulla all contribute to the body's fight-or-flight reaction by acting on the sympathetic nervous system.

Figure 11-8. The adrenal glands lie superior to each kidney. (Lightspring/shutterstock.com).

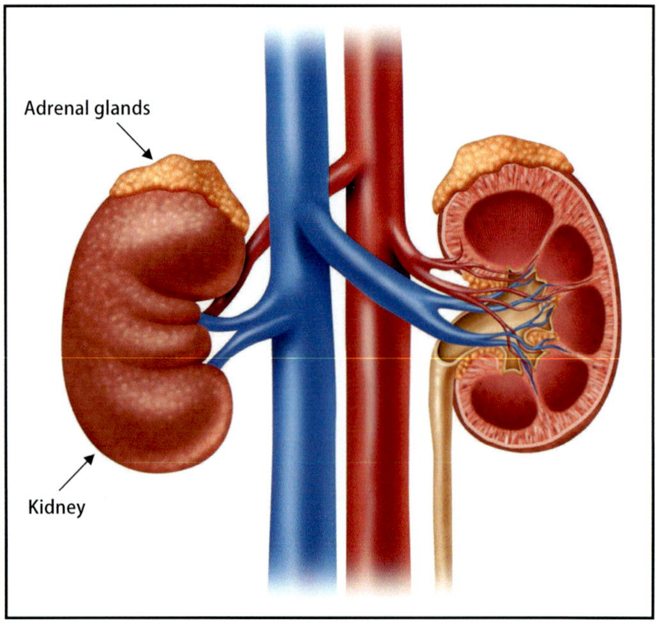

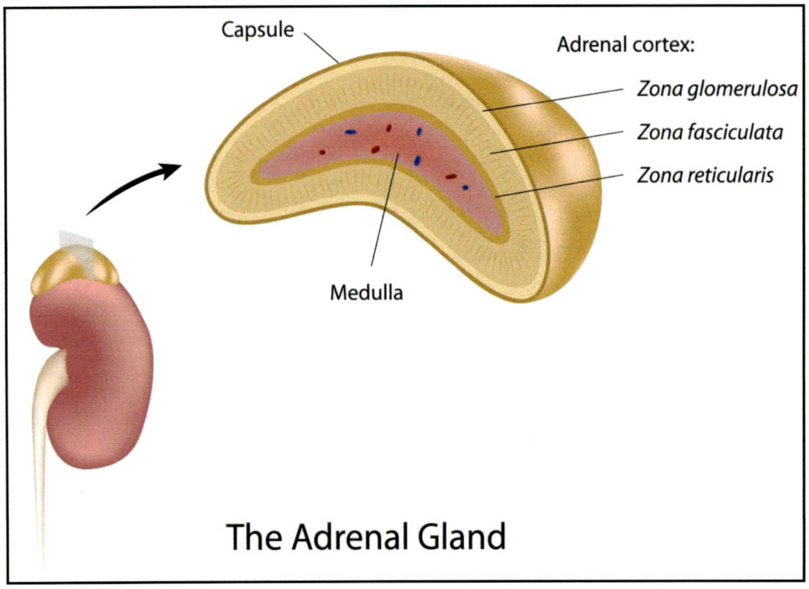

Figure 11-9. A cross-section of the adrenal gland. (Alila Medical Images/shutterstock.com)

The Gonads

The **ovaries** and **testes** are gonads (sex organs) that are also endocrine glands. The ovaries (ovari/o) lie in the lower abdomen alongside of the uterus, attached to a structure called the **broad ligament**. Each ovary is fixed to the side of the pelvis via **suspensory ligaments** (Figure 11-10). As with the adrenal glands, ovaries have two distinct areas: the outer cortex and the inner medulla. The ovarian cortex contains small sacs called **follicles** that are in one of three stages of maturity: **primary**, **growing**, or **graafian** (mature; Figure 11-11). Within the medulla lie nerves, vessels, connective tissue, and smooth muscle. The hormones associated with gonads are listed in Table 11-8.

Physiology of Ovulation

The onset of maturity in females coincides with **menarche** (the menstrual cycle) and it affects the uterus, ovaries, and breasts. Because menarche is driven by hormones, it is discussed in this chapter. Every month in between puberty and menopause, a **graafian follicle** ruptures from the cortex of the ovary, releasing an egg (**ovum**). This process is called **ovulation** and is stimulated by FSH and LH, released by the anterior lobe of the pituitary gland. Collectively, these hormones

Table 11-7
Hormones Secreted by the Adrenal Gland

ADRENAL CORTEX HORMONES	PURPOSE
aldosterone	Regulates electrolyte and water balance by promotion of sodium and chloride reabsorption and potassium secretion
androsterone	Stimulates secondary male sex characteristics
corticosterone	Carbohydrate and protein synthesis; absorbs glucose
cortisol	Carbohydrate, fat, and protein synthesis; increases blood glucose; has an anti-inflammatory effect; assists with stress management
testosterone	Stimulates secondary male sex characteristics
ADRENAL MEDULLA HORMONES	**PURPOSE**
dopamine	Dilates systemic vessels; increases blood pressure
epinephrine (also called *adrenaline*)	Vasoconstrictor; cardiac stimulator
norepinephrine (also called *noradrenaline*)	Vasoconstrictor

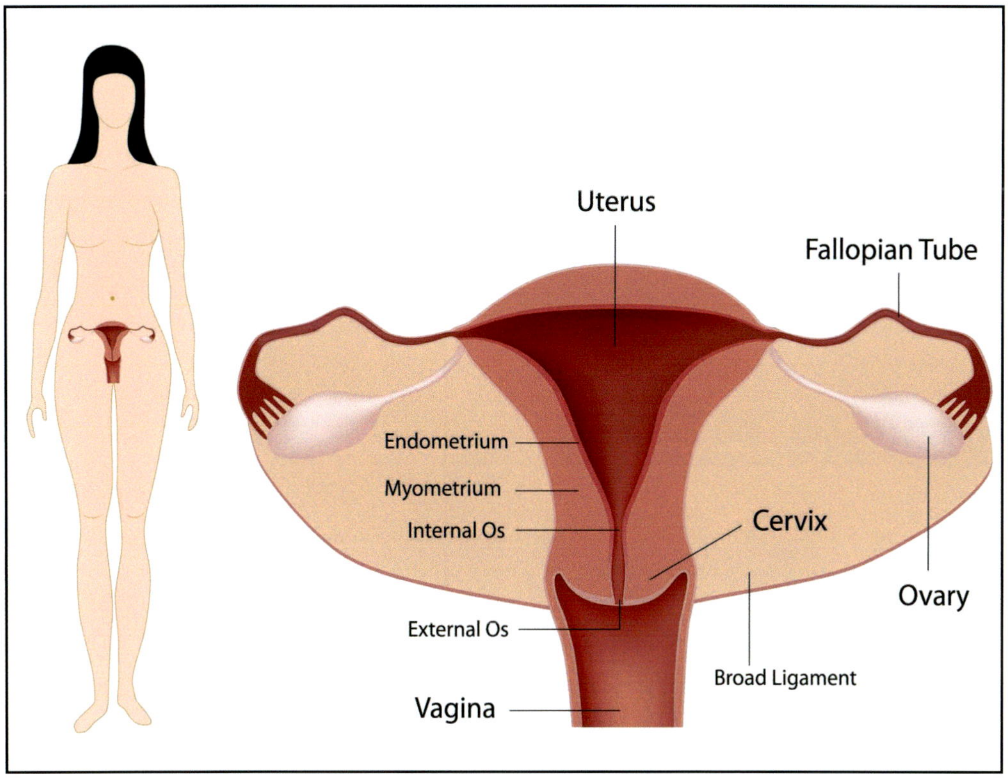

Figure 11-10. The relationship of the ovaries to the uterus. (Alila Medical Images/shutterstock.com)

are termed *gonadotrophic* (**gonad/o**—sex organ; **troph/**—development; **-ic**—pertaining to) hormones. The follicle, now termed the **corpus luteum**, then releases estrogen and progesterone, which supply negative feedback information to the pituitary gland (Figure 11-12). As estrogen levels increase, the pituitary decreases the levels of FSH secreted. Likewise, as progesterone levels in the blood increase, LH levels decrease. The phases of menstruation are presented in Table 11-9.

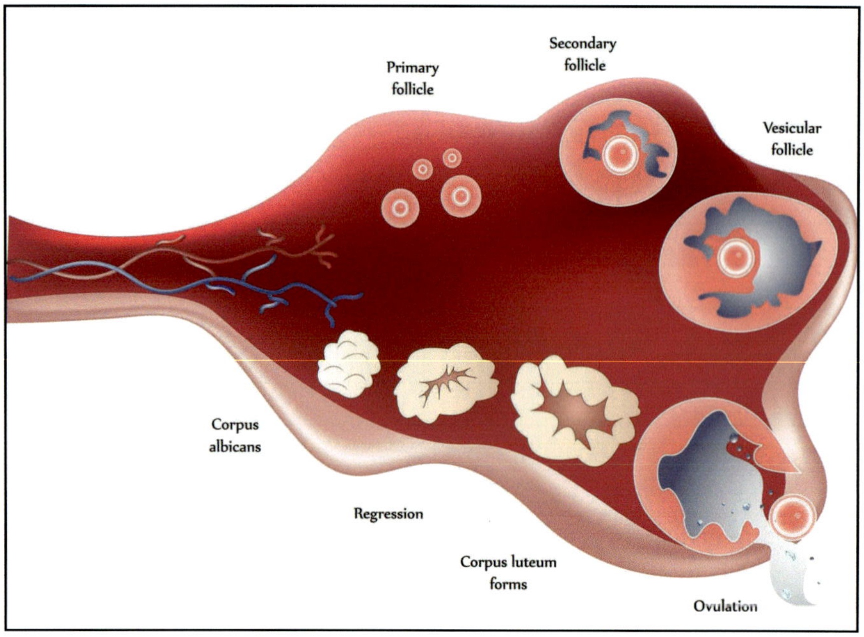

Figure 11-11. The stages of maturity in follicles within the ovarian cortex. (GRei/shutterstock.com)

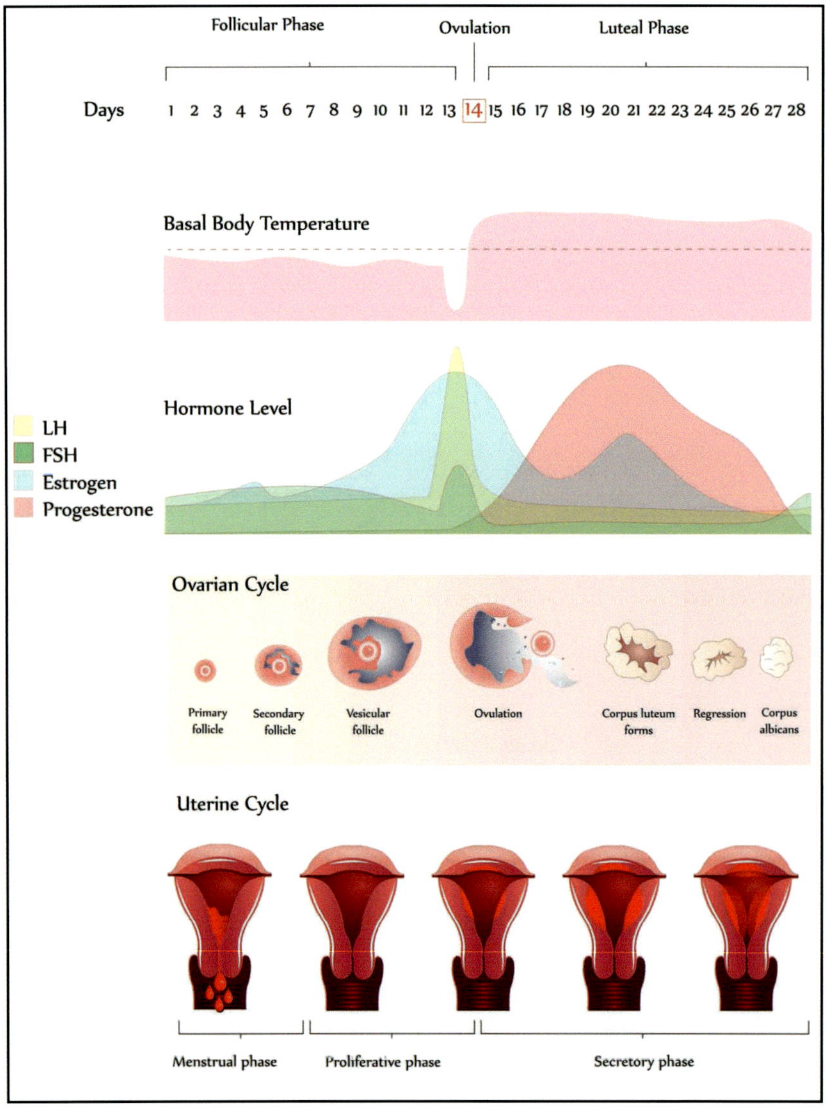

Figure 11-12. The ovulation cycle. (GRei/shutterstock.com)

Table 11-8 Hormones of the Gonads		
OVARIES HORMONES	**TARGET ORGANS**	**PURPOSE**
estrogen (estradiol, estrone, and estriol)	female sex organs, mammary glands	Development and maintenance of female sex organs and characteristics; development of mammary glands, sex drive
progesterone	uterus	Prepares the uterus for pregnancy
TESTES HORMONES	**TARGET ORGANS**	**PURPOSE**
testosterone	male sex organs	Development and maintenance of male sex organs and characteristics; penile erection

The Testes

The **testes** (combining forms for testes are **orch/o; orchi/o; orchid/o; test/o; didym/o**) are oval-shaped structures housed and suspended in the **scrotum** (**scrot/o**), a sac that keeps sperm within the testes cooler than body temperature. The scrotum is located behind the penis and descends from the perineal region of the abdomen. It separates into two regions, each supporting one testis. Superior to each testis is an **epididymis** (**epi-**—above; **didym/**—testes). Minute coils from the epididymis ascend from the distal testis along the posterior aspect of the gland to become the **vas deferens** and then join blood vessels and nerves to form the **spermatic cord** (Figure 11-13). These spermatic cords allow the testis to swing relatively freely within the protection of the scrotum. Within the testes are approximately 250 wedge-shaped lobes of fibrous tissue. Coiled inside each lobe are tiny tube-like structures called **seminiferous tubules**, which provide the location of developing sperm, or **spermatozoa** (Figure 11-14). Functioning as an endocrine gland, testes produce the hormone testosterone, which is the substance responsible for developing the secondary male sex characteristics.

A WORD ABOUT TESTICULAR CANCER

Testicular cancer is most often discovered in the 20- to 40-year-old population, and has one of the highest cure rates. Men should be encouraged to perform a testicular self-exam (TSE) on a regular basis and report unusual findings or changes to their physician.

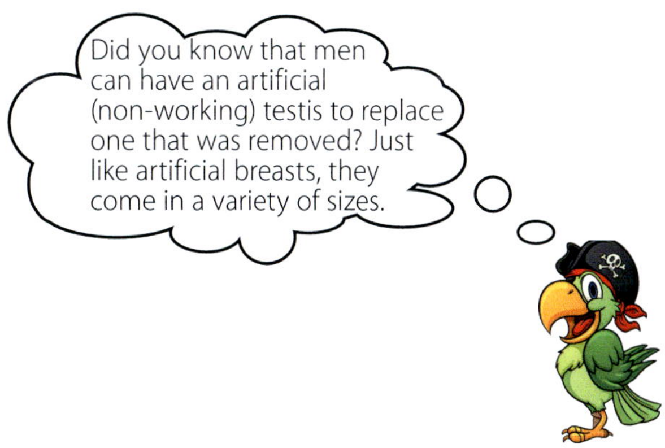
Did you know that men can have an artificial (non-working) testis to replace one that was removed? Just like artificial breasts, they come in a variety of sizes.

The Mammary Glands

All people have breasts, but only females respond to the hormone **prolactin** (secreted by the anterior pituitary), which stimulates the mammary glands to produce milk following childbirth (Figure 11-15). Insulin (from the pancreas) and hormones from the adrenal cortex also have a role in milk production. Anatomically, breasts lie anterior to the pectoralis major on either side of the sternum. They have alveolar-like structures internally, with 15 to 20 glands leading to **lactiferous glands** and **lactiferous ducts**, which produce and deliver milk. Surrounding the **nipple** is the **areola**, which is a circular, pigmented, and elevated area. There are sebaceous glands in the areola secreting an oil to keep the skin resilient (Figure 11-16). Breasts vary in shape and size, as do areolas. Body fat, heredity, and age can all factor in to breast size. It is not uncommon for one to have breasts of different sizes, as the same is true for testes. During pregnancy, the areola darken in color. Infants' suckling motion stimulates **oxytocin**, which causes uterine contractions and promotes its return to normal size following childbirth. Anyone can get breast cancer, and new or persistent lumps in the breast tissue should be investigated by a physician.

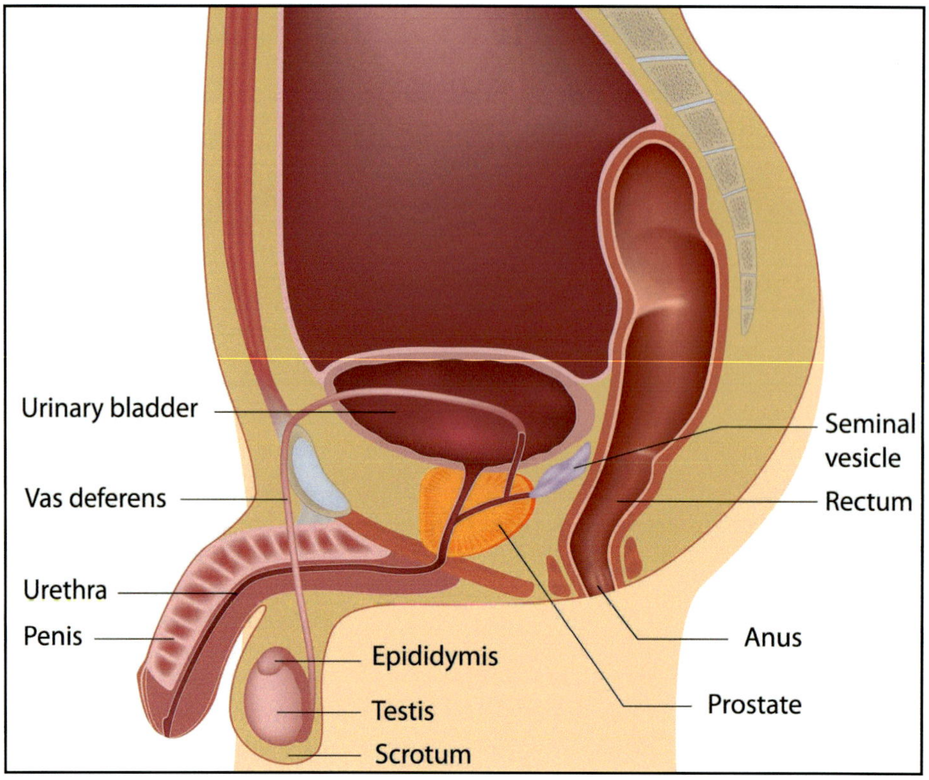

Figure 11-13. Relationship of the testis in the reproductive system. (Alila Medical Images/shutterstock.com)

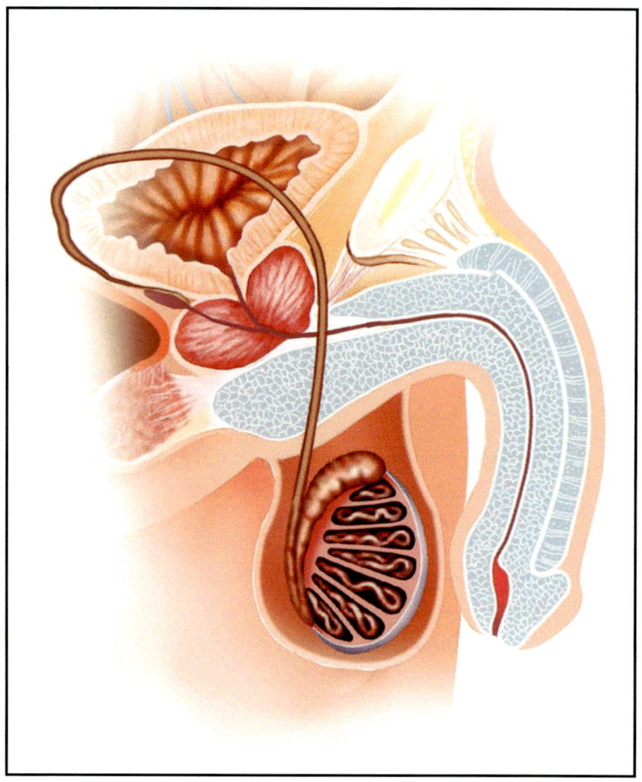

Figure 11-14. The seminiferous tubules in the testis. (Alex Luengo/shutterstock.com)

TABLE 11-9

PHASES OF THE MENSTRUAL CYCLE (28-DAY CYCLE)

PHASE	WHAT HAPPENS	LENGTH AND OCCURRENCE
follicular phase	Menstruation begins with bloody discharge from the uterus via the vagina; the endometrium (inner layer) of the uterus is shed	Begins the first day of menstruation, it lasts 4 to 7 days
ovulatory phase	Due to a release of estrogen, the endometrium thickens and becomes vascularized in preparation for implantation of a fertilized egg; the graafian follicle ruptures, releasing the ovum; if it is not fertilized within the first 48 hours, it breaks down	Begins on day 5 following menstruation, but actually only lasts 12 to 48 hours; occurs about the 14th day of the menstrual cycle
luteal phase	If fertilization does not occur, the corpus luteum develops and secretes progesterone, which in turn thickens the mucus in the cervix, making sperm less likely to enter the uterus; in the later aspects of this stage, the endometrium thickens in preparation for a fertilized egg; the breasts may swell due to increased levels of both estrogen and progesterone	Lasts 2 weeks (14 days)
premenstrual phase	Uterine arteries constrict and the endometrium shrink	Lasts about 2 days

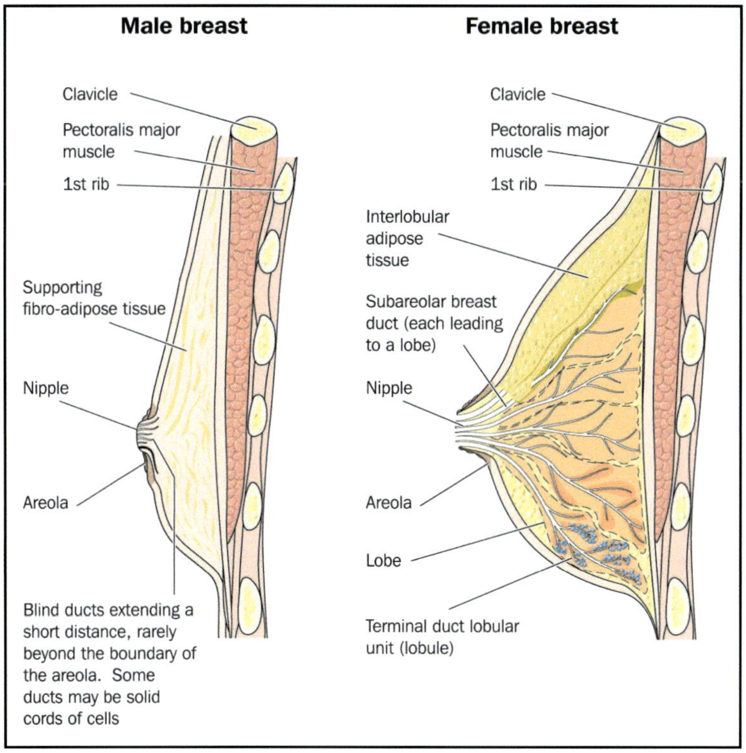

Figure 11-15. Anatomy comparison between male and female breasts. (Blamb/shutterstock.com)

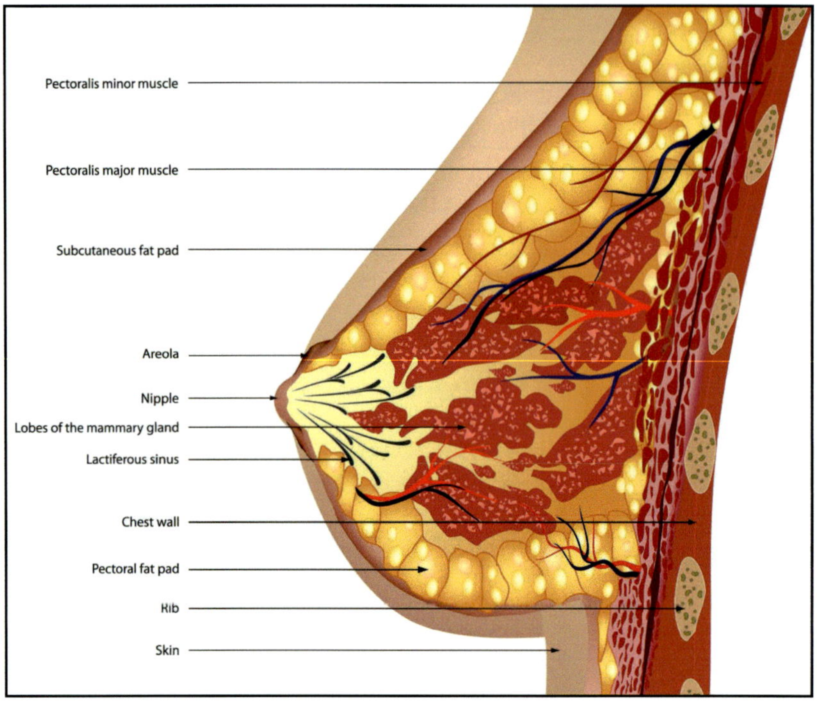

Figure 11-16. Anatomy of the female breast. (Mariya Ermolaeva/shutterstock.com)

Word Building

Table 11-10
Prefixes

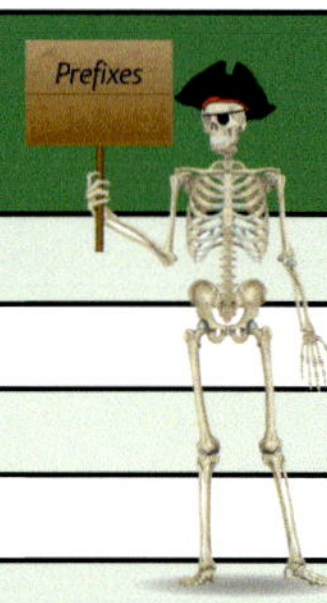

PREFIX	DEFINITION
ad-	toward (to add to the body)
an-	without; not
anti-	against
crypt-	hidden
dys-	bad; painful; difficult; abnormal
endo-	in; within
epi-	above; upon
ex-; exo-	away; away from; out; outside
hyper-	above; excessive; high; increased
hypo-	below; decreased; deficient; insufficient; low; under
pan-	all
para-	beside; near; abnormal
poly-	excessive; many; much; over
supra-	above
syn-	union; together

Table 11-11
Suffixes

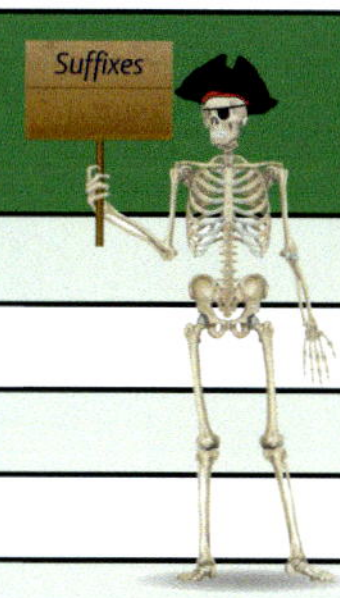

SUFFIX	DEFINITION
-al	pertaining to
-arche	beginning
-ation	process of
-cele	hernia; protrusion; swelling
-crine	to secrete; secreting
-drome	to run; running
-ectomy	excision; surgical removal
-edema	swelling
-emia	blood condition
-graphy	process of recording; the act of recording information
-ia	condition
-ic	pertaining to
-ism	condition
-itis	inflammation
-megaly	abnormally large; enlargement
-meter	an instrument used to measure
-oid	resembling
-oma	tumor
-osis	condition of
-ostomy	a surgical opening
-otomy; -tomy	incision; to cut into
-pathy	disease
-penia; -penic	decrease; deficient
-pexy	surgical fixation of
-physis	growth
-plasia	formation; growth
-plasty	reconstruction; repair; plastic surgery
-ptosis	drooping; falling; prolapse; prolapse
-rrhagia	abnormal flow
-rrhaphy	suture; surgical repair
-rrhea	discharge; excessive flow
-rrhexis	rupture
-tic	pertaining to
-troph	development; growth; nourishment
-uria	pertaining to urine

Table 11-12 Combining Forms

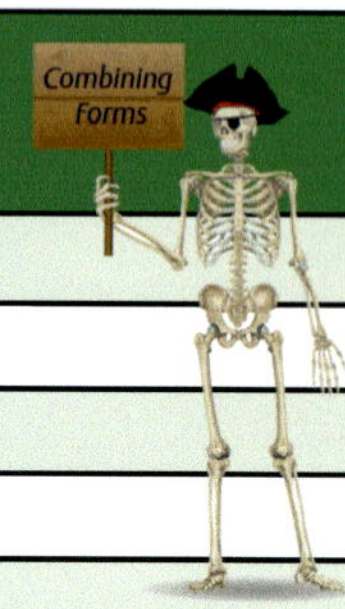

COMBINING FORM	DEFINITION
acid/o	something with a pH of 7 or less; acidic
aden/o	gland
adren/o	adrenal gland
andr/o	male
calc/i; calc/o	calcium
carcin/o	cancer
chrom/o	color; stain
cortic/o	cortex; outer portion
crin/o	to secrete
cyst/o	bladder; sac
cyt/o	cell
didym/o	testis
dips/o	thirst
galact/o	milk
gluc/o	sugar
glyc/o; glycos/o	sugar
gonad/o	gonad; sex organ
gynec/o	female; woman
hormon/o	to set in motion
hydr/o	water; fluid
hypophys/o	pituitary gland
idi/o	unknown
kal/o	potassium (the chemical symbol for potassium is K)
ket/o; keton/o	ketone
lact/o	milk
mamm/o	breast
mast/o	breast
men/o	menstrual
metr/o	uterus; measure
myx/o	mucus
nat/o	sodium (the chemical symbol for sodium is Na); birth
neur/o	nerve
oophor/o	ovary
ophthalm/o	eye
orch/o; orchi/o; orchid/o	testis; testicle
ov/i; ov/o; ovul/o	ovum (egg)

(continued)

Table 11-12 (continued)
Combining Forms

COMBINING FORM	DEFINITION
ovari/o	ovary
pancreat/o	pancreas; sweetbread
papill/o	nipple; papilla
phe/o	dark
pituitar/o	pituitary gland
prolactin/o	prolactin
pub/o	pubic bone
ren/o	kidney
scrot/o	scrotum
somat/o	body
test/o	testis; testicle
thel/e	nipple
thym/o	thymus gland
thyr/o	thyroid; shield
troph/o	development; growth; nourishment
ur/o	urine
varic/o	dilated vein; swollen vein; varicose vein

Signs and Symptoms

Table 11-13
Signs and Symptoms Related to the Endocrine System

SIGN/SYMPTOM	WORD PARTS	DEFINITION
exophthalmos	**ex-** (outside) ophthalm/o (eye)	Protrusion of the eyeball; sign of hyperthyroidisim Also termed *exophthalmia* (**-ia**—condition)
glucosuria	gluc/o (sugar) **-uria** (urine)	Presence of sugar in the urine; sign of diabetes mellitus
hypercalcemia	**hyper-** (excessive) calc/ (calcium) **-emia** (blood condition)	Excessive amounts of calcium in the blood, often from unusual amounts of calcium released from bones
hyperglycemia	**hyper-** (excessive) glyc/ (sugar) **-emia** (blood condition)	Excessive amounts of sugar in the blood, an indicator that the body is not supplying sufficient insulin or receptors; a sign of diabetes mellitus

(continued)

Table 11-13 (continued)

Signs and Symptoms Related to the Endocrine System

SIGN/SYMPTOM	WORD PARTS	DEFINITION
hypocalcemia	**hypo-** (low) calc/ (calcium) **-emia** (blood condition)	Abnormally low levels of calcium in the blood caused by low activity of the parathyroid hormone; also called *calcipenia* (**-penia**—deficient)
hypoglycemia	**hypo-** (below) glyc/ (sugar) **-emia** (blood condition)	Blood glucose is below normal, resulting in headache, blurred vision, nausea, irritability, weakness, confusion; can lead to coma and death
goiter (Figure 11-17)		Enlarged thyroid gland, displayed as a large swelling on the anterior neck; also called thyromegaly (**-megaly**—abnormally large; enlargement)
ketoacidosis	ket/o (ketone) acid/ (acid) **-osis** (condition)	Excessive production of ketones in the blood, making it more acidic; often a result of extensive breakdown of fats due to defective carbohydrate metabolism; life-threatening sign of diabetes mismanagement
ketonuria	keton/ (ketone) **-uria** (urine)	Ketones in the urine, a sign of Graves' disease and hyperthyroidism; also called *ketoaciduria*
polydipsia	**poly-** (excessive) dips/ (thirst) **-ia** (condition)	Abnormal thirst; often a sign of disorders of the pancreas or pituitary gland
polyuria	**poly-** (excessive) **-uria** (pertaining to urine)	Abnormal amounts of urine
virilism	virile (masculine) **-ism** (condition)	When a woman develops characteristics more typically associated with men

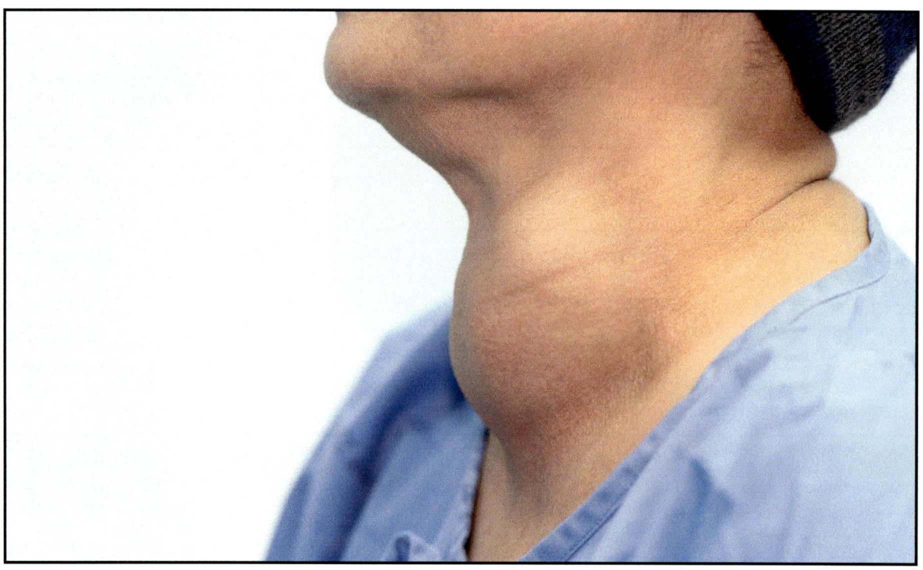

Figure 11-17. A goiter is a sign of an enlarged thyroid gland. (Love Sillhouette/shutterstock.com)

Medical Conditions

Because the endocrine system functions largely on feedback from the environment and tissues, over- or undersecretion of hormones can lead to many medical conditions.

Table 11-14

Medical Conditions Related to the Endocrine System

NAME	WORD PARTS	DEFINITION
adenitis	aden/ (gland) **-itis** (inflammation)	Inflammation of a gland
adenoma	aden/ (gland) **-oma** (tumor)	Tumor in a gland
adenopathy	aden/o (gland) **-pathy** (disease)	Disease of a gland
hyperthyroidism	**hyper-** (excessive) thyr/ (thyroid) **-ism** (condition)	Overabundant production of the thyroid hormones; most typically presented as Graves' disease
hyponatremia	**hypo-** (deficient) nat/ (sodium) **-emia** (blood condition)	Too little sodium (Na) in the blood, causing swelling and pressure on the lungs and brain
hypothyroidism	**hypo-** (deficient) thyr/ (thyroid) **-ism** (condition)	Deficient production of thyroid hormones; in children, called *congenital hypothyroidism*
myxedema	myx/ (mucus) **-edema** (swelling)	Most severe form of hypothyroidism, characterized by extreme facial swelling
panhypopituitarism	**pan-** (all) **hypo-** (deficient) pituitar/ (pituitary gland) **-ism** (condition)	Lack or deficiency of all pituitary hormones; characterized by hypotension, weakness, and weight loss; also called *Simmonds disease*
parathyrotropic	**para-** (beside) thyr/o (thyroid) troph/ (growth) **-ic** (pertaining to)	To stimulate the growth or activity rate of the parathyroid gland
pheochromocytoma	phe/o (dark) chrom/o (color) cyt/ (cell) **-oma** (tumor)	Dark-colored tumor of the adrenal medulla; typically benign

(continued)

Table 11-14 (continued)

Medical Conditions Related to the Endocrine System

NAME	WORD PARTS	DEFINITION
prolactinoma	prolactin/ (prolactin) **-oma** (tumor)	Tumor that produces oversecretion of the hormone prolactin
thymoma	thym/ (thymus) **-oma** (tumor)	Tumor of the thymus

Table 11-15

Medical Conditions Related to the Gonads and Mammary Glands

NAME	WORD PARTS	DEFINITION
anorchism	**an-** (without) orch/ (testicle) **-ism** (condition)	Born without a testicle
anovulation	**an-** (without) ovul/ (ovum [egg]) **-ation** (process of)	Without ovulation, the failure of the ovary to release an ovum
cryptorchidism	**crypt-** (hidden) orchid/ (testicle) **-ism** (condition)	Hidden testicle, one that fails to descend into the scrotum
dysmenorrhea	**dys-** (painful; difficult) men/o (menstrual) **-rrhea** (discharge)	Painful or difficult menstruation
galactorrhea	galact/o (milk) **-rrhea** (discharge)	Abnormal discharge of milk from the breasts, unassociated with childbirth or nursing
gynecomastia	gynec/o (female) mast/ (breast) **-ia** (condition)	Enlargement of breast tissue in a male, often due to hormones
hydrocele	hydr/o (fluid) **-cele** (hernia; protrusion; swelling)	Collection of fluid-like material within the scrotum
lactorrhea	lact/o (milk) **-rrhea** (discharge)	Discharge of milk
mastoptosis	mast/o (breast) **-ptosis** (drooping)	Drooping, or downward displacement, of the breasts
menopause	men/o (menstrual)	Stopping of menses due to a depletion of female sex hormones
menorrhagia	men/o (menstrual) **-rrhagia** (abnormal flow)	Excessive menstrual bleeding

(continued)

Table 11-15 (continued)
Medical Conditions Related to the Gonads and Mammary Glands

NAME	WORD PARTS	DEFINITION
metrorrhagia	metr/o (uterus) **-rrhagia** (abnormal flow)	Abnormal bleeding of the uterus in between menses
oophoritis	oophor/ (ovary) **-itis** (inflammation)	Inflammation of an ovary
orchitis	orch/ (testicle) **-itis** (inflammation)	Inflamed testicle; also termed *testitis*
polycystic ovary syndrome (PCOS) (Figure 11-18)	**poly-** (many) cyst/ (sac) **-ic** (pertaining to)	Condition where both ovaries have many cysts due to a hormone imbalance
pubarche	pub/ (pubic bone) **-arche** (beginning)	Onset of pubic and axillary hair growth
thelarche	thel/ (breast) **-arche** (beginning)	Beginning of breast development
thelitis	thel/ (nipple) **-itis** (inflammation)	Inflammation of the nipple
varicocele	varic/o (swollen vein) **-cele** (hernia; protrusion; swelling)	Varicose veins in the spermatic cord

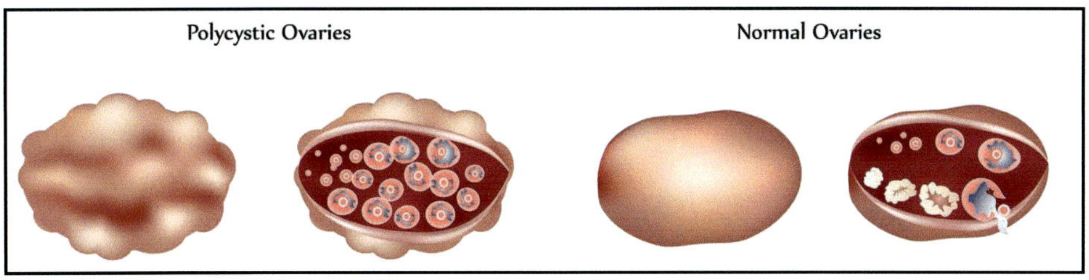

Figure 11-18. A ovary with multiple cysts (polycystic). (GRei/shutterstock.com)

Table 11-16
Endocrine System Terms Without Common Word Parts

TERM	DEFINITION
Addison's disease	Inadequate supply of cortisol secreted from the adrenal cortex; characterized by hypotension, dehydration, and gastrointestinal problems
Cushing's syndrome	Excessive secretion of cortisol from the adrenal cortex, causing obesity, hyperglycemia, and muscle atrophy; named after neurosurgeon Harvey Cushing
DiGeorge syndrome	Condition that results in being born without a thymus gland; named after pediatrician Angelo DiGeorge
Graves' disease	Form of hyperthyroidism

(continued)

Table 11-16 (continued) Endocrine System Terms Without Common Word Parts	
TERM	**DEFINITION**
Hashimoto's disease	Autoimmune disorder of the thyroid presented as an enlarged thyroid (goiter), and replacement of normal thyroid structures with lymphoid tissues; named after surgeon Hakaru Hashimoto
hirsutism	Excessive body and facial hair, especially in women; also termed *hypertrichosis*
mittelschmerz	Abdominal pain occurring midway through the menstrual cycle as a result of ovulation
Simmonds' disease	Lack or deficiency of all pituitary hormones; also called *panhypopituitarism*

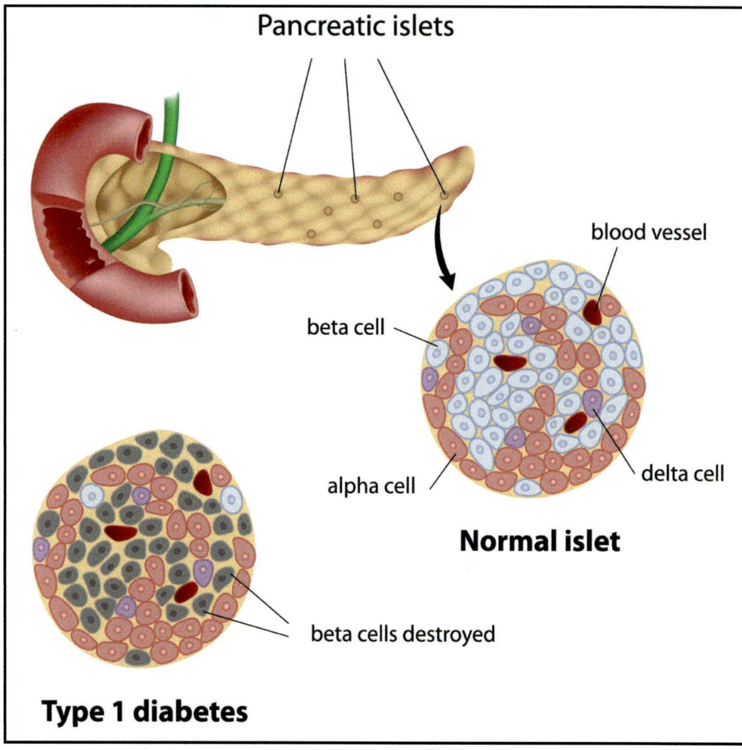

Figure 11-19. Type 1 diabetes occurs because the beta cells are destroyed or incapable of producing insulin. (Alila Medical Images/shutterstock.com)

A WORD ABOUT DIABETES

Diabetes mellitus is an endocrine disease resulting from inadequate insulin, which results in very high blood glucose levels. There are several types of diabetes mellitus. **Type 1** used to be called insulin-dependent diabetes mellitus, and has an onset at a young age (under 20). Type 1 diabetes occurs because the beta cells in the islets of Langerhans of the pancreas cannot produce insulin (Figure 11-19).

The overwhelming majority of people with diabetes mellitus have **type 2,** formerly called non-insulin-dependent diabetes mellitus. People with type 2 diabetes cannot use the insulin they produce efficiently. Whereas type 1 diabetes is thought to be an autoimmune response that destroys beta cells, type 2 most often results from obesity and sedentary lifestyles (Figure 11-20). Pregnant people are also susceptible to **gestational diabetes** during the last trimester of their pregnancy. This condition typically resolves following birth.

Two terms associated with diabetes are **hypoglycemia** and **hyperglycemia**. Hypoglycemia is low blood sugar, usually below 60 mg/dL, and hyperglycemia is a very high glucose level, over 180 mg/dL. Both can be very dangerous and either can cause many other systemic problems if prolonged. It is critical that people with diabetes monitor their blood sugar (via a **glucometer**; **gluc/o**—sugar; **-meter**—an instrument to measure) and are aware of both their food intake and activity levels (Figure 11-21). Typical blood sugar values are provided in Table 11-17.

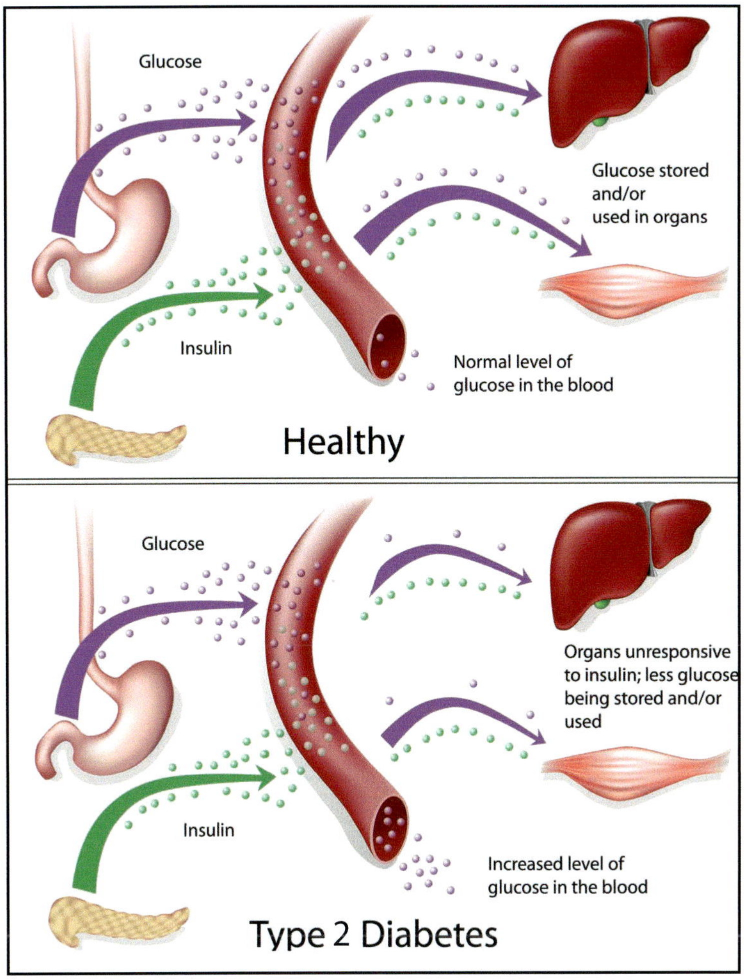

Figure 11-20. Type 2 diabetes can be brought about by a sedentary lifestyle and obesity. (Alila Medical Images/ shutterstock.com)

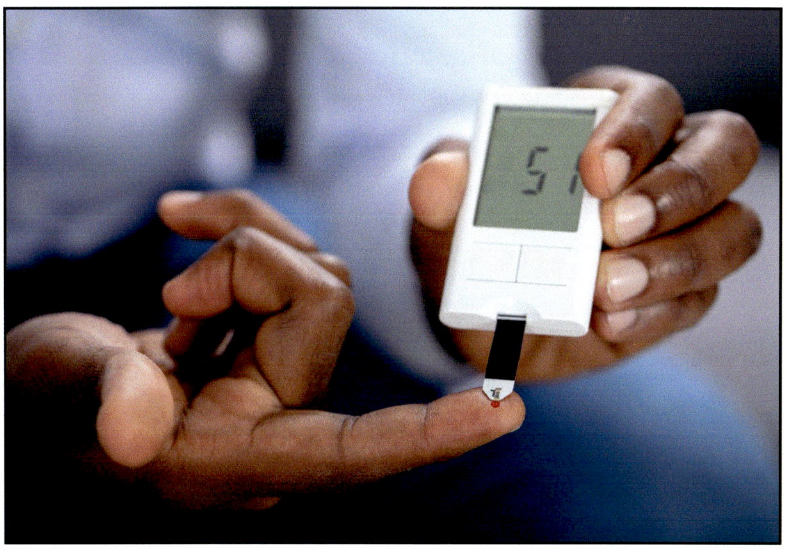

Figure 11-21. A glucometer is a device used for measuring the current blood sugar of a person with diabetes. (Andrey Popov/shutterstock.com)

Table 11-17
Blood Glucose Levels

TIME THAT BLOOD IS MEASURED	BLOOD GLUCOSE LEVEL (MG/DL)
Fasting 12 hours	60 to 80
2 to 3 hours after a meal	100 to 140
Normal, unplanned glucose reading	126 or lower

Tests and Procedures

Table 11-18
Tests and Procedures Related to the Endocrine System

NAME	PURPOSE
A1c; also called HbA1c	From a blood sample, measures the average blood sugar over the past 3 months; used to monitor how people with diabetes are managing their disease
fasting blood sugar (FBS)	Blood is analyzed following a 12-hour fast to determine what the typical blood glucose level is for that patient
glucose tolerance test (GTT)	Following consumption of glucose (or an IV with glucose) a patient has serial blood tests performed to measure their reaction to reaction to it; used to confirm the presence of diabetes mellitus
radioactive iodine (RAI)	Used in diagnosis and treatment of hyperthyroidism
radioactive iodine uptake test (RAIU)	Test that measures the amount of iodine taken up by thyroid cells by a scanner
thyroxine test	Test that measures the levels of thyroxine in the blood; used to diagnose hypo- and hyperthyroidism

In Tables 11-19 and 11-20, note that most surgical procedures identify the structure (combining form) and add a suffix to describe what was done to the organ or gland. Common surgical suffixes are:

- **-ectomy** (excision; surgical removal)
- **-ostomy** (a surgical opening)
- **-otomy** and **-tomy** (incision; to cut into)
- **-pexy** (surgical fixation of)
- **-plasty** (surgical repair; suturing)
- **-rrhaphy** (suture; surgical repair)

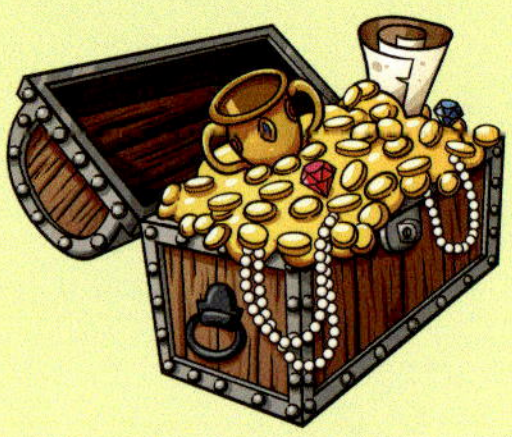

Table 11-19

Procedures Related to the Endocrine System

NAME	WORD PARTS	PURPOSE
adrenalectomy	adren/ (adrenal gland) **-al** (pertaining to) **-ectomy** (surgical excision)	Removal of the adrenal glands to stop production of their hormones
hypophysectomy	hypophys/ (pituitary gland) **-ectomy** (surgical excision)	Excision of the pituitary gland
pancreatectomy	pancreat/ (pancreas) **-ectomy** (surgical excision)	Removal of a portion or the entire pancreas gland

Table 11-20

Tests and Procedures Related to the Gonads and Mammary Glands

NAME	WORD PARTS	PURPOSE
breast self-exam (BSE) (Figure 11-22)		Examination of one's own breasts for changes (eg, swelling, lumps); the American Cancer Society (www.cancer.org) suggests women perform monthly BSEs
lumpectomy	**-ectomy** (surgical excision)	Surgical excision of a lump, typically within the breast tissue; the removed tissue is then analyzed for cancer
mammography (Figure 11-23)	mamm/o (breast) **-graphy** (process of recording)	Process of recording used to examine breast tissue for abnormalities, especially early detection of breast cancer
mammoplasty	mamm/o (breast) **-plasty** (repair)	Surgical repair of the breast
mastectomy	mast/ (breast) **-ectomy** (surgical removal)	Surgical removal of the breast
mastopexy	mast/o (breast) **-pexy** (surgical fixation of)	Reconstructive procedure lifting or fixating the breasts
oophorectomy	oophor/ (ovary) **-ectomy** (surgical removal)	Surgical removal of an ovary
orchidectomy	orchid/ (testicle) **-ectomy** (surgical removal)	Surgical removal of a testis
orchiopexy	orchi/o (testicle) **-pexy** (surgical fixation of)	Fixation of a previously undescended testicle in the scrotum so it will not retract; also termed *orchidorrhaphy*
testicular self-exam (TSE)		Examination of one's own testes for changes (eg, swelling, lumps) the American Cancer Society (www.cancer.org) suggests men perform monthly TSEs
theleplasty	thel/e (nipple) **-plasty** (repair)	Surgical/cosmetic repair of the nipple

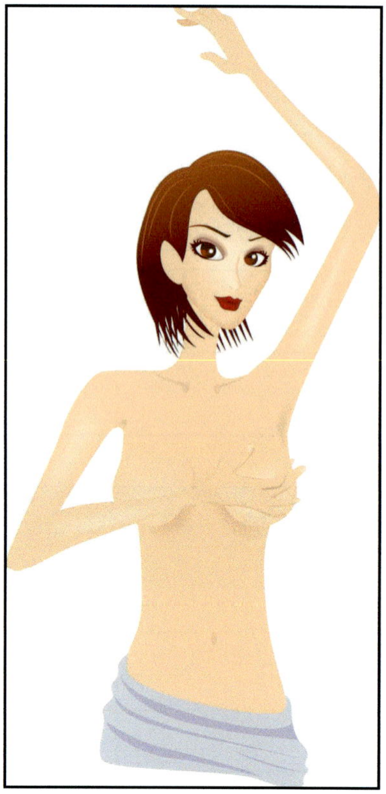

Figure 11-22. Women should perform BSEs monthly. (Lorelyn Medina/shutterstock.com)

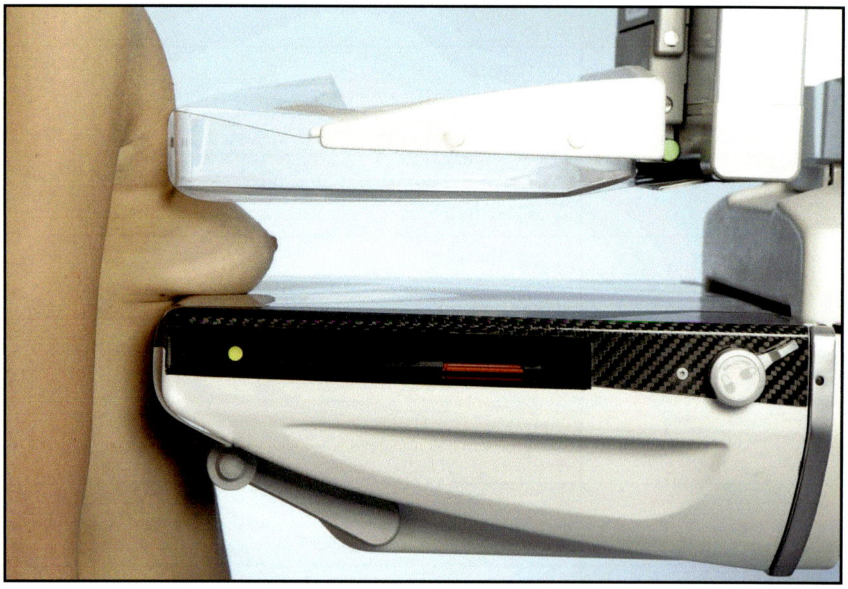

Figure 11-23. A mammogram is a machine that uses low-energy x-rays to evaluate breast tissue for abnormalities. (bart78/shutterstock.com)

Medication Classifications

Table 11-21 Medication Classifications Used in Treatment of Endocrine Conditions	
CATEGORY	**WHAT IT DOES**
antithyroids	Inhibits thyroid production
birth control pills (BCP)	Prevents ovulation
corticosteroids	Relieves inflammation
hormone replacement therapy (HRT)	Replaces lost sex hormones (eg, due to menopause, surgical removal of the ovaries) with manufactured hormones
human growth hormone	Stimulates skeletal muscle growth to promote development in children whose progression is stunted
insulin	Replaces or supplements insulin for people with diabetes mellitus
thyroid replacement	Replaces thyroid hormones for excised, diseased, or malfunctioning thyroid glands
vasopressin	Encourages water reabsorption to treat diabetes mellitus

11

Bibliography

Allan D. *Medical Language for Modern Health Care.* 4th ed. McGraw-Hill; 2019.

American Cancer Society. Key statistics for thyroid cancer. Revised January 12, 2021. Accessed August 31, 2022. https://www.cancer.org/cancer/thyroid-cancer/about/key-statistics.html

Chabner DE. *The Language of Medicine.* 12th ed. Saunders/Elsevier; 2019.

Cohen BJ, Jones SA. *Medical Terminology: An Illustrated Guide.* 9th ed. Jones & Bartlett; 2021.

Flanagan KW, Cuppett M. Systemic disorders. In *Medical Conditions in the Athlete.* 3rd ed. Human Kinetics; 2017.

Fremgen BF, Frucht SS. *Medical Terminology: A Living Language.* 7th ed. Pearson; 2019.

McCance KL, Huether SE. *Pathophysiology: The Biologic Basis for Disease in Adults and Children.* 8th ed. Mosby; 2019.

Mosby's Dictionary of Medicine, Nursing & Health Professions. 10th ed. Elsevier; 2017.

Venes D, ed. *Taber's Cyclopedic Medical Dictionary.* 24th ed. F. A. Davis; 2021.

NOTES

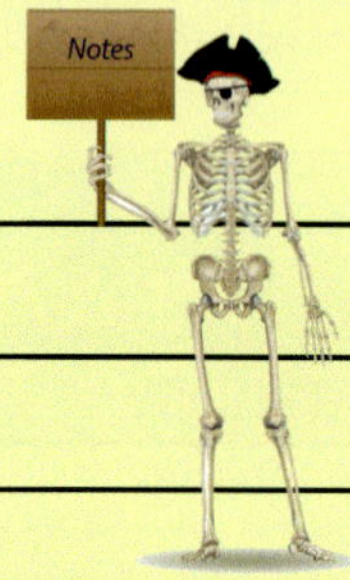

NOTES

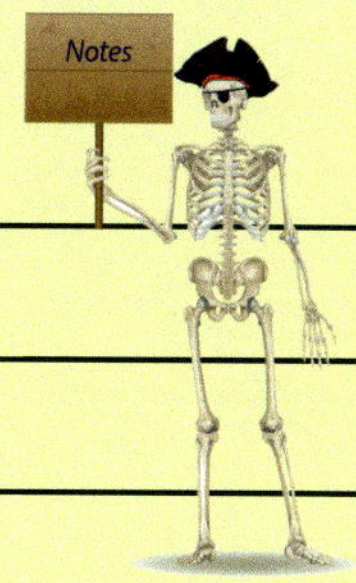

LEARNING ACTIVITIES

Name:______________________

Endocrine System

A. Label the glands of the endocrine system from the following list of words.

- ovary______________
- pancreas___________
- thymus____________
- testis______________
- pituitary___________
- thyroid____________
- hypothalamus_______
- adrenal____________
- pineal_____________

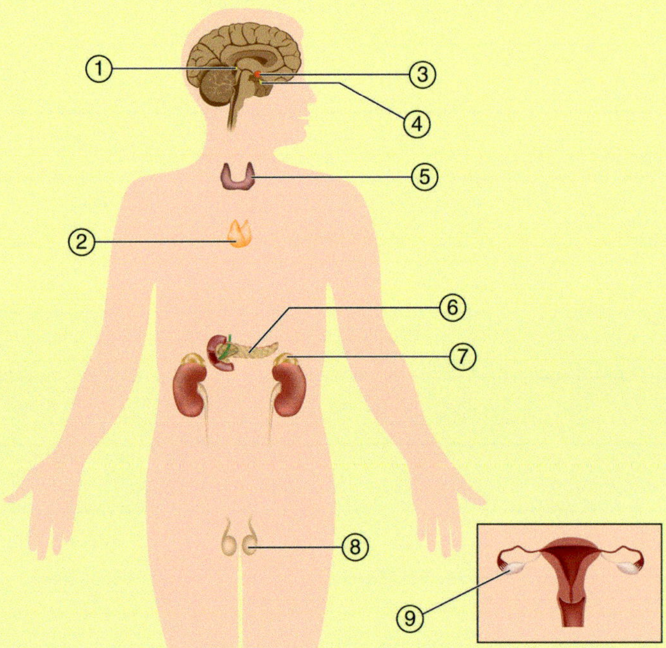

(Alila Medical Images/shutterstock.com)

B. Matching.

Match the word element with its best meaning.

1. -crine_______ a. nipple
2. oophor/o_____ b. male
3. crypt-_______ c. menstrual
4. dys-_________ d. above; upon
5. ovum_______ e. ovary
6. andr/o_______ f. egg
7. papill/o______ g. hidden
8. -cele________ h. hernia; swelling
9. epi-_________ i. bad; painful; difficult; abnormal
10. men/o_______ j. to secrete

C. For each hormone, list which gland is responsible for its secretion.

HORMONE	GLAND
thymosin	
FSH (follicle-stimulating hormone)	
glucagon	
oxytocin	
melatonin	
PTH (parathyroid hormone)	
calcitonin	
ACTH (adrenocorticotropic hormone)	

D. Build the word.

Using the word root, add the other word element and define the new word created.

1. **aden/o**
   a. -megaly____________________________
   b. -otomy____________________________
   c. -oma____________________________
   d. -itis____________________________
   e. -oid____________________________
2. -ectomy
   a. oophor/o____________________________
   b. adrenal/____________________________
   c. parathyroid/o________________________
   d. orch/i____________________________
   e. thyroid____________________________

3. **menorrhea**
    a. **a-**____________________________
    b. **oligo-**____________________________
    c. **dys-**____________________________
    d. **poly-**____________________________

E. Separate the word elements of the following terms and define them.

1. adrenocorticotropic____________________________
2. orchidorrhaphy____________________________
3. somatotropin____________________________
4. pheochromocytoma____________________________
5. adenocarcinoma____________________________
6. parathyrotropic____________________________

F. Name the gland involved in the following conditions.

1. mittelschmerz____________________________
2. Cushing's syndrome____________________________
3. hypoglycemia____________________________
4. DiGeorge syndrome____________________________
5. ovulation____________________________
6. Hashimoto's disease____________________________

G. Using your medical terminology knowledge, write the best medical word for each definition.

1. breast pain____
2. an enlarged thyroid____
3. an instrument used to measure sugar in the blood____________________
4. a male born without a testicle____
5. the onset of breast development____

Case Study

Define the numerical terms (1 to 12) and draw the alphabetical term (A) on the anatomy figure..

History, Chief Complaint

A 52-year-old judge complained of sudden weight loss, inability to sleep, and **polyuria** (1). He had been taking caffeine pills to prepare for a big court trial and thought it might be related to the caffeine in the pills, but the case has been over for 1 week and he still feels bad.

Evaluation

The judge appears tense, and hyperactive. His blood pressure is 130/90 and he had **tachycardia** (2) with 120 **bpm** (3). He denied **anorexia** (4) or **gastrodynia** (5) but had increased **eructation** (6). He appeared to have **exophthalmos** (7) and **diplopia** (8) and a **goiter** (9, A). As this condition is quite rare in men, we must also rule out **Hashimoto's disease** (10).

Diagnostic Studies

Blood was drawn to assess the **TSH** (11) levels, which were elevated. After more specific evaluation, the judge was diagnosed with **hyperthyroidism** (12) and given a medical protocol involving hypertensive and thyroid-inhibiting medications.

Terms

1. ______________________________
2. ______________________________
3. ______________________________
4. ______________________________
5. ______________________________
6. ______________________________
7. ______________________________
8. ______________________________
9. ______________________________
10. ______________________________
11. ______________________________
12. ______________________________

Anatomy

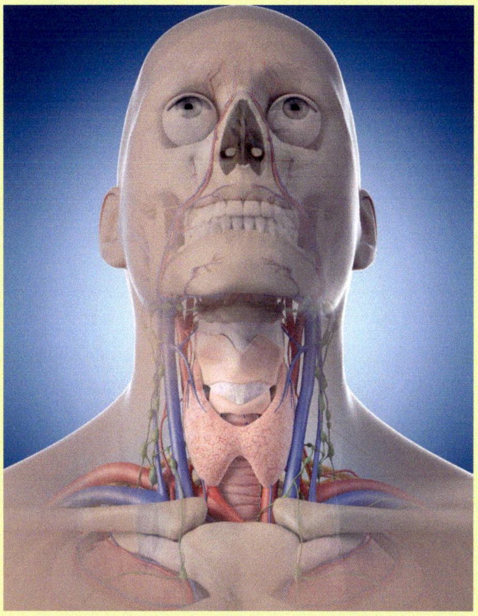

(SciePro/shutterstock.com)

11

12

Urinary System

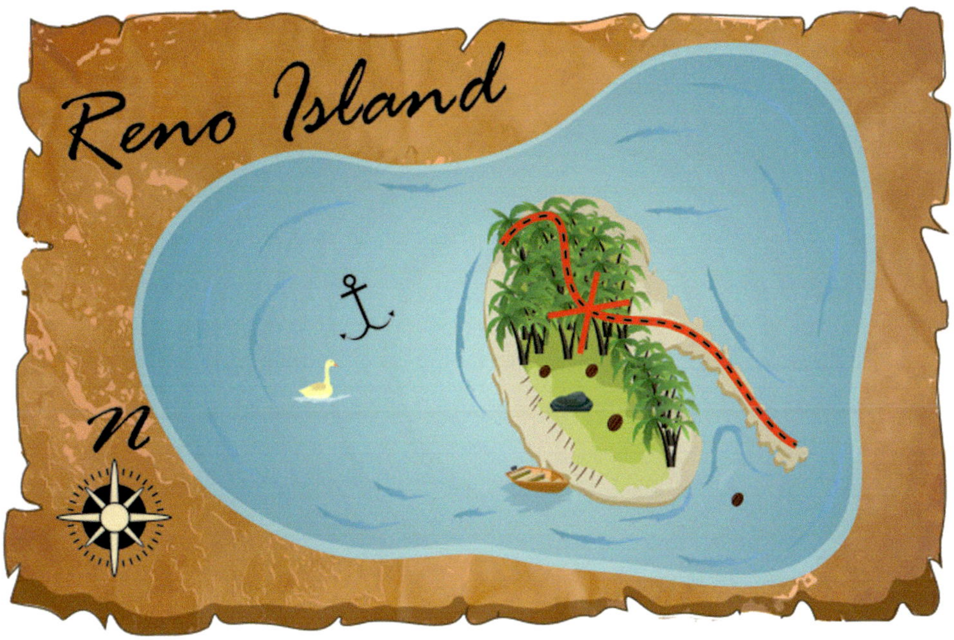

OBJECTIVES

After studying this chapter, you will be able to:

1. Identify the major components of the urinary system.
2. Describe the function of the kidneys.
3. Recall the normal attributes of urine.
4. Construct medical words pertaining to the urinary system.
5. List signs and symptoms of urinary conditions.
6. Describe basic abnormalities or conditions of the urinary system.
7. Explain diagnostic tests and procedures specific to the urinary system.

Flanagan KW.
Medical Terminology With Case Studies: A Navigated Guide to Learning for Health Care Professionals, Third Edition (pp 329-361).

Chapter Outline

- Self-assessment
- Checklist for word parts in the chapter
- Checklist of new anatomy
- Introduction
- Anatomy
- Word building
    - Prefixes
    - Suffixes
    - Combining forms
- Signs and symptoms
- Medical conditions
- Tests and procedures
- Learning activities
- Case study

Self-Assessment

Based on what you have learned so far, can you write the definition of these words?

- hematuria____________________
- nephrectomy____________________
- oliguria____________________
- anuria____________________
- renal____________________
- suprarenal____________________
- polyuria____________________
- nephrohypertrophy____________________

Checklist for Word Parts in the Chapter

Prefixes

- ☐ an-
- ☐ di-
- ☐ dia-
- ☐ dys-
- ☐ en-
- ☐ epi-
- ☐ extra-
- ☐ hydro-
- ☐ hyper-
- ☐ hypo-
- ☐ in-
- ☐ intra-
- ☐ par-
- ☐ per-
- ☐ peri-
- ☐ poly-
- ☐ re-
- ☐ retro-
- ☐ steno-
- ☐ sub-
- ☐ supra-
- ☐ trans-

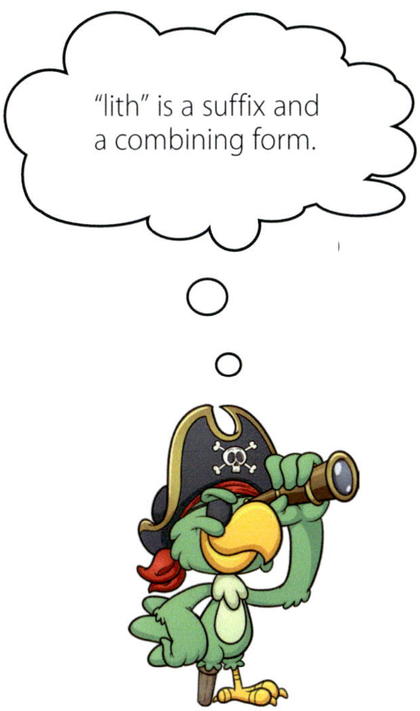

Suffixes

- ☐ -al; -ar
- ☐ -algia
- ☐ -ary
- ☐ -ation
- ☐ -cele
- ☐ -cide
- ☐ -dipsia
- ☐ -ectomy
- ☐ -emia
- ☐ -esis
- ☐ -flux
- ☐ -genesis
- ☐ -gram
- ☐ -graphy
- ☐ -ia
- ☐ -iasis
- ☐ -ic
- ☐ -ion
- ☐ -ism
- ☐ -itis
- ☐ -lith
- ☐ -lysis
- ☐ -meter
- ☐ -oma
- ☐ -osis
- ☐ -otomy
- ☐ -ous
- ☐ -pathy
- ☐ -pexy
- ☐ -plasty
- ☐ -ptosis
- ☐ -rrhagia
- ☐ -scope
- ☐ -scopy
- ☐ -sepsis
- ☐ -sis
- ☐ -spadias
- ☐ -stomy
- ☐ -thelium
- ☐ -tomy
- ☐ -tripsy
- ☐ -ure
- ☐ -uria
- ☐ -us

Combining Forms

- ☐ acid/o
- ☐ albumin/o
- ☐ bacter/i
- ☐ balan/o
- ☐ calc/i
- ☐ carcin/o
- ☐ col/o
- ☐ continence
- ☐ corpor/e
- ☐ cutan/e
- ☐ cyst/o
- ☐ excret/o
- ☐ glomerul/o
- ☐ glycos/o
- ☐ hem/o
- ☐ hemat/o
- ☐ ket/o
- ☐ keton/o
- ☐ lith/o
- ☐ meat/o
- ☐ metr/o
- ☐ micturit/o
- ☐ muc/o
- ☐ nephr/o
- ☐ noct/o
- ☐ olig/o
- ☐ ozot/o
- ☐ perine/o
- ☐ perit/o
- ☐ peritone/o
- ☐ phim/o
- ☐ py/o
- ☐ pyel/o
- ☐ ren/o
- ☐ scler/o
- ☐ son/o
- ☐ strict
- ☐ tens/o
- ☐ trigon
- ☐ ultra
- ☐ ur/o
- ☐ ureter/o
- ☐ urethr/o
- ☐ urin/o
- ☐ ven/o
- ☐ vesic/o

Checklist of New Anatomy

Kidney

- ❐ Hilum (hilus)
- ❐ Cortex
- ❐ Medulla
- ❐ Pyramids
- ❐ Minor calix
- ❐ Major calix
- ❐ Renal pelvis
- ❐ Renal artery
- ❐ Renal vein
- ❐ Nephron
- ❐ Renal corpuscle
    - ❐ Glomerulus
    - ❐ Bowman capsule
    - ❐ Afferent arteriole
    - ❐ Efferent arteriole
    - ❐ Peritubular capillaries
- ❐ Renal tubule
    - ❐ Proximate tubule
    - ❐ Loop of henle
    - ❐ Distal tubule
    - ❐ Collecting tubule

Tubes and Bladder

- ❐ Ureter
- ❐ Urinary bladder
    - ❐ Rugae
    - ❐ Apex
    - ❐ Neck
    - ❐ Trigone
    - ❐ Urothelium
    - ❐ Submucosa
    - ❐ Detrusor muscle
- ❐ Urethra
- ❐ Urinary meatus

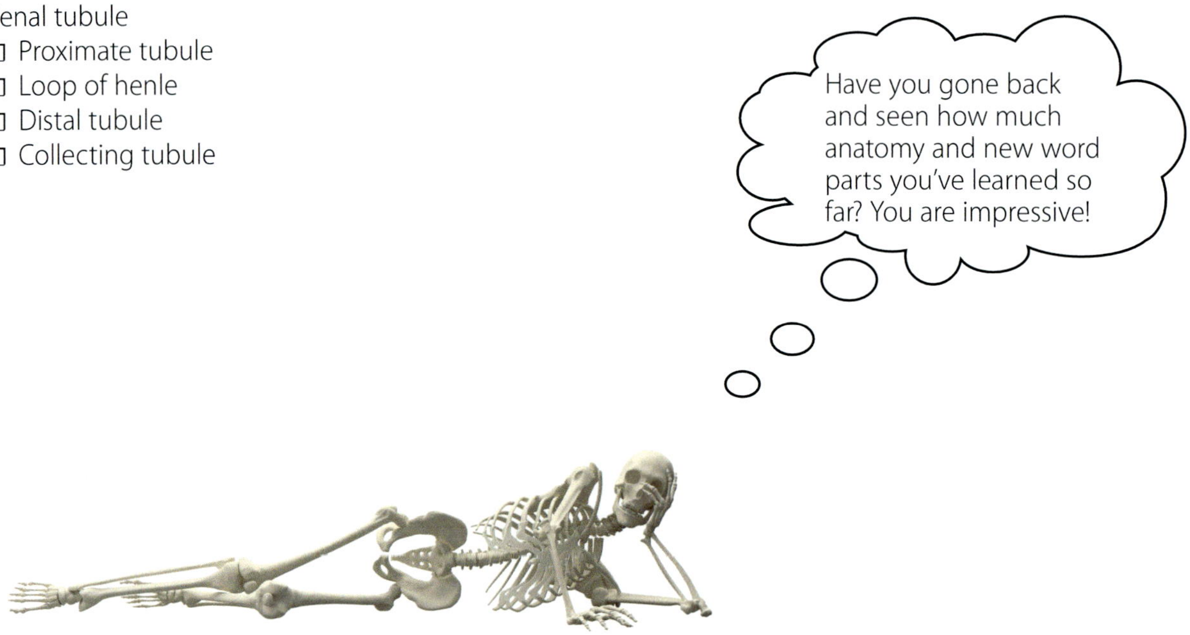
Have you gone back and seen how much anatomy and new word parts you've learned so far? You are impressive!

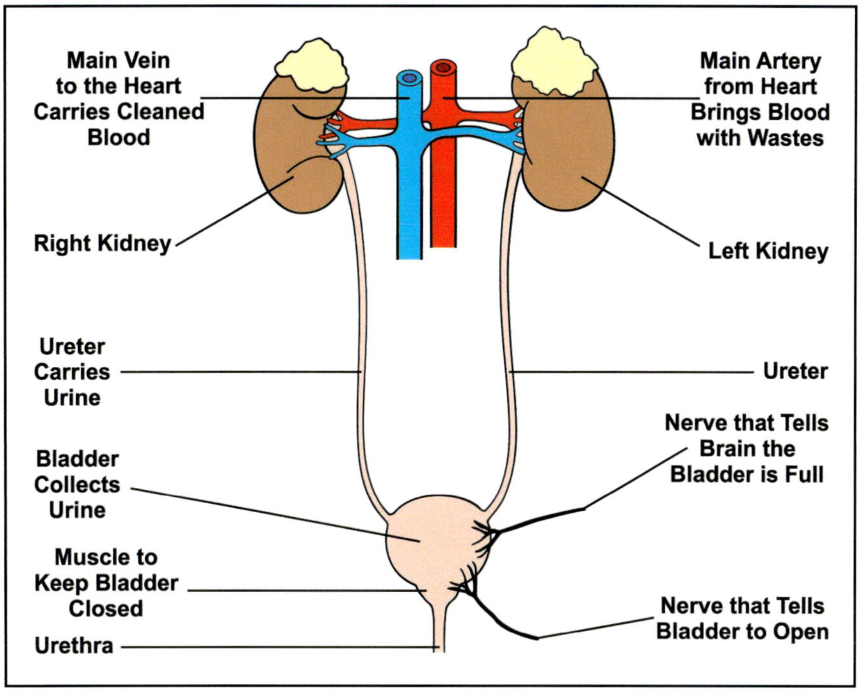

Figure 12-1. Urinary system. (udaix/shutterstock.com)

12

Introduction

Reno Island is the shape of a kidney (**ren/o**—kidney), as it represents the urinary system. The island contains word roots and combining forms distinctive to the urinary system. The urinary system has several other names—genitourinary (GU) system, urogenital (UG) system, and excretory system—but all pertain to the function of the kidneys, bladder, and structures that assist in urine production and excretion.

Anatomy

The main function of the urinary system is to filter blood and remove harmful or excessive substances through excretion in the urine. The kidneys also serve to regulate electrolytes and fluid levels in the blood. The urinary system is composed of two kidneys, a bladder, and three tubes that move waste from each kidney to the bladder, and excrete it (Figure 12-1). The highly vascular **kidneys** are the size of clenched fists and lie in the midback attached to the diaphragm. They actually move slightly upon breathing. The right kidney is slightly lower than the left, as it makes room for the liver. Both kidneys lie in the retroperitoneal (**retro-**—back, backward, behind) space (behind and outside of the peritoneal cavity of the abdomen) and are susceptible to injury. The lower (floating) ribs offer some protection from contusions, but many collision sports athletes wear additional padding to protect them (Figure 12-2). Each kidney has both a concave and convex border. In the center of the concave (medial) border lies an area called the **hilum** (also the **hilus**). It is in the hilum that the **renal artery,** vein, nerve, and lymphatic vessel pass (Figure 12-3). The **ureter** exits from the hilum as well, taking waste in the form of urine to the **urinary bladder**. As with the adrenal gland above it, kidneys have an outer layer, the **cortex**, and an inner **medulla**. A cross-section of the organ shows triangular structures called **pyramids**. An area called the **minor calix** lies at the base (pointy end) of the pyramids and expands into **major calix**, ending in the **renal pelvis**, which is a hollow chamber that collects the filtered waste and leads to the ureter.

The functional unit of the kidney that lies within the pyramids is the **nephron**, and each kidney has approximately 1 million of them. Nephrons provide the actual filtering of blood and exchange of waste, and they cross into both the renal cortex and medulla. Each nephron has two distinct aspects: the **renal corpuscle** and the **renal tubule**. The renal corpuscle is a collection of capillaries with four distinct aspects: The **glomerulus** (which is surrounded by an extension of the renal tubule called **Bowman's capsule**), large **afferent arterioles** carrying blood to the glomerulus, and smaller **efferent arterioles** that transport blood away from the glomerulus. As the efferent arterioles move away, they form the **peritubular capillaries,** named such as they surround (**peri-**—around) the tubules. Renal tubules also have four distinct sections, named by

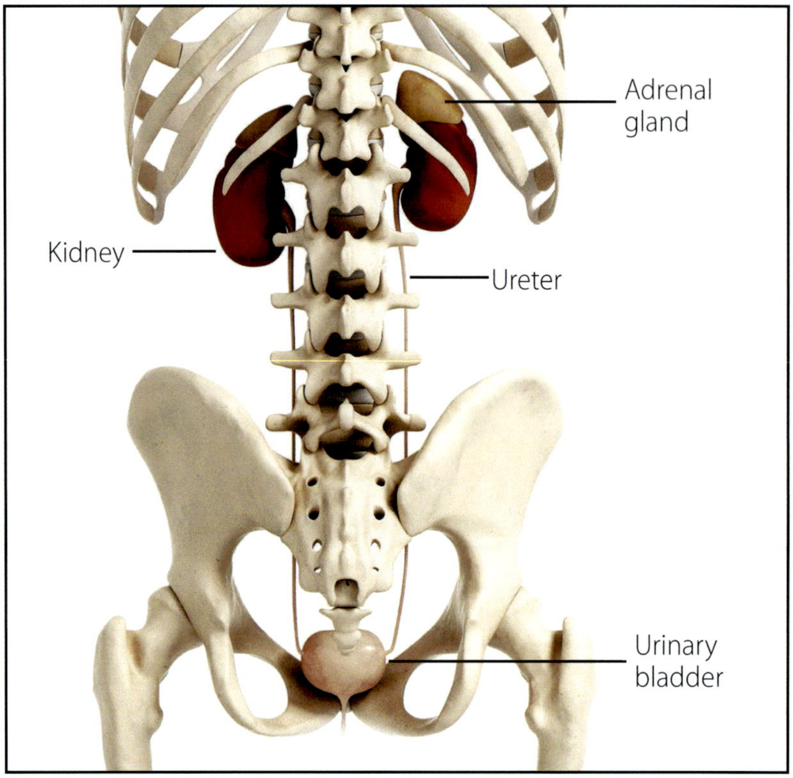

Figure 12-2. Posterior view of the urinary system with the urinary bladder hidden within pelvis. (Sebastian Kaulitzki/shutterstock.com)

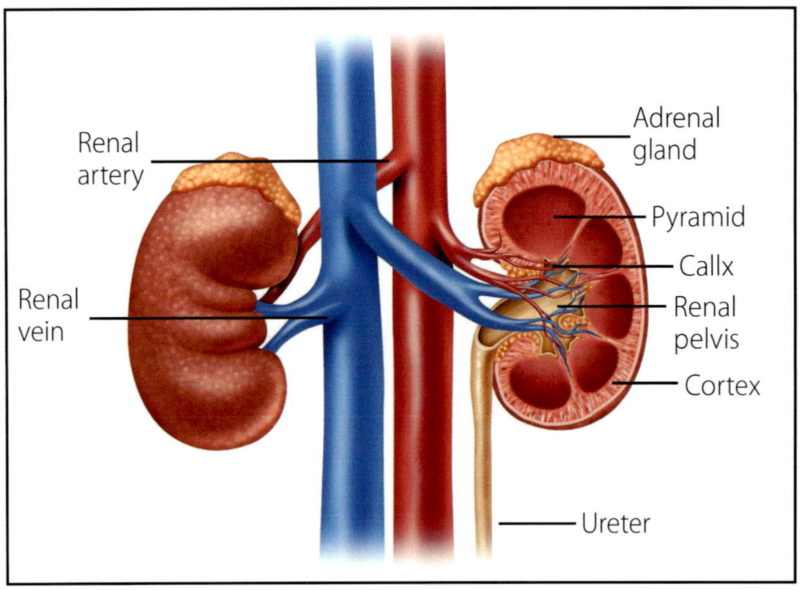

Figure 12-3. The renal artery and vein attach to the renal hilum. (Lightspring/shutterstock.com)

the location or function of the tube. **Proximal tubules** are convoluted and carry fluid into the renal medulla through the **loop of Henle**, where they interact with the peritubular capillaries, then pass back into the renal cortex forming the **distal tubules**, descending again into the cortex via the large **collecting tubule**. At the end of the collecting tubule is the renal pelvis, the collection station prior to passing into the ureter (Figure 12-4).

The two ureters drain urine via peristaltic waves from their respective kidneys to the urinary bladder. The bladder has an amazing capacity to expand and hold urine, as it is a muscular hollow sac that expands as it fills via the **rugae** (small folds in the walls that allow expansion, similar to those in the stomach). The internal layer of the bladder is called the **urothelium** (**ur/o**—urine; **-thelium**—specialized layer of cells), followed by the **submucosa** (**sub-**—under; **muc/o**—mucus) and then a muscular layer. Protecting the muscular layer is fatty tissue followed by a thin membrane shielding the bladder

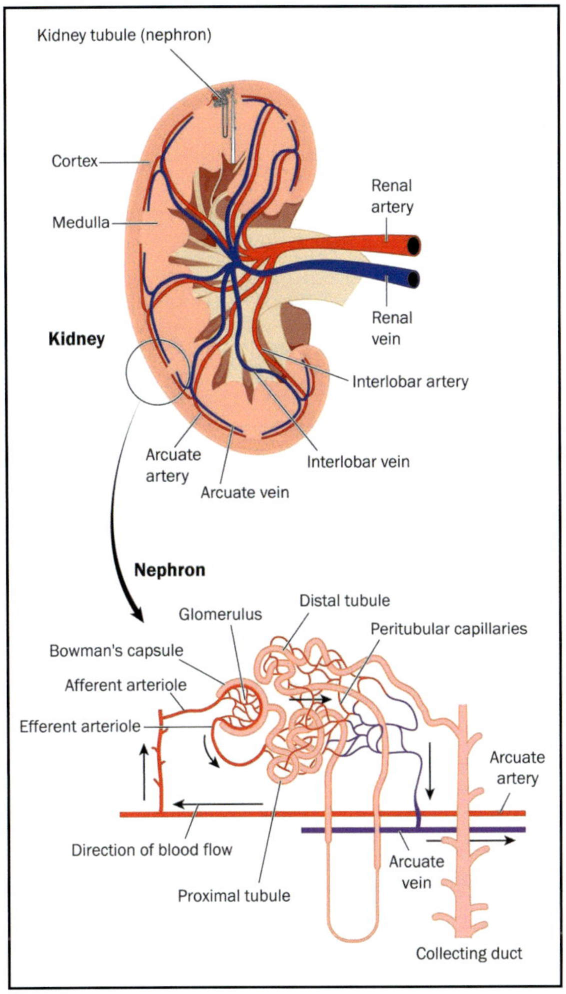

Figure 12-4. Internal structures of the kidney. (Blamb/shutterstock.com)

from the rest of the abdomen. Parasympathetic motor nerve fibers supply the **detrusor muscle** at the base of the bladder. When the bladder stretches as it fills, these nerve fibers signal the need to void (urinate). An unfilled bladder is protected behind the pubic bone of the pelvis, but swells over its protection when full, and can distend into the lower abdomen. This is why one should not drive with a full bladder, as the lap portion of a seatbelt applies pressure on a distended bladder, which can rupture it if involved in an accident. Anatomically, the bladder has an **apex** at the upper portion, and **neck** at the lower end. The triangular aspect between the entrance of the two ureters and exit of the urethra is termed the **trigone**. Neurological sensors within the bladder signal the extent of its fullness and send the urge to void to the brain. A full bladder can actually be quite painful. Bar owners know most people can hold only a finite amount of fluid in their bladders, and lure patrons into bars with extremely cheap beer, so long as no one uses the bathroom. The term most often used to promote these events is *bladder buster* (Figure 12-5).

The ure**thra** (think: it **thr**ows urine out, compared to the ureter) provides the gateway from the bladder to outside the body. The external opening is termed the **urinary meatus**. In men, the urethra is about 20 cm long and passes either urine or semen through it. The female urethra is 3 cm long and passes only urine.

Urine has many aspects (Table 12-1) and is a by product of the kidney's filtration. It is composed of 95% water with the remaining 5% solid waste, and has a slightly acidic content (6.9 pH). It can vary in color and odor depending on what was ingested and the person's overall health. Unnecessary vitamins, minerals, and other substances are passed through the urine, as is the breakdown of most medications. A urinalysis (UA) can easily provide a spot check on overall health. The average adult will void between 1000 and 1500 mL daily of urine, but the body sends an urge to void when the bladder has about 300 to 350 mL of urine within it.

One method of UA involves a specialized dipstick that is dipped into a sample of urine (Figure 12-6). Each component (eg, protein, glucose) has an indicator that reacts with the sample and turns that section of the dipstick a color. The color shade is then matched on the container holding the dipsticks for a value.

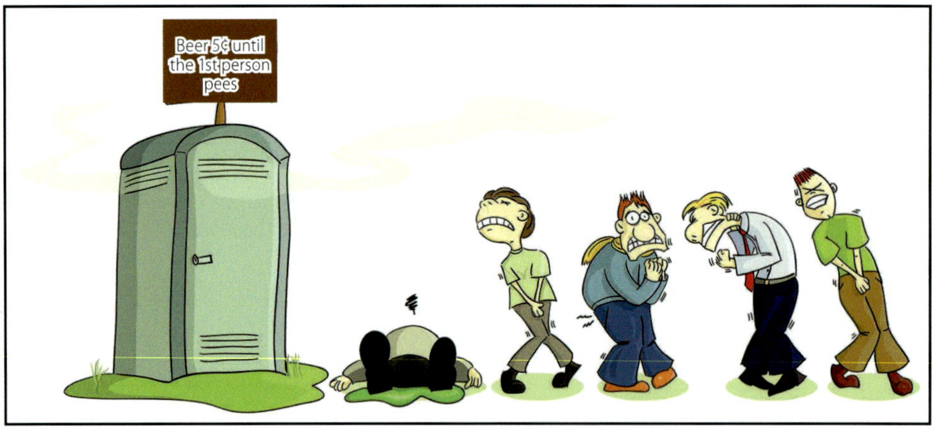

Figure 12-5. A full urinary bladder can be painful. (Hermin/shutterstock.com)

Table 12-1

Urine Values

COMPONENT	NORMAL VALUE	ABNORMAL SIGN AND IMPLICATION
appearance	Clear	Hazy: Refrigerated sample Milky: Bacteria, fat globules, pus Smoky: Blood cells
bilirubin	Negative	Positive: Biliary obstruction, congestive heart failure (CHF), liver disease
blood	Negative	Positive: Renal disease, trauma
color	Pale yellow	Greenish brown to black: Caused by bile pigments Orange: Medication induced Red/reddish: Hemoglobin in the sample *Note: Urine samples darken upon standing.*
glucose	Negative	Positive: Diabetes mellitus
ketones	Negative	Positive: High-protein/low-carbohydrate diet; uncontrolled diabetes mellitus; starvation (or fasting)
nitrates	Negative	Positive: Bacteriuria
odor	Slightly aromatic	Fruity/sweet: Acetone, associated with diabetes mellitus Unpleasant: Decomposition of alcohol, drugs, foods
protein	Negative	Positive: Renal disease
quantity	About 1000 to 1500 mL per day	High: Diabetes mellitus, diabetes insipidus, diuretics, excessive intake, nervousness Low: Acute nephritis, diarrhea, dehydration, heart disease, vomiting None: Renal failure, obstruction, pyelonephritis
reaction	Between 4.6 and 8.9 pH; average of 6.0	High acidity: Diabetic acidosis, dehydration, fever Alkaline: Renal failure, urinary tract infection (UTI)
specific gravity	Between 1.003 and 1.030	High (over 1.030: CHF, diabetes mellitus, hepatic disease Low (1.001 to 1.002): Diabetes insipidus
urobilinogen	0.1 to 1.0	Absent: Biliary obstruction Increased: Early sign of liver or hemolytic disease Reduced: Reaction to antibiotic medication

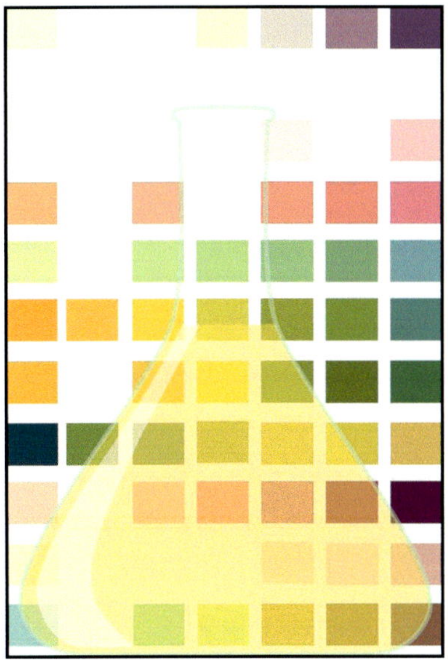

Figure 12-6. A dipstick placed in urine will react and change colors to indicate a specific value for the component tested. (lekcej/shutterstock.com)

Word Building

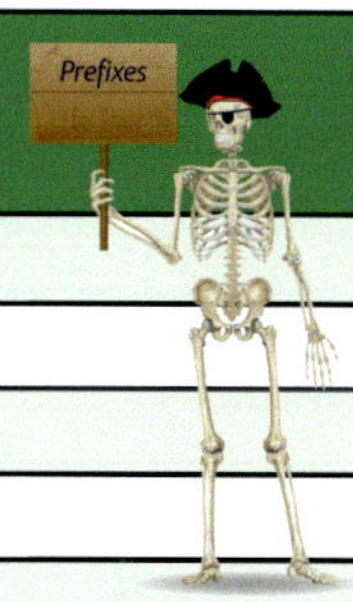

Table 12-2

Prefixes

PREFIX	DEFINITION
an-	not; without
di-; dia-	two; through; apart; across
dys-	abnormal; bad; difficult; painful
en-	within
epi-	above; upon
extra-	outside
hydro-	water
hyper-	above; excessive; high; increased
in-	not
intra-	inside; within
par-	alongside; around; beside; near
per-	through
peri-	around
poly-	excessive; many; much; over
re-	back; behind
retro-	back; backward; behind
steno-	narrow; short
sub-	under; below
supra-	above
trans-	across; through

Table 12-3

Suffixes

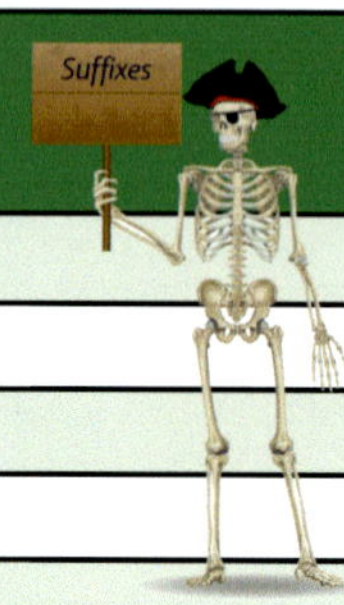

SUFFIX	DEFINITION
-al; -ar	pertaining to
-algia	pain
-ary	pertaining to
-ation	process of
-cele	hernia; protrusion; swelling
-cide	killing
-dipsia	thirst
-ectomy	excision; surgical removal
-emia	blood condition
-esis	state of
-flux	flow
-genesis	forming; producing; origin
-gram	a record
-graphy	process of recording; the act of recording information
-ia	condition
-iasis	condition; presence of
-ic	pertaining to
-ion	process; the act of
-ism	condition
-itis	inflammation
-lith	stone
-lysis	breaking down; destruction; loosening; separating; to loosen or break
-meter	instrument for measuring
-oma	mass; tumor
-osis	condition
-ous	pertaining to
-pathy	disease
-pexy	surgical fixation of
-plasty	reconstruction; repair; plastic surgery
-ptosis	drooping; falling; prolapse
-rrhagia	abnormal flow
-scope	an instrument used to view or inspect
-scopy	examination of
-sepsis	an inflammatory response to an infection
-sis	condition; state of
-spadias	fissure
-stomy	surgical opening

(continued)

Table 12-3 (continued)
Suffixes

SUFFIX	DEFINITION
-thelium	layer of specialized material
-tomy; -otomy	incision; to cut into
-tripsy	crushing
-ure	process
-uria	urine
-us	pertaining to; structure

Table 12-4
Combining Forms

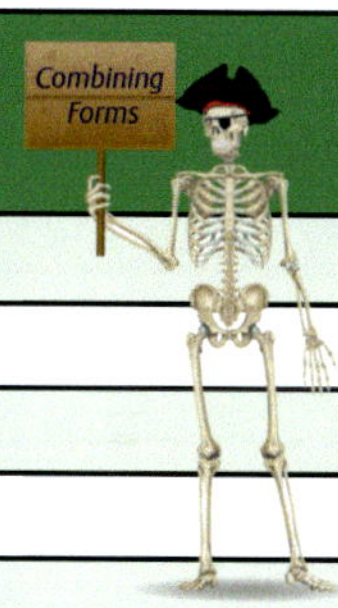

COMBINING FORM	DEFINITION
acid/o	acid
albumin/o	protein
bacter/i	bacteria
balan/o	glans penis
calc/i	calcium
carcin/o	cancer
col/o	colon
continence	to hold
corpor/e	body
cutan/e	skin
cyst/o	bladder; sac
excret/o	shifted out
glomerul/o	glomerulus; little ball
glycos/o	glucose; glycogen; sugar
hem/o; hemat/o	blood
ket/o; keton/o	ketone
lith/o	stone
meat/o	opening
metr/o	uterus
micturit/o	to urinate
muc/o	mucus
nephr/o	kidney
noct/o	night
olig/o	scanty
ozot/o	nitrogen
perit/o	peritoneum (membrane lining the abdomen)
phim/o	muzzle

(continued)

Table 12-4 (continued) Combining Forms	
COMBINING FORM	**DEFINITION**
py/o	pus
pyel/o	renal pelvis
ren/o	kidney
scler/o	hard; hardening; thick; sclera
son/o	sound
strict	tightening; contracture
tens/o	pressure; stretching
trigon	trigone
ultra	beyond; farther
ur/o	urine; urinate
ureter/o	ureter
urethr/o	urethra
urin/o	urine
ven/o	vein
vesic/o	urinary bladder

Signs and Symptoms

Table 12-5 Signs and Symptoms Related to the Urinary System		
SIGN/SYMPTOM	**WORD PARTS**	**DEFINITION**
cystalgia (Figure 12-7)	cyst/ (bladder) **-algia** (pain)	Pain in the bladder; also called *cystodynia*
dysuria	**dys-** (painful) **-uria** (urine)	Painful or difficult urination
ketoacidosis	ket/o (ketone) acid/ (acid) **-osis** (condition)	Condition indicating starvation or fasting
polydipsia	**poly-** (excessive) **-dipsia** (thirst)	Excessive thirst; can be indicative of diabetes insipidus and mellitus
urethralgia	urethr/ (urethra) **-algia** (pain)	Pain in the urethra

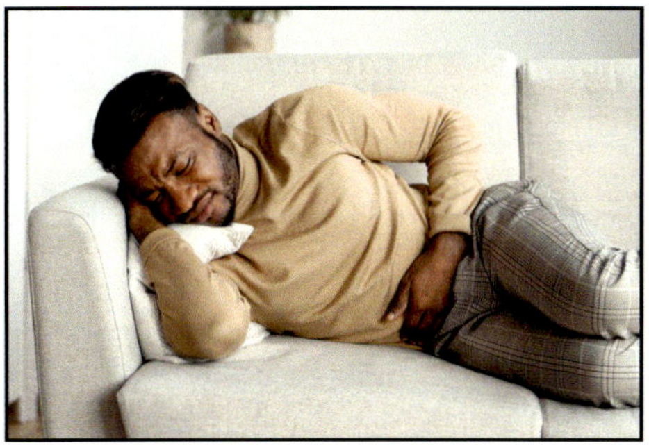

Figure 12-7. Cystalgia presents with low midabdominal pain. (Prostock-studio/shutterstock.com)

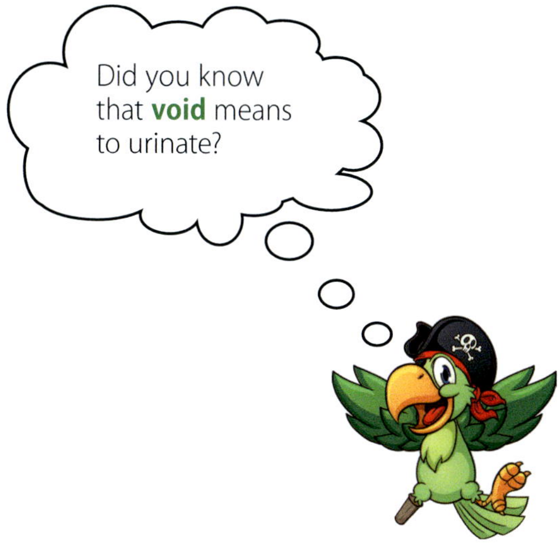

TABLE 12-6 WORDS ASSOCIATED WITH URINE OR URINATION		
WORD	**WORD PARTS**	**DEFINITION**
albuminuria	albumin/ (protein) **-uria** (urine)	Protein in the urine (can indicate renal disease)
anuria	**an-** (without) ur/ (urine) **-ia** (condition)	Lack of urine production
azoturia	azot/ (nitrogen) **-uria** (urine)	Excessive nitrogenous components in the urine
bacteriuria	bacter/i (bacteria) ur/ (urine) **-ia** (condition)	Presence of bacteria in the urine
calciuria	calc/i (calcium) ur/ (urine) **-ia** (condition)	Presence of calcium in the urine
cystorrhagia	cyst/o (bladder) **-rrhagia** (abnormal flow)	Profuse bleeding from the urinary bladder
diuresis	**di-** (through) ur/ (urine) **-esis** (state of)	Increased urine production
enuresis (Figure 12-8)	**en-** (within) ur/ (urine) **-esis** (state of)	Involuntary emission of urine; also called *nocturnal enuresis* (bedwetting at night)

(continued)

TABLE 12-6 (CONTINUED)

WORDS ASSOCIATED WITH URINE OR URINATION

WORD	WORD PARTS	DEFINITION
glycosuria	glycos/ (glucose) **-uria** (urine)	Presence of glucose in the urine
hematuria	hemat/ (blood) **-uria** (urine)	Presence of blood in the urine; can be *occult* (determined only by microscopic inspection or dipstick) or *gross* (visible to the human eye)
hesitancy		Decreased force in the urine stream, often due to an enlarged prostate or kidney stone
hypercalciuria	**hyper-** (excessive) calc/i (calcium) **-uria** (urine)	Excessive amount of calcium in the urine
incontinence	**in-** (not) continence (to hold)	Inability to hold urine; inability to control urination or defecation
ketonuria	keton/ (ketone) **-uria** (urine)	Presence of ketones in urine; caused by tissue breakdown or complication of diabetes mellitus
micturition		Act of urinating
nocturia	noct/ (night) **-uria** (urine)	Need to urinate during the night
oliguria	olig/ (scanty) **-uria** (urine)	Scanty, or diminished, amount of urine; caused by dehydration, shock, urinary obstruction, or renal failure
polyuria	**poly-** (excessive) **-uria** (urine)	Frequent urination; caused by diabetes mellitus, diabetes insipidus, renal disease, diuretic medication, excessive fluid intake
pyuria	py/ (pus) **-uria** (urine)	Pus in the urine
uremia	ur/ (urine) **-emia** (blood condition)	Retention of excessive amounts of nitrogenous compounds in the blood; also called *azotemia*
urgency		Sudden need to urinate
void		Act of urinating

Most of these words are also signs or symptoms of a urinary system condition.

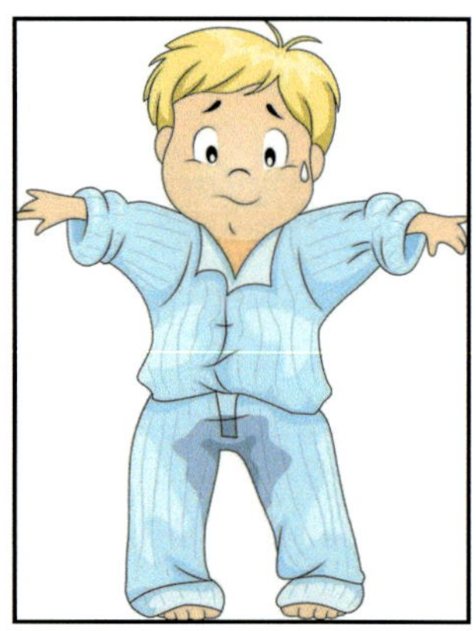

Figure 12-8. Enuresis is also known as *bedwetting*. (Lorelyn Medina/shutterstock.com)

Table 12-7
Terms Associated With Anatomical Location

TERM	WORD PARTS	DEFINITION
periurethral	**peri-** (around) urethr/ (urethra) **-al** (pertaining to)	Pertaining to around the urethra
renal	ren/ (kidney) **-al** (pertaining to)	Pertaining to the kidney
suprarenal	**supra-** (above) ren/ (kidney) **-al** (pertaining to)	Pertaining to above the kidney
transurethral procedure	**trans-** (through) urethr/ (urethra) **-al** (pertaining to)	Procedures that can be accomplished by going up (through) the urethra
urethroperineal	urethr/o (urethra) perine/ (perineum) **-al** (pertaining to)	Pertaining to the urethra and perineum

Medical Conditions

Table 12-8
Medical Conditions Related to the Urinary System

NAME	WORD PARTS	DEFINITION
calculus (Figure 12-9)	calc/ (calcium) **-us** (structure)	Stone; plural is *calculi*
carcinoma in situ (CIS)	carcin/ (cancer) **-oma** (tumor)	Cancer that is in one place and has not metastasized (spread) to other tissues/organs. This term is not specific to the urinary system
cystitis	cyst/ (bladder) **-itis** (inflammation)	Inflammation of the bladder, typically in response to a UTI
cystocele	cyst/o (bladder) **-cele** (hernia; protrusion; swelling)	Hernia of the bladder
cystolith	cyst/o (bladder) **-lith** (stone)	Stone in the bladder
glomerulitis	glomerul/ (glomerulus) **-itis** (inflammation)	Inflammation of the glomerulus
glomerulonephritis	glomerul/o (glomerulus) nephr/ (kidney) **-itis** (inflammation)	Inflammation of the kidney primarily involving the glomeruli

(continued)

TABLE 12-8 (CONTINUED)

MEDICAL CONDITIONS RELATED TO THE URINARY SYSTEM

NAME	WORD PARTS	DEFINITION
hydronephrosis	**hydro-** (water) nephr/ (kidney) **-osis** (condition)	Obstruction that causes water to accumulate in the renal pelvis, causing kidney damage and obstructing urine flow
nephritis	nephr/ (kidney) **-itis** (inflammation)	Inflammation of the kidney
nephrocystitis	nephr/o (kidney) cyst/ (bladder) **-itis** (inflammation)	Inflammation of the kidney and bladder
nephrolith	nephr/o (kidney) **-lith** (stone)	Kidney stone (calculus)
nephrolithiasis	nephr/o (kidney) **-lith** (stone) **-iasis** (condition)	Condition of having kidney stones
nephroma	nephr/ (kidney) **-oma** (tumor)	Tumor in the kidney
nephropathy	nephr/o (kidney) **-pathy** (disease)	Disease of the kidney
nephroptosis	nephr/o (kidney) **-ptosis** (prolapse)	Prolapse or sagging of a kidney
nephrosclerosis	nephr/o (kidney) scler/ (hardening) **-osis** (condition)	Hardening of the kidney
polycystic kidney disease (Figure 12-10)	**poly-** (many) cyst/ (sac) **-ic** (pertaining to)	Renal cysts caused by a genetic disorder
pyelocystitis	pyel/o (renal pelvis) cyst/ (bladder) **-itis** (inflammation)	Inflammation of the renal pelvis and bladder
pyelonephritis (Figure 12-11)	pyel/o (renal pelvis) nephr/ (kidney) **-itis** (inflammation)	Inflammation of the renal pelvis and kidney

(continued)

Table 12-8 (continued)

Medical Conditions Related to the Urinary System

NAME	WORD PARTS	DEFINITION
renal hypertension	ren/ (kidney) **-al** (pertaining to) **hyper-** (high) tens/ (pressure) **-ion** (process; the act of)	Hypertension brought about due to kidney dysfunction
stricture	strict/ (tightening) **-ure** (process)	Abnormal narrowing or tightening of a passage (eg, ureter, urethra, esophagus)
trigonitis (Figure 12-12)	trigon (trigone) **-itis** (inflammation)	Inflammation of the trigone of the bladder
ureterocele	ureter/o (ureter) **-cele** (hernia)	Hernia at the terminal end of the ureter, prolapsing into the bladder
ureteropathy	ureter/o (ureter) **-pathy** (disease)	Disease of the ureter
urethritis	urethr/ (urethra) **-itis** (inflammation)	Inflammation of the urethra
urinary tract infection (UTI)	urin/ (urinary) **-ary** (pertaining to)	Infection anywhere in the urinary system; caused most often by bacteria, but can also arise from yeast, parasites, or protozoa
urolithiasis	ur/o (urine) lith/ (stone) **-iasis** (condition)	Stones anywhere in the urinary system; also called *urinary calculi*
urosepsis	ur/o (urine) **-sepsis** (an inflammatory response to an infection)	Bacteria in the urine caused by a UTI
vesicoureteral reflux	vesic/o (urinary bladder) ureter/ (ureter) **-al** (pertaining to) **re-** (back) **-flux** (flow)	Abnormal backflow of urine from the bladder back up into the ureter

12

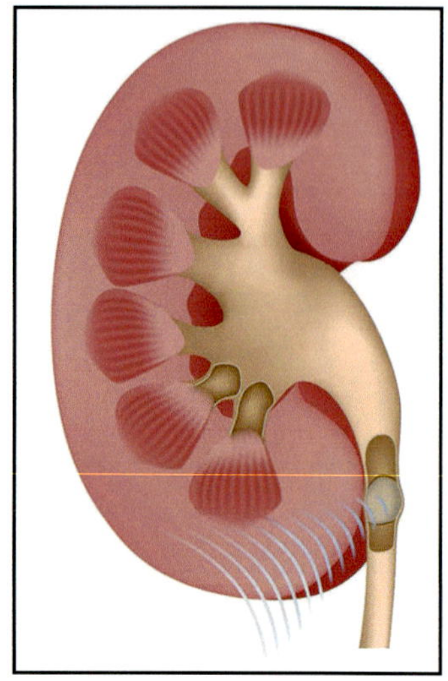

Figure 12-9. A calculus at the opening of the ureter. (Alila Medical Images/shutterstock.com)

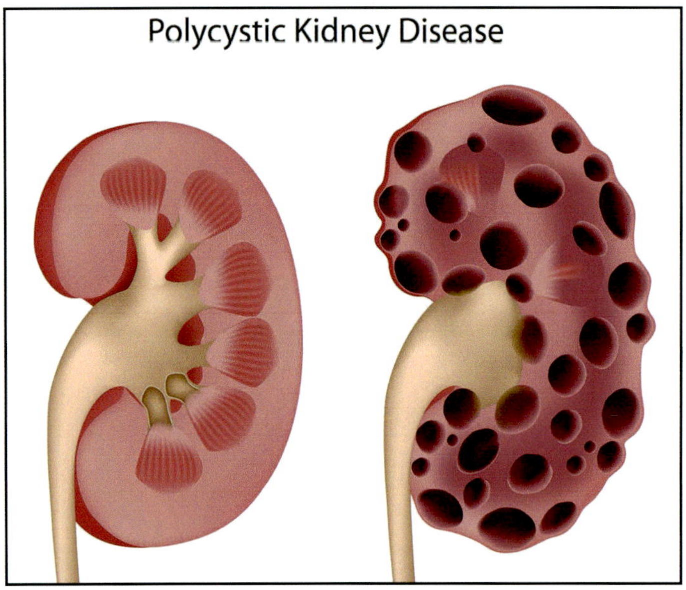

Figure 12-10. Polycystic kidney disease, compared to a healthy kidney (left). (Alila Medical Images/shutterstock.com)

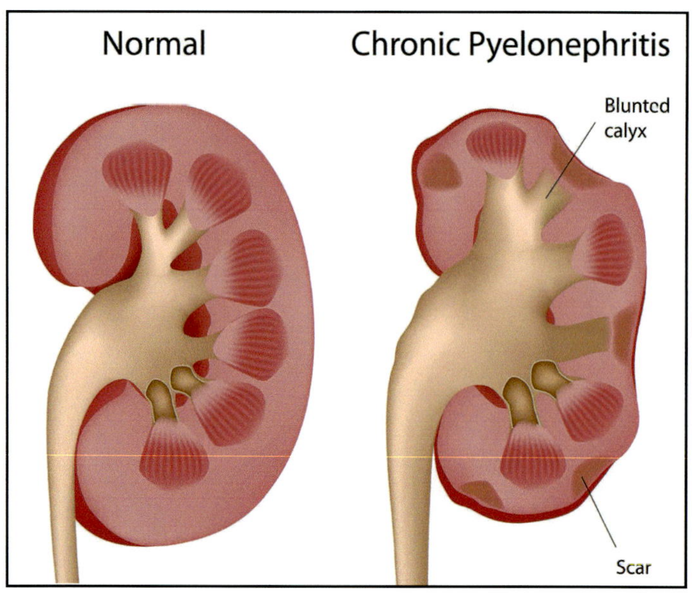

Figure 12-11. Chronic pyelonephritis. (Alila Medical Images/shutterstock.com)

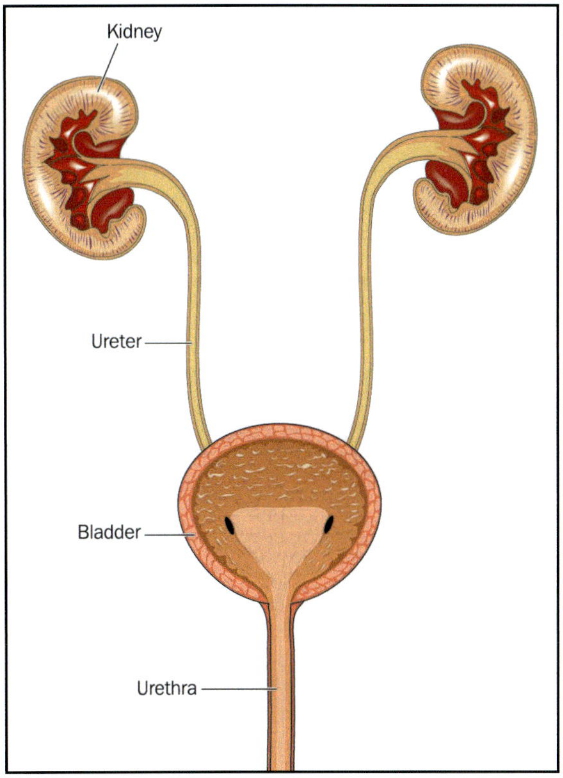

Figure 12-12. The trigone area of the bladder. (Blamb/shutterstock.com)

TABLE 12-9
MEDICAL CONDITIONS OF THE PENIS

NAME	WORD PARTS	DEFINITION
balanitis	balan/ (glans penis) **-itis** (inflammation)	Inflammation of the skin covering the glans penis
epispadias	**epi-** (above) **-spadias** (fissure)	Malformation in which the urethra opens on the upper (dorsum) aspect of the penis
hypospadias	**hypo-** (below) **-spadias** (fissure)	Malformation in which the urethra opens on the underside aspect of the penis

Tests and Procedures

Table 12-10

Tests and Procedures Related to the Urinary System

NAME	WORD PARTS	PURPOSE
cystectomy	cyst/ (bladder) **-ectomy** (surgical excision)	Surgical removal of part or all of the bladder
cystogram	cyst/o (bladder) **-gram** (a record of)	X-ray recording of the bladder
cystolithectomy	cyst/o (bladder) lith/ (stone) **-ectomy** (surgical excision)	Surgical removal of stones (calculi) from the bladder
cystometrography	cyst/o (bladder) metr/o (measure) **-graphy** (process of recording)	A test stressing the urinary bladder, assessing the pressure and volume of a saline solution inserted via catheter
cystoscope (Figure 12-13)	cyst/o (bladder) **-scope** (an instrument used to view or inspect)	Instrument used to visually inspect the bladder
cystourethroscopy	cyst/o (bladder) urethr/o (urethra) **-scopy** (examination of)	Visual examination of the urinary bladder and urethra
extracorporeal shock wave lithotripsy (Figure 12-14)	**extra-** (outside) corpor/e (body) **-al** (pertaining to) lith/o (stone) **-tripsy** (crushing)	Noninvasive medical procedure lithotripsy used to crush kidney stones
hemodialysis (Figure 12-15)	hem/o (blood) **dia-** (through) **-lysis** (separating)	Medical procedure typically performed in a special office or hospital that separates byproducts in the blood that the kidney would normally do
intravenous pyelography (IVP)	**intra-** (inside) ven/ (vein) **-ous** (pertaining to) pyel/o (renal pelvis) **-graphy** (the act of recording information)	Examination via x-rays and injectable radiographic dye used to inspect the urinary system

(continued)

Table 12-10 (continued)

Tests and Procedures Related to the Urinary System

NAME	WORD PARTS	PURPOSE
kidney, ureter, bladder (KUB) study		X-ray that shows the anatomical location of the kidneys, ureters, and bladder
lithotripsy	lith/o (stone) **-tripsy** (crushing)	Noninvasive procedure to crush a stone (gall or kidney)
meatotomy	meat/o (opening) **-tomy** (incision)	Incision into the urinary opening to widen it
nephrectomy	nephr/ (kidney) **-ectomy** (surgical excision)	Surgical removal of a kidney
nephrolithotomy	nephr/o (kidney) lith/o (stone) **-tomy** (incision)	Incision into a kidney to remove a kidney stone
nephropexy	nephr/o (kidney) **-pexy** (surgical fixation of)	Surgical fixation of a kidney
nephrostomy	nephr/o (kidney) **-stomy** (surgical opening)	Making an incision into the kidney (usually to insert a catheter)
percutaneous ultrasonic lithotripsy	**per-** (through) cutan/e (skin) **-ous** (pertaining to) ultra/ (beyond; farther) son/ (sound) **-ic** (pertaining to) lith/o (stone) **-tripsy** (crushing)	Crushing a kidney stone using sound waves via ultrasound; usually accomplished via a nephroscope
peritoneal dialysis (PD) (Figures 12-16 and 12-17)	peritone/ (peritoneum) **-al** (pertaining to) **dia-** (through) **-lysis** (separating)	Medical procedure where blood from the vessels in the peritoneal (abdominal) lining are filtered to separate byproducts; takes over for the filtering that kidney would normally do; can be done at home

(continued)

12

Table 12-10 (continued)

Tests and Procedures Related to the Urinary System

NAME	WORD PARTS	PURPOSE
pyelolithotomy	pyel/o (renal pelvis) lith/o (stone) **-tomy** (incision)	Surgical incision into the renal pelvis for the purpose of removing a kidney stone
ureterocolostomy	ureter/o (ureter) col/o (colon) **-stomy** (surgical opening)	Surgically creating a new opening of the ureter into the colon
ureteroplasty	ureter/o (ureter) **-plasty** (repair)	Surgical repair of the ureter
urethral stricture	urethr/ (urethra) **-al** (pertaining to) strict/ (tightening) **-ure** (process)	Process of narrowing or constriction of the urethra
urinary catheter (Figure 12-18)	urin/ (urine) **-ary** (pertaining to)	Flexible tube inserted in the urinary bladder to facilitate the removal of urine; an *indwelling catheter* remains in place, and a *straight catheter* is removed after urine is drained from the bladder
urinometer	urin/o (urine) **-meter** (instrument for measuring)	Instrument used to measure the specific gravity of urine
vesicotomy	vesic/o (urinary bladder) **-tomy** (incision)	Incision into the urinary bladder

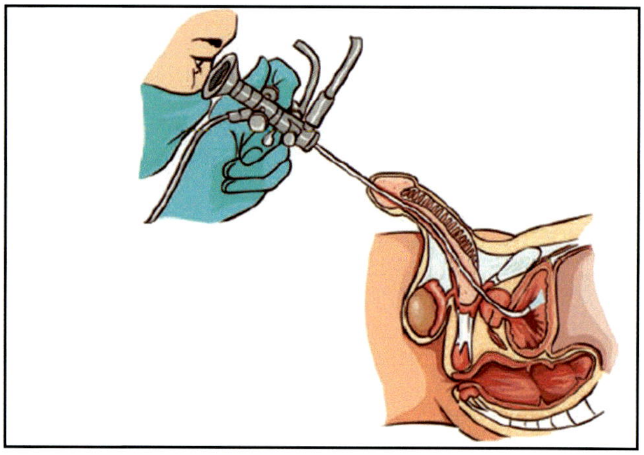

Figure 12-13. Cystoscopy is one way to view the bladder for irregularities. (hkannn/shutterstock.com)

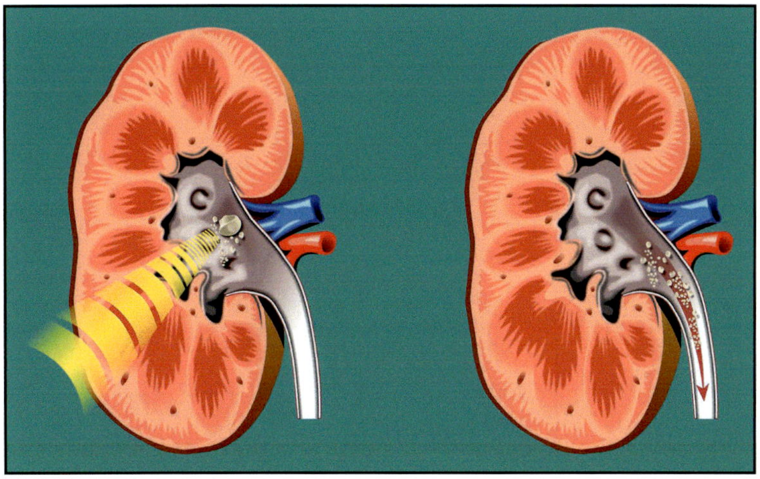

Figure 12-14. Lithotripsy allows sound waves to break up kidney stones so they may be more easily passed through the ureter and urethra. (Alexonline/shutterstock.com)

Figure 12-15. Hemodialysis involves arterial blood passing through a machine that acts as a kidney, then returning filtered blood back through a vein. (gopixa/shutterstock.com)

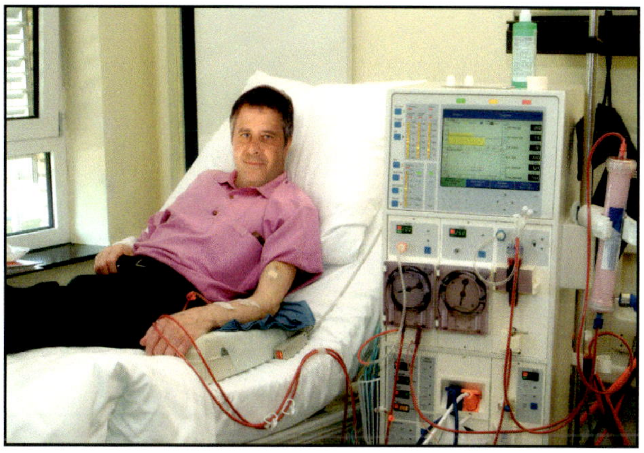

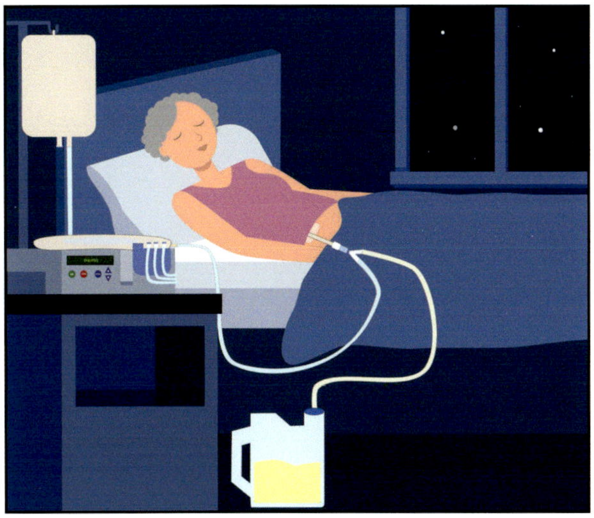

Figure 12-16. Dialysis can be accomplished at home. (Orathai Yingyould/shutterstock.com)

Figure 12-17. Continuous ambulatory peritoneal dialysis involves introducing dialysis fluid into the peritoneal cavity for removal of wastes. (Blamb/shutterstock.com)

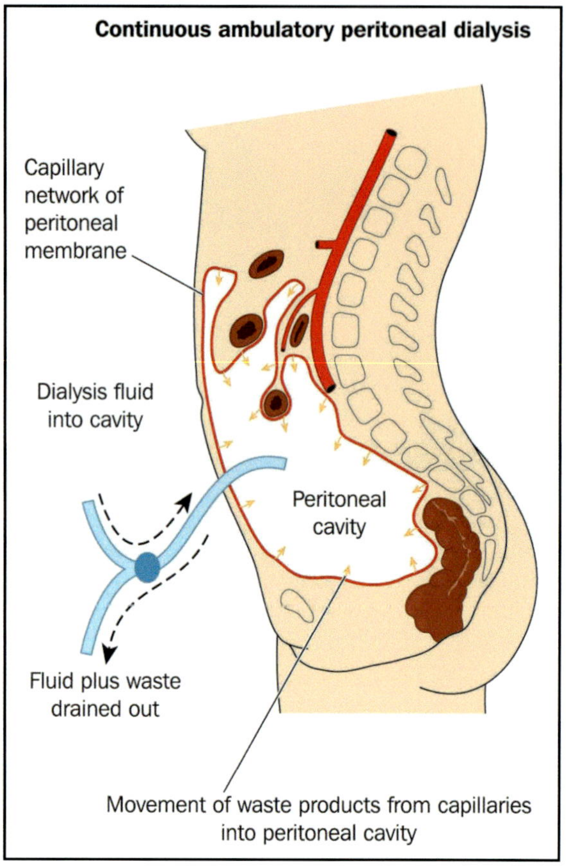

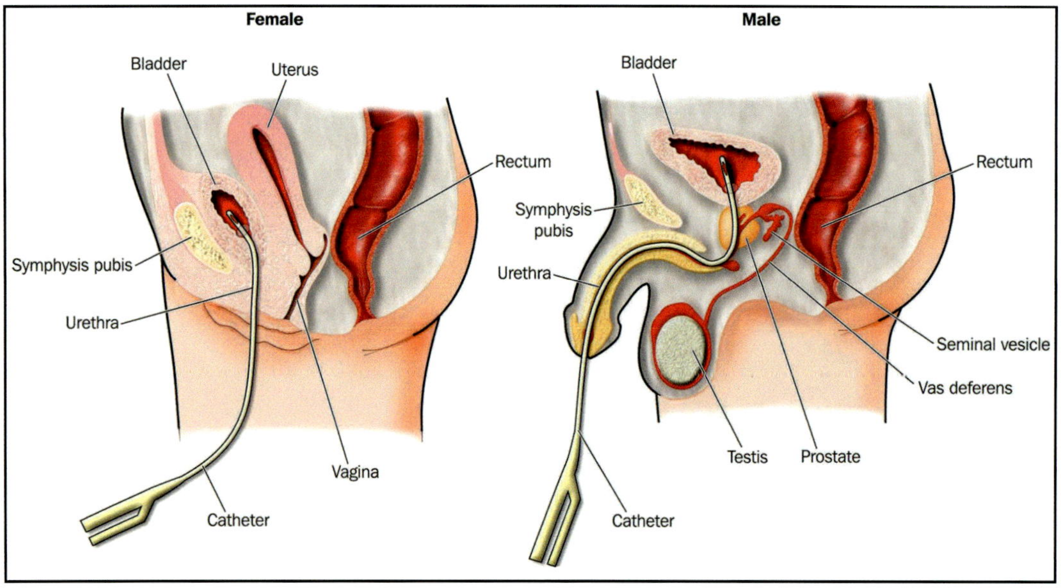

Figure 12-18. Urinary catheters inserted correctly in a female and male patient. (Blamb/shutterstock.com)

A WORD ABOUT KIDNEY AND URINARY BLADDER CANCERS

According to the American Cancer Society (www.cancer.org), new diagnoses of kidney cancer ranks seventh in men and tenth in women in 2015. Urinary bladder cancer ranks fourth in new diagnoses for men for the same time period. Whereas early stages of kidney cancer have few signs or symptoms, once diagnosed, the 5-year survival rate for both cancers is high, as long as they are **in situ** (Figure 12-19). A cancerous kidney can be excised, and people can function quite well on one kidney. Urinary bladder cancer has a more common occurrence than kidney cancer, with a 1:26 chance of it in men in their lifetime (1:87 in women). Early signs of bladder cancer include **hematuria** and increased urgency and frequency. Depending on the staging (Figure 12-20), bladder cancer treatment ranges from surgery, chemotherapy inserted directly into the bladder, or cystectomy.

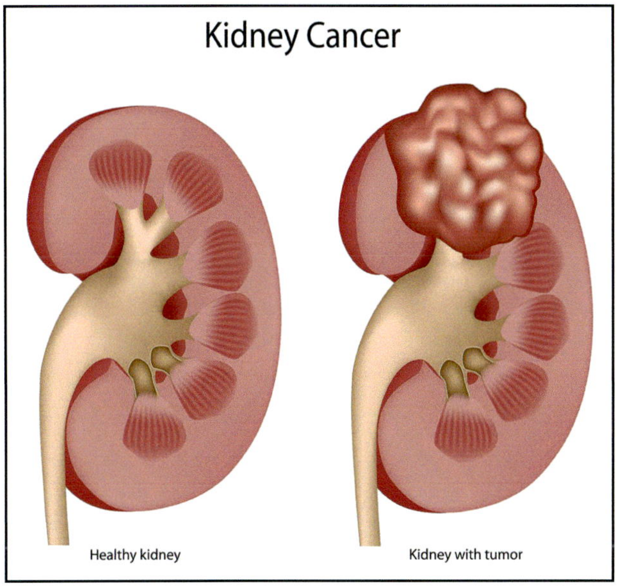

Figure 12-19. Kidney cancer on the superior aspect of the kidney cortex. (Alila Medical Images/shutterstock.com)

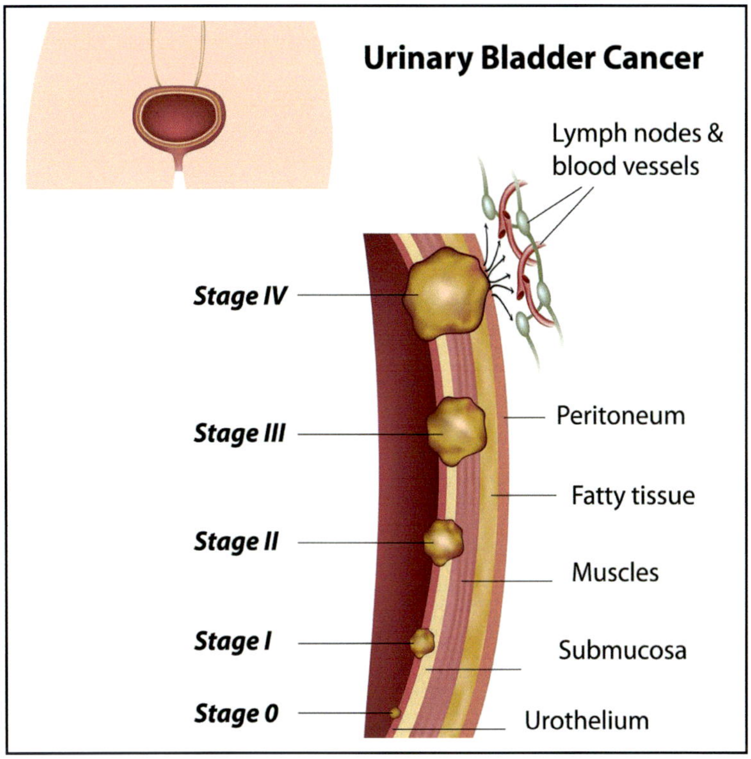

Figure 12-20. Stages of urinary bladder cancer. (Alila Medical Images/shutterstock.com)

12

Bibliography

Cancer.Net. Testicular cancer: symptoms and signs. American Society of Clinical Oncology. Published November, 2020. Accessed Devember 31, 2021. https://www.cancer.net/cancer-types/testicular-cancer/symptoms-and-signs

Flanagan KW, Cuppett M. Genitourinary and gynecological systems. In *Medical Conditions in the Athlete.* 3rd ed. Human Kinetics; 2017.

Fremgen BF, Frucht SS. *Medical Terminology: A Living Language*. 7th ed. Pearson; 2019.

Hutton A. *Medical Terminology for Health Care*. 5th ed. Churchill Livingstone; 2017.

McCance KL, Huether SE. *Pathophysiology: The Biologic Basis for Disease in Adults and Children*. 8th ed. Mosby; 2019.

Mosby's Dictionary of Medicine, Nursing & Health Professions. 10th ed. Elsevier; 2017.

Rice J. *Medical Terminology for Health Care Professionals.* 9th ed. Pearson; 2018.

Shiland BJ. *Mastering Healthcare Terminology.* 6th ed. Elsevier; 2019.

Venes D, ed. *Taber's Cyclopedic Medical Dictionary.* 24th ed. F. A. Davis; 2021.

NOTES

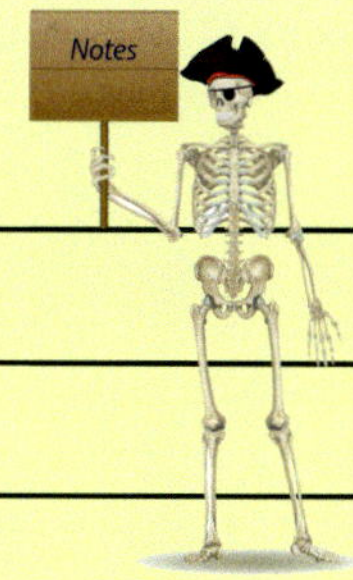

NOTES

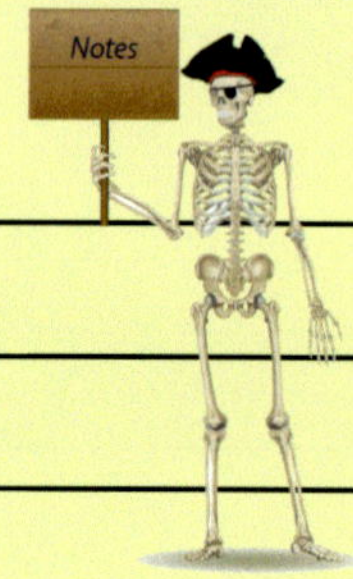

Learning Activities

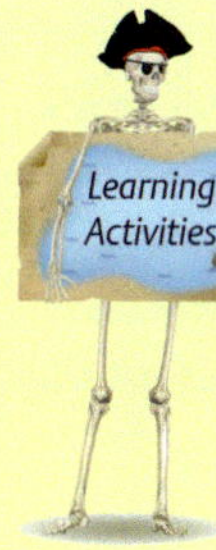

Name:______________________

Urinary System

A. Label the components of the urinary system from the following list of words.

- cortex____________
- renal artery________
- renal vein_________
- pyramids__________
- minor calix________
- major calix________
- renal pelvis________
- ureter____________

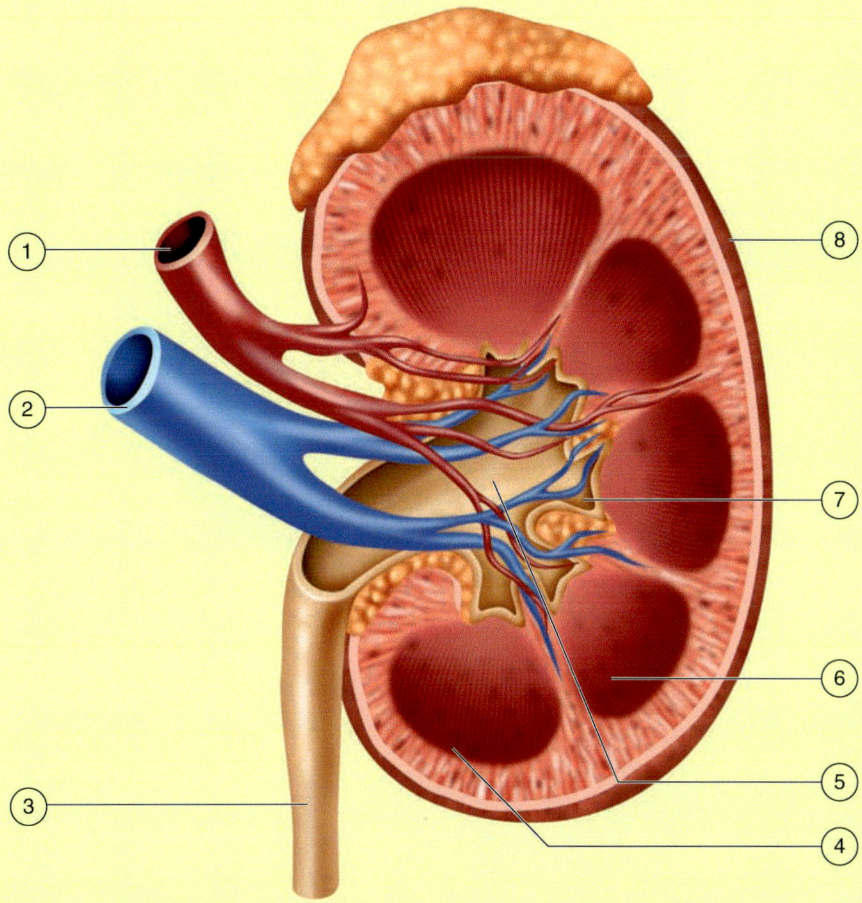

(Lightspring/shutterstock.com)

B. Indicate the anatomical structures by listing numbers on the figure next to the name listed.

- urethra____________
- ureter_____________
- bladder____________
- trigone____________
- apex______________
- neck______________
- urothelium_________
- hilus______________

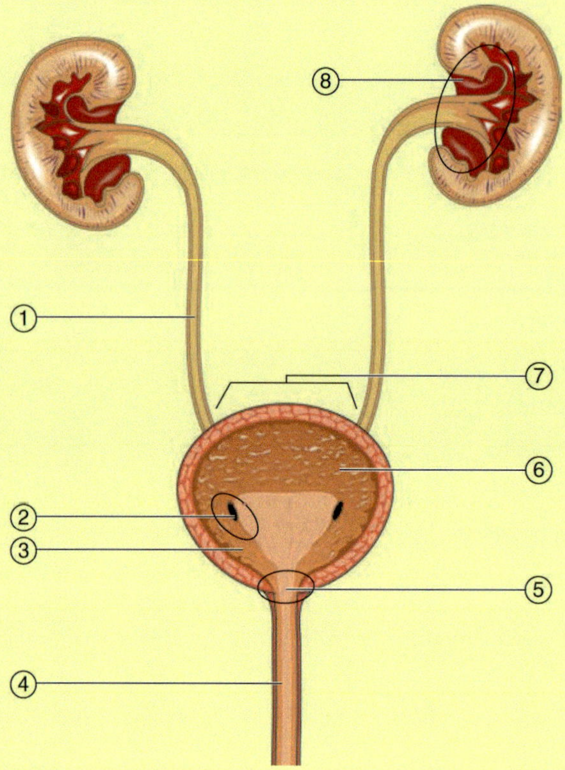

(Blamb/shutterstock.com)

C. Match the word element with its best meaning.

1. **en-**__________	a. alongside; around; beside; near
2. **-iasis**________	b. fissure
3. **peri-**________	c. pus
4. lith/o_______	d. within
5. **per-**_________	e. renal pelvis
6. **-spadias**_____	f. condition; presence of
7. py/o_________	g. around
8. pyel/o_______	h. urine
9. ur/o_________	i. through
10. **par-**________	j. stone

D. Word building: Using the word part, add the other word element and define the new word created.

1. **cyst/o**
   - a. **-scopy**____________________________
   - b. **-ectomy**____________________________
   - c. **-lith**____________________________
   - d. **poly-** + **-ic**____________________________
   - e. **-cele**____________________________
2. **nephr/o**
   - a. **-malacia**____________________________
   - b. **-algia**____________________________
   - c. **-pathy**____________________________
   - d. pyel/o + **-itis**____________________________
   - e. **-ptosis**____________________________
3. **-uria**
   - a. **poly-**____________________________
   - b. **dys-**____________________________
   - c. **glycos-**____________________________
   - d. noct/____________________________
   - e. **py-**____________________________

12

E. Separate the word elements in the following terms and define each element.

1. antidiuretic____________________________________
2. polydipsia____________________________________
3. hematuria____________________________________
4. cystorrhagia____________________________________
5. intravenous pyelography____________________________

F. Define the word element.

1. **-ectomy**____________________________________
2. **-tomy**____________________________________
3. **-stomy**____________________________________
4. **-gram**____________________________________
5. **-graphy**____________________________________
6. **-lith**____________________________________
7. scler/o____________________________________
8. olig/o____________________________________
9. ureter/o____________________________________
10. urethr/o____________________________________

Case Study

Define the numerical terms (1 to 13) and on the figure, indicate with an X where the right kidney is located. For assistance with medical abbreviations, refer to Appendix A.

History, Chief Complaint

A snowboarder presented with **gross hematuria** (1), **LBP** (2), nausea, and **oliguria** (3). She stated she has a history of **UTI** (4) and recently landed on her back during a stunt. Although she momentarily had the breath knocked out of her, she was able to finish the competition before seeking help.

Evaluation

She is **diaphoretic** (5) and **afebrile** (6). She had **dyspnea** (7), and experienced pain upon palpation on the right side of her back. She does have slight **ecchymosis** (8) in that area. Her back **ROM** (9) is normal, with the exception of flexion, which was painful.

Diagnostic Studies

Differential diagnoses are UTI, **renal calculi** (10), or a **contused** (11) kidney. **UA** (12) produced no evidence of leukocytes or nitrates but confirmed the hematuria. A **CT** (13) was performed that indicated a right bruised kidney. She completely recovered and was competing again in 2 weeks.

Terms

1. ______________________________
2. ______________________________
3. ______________________________
4. ______________________________
5. ______________________________
6. ______________________________
7. ______________________________
8. ______________________________
9. ______________________________
10. ______________________________
11. ______________________________
12. ______________________________
13. ______________________________

Anatomy

On the figure, indicate where the right kidney is located.

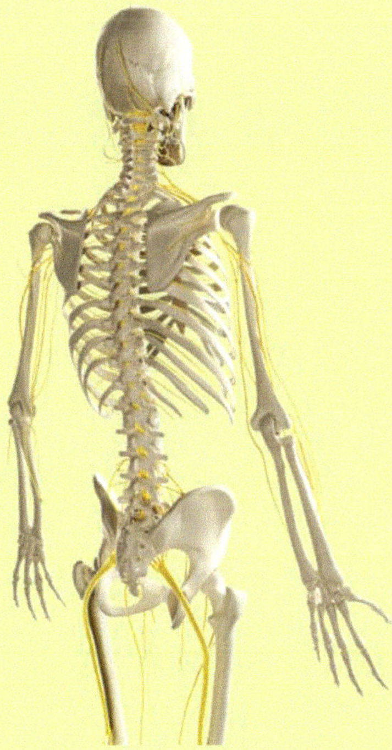

13

Reproductive System

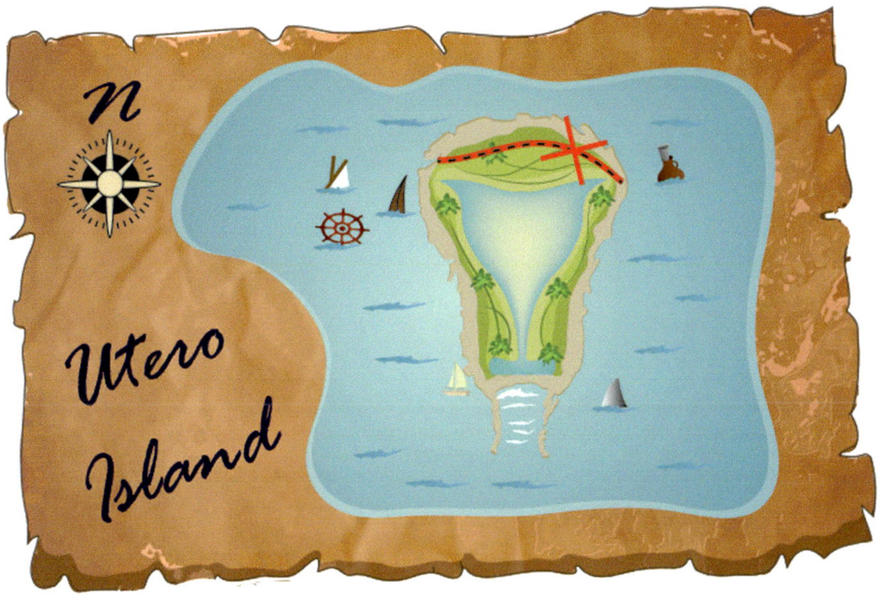

OBJECTIVES

After studying this chapter, you will be able to:

1. Identify the major components of the reproductive systems.
2. Describe anatomy and physiology of pregnancy and childbirth.
3. Identify and build words relating to the reproductive system.
4. Describe common medical conditions of the reproductive systems.
5. Differentiate between sexually transmitted infections (STIs).
6. Define words associated with pregnancy and childbirth.
7. Identify diagnostic tests and procedures specific to the reproductive system.
8. Explain surgical terms specific to the reproductive system.

Flanagan KW.
Medical Terminology With Case Studies: A Navigated Guide to Learning for Health Care Professionals, Third Edition (pp 363-399).

Chapter Outline

- Self-assessment
- Checklist for word parts in the chapter
- Checklist of new anatomy
- Introduction
- Anatomy
  - Anatomy and physiology of the male reproductive system
  - Anatomy and physiology of the female reproductive system
  - Anatomy and physiology of pregnancy and childbirth
- Word building
  - Prefixes
  - Suffixes
  - Combining forms
- Medical conditions
- Tests and procedures
- Medication classifications
- Learning activities
- Case study

Self-Assessment

Based on what you have learned so far, can you write the definition of these words?

- orchitis____________________
- ovarian____________________
- testicular____________________
- ectopic____________________
- transcutaneous____________________
- multigravida____________________

Checklist for Word Parts in the Chapter

Prefixes

- ☐ a-
- ☐ an-
- ☐ ante-
- ☐ circum-
- ☐ dys-
- ☐ ecto-
- ☐ endo-
- ☐ epi-
- ☐ hyper-
- ☐ intra-
- ☐ micro-
- ☐ multi-
- ☐ nulli-
- ☐ peri-
- ☐ post-
- ☐ pre-
- ☐ retro-
- ☐ supra-
- ☐ trans-
- ☐ ultra-

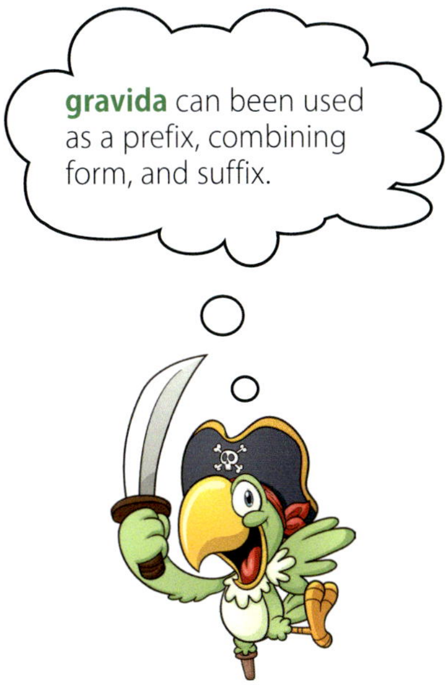

gravida can been used as a prefix, combining form, and suffix.

Suffixes

- ☐ -al
- ☐ -amnios
- ☐ -ar
- ☐ -atresia
- ☐ -cele
- ☐ -centesis
- ☐ -cision
- ☐ -cyesis
- ☐ -ectomy
- ☐ -emesis
- ☐ -gen
- ☐ -genesis
- ☐ -graphy
- ☐ -gravida
- ☐ -ia
- ☐ -iasis
- ☐ -ic
- ☐ -ine
- ☐ -ion
- ☐ -ism
- ☐ -itis
- ☐ -ium
- ☐ -lith
- ☐ -lysis
- ☐ -metry
- ☐ -oma
- ☐ -osis
- ☐ -otomy
- ☐ -para
- ☐ -partum
- ☐ -plasia
- ☐ -plasty
- ☐ -ptosis
- ☐ -rrhagia
- ☐ -rrhaphy
- ☐ -rrhea
- ☐ -rrhexis
- ☐ -salpinx
- ☐ -scopy
- ☐ -tocia
- ☐ -tomy
- ☐ -troph
- ☐ -um
- ☐ -us

Combining Forms

- ☐ aden/o
- ☐ amni/o
- ☐ arter/o
- ☐ balan/o
- ☐ carcin/o
- ☐ cephal/o
- ☐ cervic/o
- ☐ chori/o
- ☐ clitor/o
- ☐ clitorid/o
- ☐ colp/o
- ☐ crypt/o
- ☐ culd/o
- ☐ cyst/o
- ☐ embry/o
- ☐ epididym/o
- ☐ episi/o
- ☐ fet/o
- ☐ galact/o
- ☐ gravid/o
- ☐ gyn/o
- ☐ gynec/o
- ☐ hemat/o
- ☐ herni/o
- ☐ hydr/o
- ☐ hymen/o
- ☐ hyster/o
- ☐ inguin/o
- ☐ lact/o
- ☐ lapar/o
- ☐ lei/o
- ☐ leuc/o
- ☐ leuk/o
- ☐ lith/o
- ☐ men/o
- ☐ mens
- ☐ metr/i
- ☐ metr/o
- ☐ my/o
- ☐ nat/o
- ☐ olig/o
- ☐ omphal/o
- ☐ oophor/o
- ☐ orch/o
- ☐ orchi/o
- ☐ orchid/o

Combining Forms

- ❐ **osche/o**
- ❐ **ov/o**
- ❐ **ovari/o**
- ❐ **ovul/o**
- ❐ **par/o**
- ❐ **para**
- ❐ **part/o**
- ❐ **pelv/i**
- ❐ **pelv/o**
- ❐ **perine/o**
- ❐ **phim/o**
- ❐ **prim/i**
- ❐ **prostat/o**
- ❐ **pseud/o**
- ❐ **puerper/o**
- ❐ **py/o**
- ❐ **pylor/o**
- ❐ **rect/o**
- ❐ **salping/o**
- ❐ **semin/i**
- ❐ **semin/o**
- ❐ **son/o**
- ❐ **sperm/i**
- ❐ **sperm/o**
- ❐ **spermat/o**
- ❐ **stri**
- ❐ **terat/o**
- ❐ **test/o**
- ❐ **toc/o**
- ❐ **urethr/o**
- ❐ **uter/o**
- ❐ **vagin/o**
- ❐ **varic/o**
- ❐ **vas/o**
- ❐ **vesicul/o**
- ❐ **vulv/o**

Checklist of New Anatomy

Male Reproductive System

- ❐ Testes
- ❐ Seminiferous tubules
- ❐ Epididymis
- ❐ Scrotum
- ❐ Vas deferens
- ❐ Seminal vesicles
- ❐ Prostate
- ❐ Bulbourethral glands
- ❐ Urethra
- ❐ Penis
  - ❐ Glans penis
  - ❐ Prepuce
- ❐ Perineum

Female Reproductive System

- ❐ Ovaries
- ❐ Fallopian tube
  - ❐ Fimbria
- ❐ Uterus
  - ❐ Corpus
  - ❐ Fundus
  - ❐ Retrouterine pouch
  - ❐ Endometrium
  - ❐ Myometrium
  - ❐ Perimetrium
- ❐ Cervix
- ❐ Vagina
  - ❐ Bartholin glands
- ❐ Hymen
- ❐ Vulva
  - ❐ Clitoris
  - ❐ Labia minora
  - ❐ Labia majora
- ❐ Perineum

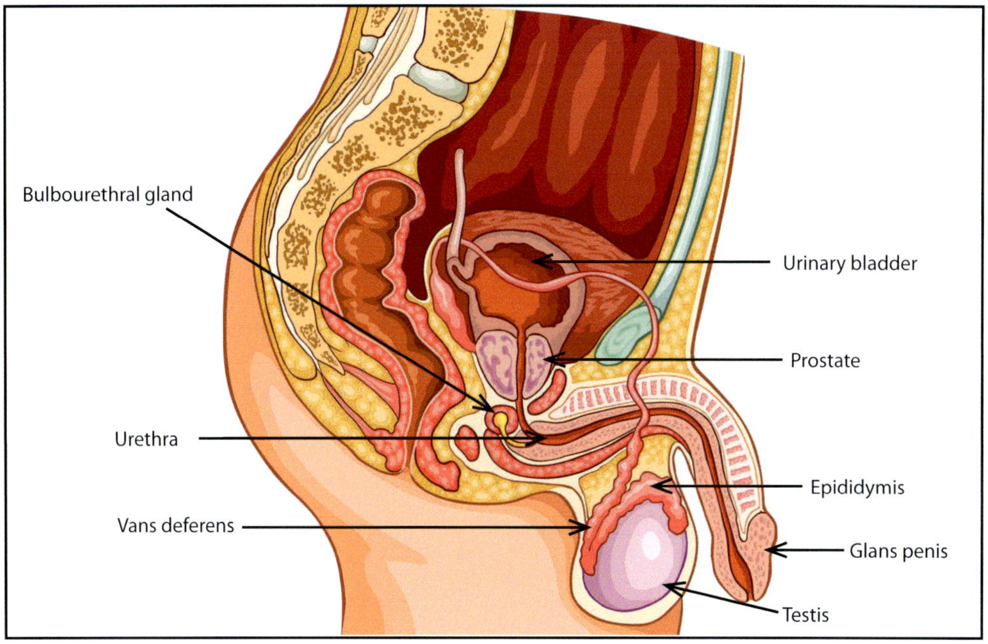

Figure 13-1. Male reproductive anatomy. (Oguz Aral/shutter stock.com)

Introduction

Welcome to Utero Island! This island has a lake shaped as a uterus and represents the reproductive systems. It contains word roots and combining forms distinctive to male and female reproductive systems as well as pregnancy and childbirth. Terms related to the testes and ovaries were discussed in Chapter 11 and are not covered in depth here.

Anatomy

13

Anatomy and Physiology of the Male Reproductive System

The majority of male reproductive anatomy was presented in Chapter 11 ("Endocrine System"), with discussion of the testes, epididymis, and scrotum. Here the discussion focuses on the prostate gland, penis, and semen. As you recall, semen is produced in the **seminiferous tubules** of the **testes**, and stored at cooler temperatures in the **epididymis** within the **scrotum**. The lower end of the epididymis becomes the **vas deferens**, which loops over the posterior bladder en route to the **seminal vesicles**. These vesicles secrete thick fluid that becomes part of semen as it passes to the **prostate** gland. The prostate also lies at the base of the urinary bladder where the **urethra** exits, and its purpose is to provide the fluid that assists in movement of sperm and in ejaculation. Just past the prostate gland are two **bulbourethral (Cowper) glands** that add an alkaline fluid to assist sperm viability. At this point, sperm joins the urethra and is ejaculated via the **penis**. The penis contains a layer of spongy erectile tissue that can become engorged with blood, harden, and cause erection. The tip of the penis is a soft **glans penis** that is covered with **prepuce** (foreskin) at birth. When this structure is cut away it is termed **circumcision**. Whereas both sperm and urine exit the urethra through the penis, a muscle constricts during intercourse to prevent micturition. As you can see in Figure 13-1, the positioning of the male reproductive system is in close proximity to both the digestive system (rectum) and urinary system. The **perineum** is an area between where the scrotum attaches to the body and the anus.

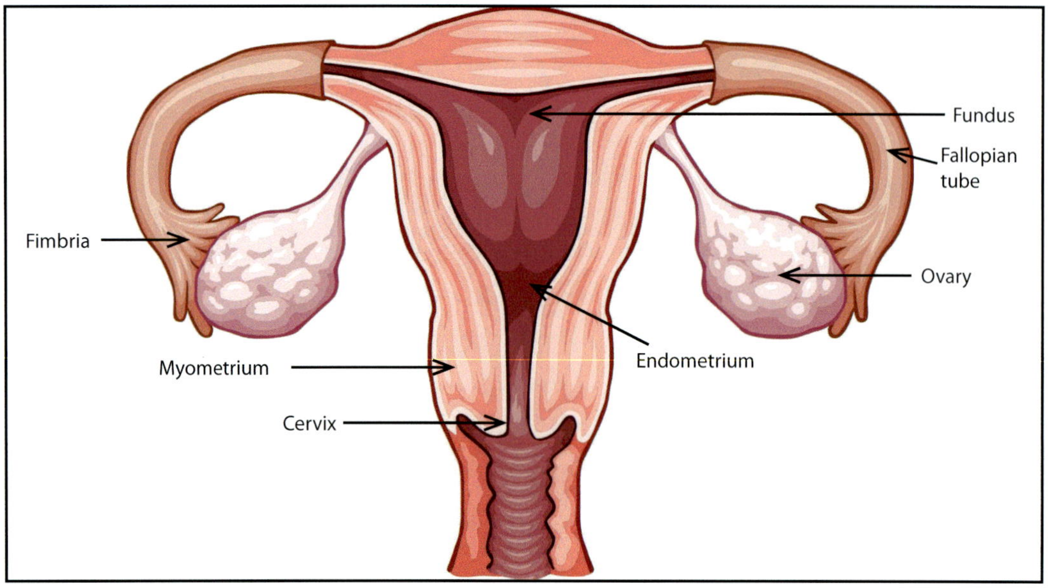

Figure 13-2. Female reproductive anatomy. (Oguz Aral/shutterstock.com)

Anatomy and Physiology of the Female Reproductive System

Female reproductive anatomy begins with the **ovaries**, which were discussed in Chapter 11. When an egg (**ovum**) is released from the ovary, it travels through the **fallopian tubes** (also called *uterine tubes*), which provide the flexible, hollow transportation system for the ovum to reach the **uterus**. There are finger-like projections (**fimbria**; plural—fimbriae) at the open end of the fallopian tubes, at the juncture where they meet the ovaries. The uterus is shaped a bit like a lightbulb, with the **corpus** (body) being more slender than the **fundus** (rounder superior portion). A **retrouterine pouch** (**retro-**—behind; **uter/o**—uterus; **-ine**—pertaining to) lies between the rectum and the posterior wall of the uterus. It is also called *Douglas cul-de-sac*. The three layers of the uterus consist of the **endometrium** (**endo-**—within; **metr/**—uterus; **-ium**—membrane), the innermost lining; the **myometrium** (**my/o**—muscle; **metr/**—uterus; **-ium**—membrane), the middle muscular layer, and the **perimetrium** (**peri-**—around), which surrounds the outer uterus. At the most distal (lower) aspect of the uterus is the cervix, which provides a gateway for menstrual blood, semen, and birthing (Figure 13-2). This structure softens and yields due to hormone release associated with childbirth, allowing passage of the fetus. The **vagina** connects the uterus to the outside world. Along the flexible vagina are **Bartholin glands** that secrete mucus to assist with the self-cleaning properties of the vagina. At its base is the **hymen**, a thin membrane that at one time (Victorian Era) was linked with virginity. External female genitalia are called the **vulva** as a group, but they are actually three structures: the **clitoris, labia minora**, and **labia majora** (Figure 13-3). The clitoris is highly erogenous and erectile and is situated anterior to the urethral meatus (opening); the labia are two different-sized lips that surround the opening of the vagina. As with men, the **perineum** is the pelvic floor, and in women it is the area between the vaginal opening and anus.

Anatomy and Physiology of Pregnancy and Childbirth

Pregnancy begins when an **ovum** is fertilized by **spermatozoa**, forming a **zygote**. This is termed **conception**, and it usually occurs in the fallopian tube. The tiny mass continues to divide cells as it travels through the fallopian tube and eventually implants on the endometrium of the uterine wall (Figure 13-4). **Implantation** takes several days, and begins about 1 week following conception. The **placenta** is a highly vascular organ that supports the life and well-being of the fetus. It arises from the endometrium and the most external layer of the developing fetus, the **chorion** (Figure 13-5). Shortly after implantation of the fertilized egg, the placenta secretes the hormone **human chorionic gonadotropin** (**hCG**) into the blood stream. The level of hCG increases steadily the first 4 months (16 weeks) after the last menstrual period (LMP); but following delivery the hormone is no longer detectable in the blood. The innermost layer of the embryonic membrane is termed the **amnion**, and it contains amniotic fluid that suspends and protects the fetus through its lifespan. When the placenta ruptures at the end of gestation, it expels amniotic fluid and is often referred to as "the water breaking," signaling the onset of labor. The **embryo** is the term for the stage of development between the zygote and weeks 8 to 12 of pregnancy; but beginning the third month following conception until birth it is termed a **fetus**. The gestational period for most pregnancies is 9 months; it is often described in trimesters (3-month intervals). The uterus expands with fetal development,

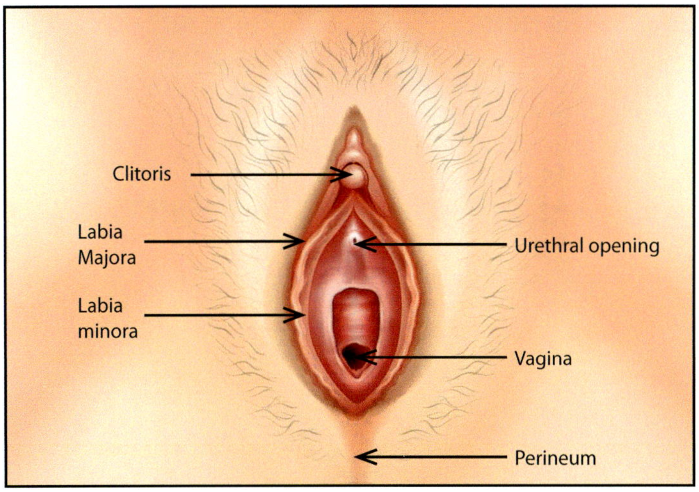

Figure 13-3. External female genital. (BlueRingMedia/shutterstock.com)

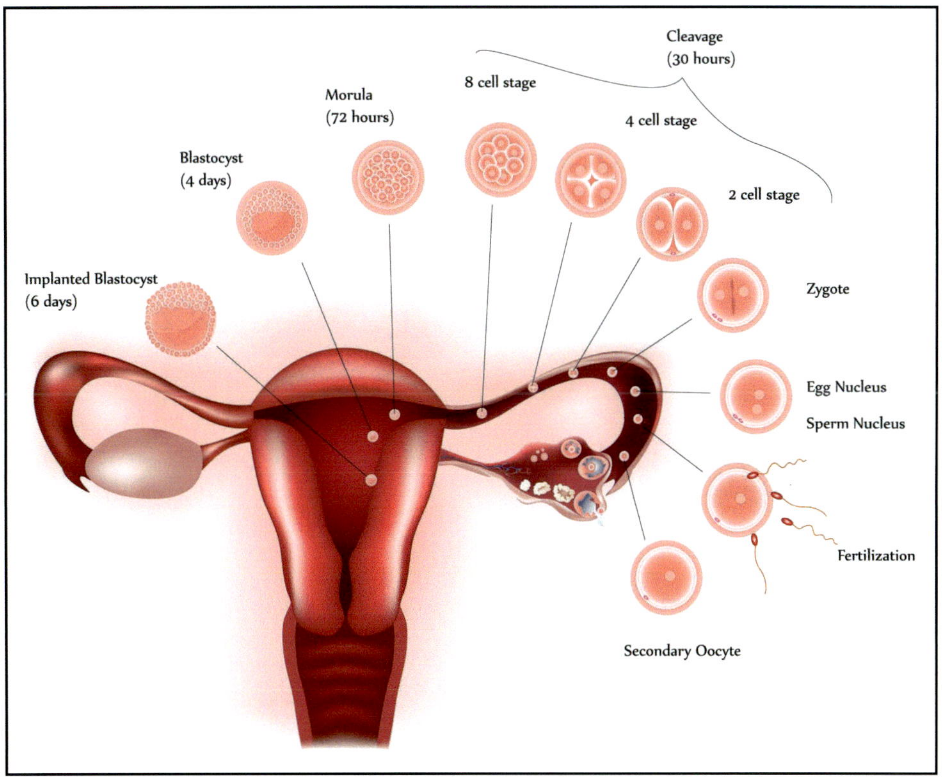

Figure 13-4. Ovulation, fertilization, cell development, and implantation. (GRei/shutterstock.com)

and occupies the majority of the abdominopelvic cavity (Figure 13-6). Labor and childbirth (termed *parturition*) begins with rhythmic contractions of the uterus and dilation of the cervix. **Braxton-Hicks contractions** are irregular tightening of the uterine muscles that can begin as early as the first trimester, and continue throughout gestation. They increase in frequency and intensity and may be confused with labor contractions later in pregnancy. After the cervix dilates at least 10 cm, delivery can begin with the typical fetus in cephalic presentation (head first in the vagina). Following birth, forceful contractions expel the placenta and attached membranes (the afterbirth).

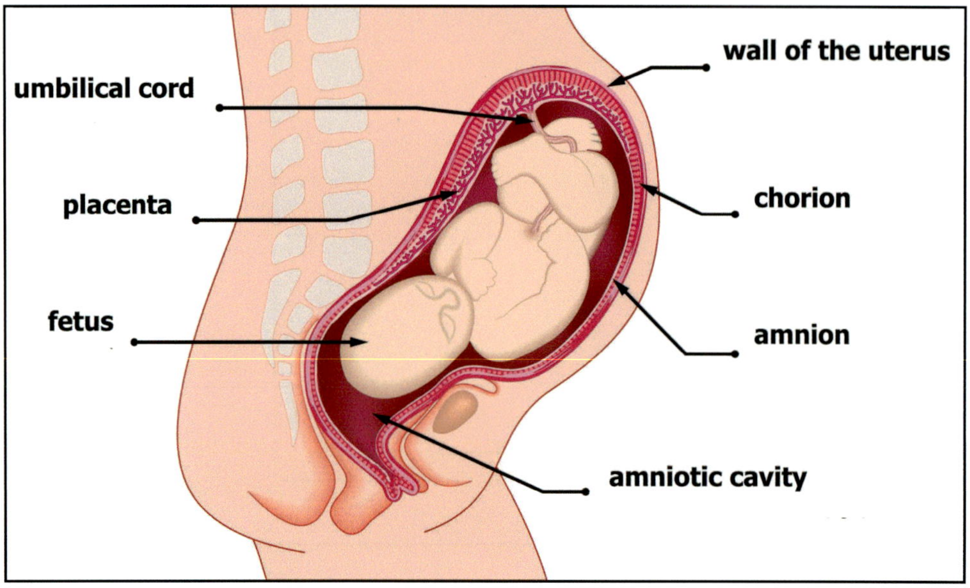

Figure 13-5. Fetus in the womb. (dr OX/shutterstock.com)

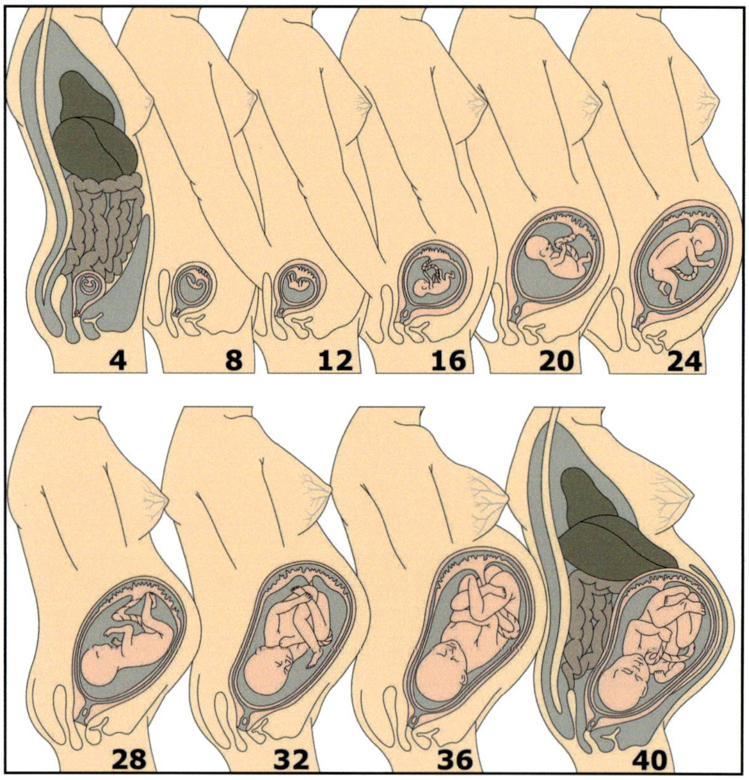

Figure 13-6. Fetal growth, in weeks. (dr OX/shutterstock.com)

Word Building

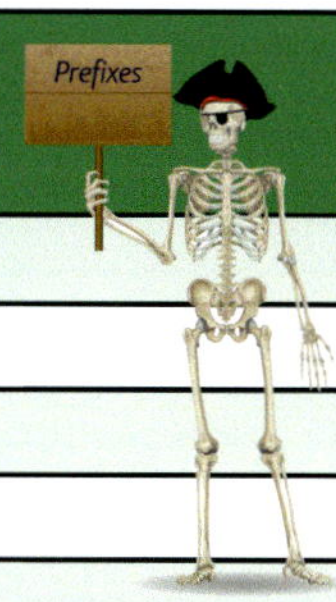

Table 13-1
Prefixes

PREFIX	DEFINITION
a-	without
an-	without; not
ante-	before; in front of
circum-	around
dys-	abnormal; bad; difficult; painful
ecto-	out; outside
endo-	in; within
epi-	above
hyper-	above; excessive; high; increased
intra-	inside; within
micro-	small
multi-	many
nulli-	none
peri-	around
post-	after; behind
pre-	before
retro-	back; backward; behind
supra-	above
trans-	across; through
ultra-	excess; beyond

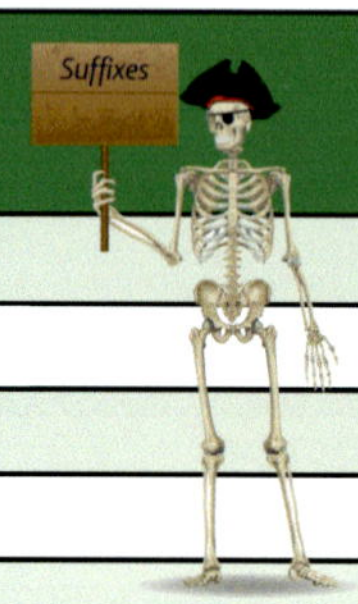

Table 13-2

Suffixes

SUFFIX	DEFINITION
-al	pertaining to
-amnios	amniotic fluid; amnion
-atresia	lacking a normal body opening; closure
-cele	hernia; protrusion; swelling
-centesis	puncture; surgical puncture
-cision	cutting
-cyesis	pregnancy
-ectomy	excision; surgical removal
-emesis	vomiting
-gen	that which produces
-genesis	forming; origin; producing
-graphy	process of recording; the act of recording information
-gravida	pregnant person
-ia	condition
-iasis	condition
-ic	pertaining to
-ine	pertaining to
-ion	process; the act of
-ism	condition
-itis	inflammation
-ium	membrane; structure
-lith	stone
-lysis	breaking down; destruction; loosening; separating; to loosen or break
-metry	measurement of
-oma	mass; tumor
-osis	condition
-para	to give birth
-partum	childbirth; labor
-plasia	formation; growth
-plasty	reconstruction; repair; plastic surgery
-ptosis	drooping; falling; prolapse
-r/rhagia	abnormal flow
-r/rhaphy	surgical repair; suturing
-r/rhea	discharge; excessive flow
-r/rhexis	rupture
-salpinx	fallopian tube
-scopy	examination of

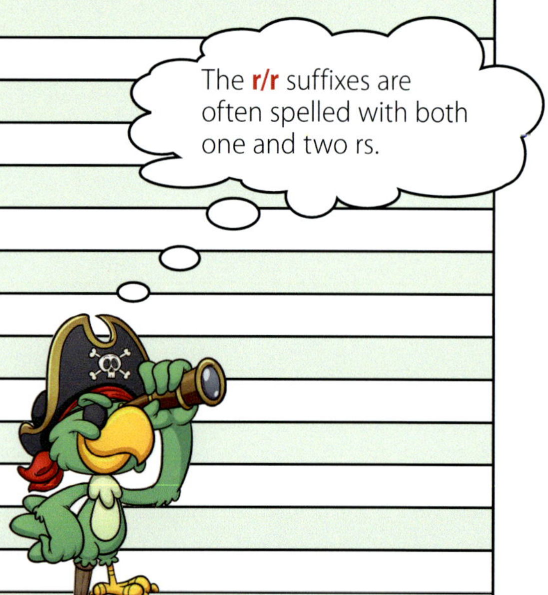
The **r/r** suffixes are often spelled with both one and two rs.

(continued)

Table 13-2 (continued)
Suffixes

SUFFIX	DEFINITION
-tocia	childbirth; labor
-tomy; -otomy	incision; to cut into
-troph	development; growth; nourishment
-um	structure; thing
-us	pertaining to; structure

Table 13-3
Combining Forms

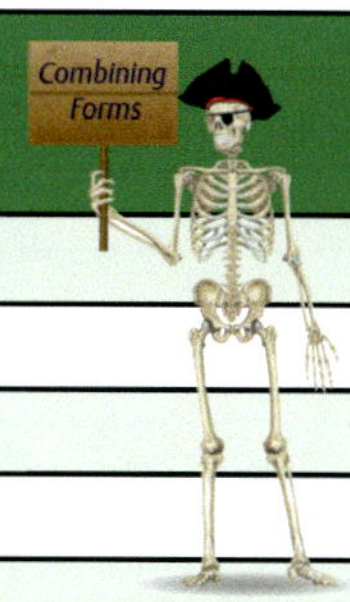

COMBINING FORM	DEFINITION
aden/o	gland
amni/o	amnion
arter/o	artery
balan/o	glans penis (head of the penis); also glans clitoris
carcin/o	cancer
cephal/o	head
cervic/o	cervix; neck
chori/o	chorion (the outermost layer of the fetal membrane)
clitor/o; clitorid/o	clitoris
colp/o	vagina
crypt/o	hidden
culd/o	retrouterine pouch
cyst/o	bladder; sac
embry/o	embryo; fetus
epididym/o	epididymis
episi/o	vulva
fet/o	fetus
galact/o	milk
gravid/o	pregnancy
gyn/o; gynec/o	female
hemat/o	blood
hydr/o	water
hymen/o	hymen
hyster/o	uterus
inguin/o	groin
lact/o	milk
lapar/o	abdomen

(continued)

Table 13-3 (continued)
Combining Forms

COMBINING FORM	DEFINITION
lei/o	smooth
leuc/o; leuk/o	white
lith/o	stone
men/o	mouth; uterus; measure
mens	mouth; menstruation
metr/i; metr/o	uterus; measure
my/o	muscle
nat/o	birth; sodium
olig/o	scanty
omphal/o	umbilicus; naval
oophor/o	ovary
orch/o; orchi/o; orchid/o	testicle; testis
osche/o	scrotum
ov/o; ovul/o	ovum (egg)
ovari/o	ovary
par/o	to give birth; labor
para	a person who has given birth
part/o	to give birth; labor
pelv/i; pelv/o	pelvis
perine/o	perineum
phim/o	muzzle
prim/i	first
prostat/o	prostate gland
pseud/o	false
puerper/o	childbirth
py/o	pus
pylor/o	gatekeeper; pylorus
rect/o	rectum; straight
salping/o	fallopian tube or eustachian tube
semin/i; semin/o	semen
son/o	sound
sperm/i; sperm/o; spermat/o	sperm; spermatozoa
stri	line; stripe
terat/o	deformity
test/o	testis; testicle
toc/o	labor

(continued)

Table 13-3 (continued) Combining Forms	
COMBINING FORM	DEFINITION
urethr/o	urethra
uter/o	uterus
vagin/o	vagina
varic/o	dilated vein; swollen vein; varicose vein
vas/o	vas deferens; vessel
vesicul/o	seminal vesicle
vulv/o	vulva

Medical Conditions

Table 13-4 Medical Conditions and Terms Related to the Male Reproductive System		
NAME	WORD PARTS	DEFINITION
anorchism	**an-** (without) orch/ (testicle) **-ism** (condition)	Missing a testicle
aspermia	**a-** (without) sperm/ (sperm; spermatozoa) **-ia** (condition)	Without sperm (in the ejaculate)
balanitis	balan/ (glans penis) **-itis** (inflammation)	Inflammation of the glans penis
balanorrhea	balan/ (glans penis) **-rrhea** (discharge)	Discharge from the penis
benign prostatic hyperplasia (BPH) (Figure 13-7)	prostat/ (prostate gland) **-ic** (pertaining to) **hyper-** (increased) **-plasia** (growth)	Nonmalignant enlargement of the prostate
circumcision	**circum-** (around) **-cision** (cutting)	Surgical removal of the prepuce
cryptorchidism	crypt/ (hidden) orchid/ (testicle) **-ism** (condition)	Undescended testicle
epididymitis	epididym/ (epididymis) **-itis** (inflammation)	Inflammation of the epididymis

(continued)

13

Table 13-4 (continued)

Medical Conditions and Terms Related to the Male Reproductive System

NAME	WORD PARTS	DEFINITION
erectile dysfunction	**dys-** (abnormal)	Lack of ability to achieve or maintain an erection until ejaculation; also termed *impotence*
hydrocele	hydr/o (water) **-cele** (hernia; protrusion; swelling)	Accumulation of fluid within a sac; most often within the scrotum
inguinal hernia	inguin/ (groin) **-al** (pertaining to)	Protrusion of the intestine or abdominal organ into the scrotum
oligospermia (Figure 13-8)	olig/o (scanty) sperm/ (sperm) **-ia** (condition)	Scanty sperm in the semen, a cause of infertility
orchitis	orch/ (testicle) **-itis** (inflammation)	Inflamed testicle
phimosis	phim/ (muzzle) **-osis** (condition)	Stenosis (narrowing) of the preputial orifice where the foreskin cannot be pulled over the penis
prostatic hyperplasia	prostat/ (prostate gland) **-ic** (pertaining to) **hyper-** (excessive) **-plasia** (growth)	Nonmalignant, excessive growth of the prostate that results in urethral constriction
prostatitis (Figure 13-9)	prostat/ (prostate gland) **-itis** (inflammation)	Inflamed prostate
prostatocystitis	prostat/o (prostate gland) cyst/ (bladder) **-itis** (inflammation)	Inflammation of the prostate gland and urinary bladder
prostatolith	prostat/o (prostate gland) **-lith** (stone)	Stone in the prostate gland
seminoma	semin/ (semen) **-oma** (tumor)	Tumor of the testis
spermatolysis	spermat/o (sperm) **-lysis** (destruction)	Destruction of sperm
varicocele	varic/o (varicose vein) **-cele** (swelling)	Varicose veins in the spermatic cord

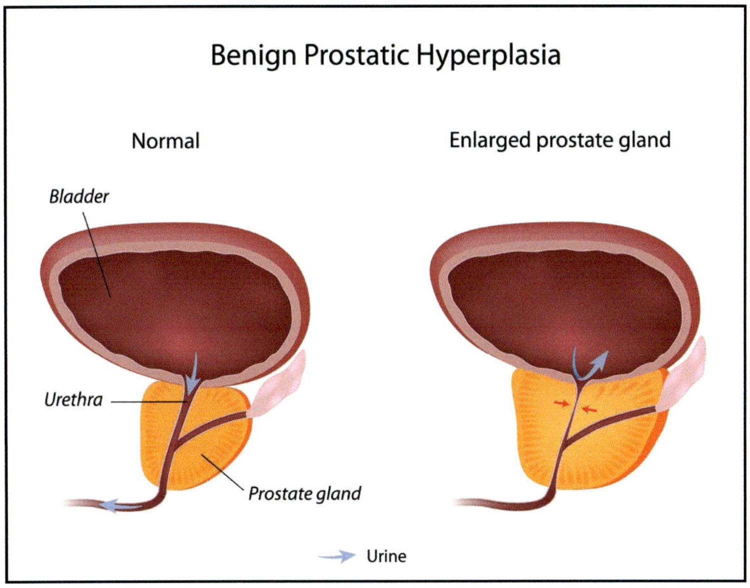

Figure 13-7. Benign prostatic hyperplasia. (Alila Medical Images/shutterstock.com)

Figure 13-8. Oligospermia (fewer/scanty sperm). (Sebastian Kaulitzki/shutterstock.com)

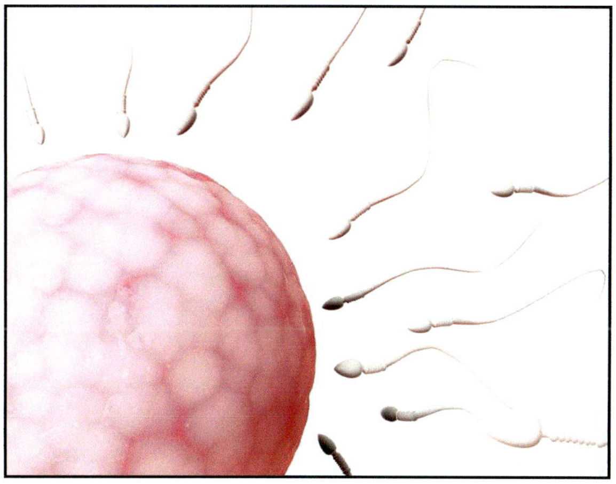

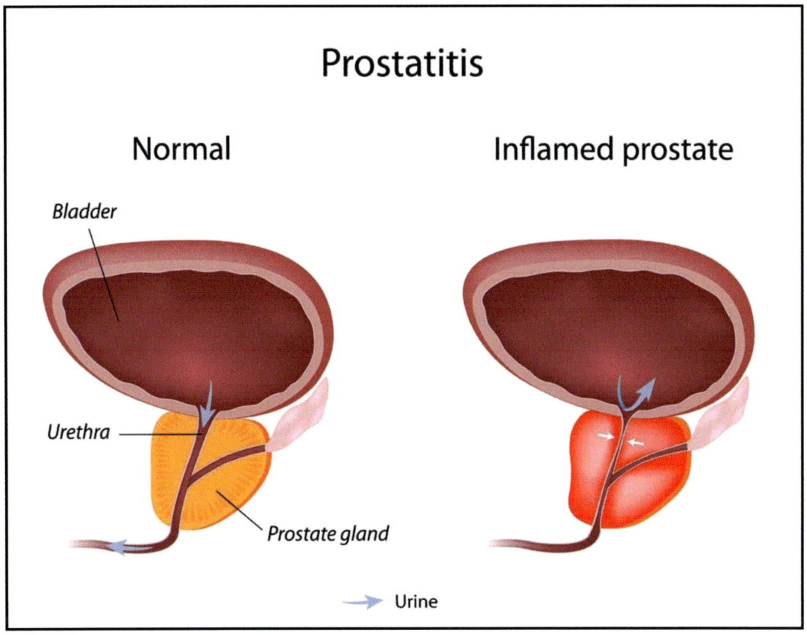

Figure 13-9. Prostatitis. (Alila Medical Images/shutterstock.com)

Table 13-5 provides terms related to the female reproduction, but it does not have terms associated with menstruation as those terms were covered in Chapter 11.

Table 13-5
Medical Conditions and Terms Related to the Female Reproductive System

NAME	WORD PARTS	DEFINITION
Bartholin adenitis	aden/ (gland) **-itis** (inflammation)	Inflammation of the Bartholin glands
cervicitis (Figure 13-10)	cervic/ (cervix) **-itis** (inflammation)	Inflammation of the cervix
cystocele (Figure 13-11)	cyst/o (bladder) **-cele** (hernia)	Herniation of the urinary bladder into the vagina
dyspareunia	**dys-** (painful) **-ia** (condition)	Painful sexual intercourse
endometriosis	**endo-** (within) metri/ (uterus) **-osis** (condition)	Endometrial tissue growing outside of the uterus
hematosalpinx	hemat/o (blood) **-salpinx** (fallopian tube)	Blood in the fallopian tube
hysteratresia	hyster/ (uterus) **-atresia** (closure)	Closure of the uterine cavity
hysteroptosis	hyster/o (uterus) **-ptosis** (prolapse)	Forward-displaced uterus, also called *prolapsed uterus*
leiomyoma	lei/o (smooth) my/ (muscle) **-oma** (tumor)	Tumor of the smooth muscle in the uterine wall; typically benign
leukorrhea	leuk/o (white) **-rrhea** (discharge)	White or yellowish discharge from the vagina
myometritis	my/o (muscle) metr/ (uterus) **-itis** (inflammation)	Inflammation of the middle layer of the uterus, the myometrium
pyosalpinx	py/o (pus) **-salpinx** (fallopian tube)	Pus in the fallopian tube
rectocele	rect/o (rectum) **-cele** (hernia)	Herniation of the rectum into the vagina, also called a *proctocele*

(continued)

Table 13-5 (continued)

Medical Conditions and Terms Related to the Female Reproductive System

NAME	WORD PARTS	DEFINITION
salpingitis	salping/ (fallopian tube) **-itis** (inflammation)	Inflammation of the fallopian tube caused by urinary tract infection or STIs; if it is a chronic condition, it can lead to infertility or an ectopic pregnancy
vaginitis	vagin/ (vagina) **-itis** (inflammation)	Inflammation of the vagina
vulvovaginitis	vulv/o (vulva) vagin/ (vagina) **-itis** (inflammation)	Inflammation of the vulva and vagina

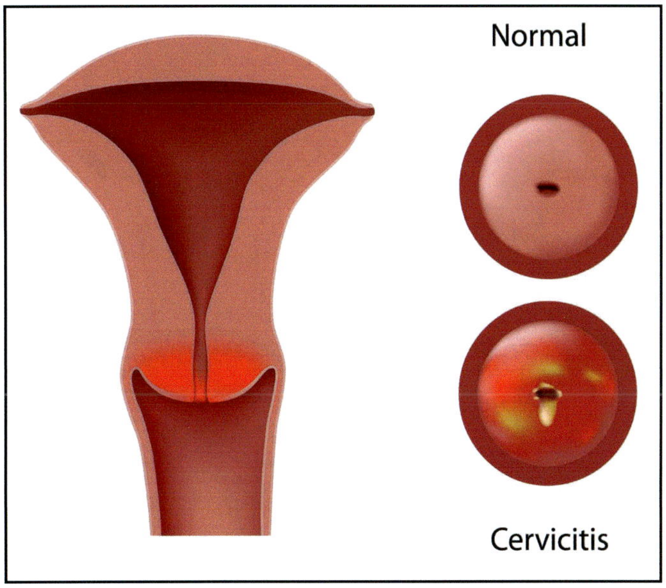

Figure 13-10. Cervicitis. (Alila Medical Images/shutterstock.com)

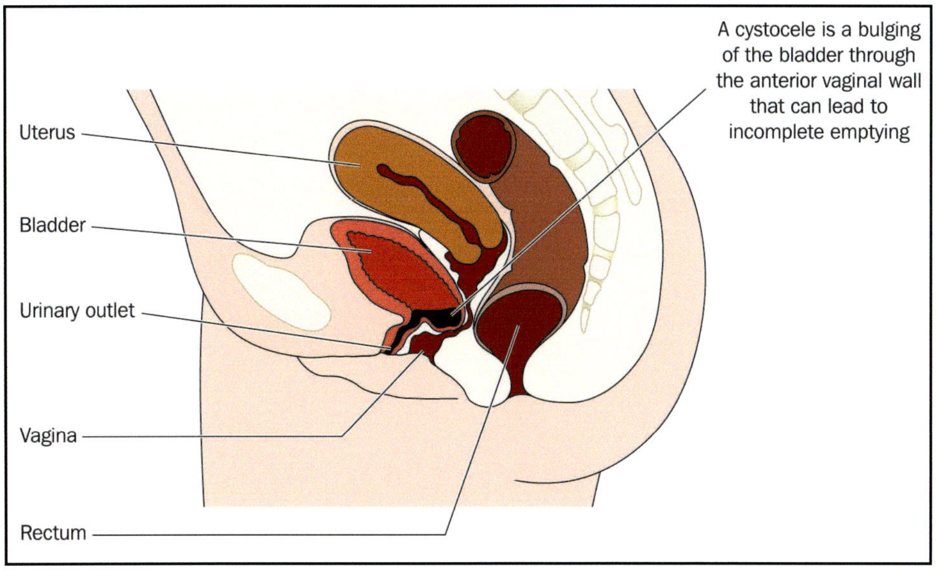

Figure 13-11. Cystocele. (Blamb/shutterstock.com)

Table 13-6 Terms With No Medical Word Parts Pertaining to the Reproductive System	
TERM	**DEFINITION**
candidiasis	Fungal infection that causes vaginitis
hydatidiform mole	Benign overdevelopment of uterine tissue
infertility	Inability to produce offspring; also called *sterility*
pelvic inflammatory disease (PID) (Figure 13-12)	Inflammation of the female reproductive organs; can have many causes and may result in infertility
priapism	Continuous erection caused by medications or spinal cord damage

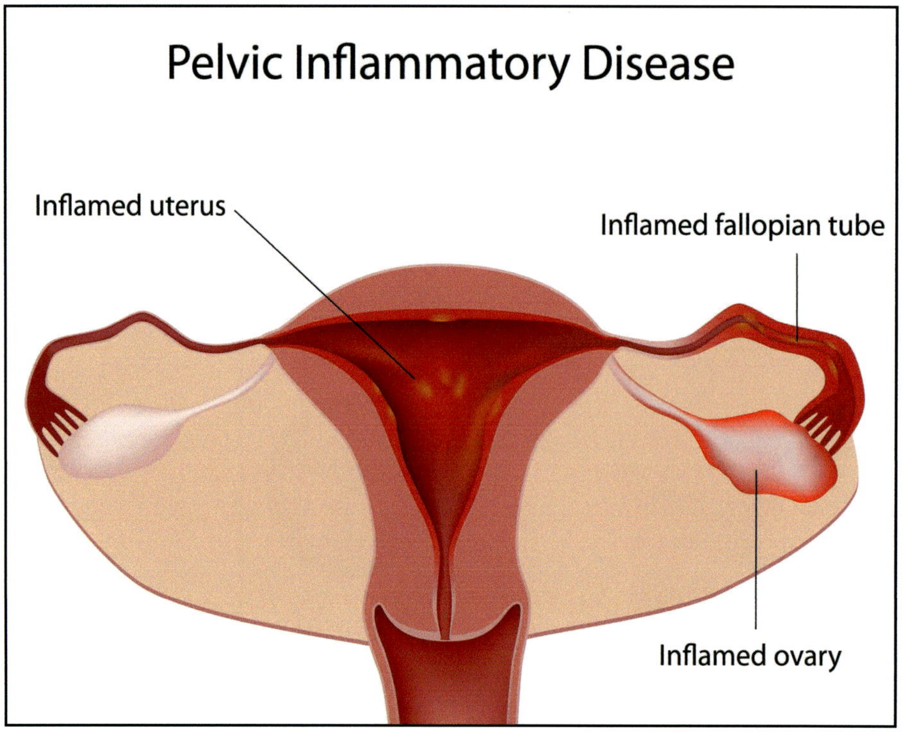

Figure 13-12. Pelvic inflammatory disease can affect all of the female reproductive organs. (Alila Medical Images/shutterstock.com)

Table 13-7
Sexually Transmitted Infections

NAME	DEFINITION
acquired immunodeficiency syndrome (AIDS)	Viral infection that attacks the T-cells in the immune system, making patients more susceptible to other infections; usually fatal
bacterial vaginosis	Vaginal infection caused by *Gardnerella vaginalis*
chlamydia	Bacterial infection that may lead to PID
condyloma acuminatum	Genital warts caused by human papillomavirus (HPV); series of vaccines available for people of all genders
genital herpes	Incurable viral infection marked by painful outbreaks of blisters
gonorrhea	Bacterial infection that causes inflammation of the reproductive and urinary tracts; can initiate systemic infection and spread to newborns
hepatitis B virus (HBV) (Figure 13-13)	Viral infection that attacks the liver and can lead to liver cancers; carriers may be unaware they have the disease; series of vaccines available for prevention
human immunodeficiency virus (HIV)	Virus that causes AIDS
HPV	Preventable STI that causes genital warts and/or cancerous growths; vaccine available for people of all genders
lymphogranuloma venereum	Swelling of the inguinal lymph nodes and scarring of genital tissues
syphilis	Three-stage bacterial infection beginning with a chancre (lesion), leading to systemic infections; syphilis has dormant stages and can cause miscarriages, stillbirths, and fetal deformities
trichomoniasis	Caused by a protozoon, this condition is also a vaginitis and presents with dyspareunia, dysuria, and itching

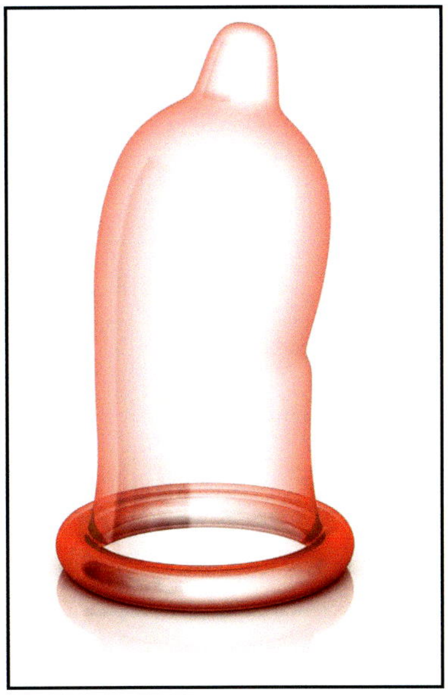

Figure 13-13. A barrier such as a condom can prevent many (but not all) sexually transmitted infections. (koya979/shutterstock.com)

Table 13-8

Terms Related to Pregnancy and Childbirth

TERM	WORD PARTS	DEFINITION
amniorrhea	amni/o (amnion) **-rrhea** (discharge)	Discharge of amniotic fluid
antepartum	**ante-** (before) **-partum** (childbirth)	In reference to the pregnant person, before childbirth
cephalopelvic disproportion	cephal/o (head) pelv/ (pelvis) **-ic** (pertaining to)	When the fetal head is larger than the pelvic opening
choriocarcinoma	chori/o (chorion) carcin/ (cancer) **-oma** (mass)	Rare malignancy in the uterus, fallopian tube; may occur following an abortion or delivery
dystocia	**dys-** (difficult) **-tocia** (childbirth; labor)	Difficult labor
ectopic pregnancy	**ecto-** (outside) **-ic** (pertaining to)	Pregnancy (implantation) outside of the uterus; most often in the fallopian tubes
embryogenic	embry/o (embryo) **-gen** (that which produces) **-ic** (pertaining to)	Producing an embryo
galactorrhea	galact/o (milk) **-rrhea** (excessive flow)	Excessive secretion of milk after breastfeeding has stopped
gravida (Figure 13-14)	**-gravida** (pregnant person)	Pregnant person, regardless of delivery of a child
hydramnios	hydr/ (water) amni/o (amnion)	Excessive amniotic fluid; also termed *polyhydramnios*
hyperemesis gravidarum	**hyper-** (excessive) **-emesis** (vomiting) gravid/ (pregnancy) **-ar** (pertaining to) **-um** (structure)	Severe nausea and vomiting during pregnancy that can be dangerous due to dehydration
intrapartum	**intra-** (within) **-partum** (labor)	Occurring during childbirth; labor
multigravida	**multi-** (many) **-gravida** (pregnant)	Many pregnancies
natal	nat/ (birth) **-al** (pertaining to)	Pertaining to the fetus
nullipara	**nulli-** (none) **-para** (to give birth)	Having never given birth

(continued)

Table 13-8 (continued)

Terms Related to Pregnancy and Childbirth

TERM	WORD PARTS	DEFINITION
oligohydramnios	olig/o (scanty) hydr/ (water) amni/o (amnion)	Deficiency of amniotic fluid
omphalitis	omphal/ (umbilicus) **-itis** (inflammation)	Inflammation of the umbilicus
patent ductus arteriosus	arteri/o (artery) **-us** (pertaining to)	Condition present at birth where there is an opening between the pulmonary artery and aorta that allows blood to pass between the two
peripartum	**peri-** (around) **-partum** (labor)	In reference to the pregnant person, occurring either in late pregnancy or within the first few months following giving birth
placenta previa	**pre-** (before) **-ia** (condition of)	Abnormal attachment of the placenta lower than normal, may cause hemorrhaging in late pregnancy
postpartum	**post-** (after) **-partum** (childbirth)	In reference to the pregnant person, following childbirth
pseudocyesis (Figure 13-15)	pseud/o (false) **-cyesis** (pregnancy)	False pregnancy; where a person believes they are pregnant
puerperal	puerper/ (childbirth) **-al** (pertaining to)	Person who has just given birth
puerperal infection	puerper/ (childbirth) **-al** (pertaining to)	Genital tract infection following childbirth
puerperium	puerper/ (childbirth) **-ium** (structure; thing)	The first 42 days following childbirth when the reproductive organs return to normal function
striae gravidarum (Figure 13-16)	stri/ (stripe) gravid/ (pregnancy) **-um** (thing)	Irregular depressions on skin that has been stretched due to pregnancy; often referred to as *stretch marks*
teratogenic	terat/o (deformity) **-gen** (that which produces) **-ic** (pertaining to)	Agent that causes malformations in a fetus

Figure 13-14. Gravida is the term for pregnancy, regardless if the person delivers a child or not. (Julia Lazebnaya/shutterstock.com)

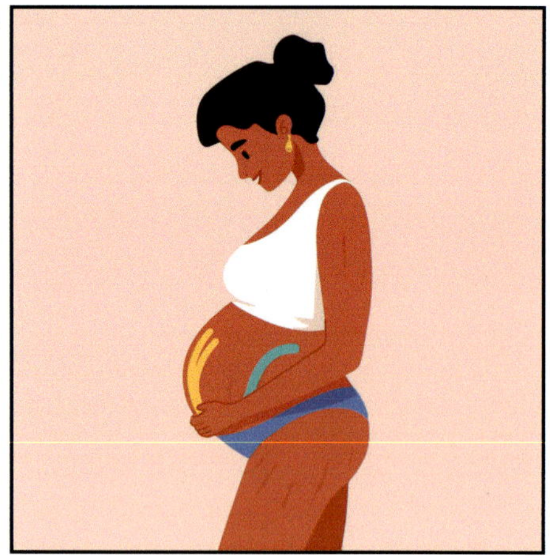

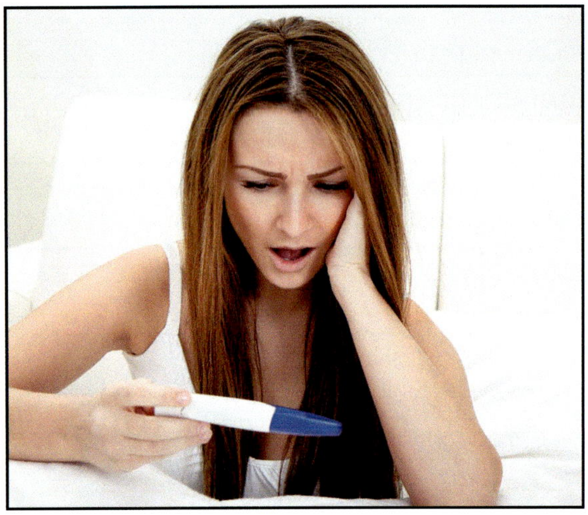

Figure 13-15. Pseudocyesis is when a person thinks they are pregnant, but they are not. (Andrey_Popov/shutterstock.com)

Figure 13-16. Stretch marks caused by pregnancy is termed *striae gravidarum*. (baipooh/shutterstock.com)

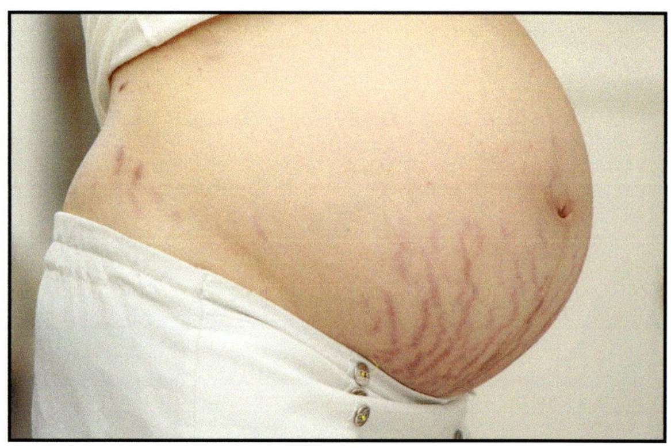

Table 13-9
Terms Related to Pregnancy and Childbirth Without Medical Parts

TERM	DEFINITION
chloasma	Brownish pigmentation appearing on the face during pregnancy; also called *melasma*
congenital disorder	Disorder present at birth
eclampsia	Life-threatening condition associated with pregnancy-induced hypertension; severe complications during or immediately following delivery
linea nigra	Dark line running from the umbilicus to the pubic bone occurring in late pregnancy
lochia	Discharge from the uterus following childbirth; combination of blood, mucus, and tissue
meconium	First feces of a newborn
parturition	Act of giving birth
placental abruption	Placenta separates prematurely
vernix caseosa	Cheese-like covering that protects the fetus

Tests and Procedures

Table 13-10
Tests and Procedures

NAME	WORD PARTS	PURPOSE
amniocentesis (Figure 13-17)	amni/o (amnion) **-centesis** (surgical puncture)	Surgical puncture into the amniotic sac to remove amniotic fluid for testing/inspection
chorionic villus sampling (CVS)	chori/ (chorion) **-ic** (pertaining to)	Prenatal testing of chorionic cells through the cervix
colposcopy	colp/o (vagina) **-scopy** (examination of)	Viewing the vagina and cervix
digital rectal examination (DRE) (Figure 13-18)	rect/ (rectum) **-al** (pertaining to)	Physician places a finger (digit) in the rectum to assess the prostate gland size and shape
pelvimetry	pelv/ (pelvis) **-metry** (measurement of)	Measurement of the pelvis, used to determine if vaginal delivery is possible
transrectal ultrasonography	**trans-** (through) rect/ (rectum) **-al** (pertaining to) **ultra-** (beyond) son/o (sound) **-graphy** (process of recording)	Using a transducer placed in the rectum, sound waves record the shape and size of the prostate gland

(continued)

13

Table 13-10 (continued)
Tests and Procedures

NAME	WORD PARTS	PURPOSE
transvaginal ultrasonography	**trans-** (through) vagin/ (vagina) **-al** (pertaining to) **ultra-** (beyond) son/o (sound) **-graphy** (process of recording)	A procedure to view the cervix, uterus, ovaries, fallopian tubes and pelvic area via an ultrasound probe placed inside the vagina

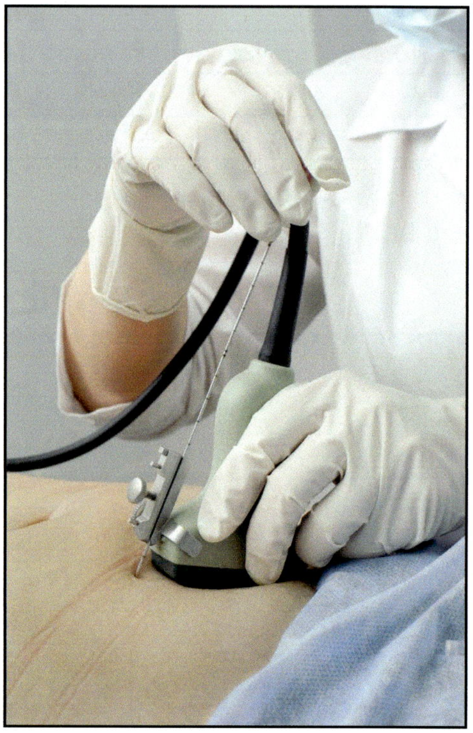

Figure 13-17. Amniocentesis using ultrasound as a guide. (Bork/shutterstock.com)

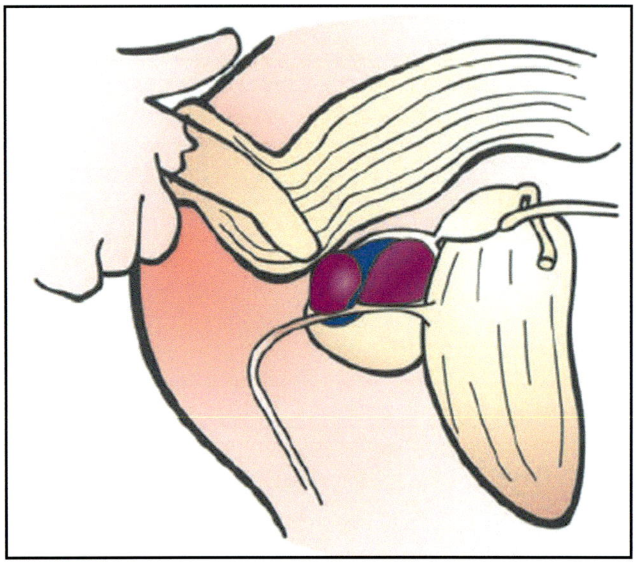

Figure 13-18. A digital rectal examination is one way to assess the prostate gland. (vikici/shutterstock.com)

Table 13-11
Surgical Procedures

NAME	WORD PARTS	PURPOSE
abortion	**-ion** (the act of)	Termination of a pregnancy prior to the fetus's ability to survive outside of the uterus
balanoplasty	balan/o (glans penis) **-plasty** (repair)	Surgical repair of glans penis
cervicectomy	cervic/ (cervix) **-ectomy** (excision; surgical removal)	Surgical excision of the cervix
colporrhaphy	colp/o (vagina) **-rrhaphy** (surgical repair; suturing)	Surgical repair of the vagina
endometrial ablation	**endo-** (within) metr/i (uterus) **-al** (pertaining to)	Destruction of specific areas of endometrial tissues; typically associated with treatment for menorrhagia
epididymectomy	epididym/ (epididymis) **-ectomy** (excision)	Excision of the epididymis
episiorrhaphy	episi/o (vulva) **-rrhaphy** (surgical repair)	Surgical repair of the vulva and/or perineum cut during child delivery
episiotomy	episi/o (vulva) **-tomy** (to cut into)	Cutting into the vulva and/or perineum to allow better passage for birth
herniorrhaphy	herni/o (hernia) **-rrhaphy** (surgical repair)	Surgical repair of a hernia
hysterectomy (Figure 13-19)	hyster/ (uterus) **-ectomy** (surgical removal)	Surgical removal of the uterus
laparoscopy	lapar/o (abdomen) **-scopy** (examination of)	Invasive procedure using an endoscope to view and sometimes perform surgery on structures within the abdomen; used when performing a tubal ligation
oophorectomy	oophor/ (ovary) **-ectomy** (excision)	Excision of an ovary
orchidectomy	orchid/ (testis) **-ectomy** (excision)	Excision of the testis

(continued)

Table 13-11 (continued)
Surgical Procedures

NAME	WORD PARTS	PURPOSE
perineorrhaphy	perine/o (perineum) **-rrhaphy** (surgical repair)	Surgical repair of the perineum
prostatectomy	prostat/ (prostate gland) **-ectomy** (surgical removal)	Surgical removal of the prostate gland
prostatolithotomy	prostat/o (prostate gland) lith/o (stone) **-tomy** (incision)	Incision into the prostate to remove a stone
radical prostatectomy (RP)	prostat/ (prostate gland) **-ectomy** (excision)	Excision of the prostate gland and all its components (capsule, seminal vesicles, vas deferens) as a treatment for prostate cancer
suprapubic prostatectomy	**supra-** (above) pub/ (pubis) **-ic** (pertaining to) prostat/ (prostate gland) **-ectomy** (surgical removal)	Removal of the prostate gland via incision into the abdomen above the pubic bone of the pelvis
transurethral incision of the prostate (TUIP)	**trans-** (through) urethr/ (urethra) **-al** (pertaining to)	Surgical widening of the urethra by incisions in the urinary bladder neck and prostate gland
transurethral resection of the prostate (TURP)	**trans-** (through) urethr/ (urethra) **-al** (pertaining to)	Portions of the prostate gland removed using a resectoscope inserted in the urethra
vasectomy (Figure 13-20)	vas/ (vas deferens) **-ectomy** (excision)	Surgical excision of a portion of the vas deferens bilaterally for sterilization purposes

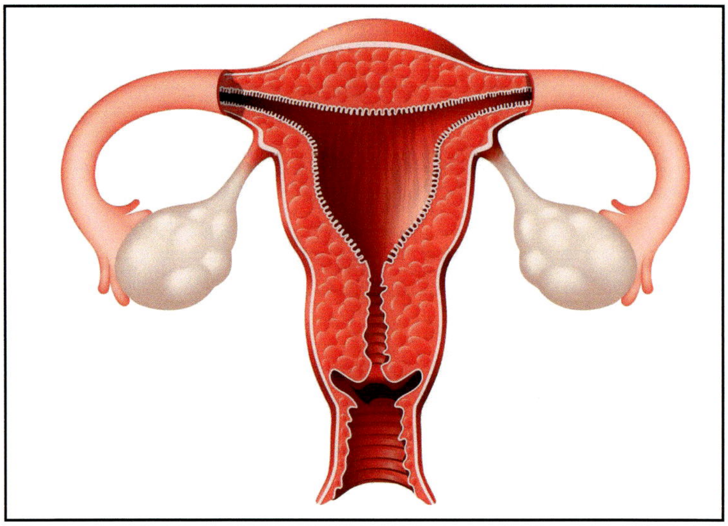

Figure 13-19. Surgical removal of the uterus (hysterectomy) does not always entail removal of the ovaries. (fixer00/shutterstock.com)

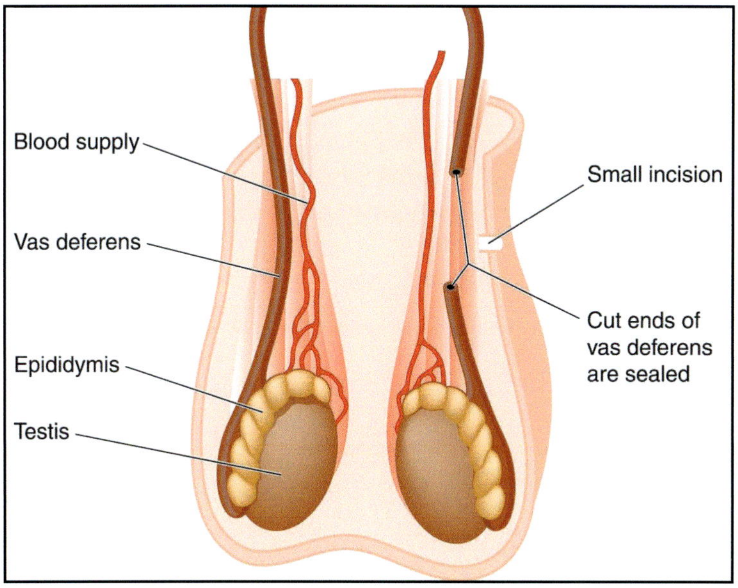

Figure 13-20. Vasectomy. (Blamb/shutterstock.com)

Table 13-12 Terms Related to Procedures Without Medical Parts	
TERM	**PURPOSE**
Apgar score	A 10-point rating system used on a newborn at 1 and 5 minutes post birth; infants with low scores require medical attention
artificial insemination (Figure 13-21)	Active semen placed into the vagina or cervix with the intention of impregnation
castration	Surgical removal of the testes or ovaries; also chemical cessation of their functions
Cesarean section	Incision into the uterus through the abdominal wall to deliver a fetus
cervical conization	Removal of a cone-shape sample from the cervix for microscopic examination; also termed *cone biopsy*
dilation and curettage (D&C)	Through a dilated cervix, the endometrial lining is scraped with a curette
dilation and evacuation (D&E)	Widening the cervix to remove conception products by suction
in vitro fertilization (IVF) (Figure 13-22)	Conception is facilitated in a lab by introducing an oocyte and zygote together and then implanting the product into the uterus
Papanicolaou smear test (Pap smear) (Figure 13-23)	Microscopic study of cells scraped from the cervix; typically performed to detect cervical cancer
semen analysis	Microscopic examination of ejaculated sperm to determine its viability in conception
tubal ligation (Figure 13-24)	Blocking (via ties, clips, bands, burning, or cutting) tubes to prevent pregnancy; not specific to the fallopian tubes

13

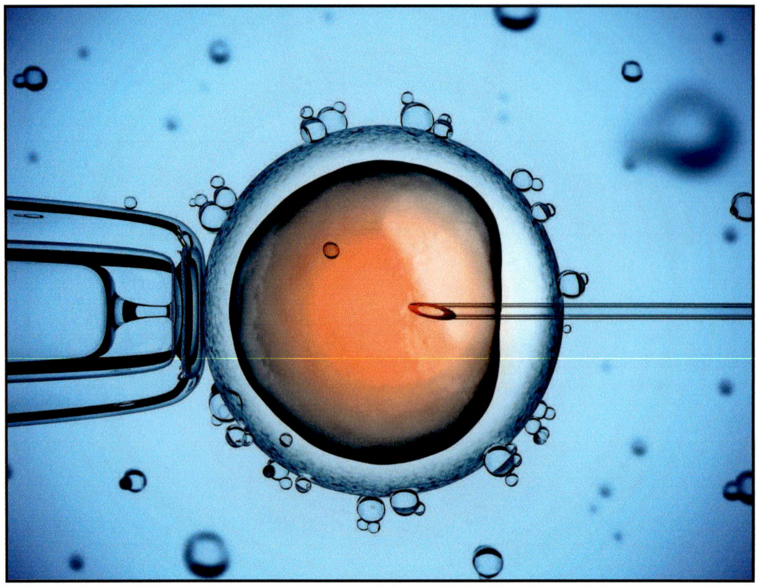

Figure 13-21. Artificial insemination involves injecting sperm into an oocyte. (koya979/shutterstock.com)

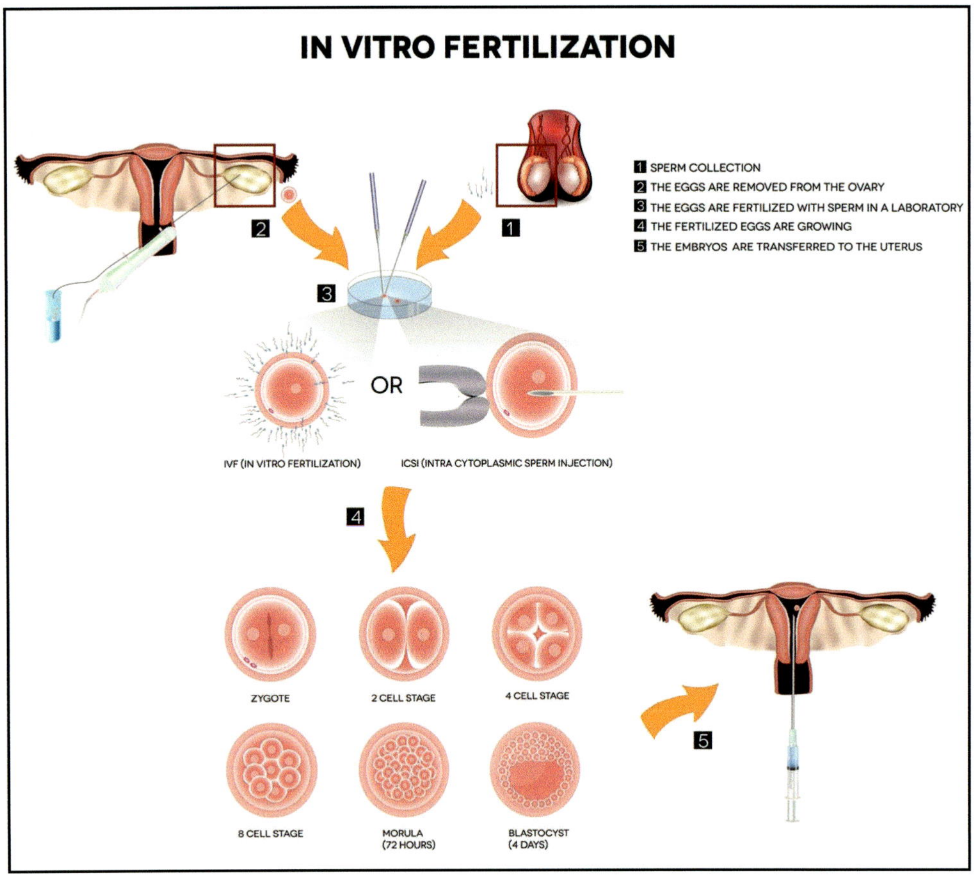

Figure 13-22. In vitro fertilization is assisted by a lab procedure. (GRei/shutterstock.com)

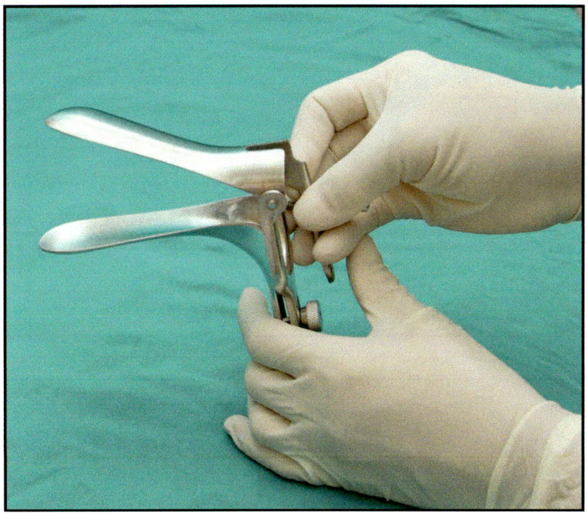

Figure 13-23. A speculum is a tool a gynecologist uses to widen the walls of the vagina to take a sample of the cervix during a Pap smear. (Praisaeng/shutterstock.com)

Figure 13-24. A tubal ligation to the fallopian tubes. (Blamb/shutterstock.com)

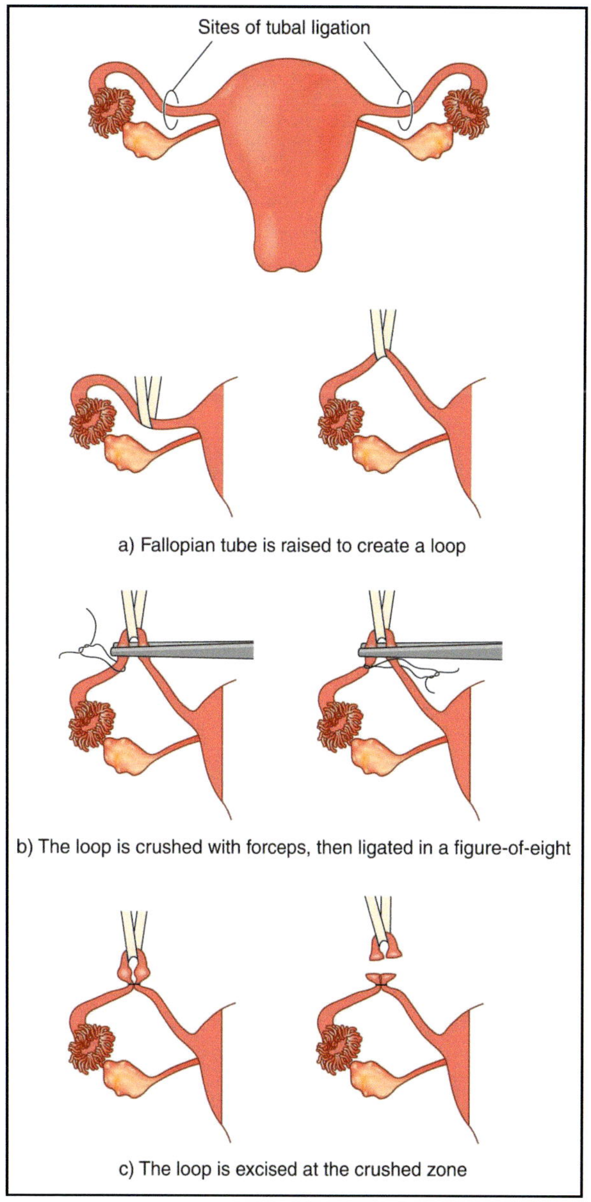

13

Medication Classifications

Table 13-13

Medication Classifications Used in Treatment of Reproductive Conditions

CATEGORY	WHAT IT DOES
abortifacient	Induces abortion
birth control pills (BCP)	Oral hormones used to prevent pregnancy
pitocin	Speeds up labor; also called *oxytocin*

Bibliography

Allan D. *Medical Language for Modern Health Care.* 4th ed. McGraw-Hill; 2019.

Farinde A. Human chorionic gonadotropin (hCG). *Medscape.* Updated November 19, 2019. Accessed December 29, 2021. https://emedicine.medscape.com/article/2089158-overview

Flanagan KW, Cuppett M. Genitourinary and gynecological systems. In *Medical Conditions in the Athlete.* 3rd ed. Human Kinetics; 2017.

Hutton A. *Medical Terminology for Health Care.* 5th ed. Churchill Livingstone; 2017.

McCance KL, Huether SE. *Pathophysiology: The Biologic Basis for Disease in Adults and Children.* 8th ed. Mosby; 2019.

Mosby's Dictionary of Medicine, Nursing & Health Professions. 10th ed. Elsevier; 2017.

Rice J. *Medical Terminology for Health Care Professionals.* 9th ed. Pearson; 2018.

Venes D, ed. *Taber's Cyclopedic Medical Dictionary.* 24th ed. F. A. Davis; 2021.

Wingerd BD. *Medical Terminology Complete!* Pearson; 2019.

NOTES

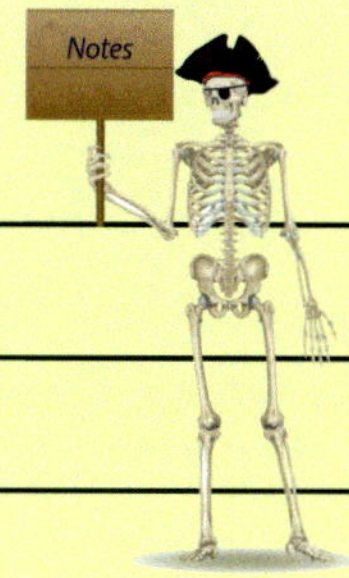

NOTES

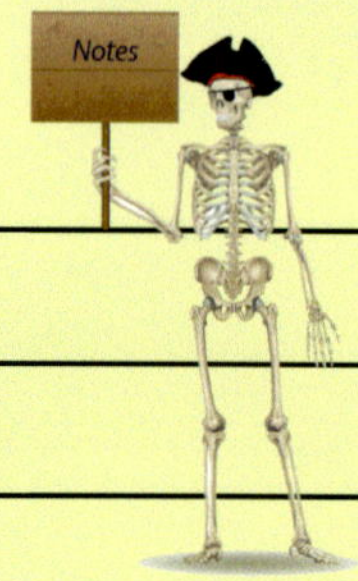

Learning Activities

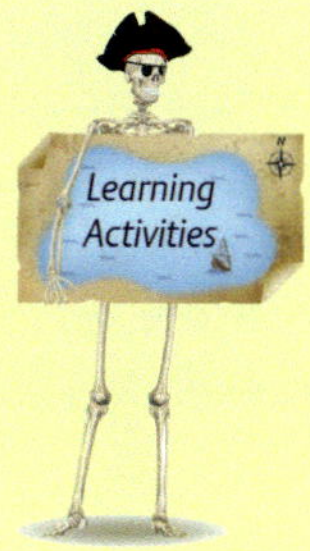

Name:______________________

Reproductive System

A. Label the components of the male reproductive system from the following list of words.

- anus______________________
- urinary bladder____________
- epididymis________________
- vas deferens_______________
- scrotum__________________
- urethra___________________
- penis_____________________
- glans penis________________
- prostate gland_____________
- testis_____________________

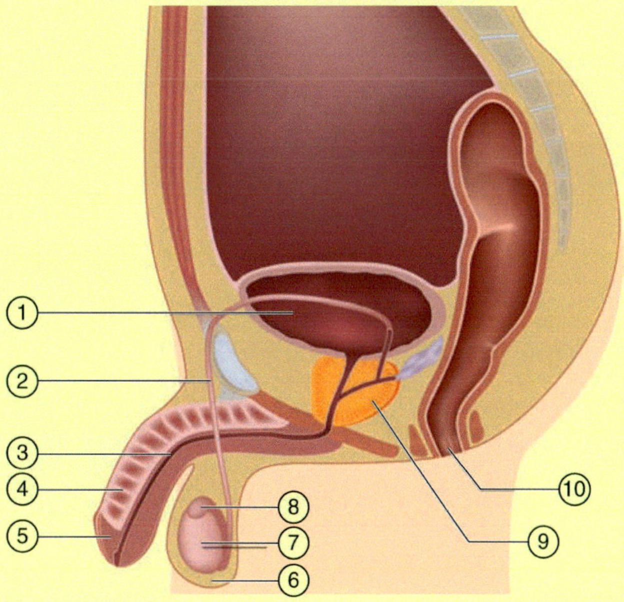

B. Label the components of the female reproductive system from the following list of words.

- anus______________________________
- urinary bladder________________________
- fimbriae____________________________
- uterus_____________________________
- vagina_____________________________
- cervix_____________________________
- urethra____________________________
- fallopian tube________________________
- ovary______________________________
- endometrium__________________________

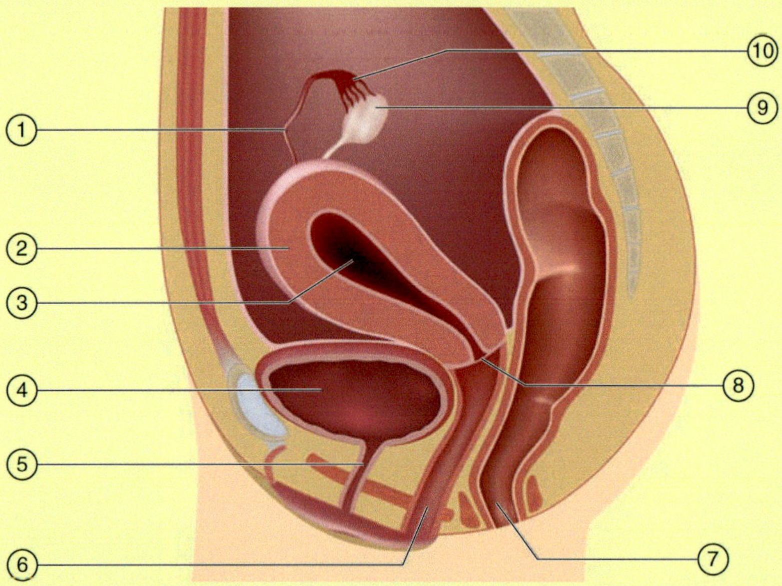

C. Match the word element with its best meaning.

1. myometrium____________	a. vagina
2. **ecto-**____________	b. vulva
3. **-emesis**____________	c. above
4. galact/o____________	d. uterus
5. episi/o____________	e. middle layer of the uterus
6. gravid/o____________	f. birth
7. metr/o____________	g. outside; outward
8. **epi-**____________	h. milk
9. nat/o____________	i. pregnancy
10. colp/o____________	j. vomiting

D. Word building: Using the word part, add the other word element and define the new word created.

1. **orchid/o**
    a. **-pexy**____
    b. **-ectomy**______________________________________
    c. **-plasty**_______________________________________
    d. **-otomy**_______________________________________
    e. **-pathy**_______________________________________
2. **salpin/**
    a. **-itis**____
    b. **-cele**____
    c. py/o____
    d. hydr/o_______________________________________
    e. hemat/o______________________________________
3. **-scopy**
    a. culd/o_______________________________________
    b. cyst/o_______________________________________
    c. hyster/o______________________________________
    d. colp/o_______________________________________
    e. lapr/o_______________________________________
4. **gravid/**
    a. **nulli-** + **-a**___________________________________
    b. **primi-** + **-a**__________________________________
    c. **multi-** + **-a**__________________________________
5. **par/**
    a. **nulli-** + **-a**___________________________________
    b. **primi-** + **-a**__________________________________
    c. **multi-** + **-a**__________________________________

E. Separate the word elements of the following terms and define them.

1. urethritis____
2. panhysterectomy__________________________________
3. prostatic hyperplasia_______________________________
4. sonohysterography_________________________________
5. hyperemesis gravidarum_____________________________

F. Indicate if the word is associated with men, women, or both.

TERM	MEN	WOMEN	BOTH
hysterectomy			
phimosis			
colposcopy			
salpingitis			
orchitis			
oophorectomy			
hydrocele			
priapism			
BPH			
D&C			

Case Study

Define the numerical terms (1 to 15).

For assistance with medical abbreviations, refer to Appendix A.

History, Chief Complaint

A freshman college student reported to the clinic with extreme fatigue, weight loss, and stomach pain. Her roommate was recently diagnosed with mononucleosis.

Evaluation

The student was **afebrile** (1), and denied **cephalalgia** (2), **cervicalgia** (3), or **pharyngitis** (4). She had no discernible **adenomegaly** (5). She complained of being **anorexic** (6) and she had lost 10 pounds in the past 3 weeks. She also mentioned she was on **BCP** (7), but had **amenorrhea** (8) for the past 3 months and **polyuria** (9). She had pain on palpation of the **RLQ** (10) of her abdomen. She admitted she experienced **syncope** (11) while moving boxes in her storage room earlier in the day.

Diagnostic Studies

At this point her **differential diagnoses** (12) were mononucleosis, appendicitis, pregnancy, **hyperthyroidism** (13), or a flu-like illness. A mono-spot was performed and was negative for mono. Abdominal evaluation revealed a slight mass near the right ovary or fallopian tube. An **ultrasound** (14) examination was inconclusive. Repeated blood tests were ordered (48 hours apart) for hCG. This blood test was positive for an ectopic pregnancy, and a **laparoscopy** (15) was scheduled to treat the condition.

Terms

1. ______________________________
2. ______________________________
3. ______________________________
4. ______________________________
5. ______________________________
6. ______________________________
7. ______________________________
8. ______________________________
9. ______________________________
10. ______________________________
11. ______________________________
12. ______________________________
13. ______________________________
14. ______________________________
15. ______________________________

13

14

Sensory System

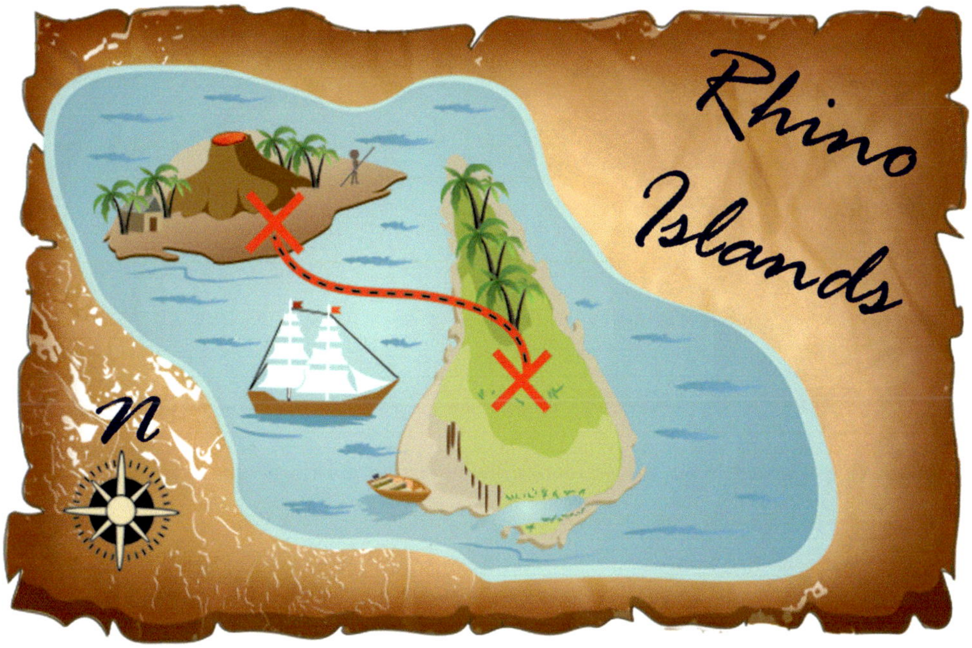

Objectives

After studying this chapter, you will be able to:

1. Identify the major anatomical components of the eyes, ears, and nose.
2. Build words relating to the eyes, ears, and nose.
3. List signs and symptoms of conditions to the eyes, ears, and nose.
4. Describe basic abnormalities or conditions of the eyes, ears, and nose.
5. Explain diagnostic tests and procedures specific to the eyes, ears, and nose.
6. Understand surgical procedures based on word parts.
7. Identify classifications of medications used to treat pathological conditions related to the eyes and ears.

Flanagan KW.
Medical Terminology With Case Studies: A Navigated Guide to Learning for Health Care Professionals, Third Edition (pp 401-436).

Chapter Outline

- Self-assessment
- Checklist for word parts in the chapter
- Checklist of new anatomy
- Introduction
- Anatomy
  - Eyes
  - Ears
  - Nose
- Word building
  - Prefixes
  - Suffixes
  - Combining forms
- Signs and symptoms
- Medical conditions
- Tests and procedures
- Medication classifications
- Learning activities
- Case study

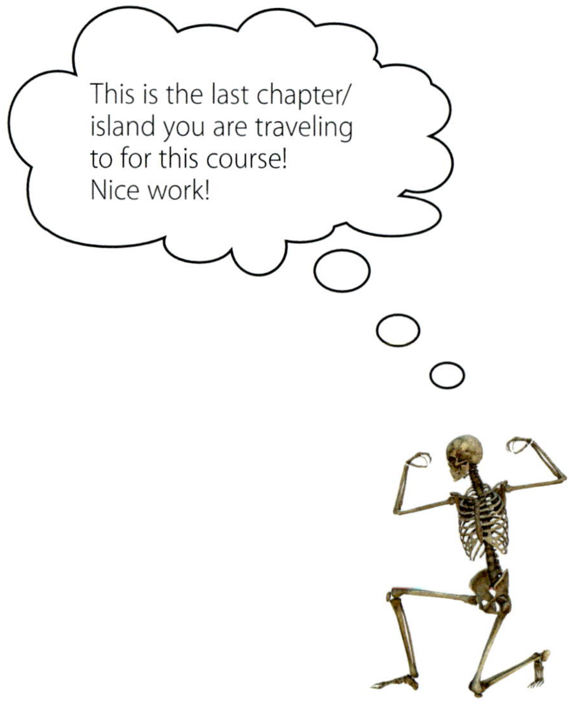
This is the last chapter/ island you are traveling to for this course! Nice work!

Self-Assessment

Based on what you have learned so far, can you write the definition of these words?

- photophobic____________________
- rhinoplasty____________________
- otoscope____________________
- nasopharyngitis____________________
- diplopia____________________

Checklist for Word Parts in the Chapter

Prefixes

- ☐ a-
- ☐ an-
- ☐ di-
- ☐ em-
- ☐ en-
- ☐ endo-
- ☐ eso-
- ☐ ex-
- ☐ exo-
- ☐ hemi-
- ☐ hyper-
- ☐ intra-
- ☐ macro-
- ☐ medi-
- ☐ micro-
- ☐ mono-
- ☐ para-

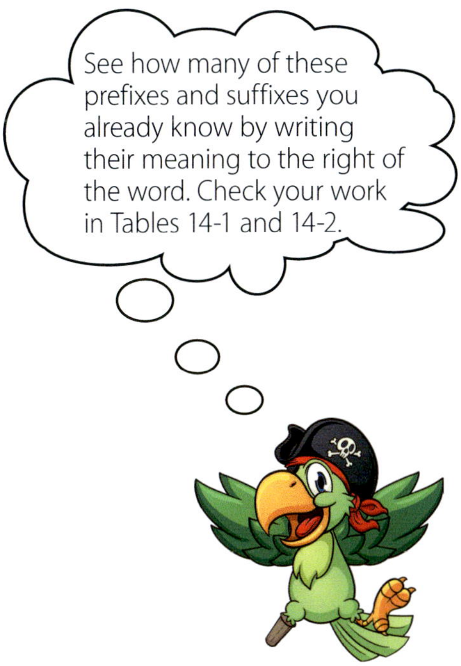
See how many of these prefixes and suffixes you already know by writing their meaning to the right of the word. Check your work in Tables 14-1 and 14-2.

Suffixes

- ☐ -acusis
- ☐ -al
- ☐ -algia
- ☐ -ar
- ☐ -asthen
- ☐ -ation
- ☐ -cusis
- ☐ -ectasia
- ☐ -ectomy
- ☐ -emia
- ☐ -gram
- ☐ -ia
- ☐ -ism
- ☐ -itis
- ☐ -lith
- ☐ -malacia
- ☐ -meter
- ☐ -metry
- ☐ -oid
- ☐ -oma
- ☐ -opia
- ☐ -opsia
- ☐ -osis
- ☐ -osmia
- ☐ -otia
- ☐ -otomy
- ☐ -pathy
- ☐ -pexy
- ☐ -phobia
- ☐ -plasty
- ☐ -plegia
- ☐ -pnea
- ☐ -ptosis
- ☐ -rrhagia
- ☐ -rrhea
- ☐ -rrhexis
- ☐ -scope
- ☐ -scopy
- ☐ -sis
- ☐ -tomy
- ☐ -trophia

Combining Forms

- ☐ acous/o
- ☐ acu/o
- ☐ aden/o
- ☐ ambly/o
- ☐ aque/o
- ☐ audi/o
- ☐ audit/o
- ☐ aur/o
- ☐ auricul/o
- ☐ blast/o
- ☐ blephar/o
- ☐ chrom/o
- ☐ chromat/o
- ☐ cochle/o
- ☐ conjunctiv/o
- ☐ cor/o
- ☐ corne/o
- ☐ cry/o
- ☐ dacry/o
- ☐ dacryocyst/o
- ☐ dipl/o
- ☐ dynam/o
- ☐ fluor/o
- ☐ fovea
- ☐ glauc/o
- ☐ heter/o
- ☐ humor
- ☐ ir/o
- ☐ irid/o
- ☐ kerat/o
- ☐ labyrinth/o
- ☐ lacrim/o
- ☐ mast/o
- ☐ mastoid/o
- ☐ metr/o
- ☐ mi/o
- ☐ myc/o
- ☐ mydr/o
- ☐ myring/o
- ☐ nas/o
- ☐ nyct/o
- ☐ ocul/o
- ☐ ophthalm/o
- ☐ opt/o
- ☐ optic/o

Combining Forms

- ☐ **oss/i**
- ☐ **ossicul/o**
- ☐ **ot/o**
- ☐ **ove/o**
- ☐ **palpebr/o**
- ☐ **papill/o**
- ☐ **phac/o**
- ☐ **phak/o**
- ☐ **phot/o**
- ☐ **phyma**
- ☐ **presby/o**
- ☐ **radi/o**
- ☐ **retin/o**
- ☐ **rhin/o**
- ☐ **salping/o**
- ☐ **scler/o**
- ☐ **scot/o**
- ☐ **sept/o**
- ☐ **spir/o**
- ☐ **staped/o**
- ☐ **stigmat/o**
- ☐ **strab/o**
- ☐ **ton/o**
- ☐ **tympan/o**
- ☐ **vestibul/o**
- ☐ **vitre/o**
- ☐ **xer/o**

Checklist of New Anatomy

The Eye

Anterior Eye

- ☐ Eyelid
- ☐ Conjunctiva
- ☐ Cornea
- ☐ Aqueous humor
- ☐ Lacrimal gland
- ☐ Lacrimal duct
- ☐ Sclera

Posterior Eye

- ☐ Uvea
  - ☐ Choroid
  - ☐ Ciliary body
  - ☐ Iris
- ☐ Lens
- ☐ Pupil
- ☐ Retina
  - ☐ Rods
  - ☐ Cones
  - ☐ Optic disc
  - ☐ Fovea
  - ☐ Macula
- ☐ Optic nerve
- ☐ Vitreous body

The Ear

Outer Ear

- ☐ Pinna (auricle)
- ☐ External auditory canal (meatus)
- ☐ Cerumen
- ☐ Tympanic membrane

Middle Ear

- ☐ Malleus
- ☐ Incus
- ☐ Stapes
- ☐ Oval window

Inner Ear

- ☐ Cochlea
- ☐ Organ of Corti
- ☐ Round window
- ☐ Semicircular canals
  - ☐ Otoliths
- ☐ Vestibulocochlear nerve (CN VIII)

The Nose

- ☐ Nares
- ☐ Septum
- ☐ Columella
- ☐ Inferior turbinate
- ☐ Middle turbinate
- ☐ Superior turbinate
- ☐ Olfactory nerve (CN I)

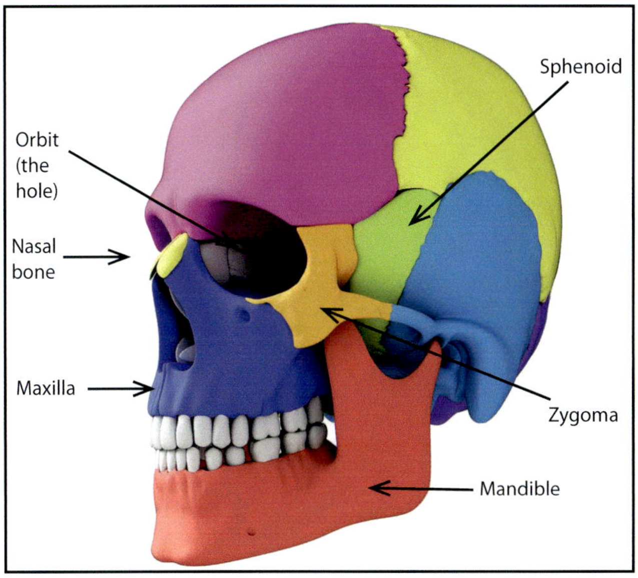

Figure 14-1. The relationship of the nasal bone to the skull and face. (Sebastian Kaulitzki/shutterstock.com)

Introduction

The last island on our sail is Rhino Island, and it represents the sensory system. The island contains combining forms distinctive to the eye, ear, and nose. This is the last stop on our medical terminology sail through the various islands, and most of the prefixes and suffixes should be reasonably familiar to you. At the conclusion of your visit to these islands, you should have gathered quite the vocabulary to assist you on your next adventure. Just remember that prefixes and suffixes are like gold and silver coins; you can carry them with you to combining forms for all different islands (body systems) and make a given word root a new word.

Anatomy

The eyes, ears, and nose are protected by the bony structures of the skull. This provides protection for the actual nervous connections that create vision, hearing, and the sense of smell (Figure 14-1).

14

Eyes

The eyes lie protected within the skeletal orbit provided by the skull. The **zygoma** and **sphenoid** bones provide lateral protection, and the **lacrimal** bone (behind the nasal bone) shelters the medial aspects (see Figure 5-3D in Chapter 5). The floor of the orbit (where the eyeball sits) is composed of the **maxilla** and **zygoma**. In the back of the orbit is an opening that allows the **optic nerve** to pass through to the brain. This is important to note, as any injury to these bones can affect vision and the overall health of the eye. In addition to the bony orbit, **eyelids** and eyelashes protect and moisten the eye, and even eyebrows are functional as they shield the eye from foreign material. A delicate, clear membrane called the **conjunctiva** lines the anterior (visible) eyeball and inner eyelids. Tears are constantly being produced to keep the eye lubricated and free of debris. They arise from the **lacrimal gland** on the upper lateral eye and drain into the nose via **lacrimal sacs and ducts** in the inner (medial) corner of the eye (Figure 14-2).

There are three main layers (tunics) of the eye. The tough outer layer (white part of the eye) is called the **sclera**. The middle layer, the **uvea**, consists of three aspects: the choroid, ciliary body, and iris. The **choroid** is a highly vascular, pigmented layer whose chief function is to provide nourishment for the retina (Figure 14-3). The **ciliary body** is a muscle that accommodates (contracts and expands), allowing the **lens** to change shape for visual focus. The last aspect of the uvea is the **iris**, which is a muscular, highly pigmented structure that determines how much light is allowed though the pupil. The iris determines the color of one's eyes, and the **pupil** is merely an opening, or hole. The iris does react to many things, including emotions. You can tell if someone is interested by watching their iris; if the pupil dilates (iris constricts, opening up the pupil), the person is attracted to you or interested in what you are saying. Patients have mydriatic drops placed in their eyes to dilate the pupil when they are examined via the ophthalmoscope (**ophthalm/o**—eye; **-scope**—an instrument used to view or inspect). This allows the examiner to view into the posterior aspects of the eye.

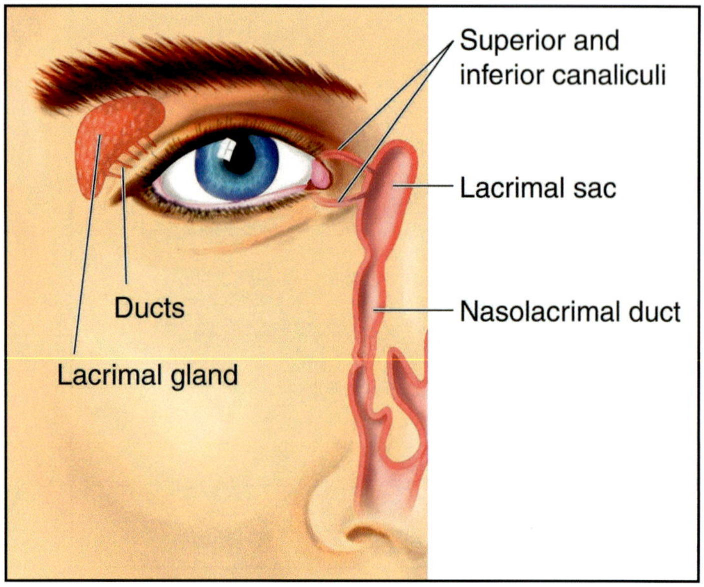

Figure 14-2. The lacrimal gland and ducts. (Blamb/shutterstock.com)

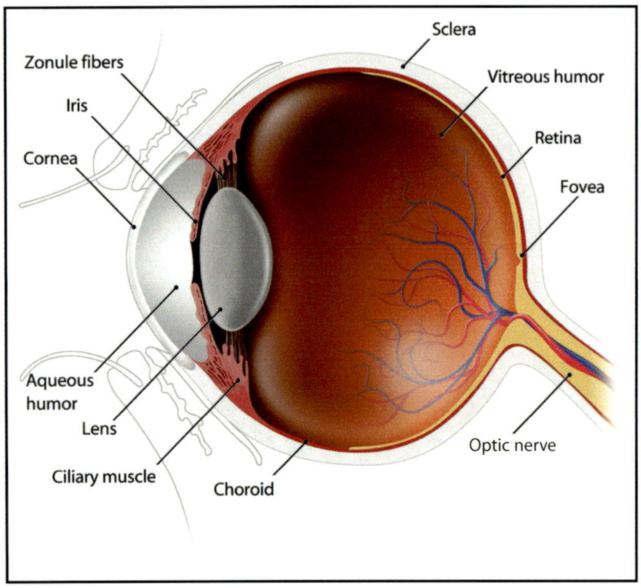

Figure 14-3. Anatomy of the eye. (kocakayaali/shutterstock.com)

The innermost layer of the eye is the **retina**, and this is where visual acuity and color is determined. The two types of specialized cells within the retina—rods and cones—have overlapping and different functions. **Rods** operate best in dim lighting and determine visual acuity (sharpness). **Cones** also address visual acuity but are most active in bright light. They are responsible for seeing color. The tunic layers are mainly in the posterior eye and adhere against the eyeball in part due to the **vitreous body** (Figure 14-4), which is a viscous, jelly-like substance that assists in keeping the globe-like shape of the eye, but also allows light to refract through it. On the most posterior aspect of the posterior chamber is the entrance/exit for the **optic nerve** and vessels. Near the opening is the **optic disc**, which is a blind spot on the retina. Finally, the **fovea** resembles a tiny dent in the retina near the optic nerve. The fovea is the focal spot for vision and is highly concentrated with cones. The area around the fovea is the **macula**.

In front of the lens is the **anterior chamber** of the eye. The **aqueous humor** plays the same role here as does the vitreous body in the posterior chamber; namely, it supports the anterior eye and maintains intraocular (**intra-**—inside, within; **ocul/o**—eye; **-ar**—pertaining to) pressure. On the visual aspect of the anterior eye, the sclera becomes a clear and highly sensitive layer, the **cornea**. Contacts sit over the cornea.

External to the eye are six muscles within the orbit (Figure 14-5) that allow the eyes to work in unison looking up, down, medial, lateral, and diagonal. The muscles are named by their attachment to the eye (superior, inferior, medial, lateral, and oblique).

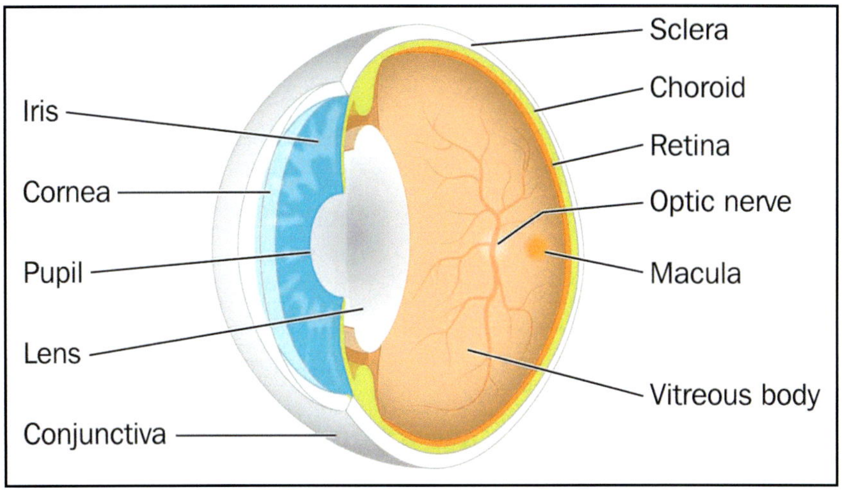

Figure 14-4. Layers of the eye. (Blamb/shutterstock.com)

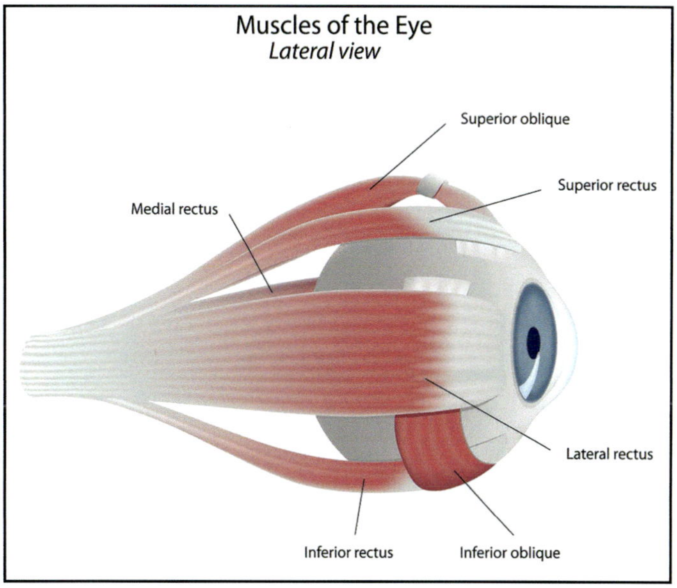

Figure 14-5. Muscles of the eye. (Alila Medical Images/shutterstock.com)

People who have longer eyeballs than normal have the images they see in front of the retina, called *nearsightedness* or **myopia**. In contrast, the shorter eyeball, where the focus would be behind the retina, is called *farsightedness* or **hyperopia**. The curvature in corrective lenses accounts for the length of the eye and can adjust the focal point so vision is more clear (Figure 14-6).

Ears

The sensory aspect of the ear is protected by the bony mastoid process of the temporal bone of the skull. There are three aspects of the ear: outer, middle, and inner. Both the middle and inner ear are encased within the skull and are typically protected from external injury. The **outer (external) ear** has a fleshy **pinna** (also called the *auricle*) that is shell shaped to catch sound waves. The pinna is merely skin over cartilage and only has a bit of fat (mainly in the earlobes). Injury to the pinna can cause permanent scarring as it has little blood supply. For this reason it is also susceptible to cold

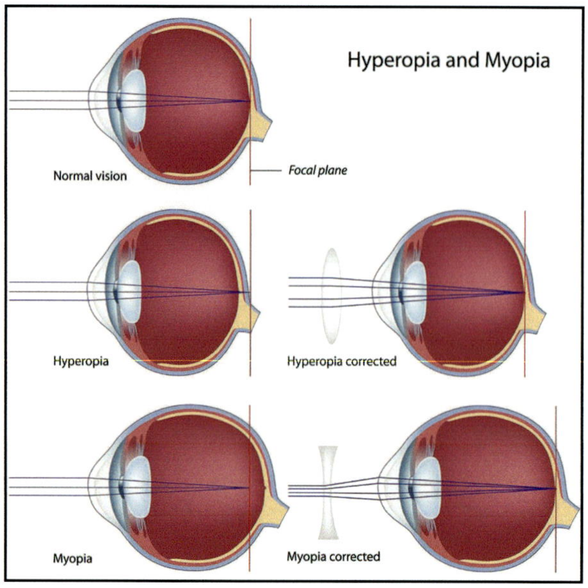

Figure 14-6. Myopia vs hyperopia. (Alila Medical Images/shutterstock.com)

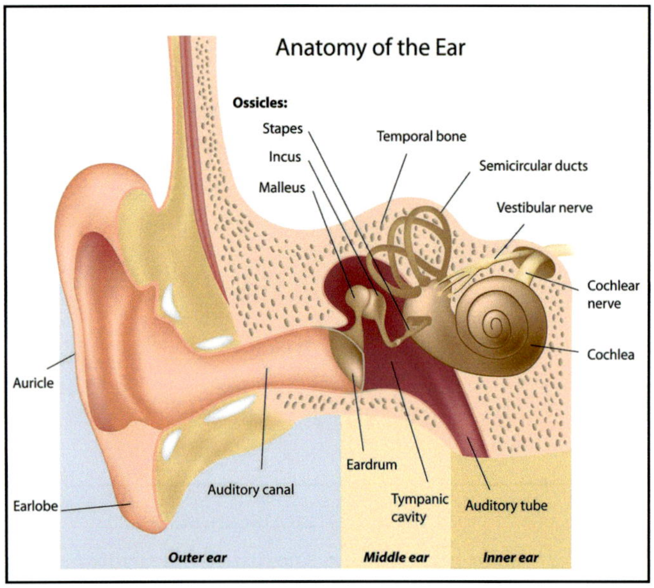

Figure 14-7. Anatomy of the ear. (Alila Medical Images/shutterstock.com)

injury. Attached to the pinna is the **external auditory canal**, also termed the *meatus*, as it is an opening. This canal is sloped slightly downward and has glands that secrete **cerumen** (earwax) to lubricate and protect it. The opening one-third of this 2.5-cm canal is flexible, and moves slightly with movement of the pinna. At the end of the external auditory canal is the **tympanic membrane**, or eardrum. This membrane vibrates with sound waves and transmits the energy to three **ossicles** (**oss/i**—bone; small bones): the **malleus** (shaped as a mallet), **incus** (anvil), and **stapes** (stirrup). The stapes rests on a structure called the **oval window**, which provides the beginning of the **inner ear**. Connecting the **middle ear** to the throat is the **eustachian tube** (also called *auditory tube*). The function of this structure is to equalize the pressure between the outer and middle ears. This is apparent when driving up a mountain, flying in a plane, or scuba diving and feeling your ears pop. That sound is equalization of pressure so the tympanic membrane does not rupture (Figure 14-7). The **inner ear** is also called the *labyrinth* (maze), as it resembles one. There are two main structures in the inner ear: the semicircular canals and the shell-shaped cochlea. The actual organ responsible for hearing is the **cochlea**, and the **organ of Corti** within it. Sound waves enter via the oval window, travel in the fluid-filled cochlea, and exit through the **round window** at the base of the cochlea.

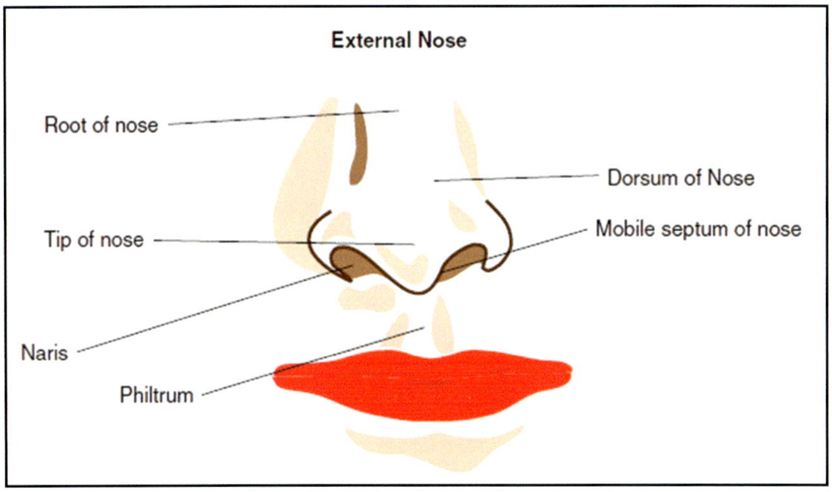

Figure 14-8. The external nose. (Alila Medical Images/shutterstock.com)

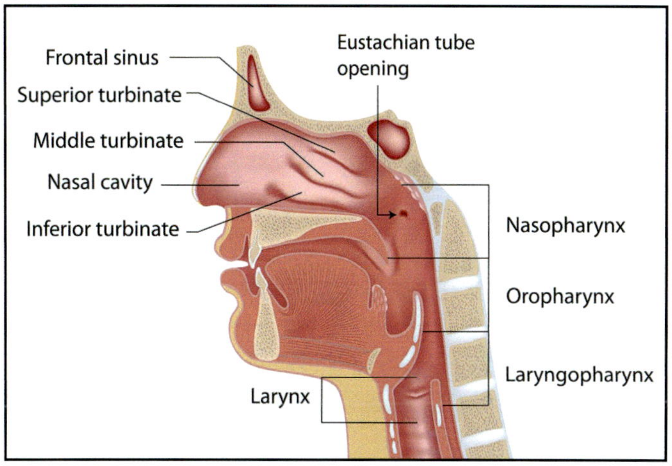

Figure 14-9. Anatomy of the nose. (Alila Medical Images/shutterstock.com)

Balance and equilibrium are also perceived within the inner ear in the **semicircular canals**. Tiny **otoliths** (**ot/o**—ear; **-lith**—stone) within the semicircular canals provide balance sensation and can be blamed for seasickness and other movement-related discomfort. The **vestibulocochlear nerve** (sound familiar from Chapter 8? It is also known as CN VIII) ends up as two separate nerves (vestibular and cochlear) as it splits and enters the respective sense organs.

14

Nose

Compared to its sensory counterparts, the nose is not well protected by the skull (see Figure 14-1). The actual nasal bone is quite small (pinch between your eyes on your nose—only the hard aspect is the nasal bone; the rest is cartilage). As air enters the nose, it passes through tiny hairs and mucous membranes. Both these hairs and mucus serve to warm, moisten, and filter the air in preparation for entry to the throat and lungs. Air enters via two **nares** (individually, naris) and is separated into right and left **anterior cavities**, separated by a nasal **septum**. Externally, the divider between the two nares is termed the **columella** (Figure 14-8). Bony separations within the nose, called **turbinates** or conchae (Figure 14-9), move the air up past the **olfactory nerve** (**CN I**) where the sense of smell occurs. These turbinates are called **inferior**, **middle**, and **superior** and are named after their location within the nasal cavity. The purpose of the turbinates is to increase the surface area for moistening and warming inhaled air. The **sphenoid sinus** and eustachian tube open into the middle turbinate and nasopharynx (**nas/o**—nose; pharynx—throat), respectfully, which is one reason why people with sinus infections or colds suffer both nasal and throat drainage.

WORD BUILDING

TABLE 14-1
PREFIXES

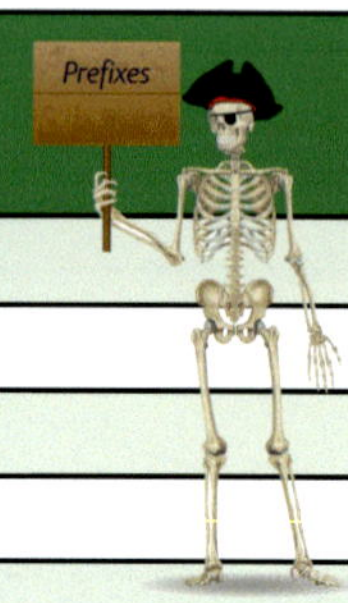

PREFIX	DEFINITION
a-; an-	not; without
di-	double
em-	in
en-; endo-	in; within
eso-	inward
ex-; exo-	away; away from; out; outside
hemi-	one half
hyper-	above; excessive; high; increased
intra-	in; within
macro-	large
medi-	middle
micro-	small
mono-	one
para-	beside; near; abnormal

TABLE 14-2
SUFFIXES

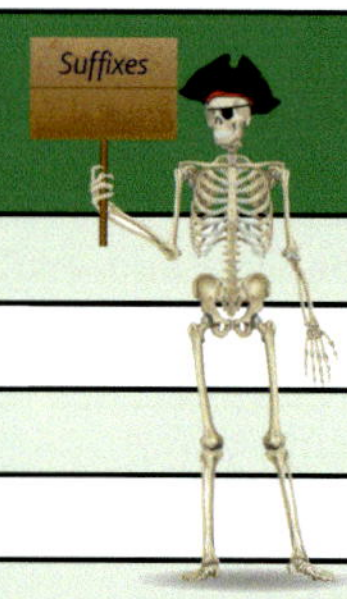

SUFFIX	DEFINITION
-acusis	hearing condition
-al	pertaining to
-algia	pain
-ar	pertaining to
-asthen	weakness
-ation	process of
-cusis	hearing
-ectasia	dilation
-ectomy	excision; surgical removal
-emia	blood condition
-gram	a record of
-ia	condition
-ism	condition

(continued)

Table 14-2 (continued)

Suffixes

SUFFIX	DEFINITION
-itis	inflammation
-lith	stone
-malacia	softening
-meter	an instrument used to measure
-metry	measurement of
-oid	resembling
-oma	mass; tumor
-opia; -opsia	vision condition
-osis	condition
-osmia	smell
-otia	ear condition
-otomy; -tomy	incision; to cut into
-pathy	disease
-pexy	surgical fixation of
-phobia	fear
-plasty	reconstruction; repair; plastic surgery
-plegia	paralysis
-pnea	breathing
-ptosis	drooping
-rrhagia	abnormal flow
-rrhea	discharge; excessive flow
-rrhexis	rupture
-scope	an instrument used to view or inspect
-scopy	examination of
-sis	state of; condition
-trophia	to turn

Table 14-3
Combining Forms

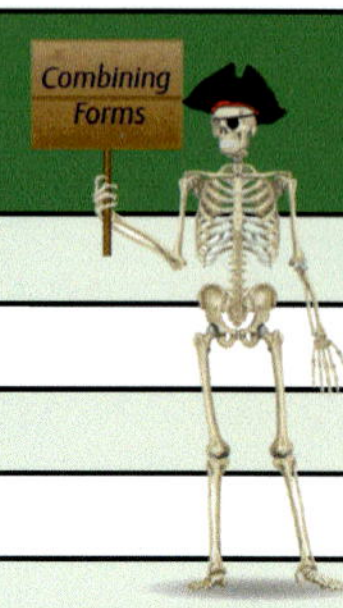

COMBINING FORM	DEFINITION
acous/o; acu/o	hearing
aden/o	gland
ambly/o	dull; dim
aque/o	water
audi/o; audit/o	hearing
aur/o; auricul/o	ear
blast/o	embryonic cell
blephar/o	eyelid
chrom/o; chromat/o	color
cochle/o	cochlea
conjunctiv/o	conjunctiva
cor/o	pupil
corne/o	cornea (covering of the eye over the iris and pupil)
cry/o	cold
dacry/o	tear; lacrimal duct/gland
dacryocyst/o	lacrimal sac (cyst/o—sac)
dipl/o	double
dynam/o	force; energy
fluor/o	luminous
fovea	small pit
glauc/o	gray
heter/o	different
humor	fluid
ir/o; irid/o	iris
kerat/o	cornea; hard; horn-like
labyrinth/o	inner ear; labyrinth
lacrim/o	tear duct or gland
mast/o	breast
mastoid/o	mastoid process
metr/o	measure; uterus
mi/o	smaller; less
myc/o	fungus
mydr/o	widen; enlarge

(continued)

Table 14-3 (continued)
Combining Forms

COMBINING FORM	DEFINITION
myring/o	eardrum; tympanic membrane
nas/o	nose
nyct/o	night
ocul/o	eye
ophthalm/o	eye
opt/o; optic/o	eye; vision
oss/i	bone
ossicul/o	ossicle
ot/o	ear
ove/o	uvea
palpebr/o	eyelid
papill/o	papilla; nipple
phac/o; phak/o	lens
phot/o	light
phyma	swelling; tumor
presby/o	old age
radi/o	root
retin/o	retina
rhin/o	nose
salping/o	eustachian or fallopian tube
scler/o	hard; hardening; thick; sclera
scot/o	darkness
sept/o	wall
spir/o	breath; breathing
staped/o	stirrup; stapes (third bone in the middle ear)
stigmat/o	point; mark
strab/o	squinting
ton/o	tension; pressure
tympan/o	eardrum; tympanic membrane
vestibul/o	vestibule
vitre/o	glassy
xer/o	dry

Signs and Symptoms

Table 14-4 Signs and Symptoms Related to the Sensory System		
SIGN/SYMPTOM	**WORD PARTS**	**DEFINITION**
amblyopia	ambly/ (dull; dim) **-opia** (vision condition)	Loss of vision, but not due to a specific disease or condition
anacusis	**an-** (without) **-acusis** (hearing)	Complete hearing loss
blepharoptosis	blephar/o (eyelid) **-ptosis** (drooping)	Drooping eyelid
diplopia	dipl/ (double) **-opia** (vision condition)	Double vision
hyperacusis	**hyper-** (excessive) **-acusis** (hearing condition)	Extremely sensitive to noise
keratoectasia	kerat/o (cornea) **-ectasia** (dilation)	Forward bulging of the cornea
otalgia	ot/ (ear) **-algia** (pain)	Ear pain, earache
otorrhagia	ot/o (ear) **-rrhagia** (abnormal flow)	Bleeding from the ear
otorrhea	ot/o (ear) **-rrhea** (discharge)	Discharge from the ear; could be cerebrospinal fluid (CSF), water, or pus
paracusis	**par-** (beside) **-acusis** (hearing condition)	Impaired hearing; partial hearing loss
PERRLA	**P**upils **E**qually **R**ound and **R**eactive to **L**ight and **A**ccommodation	Acronym used to assess pupils' reaction to light following an eye or head injury
photophobia	phot/o (light) **-phobia** (fear)	Sensitivity or fear of light
rhinitis	rhin/ (nose) **-itis** (inflammation)	Inflammation of the nose; runny nose
rhinorrhagia	rhin/o (nose) **-rrhagia** (abnormal flow)	Profuse bleeding from the nose
rhinorrhea	rhin/o (nose) **-rrhea** (discharge)	Watery discharge from the nose; if CSF, indicates a head injury
xerophthalmia	xer/o (dry) ophthalm/ (eye) **-ia** (condition)	Dry eye

Medical Conditions

Table 14-5 Medical Conditions Related to the Sensory System		
NAME	**WORD PARTS**	**DEFINITION**
achromatopsia (Figure 14-10)	**a-** (without) chromat/ (color) **-opsia** (vision condition)	Color-blindness; inability to distinguish colors
asthenopia	**-asthen** (weakness) **-opia** (vision condition)	Condition where the eyes tire easily, often due to strain on ocular muscles; also called *eye strain*
astigmatism (Figure 14-11)	**a-** (without) stigmat/ (point; mark) **-ism** (condition)	Defective curvature of the eye
blepharitis	blephar/ (eyelid) **-itis** (inflammation)	Inflammation of the eyelid
conjunctivitis (Figure 14-12)	conjunctiv/ (conjunctiva) **-itis** (inflammation)	Inflammation of the conjunctiva; also called *pink eye*
corneal abrasion	corne/ (cornea) **-al** (pertaining to)	Scratch on the cornea causing pain, tearing, and photophobia
corneoiritis	corne/o (cornea) ir/ (iris) **-itis** (inflammation)	Inflammation of the cornea and iris
dacryoadenitis	dacry/o (lacrimal gland) aden/ (gland) **-itis** (inflammation)	Inflammation of the lacrimal gland
dacryocystitis	dacrycyst/ (lacrimal sac) **-itis** (inflammation)	Inflammation of the lacrimal sac
emmetropia	**em-** (in) metr/ (measure) **-opia** (vision)	Normal vision
endophthalmitis	**endo-** (within) ophthalm/ (eye) **-itis** (inflammation)	Inflammation of the internal structures of the eye
hemianopia	**hemi-** (one half) **an-** (without) **-opia** (vision condition)	Loss of half of the visual field; most often due to brain injury or medical condition

(continued)

Conjunctivitis is very contagious and can be spread by using the same towels, sharing eye makeup, or using eye makeup that was used prior to diagnosis.

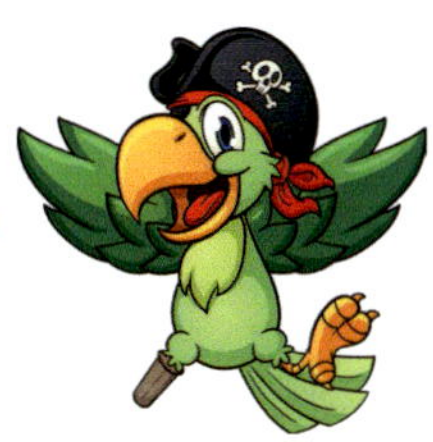

Table 14-5 (continued)

Medical Conditions Related to the Sensory System

NAME	WORD PARTS	DEFINITION
hyperopia (see Figure 14-6)	**hyper-** (above; excessive; high; increased) **-opia** (vision condition)	Reduced vision of objects that are nearby; also termed *farsightedness*
hyphema		Blood pooling into the anterior chamber of the eye due to a blow
iridoplegia	irid/o (iris) **-plegia** (paralysis)	Paralysis of the iris
iritis	ir/ (iris) **-itis** (inflammation)	Inflammation of the iris
keratitis	kerat/ (cornea) **-itis** (inflammation)	Inflammation of the cornea
keratoectasia	kerat/o (cornea) **-ectasia** (dilation)	Forward bulging of the eye
keratomalacia	kerat/o (cornea) **-malacia** (softening)	Softening of the cornea, often from a severe vitamin A deficiency
labyrinthitis	labyrinth/ (inner ear) **-itis** (inflammation)	Inflammation of the inner ear
macrotia	**macro-** (large) **-otia** (ear condition)	Having large ears
microtia	**micro-** (small) **-otia** (ear condition)	Having small ears
monochromatism	**mono-** (one) chromat/ (color) **-ism** (state of)	Only able to see one color
myopia	**-opia** (vision condition)	Reduced vision of objects that are distant; also termed *nearsightedness*
myringitis	myring/ (eardrum) **-itis** (Inflammation)	Inflammation of the eardrum, also called *tympanitis*
nyctalopia	nyct/ (night) **-al** (pertaining to) **-opia** (vision condition)	Poor vision at night or in dim lighting
oculomycosis	ocul/o (eye) myc/ (fungus) **-osis** (condition)	Fungal infection of the eye
ophthalmopathy	ophthalm/o (eye) **-pathy** (disease)	Disease affecting the eye
ophthalmorrhagia	ophthalm/o (eye) **-rrhagia** (abnormal flow)	Hemorrhage of the eye

(continued)

Table 14-5 (continued)

Medical Conditions Related to the Sensory System

NAME	WORD PARTS	DEFINITION
otitis externa (Figure 14-13)	ot/ (ear) **-itis** (inflammation) **ex-** (outside)	Inflammation of the external auditory meatus (ear canal); also termed *swimmer's ear*
otitis media (Figure 14-14)	ot/ (ear) **-itis** (inflammation) **medi-** (middle)	Inflammation of the middle ear
otosclerosis	ot/o (ear) scler/ (hardening) **-osis** (condition)	Progressive hearing loss caused by bone formation between the stapes and the oval window
photoretinitis	phot/o (light) retin/ (retina) **-itis** (inflammation)	Retina inflammation due to intense light
presbycusis	presby/ (old age) **-cusis** (hearing condition)	Age-related hearing loss
presbyopia	presby/ (old age) **-opia** (vision condition)	Age-related vision impairment
retinitis pigmentosa	retin/ (retina) **-itis** (inflammation)	Genetic condition characterized by night blindness, increasing atrophy
retinoblastoma	retin/o (retina) blast/ (embryonic cell) **-oma** (tumor)	Malignant tumor arising from the retina
rhinomycosis	rhin/o (nose) myc/ (fungus) **-osis** (condition)	Fungal infection of the nasal mucous membranes
rhinophyma	rhin/o (nose) phyma (tumor)	Deformity of the nose caused by a form of rosacea, producing swelling, increased vascularity, and redness
rhinosalpingitis	rhin/o (nose) salping/ (eustachian tube) **-itis** (inflammation)	Inflammation of the eustachian tube and nose
scleromalacia	scler/o (sclera) **-malacia** (softening)	Softening of the sclera of the eye
tympanorrhexis (Figure 14-15)	tympan/o (tympanic membrane) **-rrhexis** (rupture)	Rupture of the tympanic membrane

Swimmer's ear (**otitis externa**) is caused by moisture in the auditory canal and can occur from water trapped after swimming, showering, etc. It is treated by antibiotics.

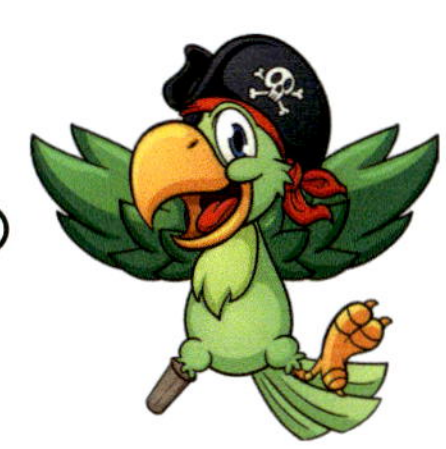

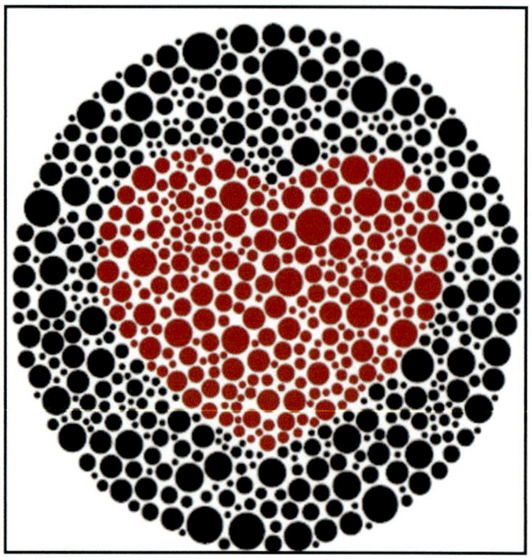

Figure 14-10. Example of a test for color blindness. (Portokalis/shutterstock.com)

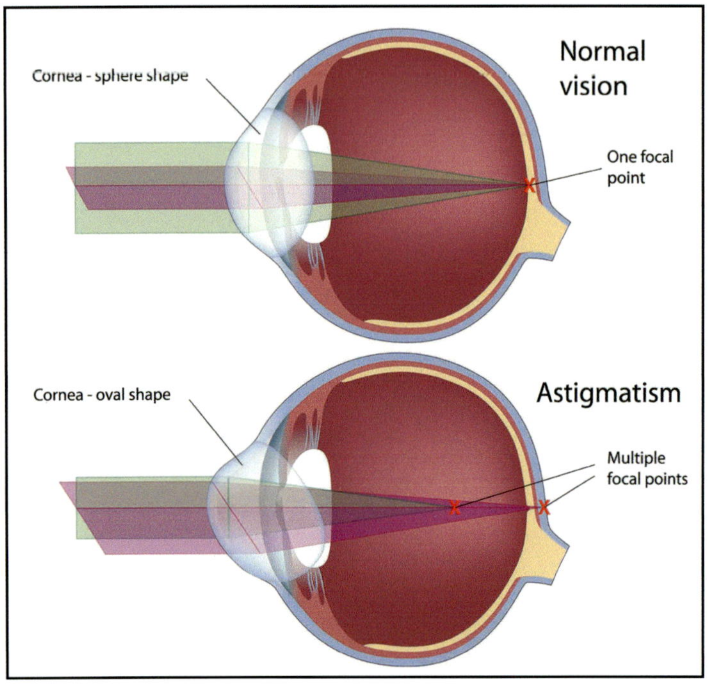

Figure 14-11. Astigmatism. (Alila Medical Images/shutterstock.com)

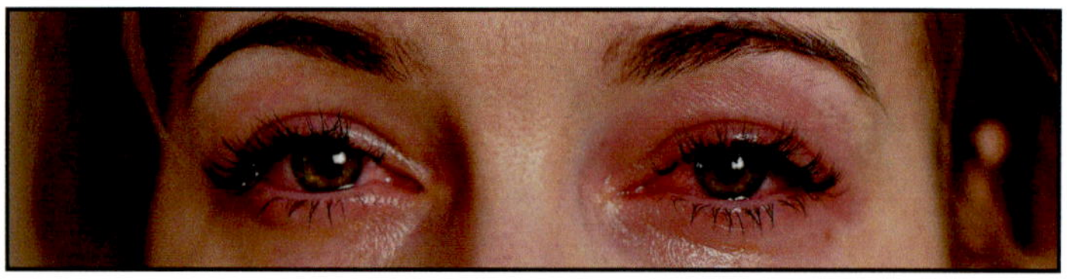

Figure 14-12. A red, weepy eye is a sign of conjunctivitis. (DROPERDER/shutterstock.com)

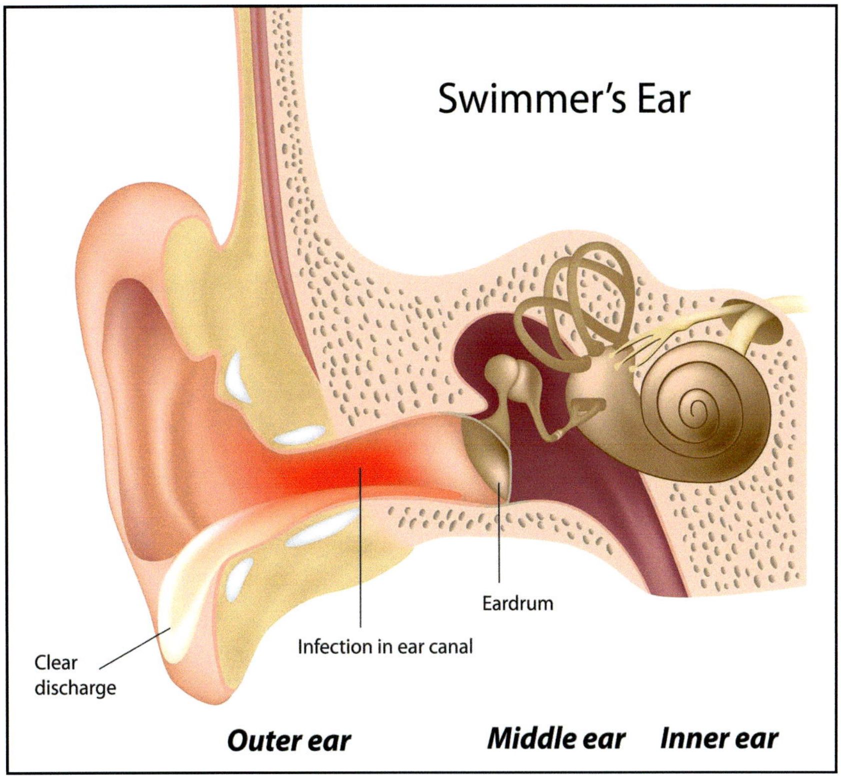

Figure 14-13. Otitis externa is another name for swimmer's ear. (Alila Medical Images/shutterstock.com)

Figure 14-14. Otitis media is common among children. (Alila Medical Images/shutterstock.com)

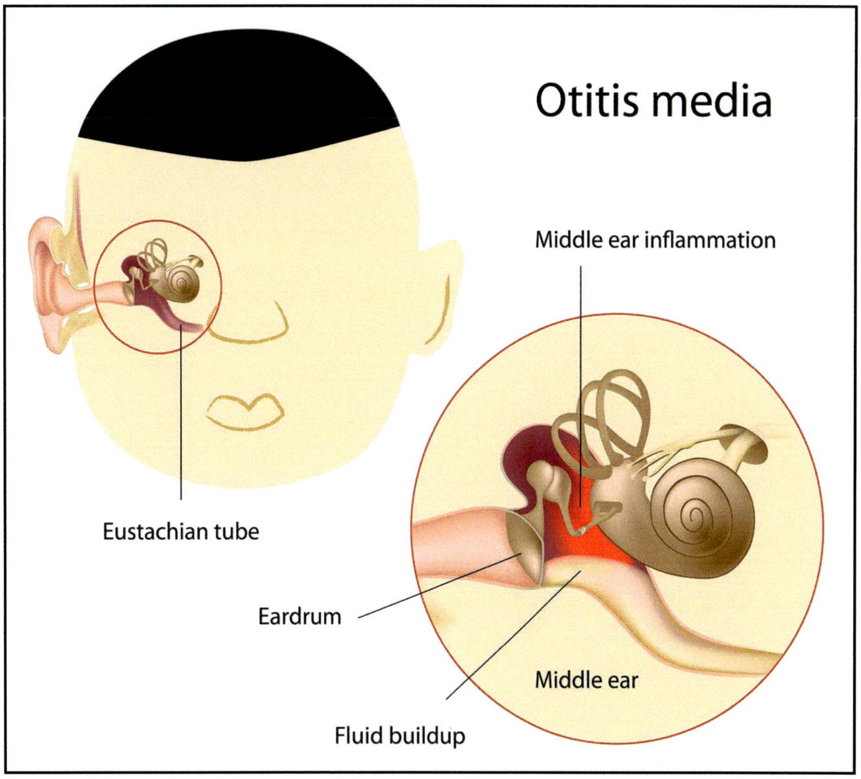

Figure 14-15. Tympanorrhexis. (Alila Medical Images/shutterstock.com)

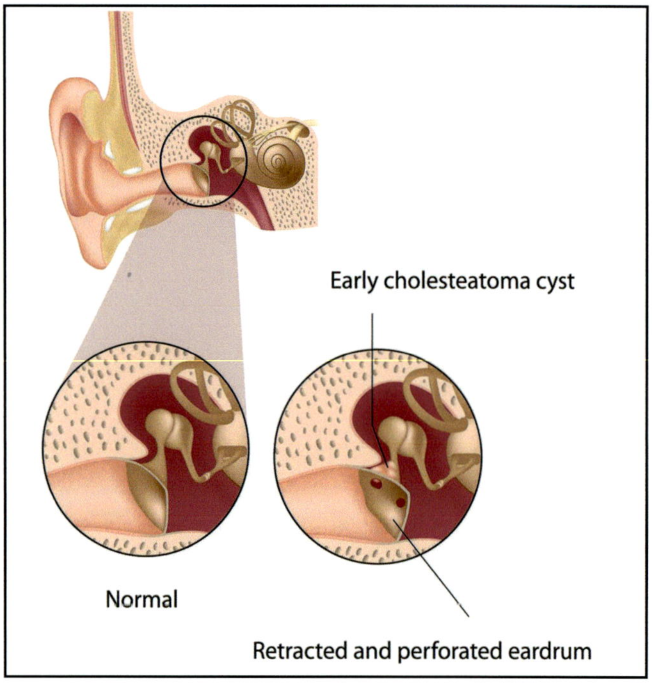

Table 14-6 Terms Related to Senses Without Medical Parts	
TERM	**DEFINITION**
cataract (Figure 14-16)	Loss of transparency of the lens
cauliflower ear (Figure 14-17)	Deformity on the pinna caused by friction, such as wrestling without ear guards; also termed *wrestler's badge*
epistaxis (Figure 14-18)	Nosebleed
glaucoma (Figure 14-19)	Vision loss due to increased intraocular pressure, which causes damage to the optic nerve
hordeolum	Infection of a sebaceous gland of the eyelash, causing localized eyelid swelling; also called a *stye*
macular degeneration (Figure 14-20)	Progressive degeneration of the retina
Ménière's disease	Chronic inner ear disease resulting in tinnitus and vertigo
nystagmus	Involuntary rhythmic movements of the eye
pterygium	Abnormal fibrous tissue between the cornea and conjunctiva
scotoma	Abnormal blind area in otherwise normal vision
strabismus (Figure 14-21)	Muscular eye weakness causing eye misalignment. The most common are: • Exotropia (one eye looking outward) • Esotropia (one eye looking inward)
tinnitus	Ringing or buzzing in the ear
vertigo	Dizziness (often due to an inner ear condition)

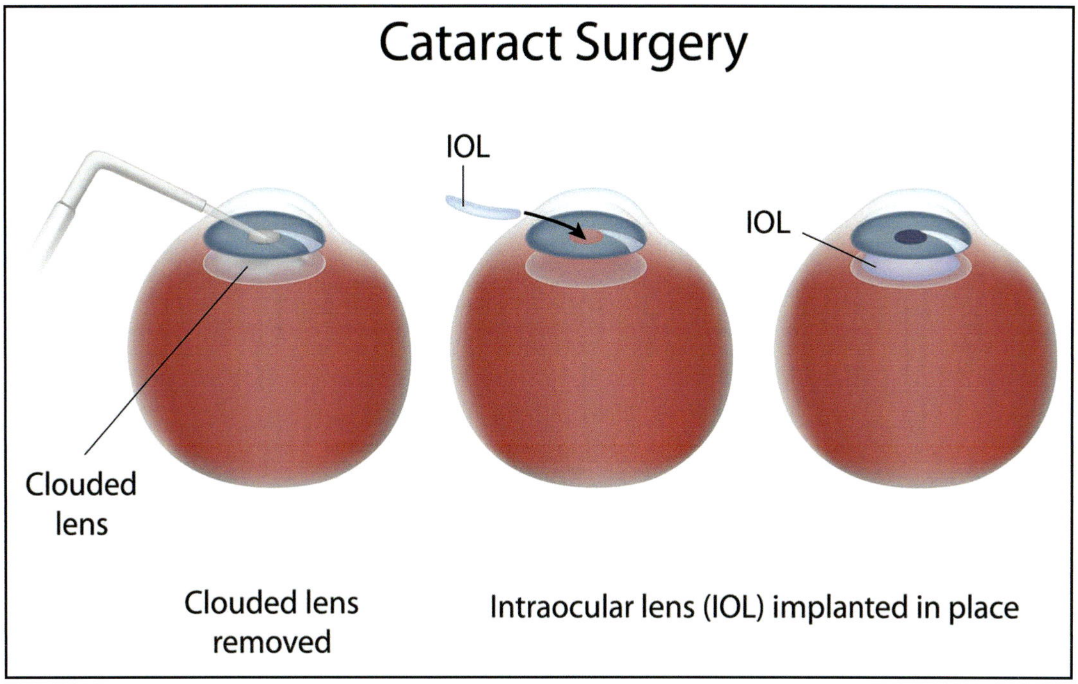

Figure 14-16. Cataract. (Alila Medical Images/shutterstock.com)

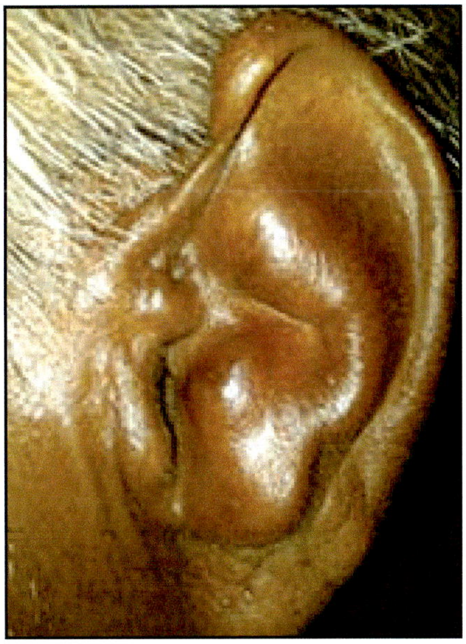

Figure 14-17. Notice the scarring of cauliflower ear on the left ear. (Featureflash/shutterstock.com)

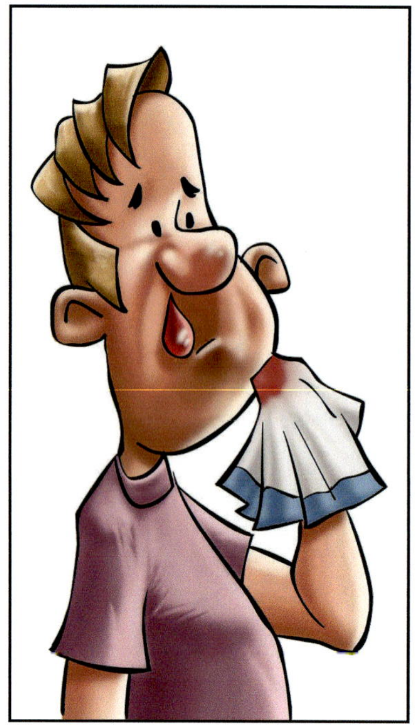

Figure 14-18. An epistaxis is a nosebleed. (Davi Sales Batista/shutterstock.com)

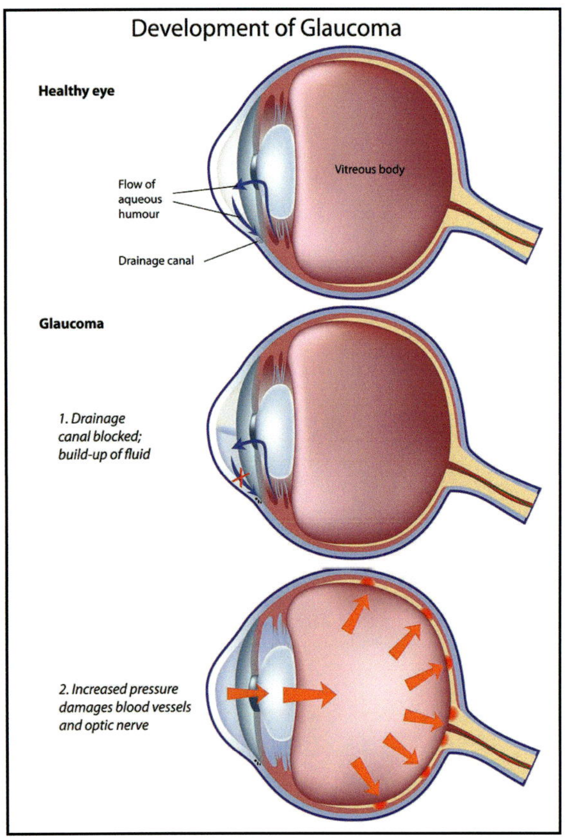

Figure 14-19. Glaucoma. (Alila Medical Images/shutterstock.com)

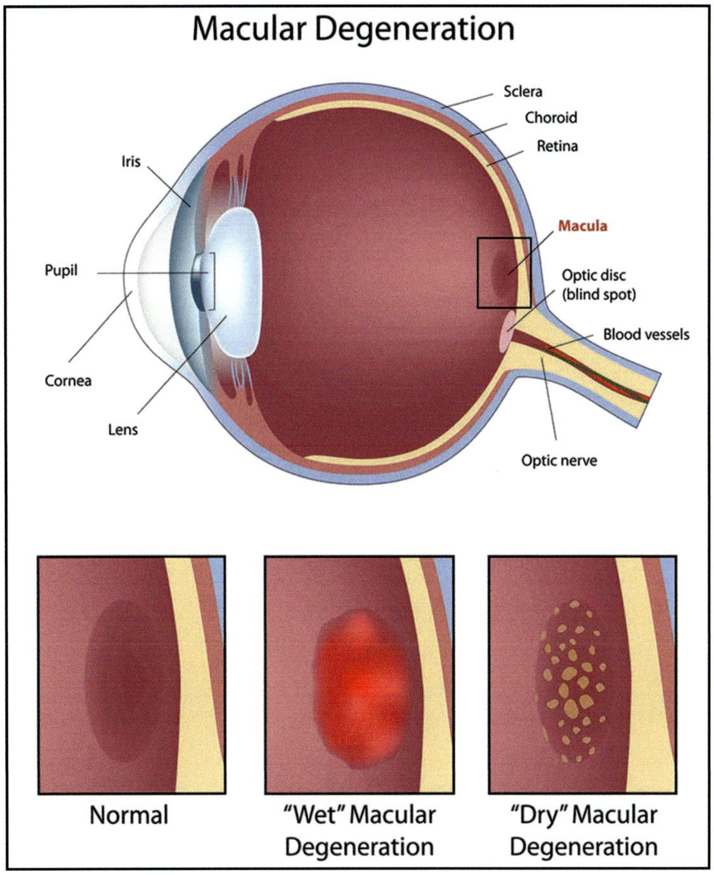

Figure 14-20. Different forms of macular degeneration. (Alila Medical Images/shutterstock.com)

Figure 14-21. Different forms of strabismus. (Alila Medical Images/shutterstock.com)

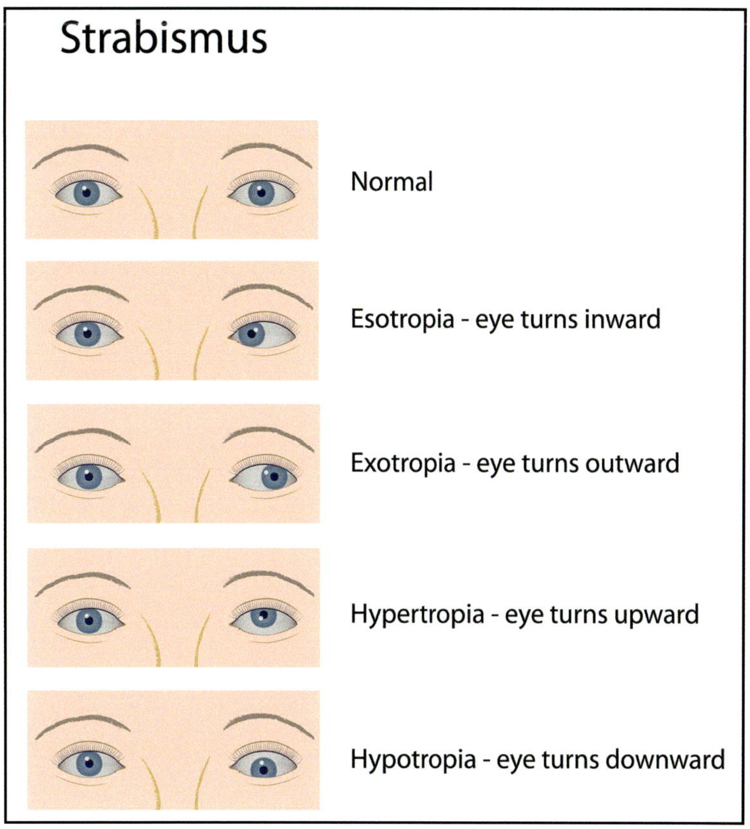

Tests and Procedures

Table 14-7 Tests and Procedures Related to the Sensory System		
NAME	**WORD PARTS**	**PURPOSE**
acoumetry	acous/ (hearing) **-metry** (measurement of)	Hearing test to measure sound ranges
audiogram	audi/o (hearing) **-gram** (a record of)	Record of the measurement of hearing; an audiometer is used to perform this test
audiometry	audi/o (hearing) **-metry** (measurement of)	Test to determine the range of intensity (in decibels) and frequency (hertz) in hearing a person can distinguish
fluorescein stain	fluor/ (luminous)	Fluorescent dye applied to the eyeball to view corneal abrasions or ulcers
keratometry	kerat/o (cornea) **-metry** (measurement of)	Measurement of corneal curvature
ophthalmoscope	ophthalm/o (eye) **-scope** (an instrument used to view or inspect)	Instrument used to view the internal structures of the eye
ophthalmodynamometry	ophthalm/o (eye) dynam/o (force; energy) **-metry** (measurement of)	Measurement of the blood pressure in the retinal vessels of the eye
otoscope (Figure 14-22)	ot/o (ear) **-scope** (an instrument used to view or inspect)	Instrument used to view the tympanic membrane of the ear
rhinoscopy	rhin/o (nose) **-scopy** (examination of)	Visual examination of the nose with a rhinoscope
tonometer	ton/o (pressure) **-metry** (measurement of)	Instrument used to measure the intraocular pressure for glaucoma
tympanometer	tympan/o (typmanic membrane) **-meter** (an instrument used to measure)	Instrument used to measure the movement of the tympanic membrane; good indicator of middle ear pressure
visual acuity test (Figure 14-23)		Assessment of vision based on norms; a visual acuity chart is used to determine distance eyesight

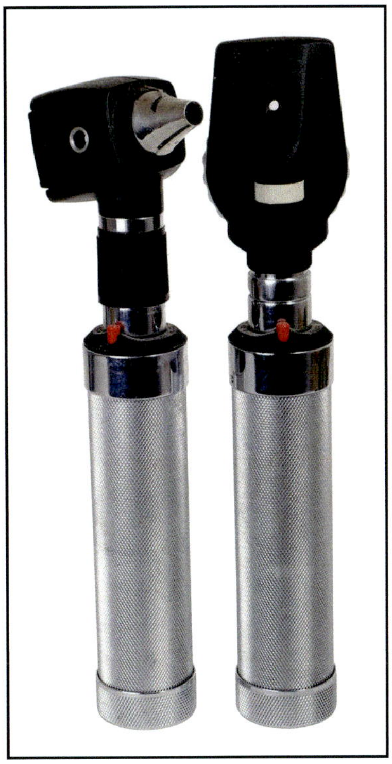

Figure 14-22. Otoscope on left, ophthalmoscope on right. (Nancy Hixson/shutterstock.com)

A WORD ABOUT VISION

What does 20/20 mean? Using a **Snellen chart** (or similar device), a person stands 20 feet from it and, using one eye at a time, reads aloud the letters/numbers on the chart. 20/20 means the person can read from 20 feet what a person with normal vision can also read from 20 feet. 20/200 indicates a person can read from 20 feet what a person with normal vision can read from 200 feet. 20/200 is legal blindness.

Figure 14-23. A Snellen visual acuity chart. (Hibrida/shutterstock.com)

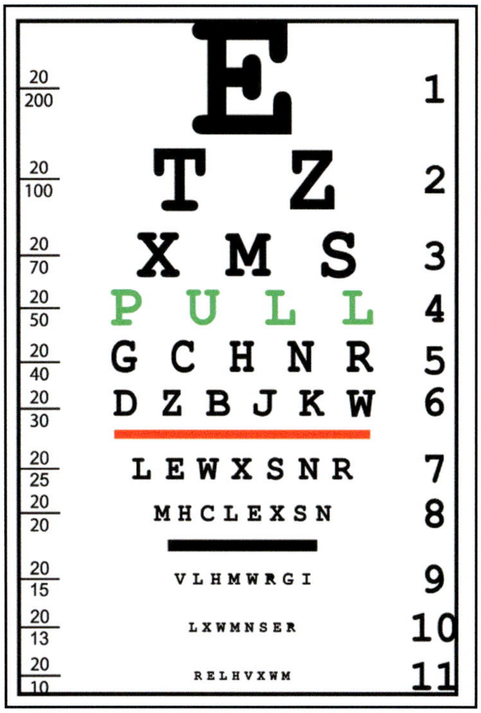

Table 14-8
Surgical Procedures Related to the Sensory System

NAME	WORD PARTS	PURPOSE
blepharoplasty	blephar/o (eyelid) **-plasty** (plastic surgery)	Surgical repair/plastic surgery of the eyelid
cochlear implant	cochle/ (cochlea) **-ar** (pertaining to)	Implanted external device that converts sound waves to magnetic impulses picked up by the vestibularcochlear nerve
cryoretinopexy	cry/o (cold) retin/o (retina) **-pexy** (surgical fixation of)	Surgical fixation of the retina using cold
enucleation	nucle/ (nucleus) **-ation** (process of)	Removal of an eyeball from its orbit (note that Skully has enucleation)
intraocular lens transplant	**intra-** (inside) ocul/ (eye) **-ar** (pertaining to)	Replacing a defective lens with an artificial one
iridosclerotomy	irid/o (iris) scler/o (sclera) **-tomy** (incision)	Incision into the iris and sclera
iridotomy	irid/o (iris) **-tomy** (incision; to cut into)	Incision into the iris to allow the anterior chamber to equalize pressure; often a treatment for glaucoma
keratoplasty	kerat/o (cornea) **-plasty** (reconstruction; repair; plastic surgery)	Corneal transplant
labyrinthectomy	labyrinth/ (labyrinth) **-ectomy** (excision)	Excision of the labyrinth from the ear
lacrimotomy	lacrim/o (tear gland) **-tomy** (incision)	Incision into the lacrimal gland
laser-assisted in situ keratomileusis (LASIK) (Figure 14-24)	kerat/o (cornea) **-sis** (state of; condition)	Using a laser to resurface the cornea to correct visual acuity
mastoidectomy	mast/ (breast) **-oid** (resembling) **-ectomy** (excision)	Excision of the mastoid process of the temporal bone; performed to treat nonresponsive otitis media
myringoplasty	myring/o (tympanic membrane) **-plasty** (repair)	Surgical repair of the tympanic membrane

(continued)

Table 14-8 (continued)

Surgical Procedures Related to the Sensory System

NAME	WORD PARTS	PURPOSE
myringotomy	myring/o (tympanic membrane) **-tomy** (incision)	Incision into the tympanic membrane
otoplasty	ot/o (ear) **-plasty** (plastic surgery)	Surgical repair or plastic surgery on the external ear
phacoemulsification	phac/o (lens) **-ation** (process of)	Using ultrasound to break up (emulsify) cataracts; the smaller portions are then removed
photorefractive keratectomy (PRK) (Figure 14-25)	phot/o (light) kerat/ (cornea) **-ectomy** (excision)	Corrective measure for those with myopia using a laser to flatten the cornea
radial keratotomy (RK)	kerat/o (cornea) **-tomy** (incision)	Corrective measure for those with myopia involving cutting spoke-like incisions in the cornea to flatten it
rhinoplasty	rhin/o (nose) **-plasty** (plastic surgery)	Surgical repair (plastic surgery) of the nose
salpingotomy	salping/o (eustachian tube) **-tomy** (incision)	Incision into the eustachian tube
stapedectomy	staped/ (stapes) **-ectomy** (excision)	Excision of the stapes bone in the inner ear
strabotomy	strab/o (squinting) **-tomy** (incision)	Incisions into one or more of the eye muscles to correct crossed eyes (strabismus)
tympanoplasty	tympan/o (tympanic membrane) **-plasty** (repair)	Surgical repair of the tympanic membrane
tympanotomy	tympan/o (tympanic membrane) **-tomy** (incision)	Incision into the tympanic membrane; often to place tubes in children to equalize pressure on both sides of the eardrum

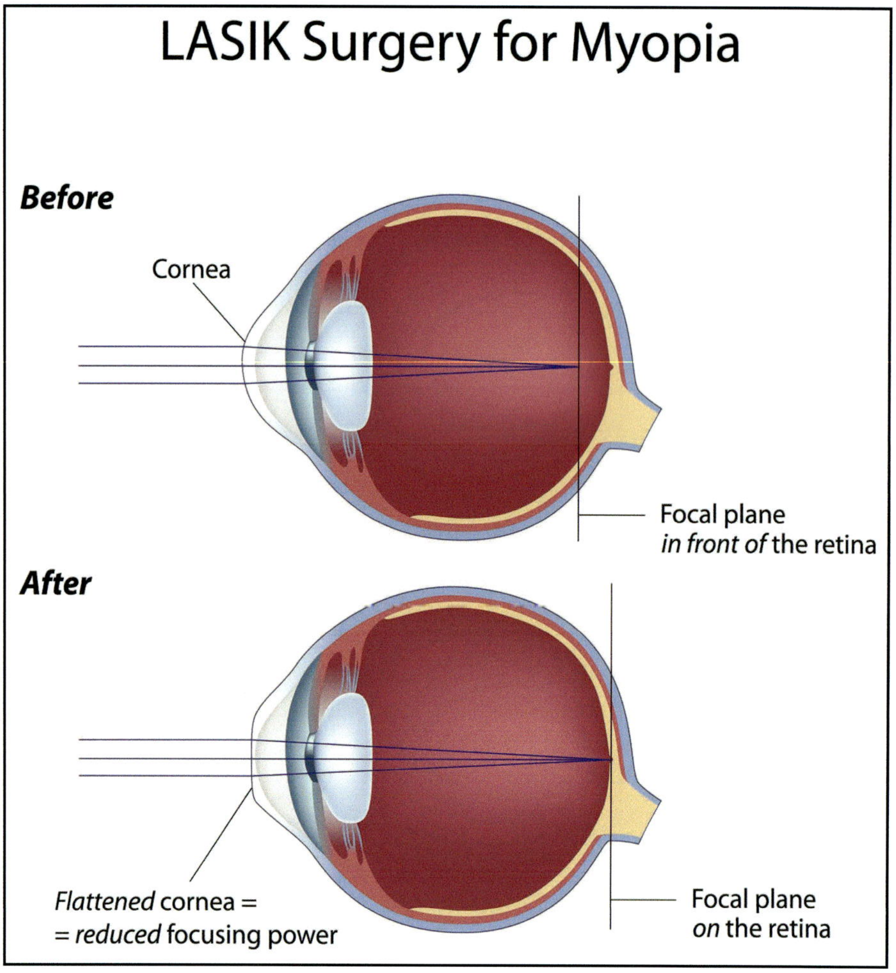

Figure 14-24. LASIK surgery for visual correction. (Alila Medical Images/shutterstock.com)

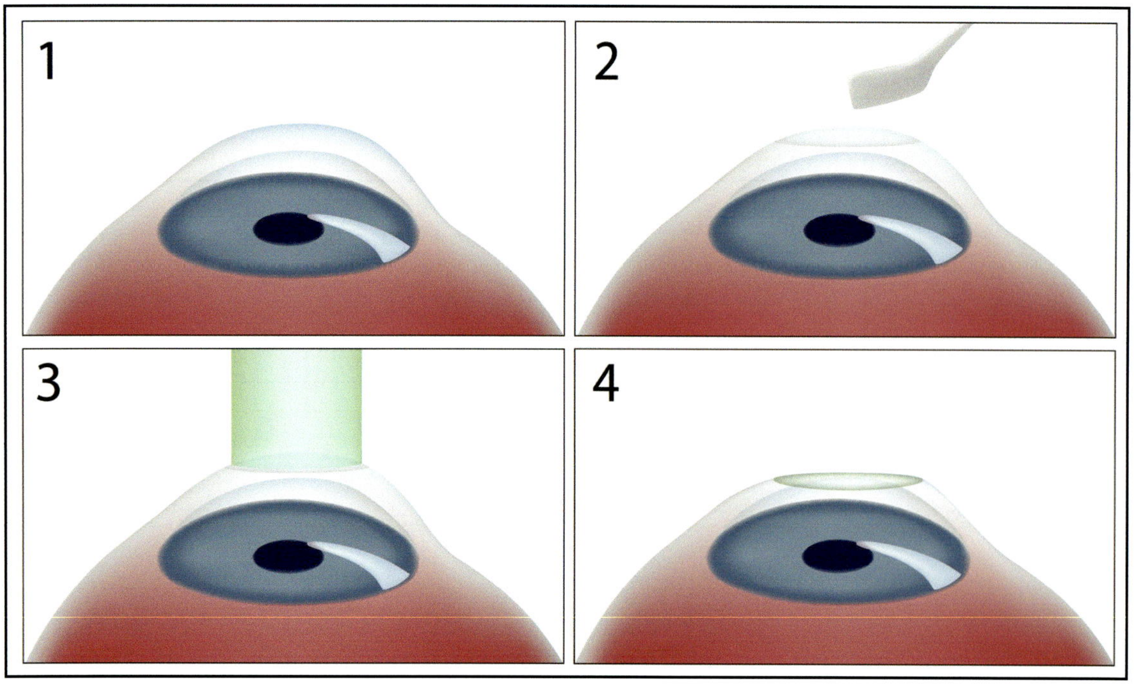

Figure 14-25. Photorefractive keratectomy surgery for visual acuity. (Alila Medical Media/shutterstock.com)

Medication Classifications

Table 14-9 Medication Classifications Used in Treatment of Sensory Conditions	
CATEGORY	**WHAT IT DOES**
anesthetic ophthalmic solution	Relief of eye pain
antibiotic ophthalmic solution	Treatment of bacterial conditions of the eye
antibiotic otic solution	Treatment for otitis media
antiglaucoma medication	Reduces intraocular pressure
antiemetics	Treats nausea (vertigo can cause nausea)
anti-inflammatory otic solution	Reduces inflammation, itching, and edema caused by otitis externa
miotic solution	Constricts the pupil
mydriatic solution	Dilates the pupil
ophthalmic decongestants	Reduces eye redness and itching by constricting ocular arterioles
wax emulsifiers	Softens earwax to prevent buildup in the external auditory canal

Bibliography

Allan D. *Medical Language for Modern Health Care.* 4th ed. McGraw-Hill; 2019.
Basco R, Allan B. *Medical Language for Modern Health Care.* 5th ed. McGraw-Hill; 2023.
Cohen BJ, Jones SA. *Medical Terminology: An Illustrated Guide.* 9th ed. Jones & Bartlett; 2021.
Flanagan KW, Cuppett M. Ear, nose, throat and mouth. In *Medical Conditions in the Athlete.* 3rd ed. Human Kinetics; 2017.
Flanagan KW, Cuppett M. The eye. In *Medical Conditions in the Athlete.* 3rd ed. Human Kinetics; 2017.
Fremgen BF, Frucht SS. *Medical Terminology: A Living Language.* 7th ed. Pearson; 2019.
McCance KL, Huether SE. *Pathophysiology: The Biologic Basis for Disease in Adults and Children.* 8th ed. Mosby; 2019.
Mosby's Dictionary of Medicine, Nursing & Health Professions. 10th ed. Elsevier; 2017.
Shiland BJ. *Mastering Healthcare Terminology.* 6th ed. Elsevier; 2019.
Venes D, ed. *Taber's Cyclopedic Medical Dictionary.* 24th ed. F. A. Davis; 2021.

NOTES

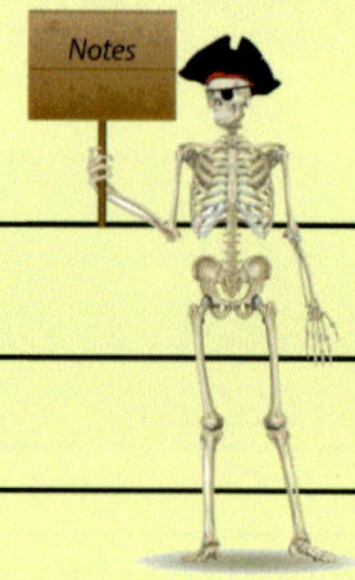

NOTES

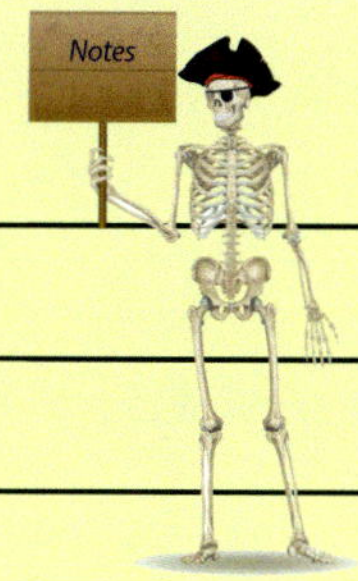

Learning Activities

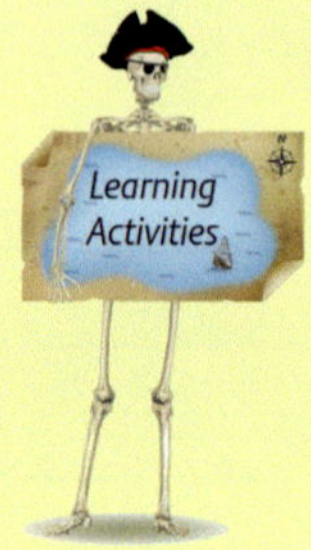

Name:______________________

Sensory System

A. Label the components of the eye from the following list of words.

- iris______________________
- optic nerve________________
- retina____________________
- cornea___________________
- sclera____________________
- ciliary muscle______________
- pupil_____________________
- anterior chamber___________

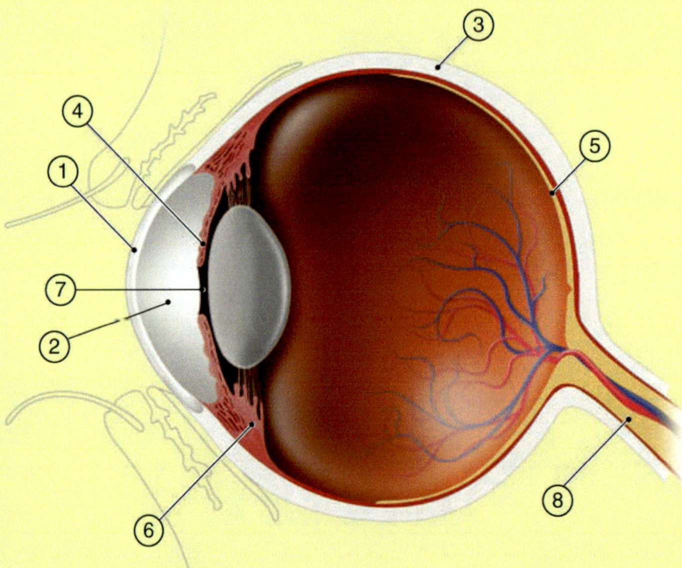

(kocakayaali/shutterstock.com)

B. Label the components of the nose from the following list of words.

- frontal sinus______________________
- eustachian tube opening______________
- superior turbinate__________________
- nasopharnyx______________________
- inferior turbinate__________________
- nasal cavity______________________
- middle turbinate___________________
- naris____________________________

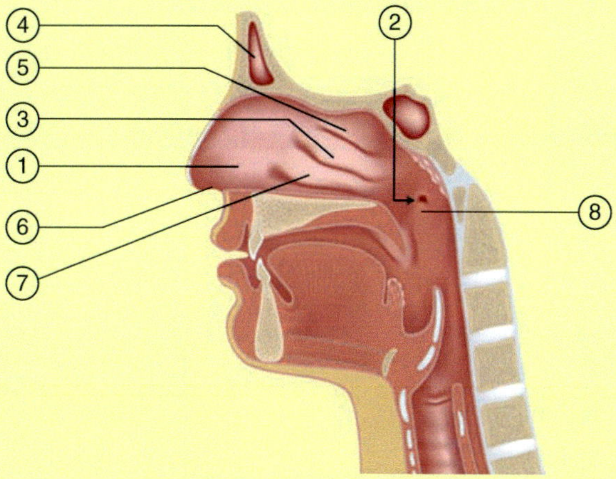

(Alila Medical Images/shutterstock.com)

C. Place the following terms for the ear in the proper order, from the external ear inward.

- cochlea______________________________
- stapes_______________________________
- tympanic membrane_____________________
- pinna________________________________
- external auditory canal_________________
- oval window__________________________
- incus________________________________
- vestibulocochlear nerve (CN VIII)__________
- malleus______________________________

D. Match the word element with its best meaning.

1. **-oid**______________	a. hearing
2. **-rrhexis**___________	b. dull; dim
3. ambly/o____________	c. rupture
4. **eso-**______________	d. vision condition
5. blephar/o___________	e. resembling
6. dacry/o____________	f. hearing
7. **-cusis**____________	g. eyelid
8. nyct/i______________	h. inward
9. aur/o______________	i. night
10. **-opsia**____________	j. tear; lacrimal duct/gland

E. Word building: Using the word part, add the other word element and define the new word created.

1. **-itis**
   a. scler/o + kerat/____________________________
   b. rhin/____________________________
   c. phot/o + retin/____________________________
   d. conjunctiv/____________________________
   e. ot/____________________________
2. **ot/o**
   a. **-itis** + media____________________________
   b. **-rrhagia**____________________________
   c. scler/ + **-osis**____________________________
   d. **-plasty**____________________________
   e. **-lith**____________________________

F. Separate the word elements of the following terms and define them.

1. ophthalmalgia____________________________
2. aqueous____________________________
3. extraocular____________________________
4. otorhinolaryngology____________________________
5. corneal____________________________
6. anesthetic ophthalmic solution____________________________
7. binaural____________________________
8. leukocoria____________________________
9. stapedectomy____________________________
10. rhinosalpingitis____________________________

G. What are the medical words for the following?

1. ear pain____________________________
2. normal vision____________________________
3. discharge of pus from the ear____________________________
4. plastic surgery on the nose____________________________
5. hardening of the ear____________________________

H. Using the medical condition strabismus, what are the terms for the following?

1. one eye looking inward____________________________
2. one eye looking outward____________________________

Case Study

Define the numerical terms (1 to 10) and draw the alphabetical terms (A to D) on the anatomy figure..
For assistance with medical abbreviations, refer to Appendix A.

History, Chief Complaint

A male rodeo athlete (bull rider) came to the first aid tent complaining of **diplopia** (1) and **HA** (2) following his last ride on a bull named *Insanity*. He explained that Insanity threw his head back as the rider was falling forward, and his face hit Insanity's head. He did not recall if he had **LOC** (3) or not.

Evaluation

The bull rider had mild discoloration where Insanity hit him. He had **rhinorrhea** (4), and **PERRLA** (5) was **WNL** (6). His eye **ROM** (7) was normal with the exception of the inability to look up with his right eye. He complained of numbness over his right **zygoma** (A), and had no pain and normal sensation over the **nasal bone** (B), **maxilla** (C), and **mandible** (D). He did not have **nystagmus** (8), **tinnitus** (9), or **vertigo** (10).

Diagnostic Studies

A CT was ordered and revealed a right orbital blowout fracture. He had surgery to place a plate in the floor of the orbit and returned to bull riding 2 months later.

Terms

1. ______________________
2. ______________________
3. ______________________
4. ______________________
5. ______________________
6. ______________________
7. ______________________
8. ______________________
9. ______________________
10. ______________________

Anatomy

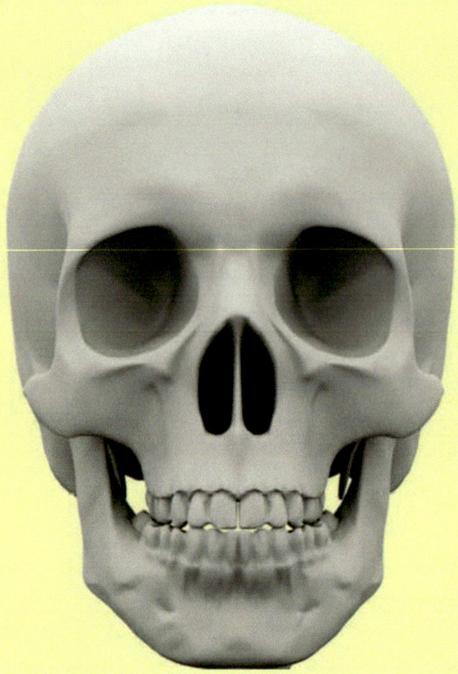

Section III

Appendices

A

Medical Abbreviations

Why Medical Abbreviations Are Used

Medical abbreviations are widely recognized shortcuts to the written medical record. The next time you see a prescription written for medications, look at it carefully (Figure A-1). For example, a drug that is to be taken once daily has "od" written by the physician on the prescription, which is then taken (or delivered electronically) to a pharmacist. Another abbreviation, qid, tells the pharmacist to produce a label that instructs the patient to take the medication four times per day. The abbreviations allow the prescribing health care provider to be clear while not spending time writing out long instructions to the pharmacist.

Flanagan KW.
Medical Terminology With Case Studies: A Navigated Guide to Learning for Health Care Professionals, Third Edition (pp 439-453).

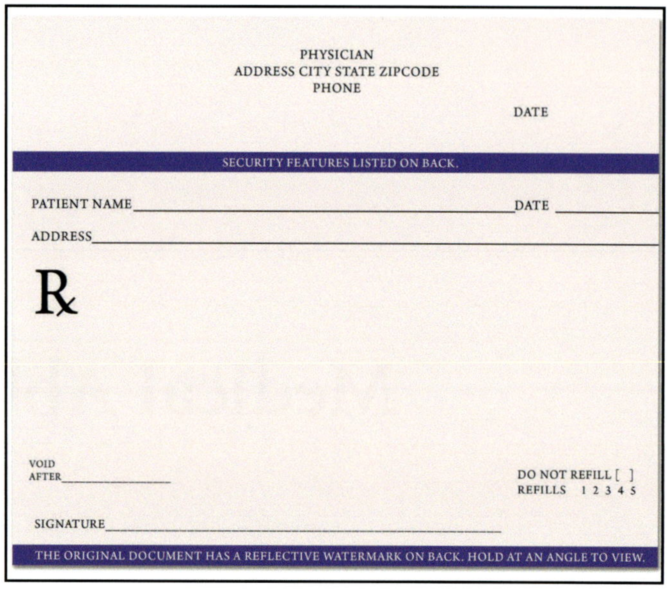

Figure A-1. Medical abbreviations assist physicians when communicating clearly with pharmacists regarding patient's instructions for taking medications.

Many health care providers use medical abbreviations as a means to chart information and inform others working with the same patient about their condition or status. Athletic trainers are health care providers who work with active people, including athletes. Often they use medical abbreviations to discuss any therapy, exercises, or improvement in their patient's progress.

Some practices/facilities create abbreviations unique to their setting; for example, *RTP* is a common abbreviation in athletic training that denotes "return to play/participation." It is merely a shortened way to communicate without having to write the entire word long hand. Symbols or abbreviations unique to a setting or facility often find their way to other similar employment settings as employees share the information as they move between jobs. In this appendix, only the most widely utilized medical abbreviations are provided.

Pay attention to the capitalization of medical abbreviations.

PT is an abbreviation for physical therapist, whereas pt means patient.

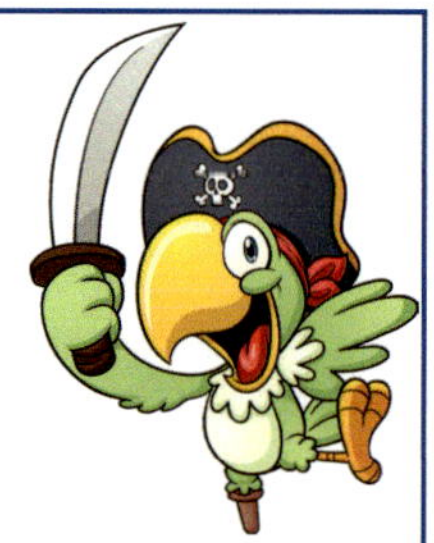

Common Medical Abbreviations and Symbols

The abbreviations listed in this appendix are not to be memorized, but to be a reference. As you progress through this text and in your career, many of these shortened terms will make their way into your daily vocabulary. If you watch medical dramas on television, many of these abbreviations are said throughout the show. In fact, watching such a show is a good way to determine if you are learning and understanding medical terminology. Throughout this text, you will see some of these abbreviations listed in this section.

NOTE: The information in the parentheses following the definition is a rough simplification of the term.	
A:	assessment
AAROM	active assistive range of motion
abd	abduction
ac	before meals
AC joint	acromioclavicular joint (a joint in the shoulder)
ACL	anterior cruciate ligament (knee)
ACTH	adrenocorticotropic hormone
A.D.	right ear (Latin: *auris dextra*)
AD	Alzheimer's disease
ad lib	at discretion
add	adduction
ADD	attention-deficit disorder
ADHD	attention-deficit/hyperactivity disorder
ADL	activities of daily living
adm	admission
ADR	adverse drug reaction
AE	above the elbow
AED	automatic external defibrillator
AFO	ankle-foot orthosis
AIDS	acquired immunodeficiency syndrome
AIIS	anterior inferior iliac spine (on the pelvic bone)
AJ	ankle jerk (a reflex)
AK	above the knee; actinic keratosis
ALL	acute lymphocytic leukemia
ALS	amyotrophic lateral sclerosis (Lou Gehrig's disease)
a.m.	morning
AMA	against medical advice; American Medical Association
amb	ambulate, ambulatory
AMD	age-related macular degeneration (an eye disorder)
AMI	acute myocardial infarction (heart attack)
AML	acute myelogenous leukemia
ANS	autonomic nervous system
ant	anterior
AP	anterior-posterior
A&P	auscultation and percussion (using a stethoscope)
ARC	AIDS-related complex
AROM	active range of motion
A.S.	left ear (Latin: *auris sinister*)
ASA	acetylsalicylic acid (aspirin)
ASAP	as soon as possible
	(continued)

NOTE: The information in the parentheses following the definition is a rough simplification of the term.	
ASIS	anterior superior iliac spine (on the pelvic bone)
ASL	American Sign Language
assist.	assistance
AT	athletic trainer (credentialed health care provider); athletic training
AU	both ears (Latin: *auris uterque*)
A&W	alive and well
AV node	atrioventricular node
BBB	blood-brain barrier
BCC	basal cell carcinoma
BCP	birth control pills
BE	barium enema; below elbow
bid; b.i.d.	twice per day
bilat	bilaterally (both sides)
BK	below the knee
BKA	below-the-knee amputation
BM	bowel movement
BMD	bone mineral density
BMI	body mass index (a measure of body fat based on height and weight)
BMR	basal metabolic rate
BMT	bone marrow transplantation
BP	blood pressure
BPH	benign prostatic hyperplasia
bpm	beats per minute (heart)
BRP	bathroom privileges
bs	blood sugar; breath sounds
BS	beside
BSE	breast self-examination
BT	bleeding time
bw; BW	birth weight
Bx; bx	biopsy
C	Centigrade; carbon; calorie
C°	degrees Celsius
C1, C2, etc	first cervical vertebra, second cervical vertebra, etc (cervical = neck)
Ca	calcium (also written as Ca^{2+})
CA	cancer; carcinoma
CABG	coronary artery bypass graft
CAD	coronary artery disease (in the heart)
Cap	capsule
CAPD	continuous ambulatory peritoneal dialysis
Cath	catheter; catheterization
	(continued)

NOTE: The information in the parentheses following the definition is a rough simplification of the term.	
CBC	complete blood count
cc	cubic centimeter
CC; C/C	chief complaint
CCU	critical care unit; coronary care unit
CDC	Centers for Disease Control and Prevention
CF	cystic fibrosis
CHD	coronary/chronic heart disease
chemo	chemotherapy
CHF	congestive heart failure
Chol	cholesterol
chr	chronic
CIS	carcinoma in situ (pertaining to cancer)
CLL	chronic lymphocytic leukemia
CML	chronic myelogenous leukemia
CNS	central nervous system (the brain and spinal cord)
CO	carbon monoxide
CO_2	carbon dioxide
c/o	complains of
COLD	chronic obstructive lung disease
cont.	continue
COPD	chronic obstructive pulmonary disease
CP	cerebral palsy; chest pain
CPAP	continuous positive airway pressure
CPM	continuous passive movement (a machine that moves joints)
CPR	cardiopulmonary resuscitation
CRPS	complex regional pain syndrome
CPT	Current Procedural Terminology
C-section	Cesarean section (non-vaginal birth)
CSF	cerebrospinal fluid
C-spine	cervical vertebra (usually x-rays)
ct.	count
CT scan	computed tomography scan
CTS	carpal tunnel syndrome (in the wrist)
CV	cardiovascular (heart and vessels)
CVA	cerebrovascular accident (stroke)
CVS	chorionic villus sampling
c/w	consistent with; compare with
CWI	crutch walking instructions
D/C; D/c	discontinue
D&C	dilatation and curettage
	(continued)

NOTE: The information in the parentheses following the definition is a rough simplification of the term.	
DCIS	ductal carcinoma in situ (cancer in a duct)
Dd	differential diagnosis (two or more conditions that have similar signs/symptoms)
DD	discharge diagnosis
DDS	doctor of dental surgery
D&E	dilation and evacuation
DIP; DIPJ	distal interphalangeal joint (pertaining to fingers and toes)
DM	diabetes mellitus
DNR	do not resuscitate
DO	doctor of osteopathy
DOA	dead on arrival
DOB	date of birth
DOE	dyspnea on exertion (difficulty breathing with exercise)
DRE	digital rectal examination
DTR	deep tendon reflexes
DVT	deep vein thrombosis (blood clot in a vein)
Dx	diagnosis
EBV	Epstein-Barr virus (cause of mononucleosis and other disorders)
ECF	extended care facility
ECG; EKG	electrocardiogram (electrical recording of the heart)
ECHO	echocardiogram (recording of the heart using sound waves)
ED	emergency department; erectile dysfunction
EEG	electroencephalogram (electrical recording of the brain)
EENT	ears, eyes, nose, and throat
EGD	esophagogastroduodenoscopy
EIA	exercise-induced asthma
EMG	electromyogram (recording of electrical activity in muscles)
EMR	electronic medical record
EMS	electrical muscle stimulation
EMT	emergency medical technician
ENT	ears, nose, throat (otorhinolaryngologist)
EP	evoked potential
EPS	intracardiac electrophysiology study
ER	emergency room
ERT	estrogen replacement therapy
ETT	exercise tolerance test
eval.	evaluation
ext.	extension (of a joint)
F	fair (muscle strength, balance)
F°	degrees Fahrenheit
FB	foreign body
	(continued)

NOTE: The information in the parentheses following the definition is a rough simplification of the term.	
FBS	fasting blood sugar
FDA	US Food and Drug Administration
FEV^1	forced expiratory volume (a test for lung capacity)
FH	family history
FHR	fetal heart rate
flex	flexion
FROM	full range of motion
FSH	follicle-stimulating hormone
ft.	foot (measurement)
F/U	follow up
FUO	fever, unknown origin
FWB	full weight bearing
Fx; fx	fracture
G	gravida (pregnant)
G; gm	gram
GB	gallbladder
GBS	gallbladder series; Guillain-Barré syndrome
Gd	gadolinium (a dye [contrast agent] used in MRI scans)
GERD	gastroesophageal reflux disease (pertaining to the stomach and esophagus)
GI	gastrointestinal (pertaining to the digestive system; stomach and intestines)
GP	general practitioner (a physician)
GU	genitourinary (pertaining to the urinary system)
GYN; gyn	gynecology
h; hr.	hour
HA; H/A	headache
Hb; Hgb	hemoglobin (protein-iron in the blood)
HBOT	hyperbaric oxygen therapy
HBV	hepatitis B virus
hCG	human chorionic gonadotropin
HCL	hydrochloric acid
HCM	hypertrophic cardiomyopathy
HCV	hepatitis C virus
HCVD	hypertensive cardiovascular disease
HDL	high-density lipoprotein (blood cholesterol)
HEENT	head, eyes, ears, nose, and throat
HEP	home exercise program
H & H; H/H	hematocrit and hemoglobin (in the blood)
HI	head injury
HIPAA	Health Insurance Portability and Accountability Act (medical information privacy act)
HIV	human immunodeficiency virus

(continued)

NOTE: The information in the parentheses following the definition is a rough simplification of the term.	
HNP	herniated nucleus pulposus (a herniated disc)
h/o	history of
HOB	head of bed
H&P	history and physical
HPI	history of present illness
HPV	human papillomavirus (a virus that causes warts and other aliments)
hr	hour
HR	heart rate
HRT	hormone replacement therapy
hs	half strength
h.s.	at bedtime (Latin: *hora somni*)
HSV	herpes simplex virus
HSV-2	genital warts
ht.	height
Htn; HTN	hypertension (high blood pressure)
Hx	history
IBD	inflammatory bowel disease (gastrointestinal system)
IBS	irritable bowel syndrome
ICD	implantable cardioverter-defibrillator (automatically restarts the heart); *International Classification of Diseases*
ICP	intracranial pressure (within the skull)
ICU	intensive care unit
ID	infectious disease
I&D	incision and drainage
IHD	ischemic heart disease
IM	intramuscular
imp.	impression (a possible diagnosis)
in	inches
inf	inferior
I&O	intake and output
IQ	intelligence quotient
IUD	intrauterine device (a birth control device)
IV	intravenous
IVF	in vitro fertilization
IVP	intravenous pyelogram (a test of the urinary system)
K	potassium (K is the chemical symbol for potassium)
kg	kilogram
KJ	knee jerk (reflex)
KS	Kaposi's sarcoma
KUB	kidney, ureters, bladder

(continued)

NOTE: The information in the parentheses following the definition is a rough simplification of the term.	
Ⓛ	left
L1, L2, etc	first lumbar vertebra; second lumbar, etc (lumbar = bones in the low back)
lb	pound
LBP	low back pain
LCL	lateral collateral ligament (elbow, knee)
LDL	low-density lipoprotein
LE	lupus erythematosus; lower extremity
LES	lower esophageal sphincter
LH	luteinizing hormone
LLQ	left lower quadrant (abdomen)
LMP	last menstrual period
LOC	loss of consciousness
LOS	length of stay (hospital)
LP	lumbar puncture
LS	lumbosacral spine
LTC	long-term care
LUQ	left upper quadrant (abdomen)
LV	left ventricle (heart)
L&W	living and well
MA	mental age
max	maximum
MCL	medial collateral ligament (elbow, knee)
MD	medical doctor
MDI	metered-dose inhaler (for breathing disorders)
MDR	minimum daily requirement
ME	medical examiner
MG	myasthenia gravis (a condition involving chronic fatigue of the body)
MH	mental history; marital history
MI	myocardial infarction (heart attack)
MMR	measles–mumps–rubella vaccine
MMT	manual muscle testing
mod	moderate
MR	magnetic resonance; mitral regurgitation
MRA	magnetic resonance angiography
MRI	magnetic resonance imaging
MS	multiple sclerosis
MVP	mitral valve prolapse (in the heart)
N	normal
NA; N/A	not applicable
NB	newborn
	(continued)

NOTE: The information in the parentheses following the definition is a rough simplification of the term.	
NCHS	National Center for Human Statistics
NCS	nerve conduction study
ND	normal development; normal delivery (pertaining to birth)
NDT	neurodevelopment treatment (pertaining to the brain)
NED	no evidence of disease
neg.	negative
NG tube	nasogastric tube (from the nose to the stomach)
NH	nursing home
NHL	non-Hodgkin's lymphoma
NICU	neonatal intensive care unit (intensive care for infants)
NKA	no known allergies
NKDA	no known drug allergies
noc	at night
NPO; npo	nothing by mouth
NSAID	nonsteroidal anti-inflammatory drug
NSR	normal sinus rhythm (pertaining to the normal heart rate and SA node)
NWB	non–weight bearing
O; O_2	oxygen
OA	osteoarthritis
OB	obstetrics
OB/GYN	obstetrics and gynecology
OCD	obsessive-compulsive disorder
OCPs	oral contraceptive pills (birth control pills)
o.d.	right eye (Latin: *oculus dexter*)
O.D.	doctor of optometry
OD	overdose
OMT	osteopathic manipulative treatment
OR	operating room
ORIF	open reduction, internal fixation (one way to fix a fractured bone)
OS; o.s.	left eye (Latin: *oculus sinister*)
OT	occupational therapy; occupational therapist
OTC	over-the-counter medication (not requiring a prescription)
OU	both eyes (Latin: *oculus uterque*)
$\bar{p}$	after
P	posterior; pulse; pressure; pupil; poor
P:	plan
PA	physician assistant; posterior-anterior
P&A	percussion and auscultation
PAC	premature atrial contraction (of the heart)
PAD	peripheral arterial disease
	(continued)

NOTE: The information in the parentheses following the definition is a rough simplification of the term.	
palp.	palpation
PALS	pediatric advanced life support
Para	paraplegia (paralysis)
p.c.	after meals (Latin: *post cibum*)
PCR test	polymerase chain reaction test
PCOS	polycystic ovary syndrome
PD	peritoneal dialysis
PE	pulmonary embolism; physical education
per os	by mouth
PERRLA	pupils equally round and reactive to light and accommodation
PET scan	positron emission tomography scan (a scan for metabolic activity of tissues)
PFT	pulmonary function test
PH	past history
PI	present illness
PID	pelvic inflammatory disease
PIP; PIPJ	proximal interphalangeal joint (knuckle of the fingers and toes)
PMH	past medical history
PMS	premenstrual syndrome
PNF	proprioceptive neuromuscular facilitation (a stretching technique)
PNS	peripheral nervous system
PNI	peripheral nerve injury
PO; p.o.	by mouth
p/o	postoperative
POP	pain on palpation
pos	positive
poss.	possible
post	posterior
post-op	after surgery
PPI	proton pump inhibitor
PRE	progressive restive exercise
p.r.n.	as necessary
PRO	patient-reported outcomes
PROM	passive range of motion
PSIS	posterior superior iliac spine (on the pelvic bone)
pt	patient
PT	physical therapist; physical therapy
PTA	prior to admission
PTCA	percutaneous transluminal coronary angioplasty
PTSD	posttraumatic stress disorder
PU	pregnancy urine

(continued)

NOTE: The information in the parentheses following the definition is a rough simplification of the term.	
PVC	premature ventricular contraction (of the heart)
PVD	peripheral vascular disease
PWB	partial weight bearing
Px	prognosis; pneumothorax (collapsed lung)
NOTE: The abbreviations listed in the "Q" section as well as those with Latin meaning (eg, t.i.d, OD, and OS) have been recommended by The Joint Commission to be discontinued, as their intentions should be written out.	
q	every
q am	every morning
qd	every day
qh	every hour
q2h; q.2h.	every two hours
q3h; q.3h.	every three hours
qid	four times per day
qn	every night
Ⓡ	right
RA	rheumatoid arthritis
RAI	radioactive iodine
RAIU	radioactive iodine uptake
RBC	red blood cell; red blood count
RD; R.D.	registered dietician
RDDA	recommended daily dietary allowance
RDS	respiratory distress syndrome
re:	regarding
REM	rapid eye movement
reps	repetitions
resp	respiration; respiratory
RLQ	right lower quadrant (abdomen)
RN	registered nurse
R/O	rule out
ROM	range of motion
ROS	review of systems
RP	radical prostatectomy
RR	respiratory rate
RROM	resistive range of motion
RRR	regular rate and rhythm (heart)
R.T.	respiratory therapist; respiratory therapy
RUQ	right upper quadrant (abdomen)
Rx	prescription; treatment; therapy
$\bar{s}$	without
S1, S2, etc	first sacral vertebra, second sacral vertebra, etc (sacral = tailbone)
	(continued)

NOTE: The information in the parentheses following the definition is a rough simplification of the term.	
SA node	sinoatrial node (in the heart)
SAD	seasonal affective disorder
SARS	severe acute respiratory syndrome
SCC	squamous cell carcinoma
SCI	spinal cord injury
sec.	seconds
SI	sacroiliac joint (where the pelvis and spine meet)
SIDS	sudden infant death syndrome
SIRS	systemic inflammatory response syndrome
SLE	systemic lupus erythematosus
SLR	single leg raise; straight leg raise
SNF	skilled nursing facility
SOAP	subjective, objective, assessment, plan (one type of medical record)
SOB	shortness of breath
S/P	status post (following procedure, condition)
SPECT	single photon emission computed tomography
SQ	subcutaneous (under the skin)
S/S	signs and symptoms
SSCP	substernal chest pain (under the breast bone)
stat; STAT	immediately
STD	sexually transmitted disease
STI	sexually transmitted infection
subcu; sub-Q	subcutaneous (under the skin)
Sx	symptoms
Sz	seizure
T	trace (muscle strength); temperature; time
T1, T2, etc	first thoracic vertebra, second thoracic vertebra, etc (in the thorax)
tab	tablet
TB	tuberculosis
TBI	traumatic brain injury
TENS	transcutaneous electrical nerve stimulator
THR	total hip replacement
TIA	transient ischemic attack (mini stroke)
tid; t.i.d.	three times per day
TKR	total knee replacement
TLC	total lung capacity
TM	tympanic membrane (eardrum)
TMJ	temporomandibular joint
TNR	tonic neck reflex
t.o.	telephone order
	(continued)

NOTE: The information in the parentheses following the definition is a rough simplification of the term.	
TPR	temperature, pulse, and respiration
TSE	testicular self-examination
TSE	testicular self-examination
TSH	thyroid-stimulating hormone
TSS	toxic shock syndrome
TUIP	transurethral incision of the prostate
TURP	transurethral resection of the prostate
Tx	treatment
UA	urinalysis; unstable angina (chest pain)
UAO	upper airway obstruction
UC	uterine contraction
UE	upper extremity
UES	upper esophageal sphincter
UG	urogenital
UGI	upper gastrointestinal
umb.	umbilicus
UMN	upper motor neuron
URI	upper respiratory infection (eg, a sinus infection)
US	ultrasound
UTI	urinary tract infection
UV	ultraviolet
VA	visual acuity
VATS	video-assisted thoracic surgery
VC	vital capacity (lungs)
VD	venereal disease (same as STD/STI)
VF	ventricular fibrillation; visual field
v.o.	verbal orders
V/S; v.s.; vs	vital signs
VSD	ventricular septal defect (of the heart)
VT	ventricular tachycardia (of the heart)
WBC	white blood cell; white blood count
w/c	wheelchair
W/cm^2	watts per centimeters squared (ultrasound)
WDWN	well developed; well nourished
WHO	World Health Organization
wk	week
WNL	within normal limits

(continued)

NOTE: The information in the parentheses following the definition is a rough simplification of the term.	
w/o	without
wt	weight
x	number of times performed (x2 = twice)
XRT	radiation therapy
y/o	years old

Symbols

♂	male	<	less than
♀	female	=	equal
↓	down; downward; decreased; diminished	+; (+)	plus; positive
↑	up; upward; increased	−; (−)	minus; negative
c̄	with	#	number; pounds
s̄	without	/	per
p̄	after	+; &	and
ā	before	1°	primary
~	approximately	2°	secondary; secondary to
@	at	Ⓡ	right
Δ	change	Ⓛ	left
>	greater than		

Bibliography

Kettenback G, Schlomer SL, Fitzgerald, J. *Writing Patient/Client Notes: Ensuring Accuracy in Documentation.* 5th ed. F. A. Davis; 2016.
Morreale MJ. *The OTA's Guide to Documentation: Writing SOAP Notes.* 5th ed. SLACK Incorporated; 2023.
Sullivan DD. *Guide to Clinical Documentation.* 3rd ed. F. A. Davis; 2019.
Venes D, ed. *Taber's Cyclopedic Medical Dictionary.* 24th ed. F. A. Davis; 2021.

B

ICD/CPT Coding

Jill Walker Dale, MS, ATC, LAT

International Classification of Diseases

ICD is an abbreviation for ***International Classification of Diseases***. It is a classification system that was developed by the World Health Organization (WHO) as a unique system to track and report morbidity and mortality. This document is updated periodically, and is currently in its 10th revision (ICD-10).

ICD-10-CM was developed as a clinical modification to ICD-10 by the National Center for Human Statistics (NCHS) as a unique system for use in the United States and pertains to all health care settings. ICD-10-PCS is another unique code set that pertains specifically to inpatient procedures in US hospital settings.

The ICD-10-CM is an alphanumeric classification. The first character of a category is always a letter. The second character is always numeric. The third to seventh characters may be alpha or numeric. Subcategories are either four or five characters and may be either letters or numbers. Codes may be four, five, or six characters in length. An "**X**" may be used as a place-holder to allow for further expansion and greater detail, and certain categories require a seventh character extension at the end of the code.

ICD-10-CM allows for a high level of specificity and requires details such as laterality (left or right), traumatic vs non-traumatic injury, dominant side vs nondominant side, single condition or bilateral condition, cause of traumatic injury, activity patient was performing when injury occurred, place of occurrence when injury occurred, initial encounter vs subsequent encounter, and injuries/conditions that are sequelae or the direct result of another condition or injury.

ICD-10 codes are required for documentation and billing purposes in all health care settings.

As an example of how a specific injury might be coded:

An athlete who sustained a right knee anterior cruciate ligament (ACL) sprain during a high school soccer game via contact with another player presents on crutches, PWB with pain and swelling. The following codes may be used:

- **S83.511A** (sprain of the ACL of the right knee, initial encounter)
- **W51.XXXA** (accidental striking against by another person, initial encounter)
- **Y92.322** (athletic field—soccer field)
- **R26.2** (difficulty walking)
- **M25.561** (pain in the right knee)
- **M25.461** (edema of the right knee)

Flanagan KW.
Medical Terminology With Case Studies: A Navigated Guide to Learning for Health Care Professionals, Third Edition (pp 455-458).

Examples of ICD-10 Codes

Morbidity (illness or injury) due to:

- **W56.01** Bitten by a dolphin (not to be confused with W56.02 Struck by a dolphin)
- **W61.33** Pecked by a chicken
- **V97.33** Sucked into a jet engine
- **V96.01** Balloon crash injuring occupant
- **V92.20** Drowning and submersion due to being washed overboard from a merchant ship
- **Y90.8** Evidence of alcohol involvement as determined by blood alcohol level of 240 mg/100 mL or more

External cause of morbidity caused by:

- **W22.02** Walked into a lamppost
- **W21.01** Being struck by a football
- **Y93.34** Hang gliding
- **Y93.J1** Playing the piano
- **Y93.C1** Computer keyboarding
- **Y93.82** Spectator at an event
- **V91.16** Crushed between two non-powered inflatable crafts and other watercraft or other object due to collision
- **V80.920** Occupant of animal-drawn vehicle injured in transport accident with military vehicle

Current Procedural Terminology

CPT is an abbreviation for ***Current Procedural Terminology***. It is a set of numerical codes, description, and guidelines used to accurately describe procedures performed and services rendered by health care providers. This document is maintained by the American Medical Association (AMA), updated each October and published annually. The primary use of the CPT is to accurately describe a procedure, service or intervention that was performed by a health care professional for billing purposes. Insurance reimbursement to the health care provider for a service is typically determined by or based on CPT codes. The CPT utilizes a five-digit code that is tied to a description or definition of a service or medical procedure. There are currently six sections of the CPT:

1. **Evaluation and Management**
2. **Anesthesiology**
3. **Surgery**
4. **Radiology**
5. **Pathology and Laboratory**
6. **Medicine**

Each of the six sections is further divided into more specific subsections that are applicable to that section. Specific guidelines regarding the handling of unlisted services, terms, and definitions that are unique to that particular section are outlined at the beginning of each section.

A list of modifiers that includes the definition and use of each one is also included in the appendix of the CPT. A modifier provides the means to report or indicate that a service or procedure that has been performed has been modified by some specific circumstance but has not changed the definition or code itself. Modifiers are often used to further define or clarify an event such as a procedure that was performed bilaterally or performed by more than one physician.

CPT categories that pertain to athletic training services are located under the Medicine/Physical Medicine and Rehabilitation section. This section is further divided into Modalities (supervised and constant attendance), Therapeutic Procedures, Active Wound Care Management, and Tests and Measurements. The codes are further broken down into timed codes (each 15 minutes) and untimed codes.

For Athletic Training specifically:

- 97005—Athletic training evaluation
- 97006 —Athletic training re-evaluation

Examples of codes utilized by multiple professions to document or bill for therapeutic modalities and therapeutic procedures include:

- 97022—Whirlpool
- 97110—Therapeutic exercise (each 15 minutes)
- 97035—Ultrasound (each 15 minutes)
- 97140—Manual therapy (each 15 minutes)

Examples of Treatment and Surgical Codes for the Knee

THERAPEUTIC CODES* (TYPICALLY 15-MINUTE INCREMENTS)	SURGICAL CODES
Therapeutic exercise (exercises that regain strength or range of motion): **97110**	*Arthroscopy of the knee* For diagnosis purposes: **29870** For surgical purposes: **20866-20868**
Ultrasound: **97035**	*Reconstruction of the knee* Ligament reconstruction: **27427-27438** Ligament prosthesis: **27445**
Neurological re-education (ie, balance training): **97112**	*Repair of the knee* Cruciate ligament reconstruction: **27427** Arthrotomy with meniscus repair: **27403** Arthroscopy with meniscus repair: **29882**
Gait training (including crutch/cane instructions): **97116**	*Fracture* Open tibia fracture with internal fixation: **27535**
Manual therapy passive range of motion, soft tissue and joint mobilization: **97140**	
*Therapy codes are not body-part specific.	

Bottom Line

- ICD relates to diagnosis and classification of a given disease or condition.
- CPT relates to procedures performed or services provided by a health care professional and it is utilized primarily for billing purposes.
- Use of each one of these resources requires training and review of the full document or book.

Bibliography

Coders' Desk Reference for ICD-10-CM Diagnoses 2022. Optum 360; 2021.

CPT (Current Procedural Terminology). American Medical Association. Accessed November 16, 2022. https://www.ama-assn.org/amaone/cpt-current-procedural-terminology

ICD-10 Version:2019. World Health Organization. Accessed November 16, 2022. https://icd.who.int/browse10/2019/en

C

Pharmacology Terms

The major terms that are in common use in the field of pharmacology (preparation and dispensation of medicines) are provided. The pronunciation guide and definition of each term is included.

abortifacient (a bor tih fay shent): Agent that terminates pregnancy as part of a therapeutic abortion.

absorption (ab sorp shun): The process of taking in, in which a drug moves into the body toward the target organ or tissue.

ACE inhibitor (ays * in hib ih tor): Angiotensin-converting enzyme inhibitor; a category of antihypertensive drugs that suppress the renin pathway to reduce blood pressure.

administration (ad min ih stra shun): Providing a drug treatment to a patient.

adverse reaction (ad vers * re ak shun): A harmful reaction to a drug that was administered at the proper dosage.

ampule (am pyool): A sealed container that contains a sterile solution to be used for injection.

analgesic (an al jee zik): Compound that produces a reduced response to painful stimuli.

androgen (an droh jen): Clinical use of male hormones to treat male patients with abnormally low levels.

anesthetic (an ess tet ik): A compound that depresses neuronal function, resulting in a loss of the ability to perceive pain and other sensations.

anorexiant (an oh reks ee ant): An agent that suppresses appetite.

antacid (ant ass id): A substance that neutralizes or buffers an acid; usually taken orally to reduce hydrochloric acid in the stomach.

antianemic (an tee a nee mik) **agent**: A drug that is used to treat or prevent anemia.

antianxiety (an tee ang zi eh tee) **agent**: A drug that is used to treat anxiety, such as fear, worry, or apprehension; usually a sedative or minor tranquilizer.

antiarrhythmic (an tee a rith mik): A drug that is used to treat cardiac arrhythmia.

antibiotic (an tee bye ott ik): A chemical substance derived from a biological source (a mold or bacteria) that inhibits the growth of other microorganisms.

Flanagan KW.
Medical Terminology With Case Studies: A Navigated Guide to Learning for Health Care Professionals, Third Edition (pp 459-464).

anticoagulant (an tye koh ag yoo lant): A drug that prevents or delays blood coagulation.

anticonvulsant (an tee kon vul sant): A drug that reduces or prevents convulsive disorders, such as epilepsy.

antidepressant (an tee dee press ant): A drug that counteracts depression.

antidiabetic (an tee dye ah bet ik): A drug that reduces the amount of glucose in the blood; also called *hypoglycemic.*

antidiarrheal (an tee dye ah ree al): A drug that relieves the symptoms of diarrhea, usually by absorbing water from the large intestine and altering intestinal motility.

antidiuretic (an tee dye yoor eh tik): A drug that reduces the formation and excretion of urine.

antiemetic (an tye ee meh tik): A drug that is used to prevent or reduce nausea and vomiting.

antifungal (an tee fung ahl): An agent that kills fungi as an antiseptic.

antiglaucoma (an tye glaw koh mah): An agent that reduces intraocular pressure by lowering the volume of aqueous humor in the eye by inhibiting its production or increasing its return to the bloodstream.

antihistamine (an tih hiss tah meen): A class of drugs that suppress the action of histamines in order to counter the effects of inflammation.

antihormones (an tee hor mohnz): Substances that inhibit or otherwise prevent the normal effects of certain hormones.

antihypertensive (an tee high per ten sihv): A drug or treatment that reduces high blood pressure.

anti-inflammatory (an tee in flam ah tor ee): A drug or treatment that reduces inflammation by acting on body function.

anti-inflammatory otic (an tye in flam ah tor ee * oh tik): An agent that reduces inflammation, edema, and pruritus associated with otitis externa.

antilipidemic (an tye lip ih dem ik): An agent that reduces levels of cholesterol and lipids in the bloodstream.

antimutagenic (an tee myoo tah jen ik): A drug or treatment that reduces a substance's ability to form mutations in cells.

antineoplastic (an tee nee oh plass tik): A drug that is used to destroy or inhibit cancer cells, usually by inhibiting the synthesis of DNA.

antiparasitic (an tee pair ah sih tik): An agent that kills arthropod parasites, such as mites or lice.

antiprostatic (an tye pross tat ik): An agent that reduces inflammation of the prostate gland in benign prostatic hyperplasia.

antipruritic (an tee proo rih tik): An agent that reduces itching and inflammation.

antipsychotic (an tee sigh koh tik): A drug that counteracts the symptoms of psychosis, such as schizophrenia and major behavioral disorders.

antiseptic (an tih sep tik): A substance that prevents infection by inhibiting the growth of microorganisms.

antispasmodic (an tee spaz mod ik): A drug or treatment that inhibits muscle contractions to relieve convulsions or spasms; also known as *skeletal muscle relaxant.*

antithyroid (an tye thigh royd): An agent that inhibits thyroid hormone production to treat hyperthyroidism.

antitoxin (an tee tahks inn): An antibody that forms in response to antigenic poisonous substances; the antibody is often collected from its biological origin and concentrated for use in treatment against the antigenic toxin.

antitussive (an tee tuss iv): A drug or treatment that relieves coughing.

antiviral (an tee vye rail): An agent that inactivates viruses, such as herpes simplex virus.

bactericidal (bak teer ih ee sigh dal): A drug or treatment that destroys bacteria.

barbiturate (barr bihch yoor aht): A derivative of barbituric acid, which acts as a depressant on the central nervous system; usually used as tranquilizers and hypnotics.

beta blocker (bay ta block er): An agent that suppresses the rate and force of heart contractions by inhibition of beta adrenergic receptors.

bioavailability (bye oh ah vayl ah bill ih tee): The percentage of a drug that is available to the target organ or tissue.

biological agent (immunotherapy agent): An agent that boosts the immune response against cancer cells by triggering the body's defense mechanisms.

biotoxin (bye oh tahks inn): Any toxic substance formed in a living organism.

biotransformation (bye oh trans for may shun): The changes that occur to a chemical due to biological action within the body.

bronchodilator (bron koh dye lay tor): An agent that expands bronchial airways by relaxing muscle spasms in the bronchial walls; aerosols are used to treat asthma.

calcium channel blockers: A class of drugs that inhibit the movement of calcium ions into muscle cells, which thereby inhibit muscle contraction; useful in the treatment of heart disease that involves coronary spasms.

capsule (kap suhl): A small container that is soluble in water; used for the oral administration of a dose of medication; abbreviated *cap*.

carcinogen (kar sin oh jinn): Any substance that causes cancer.

cardiotonic (kar dee oh tohn ik): A substance that exerts a favorable effect upon the action of the heart by increasing the force and efficiency of its contractions.

catabolic (kat ah bohl ik): Relating to catabolism, which is the metabolic breakdown of chemicals to produce energy in the form of ATP.

cerumen emulsifier (seh roo men * ee mull sih fye er): Ear drops that soften earwax to prevent compaction in the external ear canal.

chemotherapeutic (kee moh thair ah pyoo tik): Agent that destroys metabolically active cells on the principle that cancer cells are more metabolically active than most healthy cells.

chemotherapy (kee moh thair ah pee): Treatment of disease by the use of chemical agents; the term is usually used to describe agents used in the treatment of cancer.

contraindication (kon trah in dih kay shun): A symptom or circumstance that renders the administration of a drug to be inadvisable.

corticosteroid (kor tih coh stair oid): An agent that inhibits inflammation to treat chronic inflammatory diseases, such as rheumatoid arthritis and Addison's disease.

corticosteroid (kor tih coh stair oid) **cream**: Topical cream that reduces inflammation.

decongestant (dee kon jess tant): An agent that reduces congestion in the sinuses and airways.

detoxify (dee tahk sih fye): To diminish or remove the poisonous quality of a substance or pathogen.

disinfectant (diss in fek tant): A chemical that destroys microorganisms and is thereby often used to sanitize objects and surfaces.

distribution (diss trih byoo shun): The pattern of absorption of drug molecules by the body once the drug has been administered.

diuretic (dye yoor eh tik): A drug that increases the production of urine by increasing water reabsorption within the kidneys; often prescribed to reduce water retention by the body, which reduces blood pressure, edema, and congestive heart failure.

dopaminergic (dope ah min er jik): An agent that substitutes or enhances the effect of the neurotransmitter dopamine as a treatment for Parkinson's disease.

dose: The quantity of a drug that is to be administered at one time.

drug: A therapeutic agent; any substance (other than food) that is used in the diagnosis, prevention, or treatment of a disease.

drug clearance: The elimination of a drug from the body, usually through excretion by the kidneys, lungs, liver, or intestinal tract.

drug fast: Microorganisms that become tolerant or resistant to an antimicrobial drug treatment; the modification of a drug that results from the drug interacting with itself or with other drugs, components of the diet, or other chemicals that are administered; the modification can be either desirable or undesirable effect; the biological effect of the administration of a particular drug; the effect may be local, if it is confined to the site of administration, or systemic, if the effect is more widespread.

effect: The biological effect of the administration of a particular drug; the effect may be **local**, if it is confined to the site of administration, or **systemic**, if the effect is more widespread.

enteral (ent er ahl): Administration of a drug by the oral route (by way of the intestines), as distinguished from parenteral; enteral administration is the most common route.

erectile dysfunction (ee rek tile * diss funk shun) **agent**: A drug that produces temporary erection as a treatment for erectile dysfunction.

expectorant (ek spek toh rant): An agent that hydrolyzes mucus to improve the ability to remove it by coughing.

fertility agent: Stimulates ovulation to promote successful fertilization.

Food and Drug Administration (FDA): The federal agency responsible for evaluation and regulation of pharmaceuticals in the United States; the FDA also enforces regulations that deal with the manufacture and distribution of food and cosmetics; the mission of the FDA is the protection of US citizens from the sale of impure or unhealthy substances.

formula (for myoo lah): A prescription that includes directions for the compounding of a medical preparation.

formulary (for myoo lair ree): A compilation of drugs and other relevant information that is used as a reference library by health professionals to prescribe treatment.

genotoxic (jee noh tahk sik): A substance that is capable of damaging DNA and therefore may cause mutation or cancer.

grain: A minute hard particle of any substance or a unit of weight equivalent to 1/60 of a dram (1/437:5 ounce).

gram: A unit of mass in the metric system equivalent to 15:432 grains.

granule (grahn yool): A very small pill that is usually gelatin or sugar coated.

H2-receptor antagonists: An agent that reduces levels of hydrochloric acid by blocking proton receptors in the gastric mucosa to treat peptic ulcers and gastroesophageal reflux disease.

homeopathy (hoh mee opp ah thee): A system of medical treatment centered on the theory that large doses of a certain drug given to a healthy person will produce conditions that are relieved by the same drug in small doses during a diseased state.

hormone (hor mohn): A chemical substance, usually a protein or steroid, that is secreted by an endocrine gland and transported by the circulatory system throughout the body; upon making physical contact with a target cell, the hormone enters the cell and induces changes in metabolism, growth rate, protein synthesis, or synthesis of other compounds; the changes the hormone induces can have profound effects on body function.

hormone (hor mohn) **replacement therapy (HRT)**: Replaces estrogen production during menopause or following surgical removal of the ovaries, which returns the benefits of estrogen. (Author's note: Hormone therapy is also used when gender identity does not align with birth assignment.)

hormone (hor mohn) **therapy agent**: Prevents the growth, spread, and recurrence of certain glandular cancers, such as breast cancer.

human growth hormone (hor mohn) **therapy** (HGH): Hormone replacement therapy using HGH to stimulate skeletal muscle growth as a treatment for slow growth in children.

hypnotics (hip nott iks): Drugs that depress central nervous system function, resulting in drowsiness; used as sedatives and to produce sleep.

immunodeficiency (im yoo noh dee fish ehn see): A condition that results from defective immune mechanisms; characterized by a frequent and rapid onset of infectious diseases.

immunosuppressant (im yoo noh suh press ant): An agent that inhibits the immune response; useful in reducing rejection of organ transplants.

infusion (inn fyoo zhun): The introduction of a fluid (other than blood) directly into a vein.

inhalation (inn hah lay shun): A treatment that involves breathing in a spray or vapor; the medication, known as the inhalant, is absorbed through capillaries in the mucous membranes of the upper respiratory tract.

injection (inn jehk shun): Introduction of a substance into the body with the use of a hollow needle; the injection may be beneath the skin (**subcutaneous** or **hypodermic**), into muscular tissue (**intramuscular** [**IM**]), into a vein (**intravenous** [**IV**]), or into the rectum (**rectal**).

insulin (in soo lin) **therapy**: Replacement for dysfunctional or insufficient insulin to treat diabetes type 1 and, in some cases, type 2.

laxative (lax ah tiv): A substance that promotes bowel movement without pain or violent action; laxatives work by softening the stool (decreasing water reabsorption), increasing the bulk of the feces, or lubricating the intestinal wall.

miotic (my ot ik): An agent that causes a pupil of the eye to constrict; may also be used to treat glaucoma.

muscle relaxant: A drug that reduces muscle contraction (see **antispasmodic**).

mydriatic (mid ree at ik): An agent that causes a pupil of the eye to dilate by paralyzing the iris and/or ciliary muscles; often used prior to eye exams and eye surgery.

nonprescription drugs: Drugs that are not required (by the FDA) to be sold with a medical prescription; also called *over-the-counter (OTC) drugs*.

non-steroidal anti-inflammatory drugs (NSAIDs): A class of drugs that reduce the symptoms of inflammation (swelling, redness, and pain) and are not steroidal compounds; the most common NSAID is aspirin (salicylic acid).

ointment (oynt ment): A semisolid, medicated mixture that is topically (externally) applied.

oral (or ahl): The mouth, the most common route of drug administration.

oral (or ahl) **contraceptive pill**: Agent that prevents conception by the use of low doses of estrogen or estrogen/progesterone, which block ovulation.

oxytocin (ox ee toh sin): Agent that increases uterine contractions to assist vaginal labor and delivery.

parenteral (pah rent er ahl): Introduction of medication through a route other than the oral (intestinal) or inhalation (lungs) routes; involves injection that may be subcutaneous, intravenous, intramuscular, or rectal.

pharmaceutical (far mih soo tih kal): A chemical used in the treatment of disease; commonly called a *medication* or *drug*.

pharmacist (farm ah sist): A health professional formally trained to formulate and dispense prescription drugs and other medications.

pharmacodynamic (farm ah koh dye nam ik): Relating to drug action.

pharmacology (farm ah kall oh jee): The science of drugs and their sources, chemistry, action within the body, and uses.

pharmacotherapy (farm ah koh thair ah pee): The treatment of disease by means of drugs.

pharmacy (farm ah see): The practice of preparing and dispensing drugs; also, a place where drugs are prepared and dispensed.

placebo (plah see boh): A neutral, ineffective substance that is identical to a known drug, which is administered to a patient for the suggestive effect or during blind testing.

potency (poh ten see): The pharmacological activity of a drug; used to determine the amount of a drug to be administered in order to cause the desired effect.

prescription (pree skrip shun): A written order for pharmacotherapy, which is provided by an authorized health professional.

protease inhibitor (proh tee ays * in hih bih tor): An agent that inhibits protease, an enzyme required by viruses to reproduce, as a part of an AIDS treatment plan.

proton pump inhibitors: An agent that inhibits the production of hydrochloric acid by the stomach mucosa to treat peptic ulcers and gastroesophageal reflux disease.

reverse transcriptase inhibitor (ree vers * trans krip tase * in hih bih tor): An agent that inhibits reverse transcriptase, an enzyme required by viruses to reproduce, as a part of an AIDS treatment plan routes of administration. The drug may be administered in various ways, including the subcutaneous injection, intravenous injection, intramuscular injection, rectal injection, oral, vaginal, rectal, or topical.

sedative (sed ah tiv): An agent that reduces central nervous system activity, producing a calming, quieting effect; usually used to treat anxiety side effects. A reaction by the body resulting from a treatment program that is a diversion from the desired effects; the reaction can be beyond the desired effects and is usually undesirable.

solution (suh loo shun): A chemical mixture that includes a dissolved substance (solute) in a liquid medium (solvent).

spermatocide (sper mah toh side): An agent that destroys sperm as a form of contraception.

stimulant (stihm yool ant): An agent that increases the rate of activity of a body function.

superscription (soo per skrip shun): The beginning of a prescription, consisting of the command recipe "take."

suppository (suh poz ih tor ee): A medication that is introduced into one of the body orifices (other than the mouth), such as rectum, vagina, or urethra; usually a solid mass that melts at body temperature.

suspension (suh spen shun): A mixture of solid particles in a liquid medium that do not dissolve; the solid particles are usually dispersed through the liquid by blending.

tablet (tab let): A small solid that contains medication for oral administration; tablets may be designed to be swallowed whole, chewed, or dissolved prior to administration.

thrombolytic (throm boh lih tik): An agent that dissolves blood clots to treat thrombosis and embolism.

thyroid replacement therapy: Hormone replacement therapy with thyroid hormone to treat hypothyroidism or for patients who have had a thyroidectomy.

topical (tahp ih kuhl): Administration of a drug onto the surface of the skin.

toxicity (tahk siss ih tee): The state of being poisonous; the level at which a drug's concentration in the body produces serious adverse effects.

toxicology (tahk sih kall oh jee): The science of poisons in which the source, chemical properties, and body responses to poisonous substances are studied.

trade name: The name provided to a drug by its manufacturer and commonly used by the health community to identify the drug.

tranquilizer (tran kwiil eye zer): A drug that brings tranquility, or a calming effect, to the mind without depression; abbreviated *trank*.

transdermal (trans derm al): Administration of a drug topically to unbroken skin for its absorption into deeper tissues.

***United States Pharmacopeia* (USP)** (farm ah kop ee ah): A reference text approved by the federal Food, Drug, and Cosmetic Act that contains specifications for drugs, such as chemical properties, uses, recommended dosage levels, contra indications, and adverse side effects

vasoconstrictor (vay zoh kon strik tor). A chemical that causes blood vessels to constrict, which reduces blood flow and elevates blood pressure; also called *vasopressors*.

vasodilator (vay zoh dye lay tor): A chemical that causes blood vessels to relax, resulting in dilation that increases blood flow and lowers blood pressure; due to their effect, they are in common use for acute heart failure.

vasopressin (vay zoh press in): Enzyme that promotes water reabsorption in the kidneys to treat diabetes insipidus.

vitamin (vye tah min): An organic compound that is required for normal function of cells; most vitamins are produced by the body, but those that are not are known as *essential vitamins* and must be included in the diet.

Section IV

Learning Activity and Case Study Answers

Worksheet Answers

Chapter 2: Word Building: An Introduction to Prefixes and Suffixes

A. Matching: Combining forms.

1. g
2. e
3. i
4. j
5. h
6. a
7. f
8. b
9. c
10. d

B. Matching: Prefixes.

1. h
2. d
3. j
4. a
5. i
6. e
7. b
8. c
9. f
10. g

C. Matching: Suffixes.

1. e
2. i
3. a
4. g
5. h
6. j
7. d
8. b
9. c
10. f

D. Locate and define the prefix for the following words.

1. **peri**/carditis—around (around the heart)
2. **hypo**/dermic—below (pertaining to below the skin)
3. **tetra**/logy—four (group of four)
4. **intra**/articular—within (within the joint)
5. **cyan**/otic—blue (pertaining to blue)
6. **a**/pnea—without (without breathing)
7. **extra**/pulmonary—outside (outside of the lungs)
8. **supra**/condylar—above (above the condyle)
9. **sub**/sternal—below (below the sternum)
10. **epi**/gastric—above (above the stomach)

E. Locate and define the suffix for the following words.

1. hemat/**oma**—tumor (blood tumor; a bruise)
2. card/**itis**—inflammation (inflammation of the heart)
3. chemo/**therapy**—treatment (treatment using chemicals)
4. phago/**cyte**—cell (a cell that eats others)
5. macrocy/**tic**—pertaining to (a cell larger than normal)
6. ceph/**algia**—pain (head pain)
7. glyco/**lysis**—destruction (breakdown of sugar)
8. diet/**ary**—pertaining to (diet)
9. dia/**rrhea**—discharge (loose, watery stools)
10. cyto/**plasm**—formation (cell formation)

F. For the following words, separate the combining form from the prefix or suffix and write out the meaning.

1. orbito/**pathy** (disease affecting the orbit of the eye)
2. osteo/**cyte** (bone cell)
3. my/**algia** (muscle pain)
4. rhino/**rrhea** (discharge from the nose)
5. **peri**/arteri/**al** (around the artery)
6. orth/odont/**ic** (pertaining to straightening the teeth)
7. encephal/itis (swelling of the brain)
8. **supra**/orbit/**al** (above the eye)
9. orchid/**ectomy** (surgical removal of one or both testes)
10. **ecto**/morph (slender physique)

Chapter 3: Body Organization and Anatomical Directions

A. Matching: Combining forms.

1. j
2. i
3. h
4. g
5. b
6. d
7. e
8. a
9. c
10. f

Flanagan KW.
Medical Terminology With Case Studies: A Navigated Guide to Learning for Health Care Professionals, Third Edition (pp 467-487).

B. Match the correct directional terms from the following list.

1. medial
2. lateral
3. anterior
4. proximal
5. superior
6. posterior
7. distal
8. inferior

C. Label the correct plane.

1. transverse
2. coronal
3. sagittal

E. Separate the combining form from the prefix or suffix and define the following words.

1. neuro/**genesis** (formation of a nerve cell)
2. **epi**/cardium (pertaining to above the heart; outermost layers)
3. bronch/**itis** (inflammation of the bronchial tubes)
4. ceph/**algia** (pain in the head)
5. oto/**rrhea** (discharge from the ear)
6. **peri**/umbilic/**al** (pertaining to around the umbilicus)
7. **extra**/ocul/**ar** (outside of the eye)
8. **erythro**/derma (red skin)
9. pulmon/**ologist** (one who studies the lungs)
10. hemat/**oma** (blood tumor—a bruise)

D. Using this list, place the tissues in the correct row identified by system.

SYSTEM	TISSUE	TISSUE	TISSUE
endocrine	thyroid	pancreas	pituitary
reproductive	fallopian tube	ovaries	prostate gland
integumentary	hair	sebaceous glands	skin
respiratory	lungs	pharynx	trachea
neurological	brain	nerves	spinal cord
gastrointestinal	gallbladder	liver	tongue
urinary	kidneys	ureter	urinary bladder
musculoskeletal	bones	ligaments	muscles
cardiovascular	heart	spleen	thymus

Chapter 4: Therapeutic and Diagnostic Procedures

A. Matching.

1. e
2. j
3. a
4. f
5. h
6. c
7. b
8. g
9. d
10. i

B. SOAP notes: Fill in the blanks using medical abbreviations.

The S portion of the SOAP note would include the patient's CC and HPI. The O portion of the note contains TPR and VS. The A portion has a list of Dd.

C. Define the following words/medical abbreviations.

1. therapy using heat
2. fasting blood sugar
3. a classification to sort patients for treatment
4. magnetic resonance imaging (using magnetic radio waves to view internal structures of the body)
5. crushing stones (usually gall or kidney stones)
6. preventing the spread of disease
7. a process for categorizing malignant tumors
8. cutting into bone
9. fainting
10. complete blood count (microscopic examination of blood components)

D. Add the suffix -scope to each of the following combining forms and define the word created.

1. cysto**scope**—an instrument used to view the urinary tract
2. nephro**scope**—an instrument used to view the kidney
3. ophthalmo**scope**—an instrument used to examine the internal structures of the eye
4. endo**scope**—an instrument used to view within a cavity
5. micro**scope**—an instrument used to view very small things

E. Add the suffix -scopy to each of the following combining forms and define the word created.

1. arthro**scopy**—viewing within a joint
2. laparo**scopy**—viewing the internal structures of the abdomen and pelvis
3. colono**scopy**—viewing the colon
4. laryngo**scopy**—viewing the larynx (vocal cord)
5. broncho**scopy**—viewing the bronchial tubes

F. Write out the medical word that means the following.

1. tonsillectomy
2. otopexy
3. colostomy
4. electroencephalogram
5. blepharoplasty

G. For each of the following conditions, determine if it is a sign or symptom.

1. sign
2. symptom
3. symptom
4. sign
5. sign
6. sign
7. symptom
8. sign
9. sign
10. symptom

Chapter 5: Musculoskeletal System

Self-Assessment

- oste/o/arthr/**itis** (bone/joint/inflammation)
- orth/o/ped/**ic** (pertaining to straightening)
- my/**algia** (muscle pain)
- oste/o/chondr/**oma** (bone/cartilage/tumor—benign tumor containing bony and cartilage elements within a bone)
- myos/**itis** (inflammation of a muscle)
- arthr/o/**scope** (an instrument used to view inside of a joint)
- oste/**ology** (the study of bones)
- my/o/**tomy** (cutting a muscle)
- arthr/o/**plasty** (surgical reconstruction of a joint)
- my/o/cardi/**al** (pertaining to the heart muscle)

A. Label parts of the joints from the following list.

1. diarthrosis
2. amphiarthrosis
3. synarthrosis

B. Label parts of a long bone from the following list.

1. proximal epiphysis
2. diaphysis
3. distal epiphysis
4. spongy bone
5. endosteum
6. medullary cavity
7. periosteum
8. articular cartilage

C. Match the word part with its meaning.

1. e
2. d
3. h
4. i
5. j
6. g
7. b
8. f
9. c
10. a

D. Using word parts from previous chapters as well as new ones presented in this chapter, separate the prefix and suffix from the word root and define the following words.

1. intercostal (**inter**/cost/**al**—between the ribs)
2. osteomyelitis (osteo/myel/**itis**—inflammation of the bone marrow)
3. osteocarcinoma (osteo/carcin/**oma**—cancerous tumor of a bone)
4. rachigraph (rachi/**graph**—an instrument used to measure the curvature of the spine)
5. periosteoedema (**peri**/osteo/**edema**—swelling around a bone)
6. radial (radi/**al**—pertaining to the radius)
7. subcostal (**sub**/cost/**al**—under the rib)
8. atrophy (**a**/**trophy**—without nourishment or development)
9. dactylospasm (dactylo/**spasm**—spasm of the finger or toe)
10. myomalacia (myo/**malacia**—softening of the muscle tissue)

E. Label the bones of the body from the following list.

1. cervical spine
2. scapula
3. lumbar spine
4. ilium
5. femur
6. maxilla
7. mandible
8. clavicle
9. sternum
10. humerus
11. ulna
12. patella

F. Build the word: Using the word root, add the other word element and define the new word created.

1. **arthr/o**
    a. **-centesis** (athrocentesis—a surgical puncture of a joint to remove fluid)
    b. **-gram** (arthrogram—a recording of a joint via dye and x-ray)
    c. **-desis** (arthrodesis—surgical fixation of a joint)
    d. **-scopy** (arthroscopy—process of viewing a joint cavity)
    e. **-algia** (arthralgia—pain in a joint)
2. **chondr/o**
    a. **-oma** (chondroma—tumor of the cartilage)
    b. **-malacia** (chondromalacia—softening of the cartilage)
    c. **-cyte** (chondrocyte—a cell that forms cartilage)
    d. cost + **-al** (chondrocostal—pertaining to the cartilage and ribs)
    e. **-clast** (chondroclast—a cell that reabsorbs [breaks down] cartilage)
3. **ten/o**
    a. **-rrhaphy** (tenorraphy—suturing a tendon)
    b. **-otomy** (tenotomy—incision into a tendon)
    c. **-plasty** (tenoplasty—surgical repair of a tendon)
    d. **-itis** (tendinitis—inflammation of a tendon)
    e. **-pathy** (tendinopathy—disease of a tendon)
4. **oste/o**
    a. **-clasis** (osteoclasis—surgically breaking a bone)
    b. **-ology** (osteology—study of bones)
    c. **-necrosis** (osteonecrosis—death and destruction of bone tissue)
    d. **-genesis** (osteogenesis—formation of bone)
    e. **-plasty** (osteoplasty—removal of damaged bone)

G. Label the muscles of the body from the following list.

1. tibialis anterior
2. rectus femoris
3. tensor fasciae latae
4. serratus anterior
5. biceps
6. deltoid
7. pectoralis major
8. rectus abdominis
9. sartorius
10. gastrocnemius

H. Recall: Using the skeleton, label the directions from the following list.

1. superior
2. anterior
3. distal
4. proximal
5. inferior
6. posterior

I. Label the skull from the following list.

1. nasal
2. mandible
3. parietal
4. zygoma
5. mandible
6. occipital
7. frontal
8. temporal
9. maxilla

J. Recall terms relating to movement and anatomical directions from Chapter 3. Define the following words.

1. to move an arm or leg toward the body
2. bending a joint, moving two bones closer together
3. to point the toes down
4. moving the thumb side of the wrist away from the body
5. in the forearm/hand, to turn the hand upward
6. lying on the front, the abdomen
7. pertaining to the palms of hands
8. straightening a joint, increasing the angle between two bones
9. to bend the trunk sideways
10. lying on the back facing up

Case Study

Terms

1. to turn the ankle by rolling the sole of the foot inward
2. to roll the heel of the foot inward
3. swelling
4. bruising
5. non–weight bearing
6. stretched or torn ligament

Anatomy

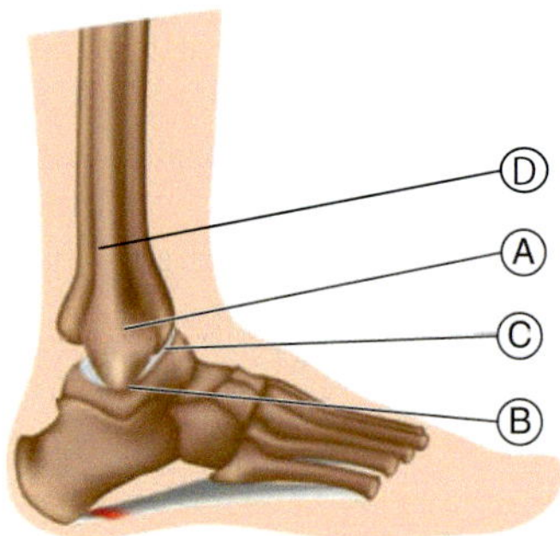

Chapter 6: Cardiovascular System

Self-Assessment

- **peri**/cardi/**um** (surrounding the heart)
- cardi/o/**megaly** (abnormally large heart)
- **cyan**/**osis** (condition of blue; bluish skin)
- **tachy**/cardi/a (a fast heartbeat)
- my/o/cardi/**um** (heart muscle)
- **a**/rrhythm/**ia** (a loss of rhythm in the heartbeat)
- **endo**/card/**itis** (inflammation within the heart)
- erythr/o/**cyte** (red blood cells)

A. Label parts of the heart from the following list.

1. right atrium
2. left atrium
3. right ventricle
4. left ventricle
5. tricuspid valve
6. pulmonary artery
7. mitral valve
8. aortic valve
9. myocardium
10. interventricular septum

B. Using the following list, number the anatomical parts of the heart in the correct order that blood flows through the heart.

_11_ aortic valve
_2_ right atrium
_5_ pulmonary valve
_6_ pulmonary artery
_9_ mitral valve
_10_ left ventricle
_1_ inferior vena cava
_12_ aorta
_3_ tricuspid valve
_4_ right ventricle
_8_ left atrium
_7_ pulmonary vein

C. Define the following medical abbreviations.

1. coronary artery disease
2. myocardial infarction
3. cerebrovascular accident
4. hypertrophic cardiomyopathy
5. peripheral artery disease
6. hypertension
7. congestive heart failure
8. mitral valve prolapse
9. deep vein thrombosis
10. pulmonary embolism

D. Match the medical word part with its meaning.

1. d
2. g
3. a
4. j
5. h
6. i
7. b
8. e
9. c
10. f

E. Build the word: Using the word root, add the other word element and define the new word created.

1. **angi/o**
    a. **-poiesis** (angiopoiesis—the process of forming a blood vessel)
    b. **-plasty** (angioplasty—reconstruction of a blood vessel)
    c. **-oma** (angioma—a tumor filled with blood vessels)
    d. **-scope** (angioscope—a microscope that views into a vessel)
    e. **-pathy** (angiopathy—disease of a blood vessel)
2. **cardi/o**
    a. vers/o + **-ion** (cardioversion—to turn the heart; reset it with an AED)
    b. **-itis** (carditis—an inflammation of the heart)
    c. **-rrhaphy** (cardiorrhaphy—suturing the heart; its muscle)
    d. **-megaly** (cardiomegaly—an enlarged heart)
    e. vascul/o + **-ar** (cardiovascular—pertaining to the heart and blood vessels)
3. **lymph/o**
    a. **-cyte** (lymphocyte—a lymph cell)
    b. aden/o + **-itis** (lymphadenitis—inflammation of a lymph node)
    c. sarc/o + **-oma** (lymphosarcoma—cancer of the lymph tissue)
    d. **-edema** (lymphedema—swelling in the lymph system; accumulation of lymph in the tissues)
    e. **-blast** (lymphoblast—an immature lymph cell)

F. Label the glands and nodes of the lymphatic system from the following list.

1. cervical nodes
2. thymus
3. palatine tonsils
4. axillary nodes
5. spleen
6. inguinal nodes

G. Using word parts from previous chapters as well as new ones presented in this chapter, separate the prefix and suffix from the word root and define the following words.

1. glycopenia (glyc/o/**penia**—deficient sugar in the body)
2. plasmapheresis (plasma/**pheresis**—removal of plasma
3. angiogram (angi/o/**gram**—a recording of a blood vessel)
4. hemorrhage (hemo/**rrhage**—uncontrollable bleeding)
5. valvotomy (valv/**otomy**—an incision into a valve)
6. hemoptysis (hemo/**ptysis**—spitting blood)
7. hypocalcemia (hypo/calc/**emia**—deficiency of calcium in the blood)
8. splenopexy (spleno/**pexy**—surgical fixation of the spleen)
9. pericardiocentesis (peri/cardio/**centesis**—a surgical puncture of the sac surrounding the heart
10. phagocytosis (phago/cyt/**osis**—process of cells consuming other cells)

Case Study

Terms

1. rapid heartbeat
2. chest pain due to lack of oxygen in the blood
3. difficulty breathing
4. irregular/abnormal heartbeat
5. contraction of the heart
6. relaxation of the heart
7. 180/100
8. a blood test measuring different fats in the blood
9. a test using sound waves to see internal structures of the heart
10. a method of recording electrical activity of the heart
11. disease to the heart muscle
12. an x-ray recording the heart and blood vessels using radiopaque dye
13. partially blocked coronary artery
14. fatty substance attaching to the vessel, narrowing the ability for blood to flow through

Chapter 7: Respiratory System

Self-Assessment

- **a**/pnea (not breathing)
- trache/**otomy** (an incision into the trachea)
- tonsil/l/**itis** (inflammation of the tonsils)
- steth/o/**scope** (an instrument to view [hear] the chest)
- pulmon/o/**logist** (one who specializes in the lung)
- bronch/o/**scopy** (examination of the bronchioles)
- or/o/pharyng/**eal** (pertaining to the mouth and pharynx)
- **dys**/**phasia** (difficulty swallowing)

A. Label the upper airway anatomy from the following list.

1. pharyngeal tonsils
2. tongue
3. pharynx
4. epiglottis
5. larynx
6. esophagus
7. trachea
8. nasal cavity
9. nares

B. Label the aspects of the chest cavity from the following list.

1. parietal pleura
2. pleural cavity
3. visceral pleura
4. mediastinum

C. Label the sinuses from the following list.

1. frontal sinuses
2. ethmoidal sinuses
3. maxillary sinuses

D. Matching.

1. j
2. i
3. h
4. g
5. f
6. a
7. e
8. c
9. d
10. b

E. Fill in the table.

WORD PART	COMBINING FORM	NEW WORD	DEFINITION
tachy-	pnea	**tachy**pnea	rapid breathing
dys-	phonia	**dys**phonia	abnormal voice (hoarseness)
-ptysis	hem/o	hemo**ptysis**	spitting blood
-dynia	pleur/o	pleuro**dynia**	pain in the pleura
-stenosis	trache/o	tracheo**stenosis**	narrowing of the trachea
-meter	ox/i	oxi**meter**	a device used to measure oxygen content in the blood
-otomy	sinus/o	sinus**otomy**	cutting into the sinus
-ectomy	laryng/o	laryng**ectomy**	surgical removal of the larynx
hem/o + pneum/o	thorax	hemopneumothorax	blood and air in the chest
pan- + **-itis**	sinus	**pan**sinus**itis**	inflammation in all of the sinuses

F. Fill in the table with the common name.

MEDICAL WORD	COMMON NAME
thyroid cartilage	Adam's apple
palatine tonsils	tonsils
coryza	the common cold
influenza	the flu
pertussis	whooping cough

G. Define the following abbreviations.

1. URI (upper respiratory infection)
2. SARS (severe acute respiratory syndrome)
3. CF (cystic fibrosis)
4. RDS (respiratory distress syndrome)
5. PFT (pulmonary function test)
6. PE (pulmonary embolism)
7. COPD (chronic obstructive pulmonary disease)
8. CPAP (continuous positive airway pressure)
9. TB (tuberculosis)
10. Tdap (tetanus, diphtheria, and pertussis [a vaccination])

H. Write out the plural forms of the following words.

SINGULAR	PLURAL
alveolus	alveoli
pleura	pleurae
bronchus	bronchi

I. Describe what the following medications do.

1. mucolytic (loosens mucous)
2. decongestant (relieves congestion)
3. antihistamine (prevents reaction to histamine)
4. bronchodilator (dilates the bronchioles)
5. antitussive (prevents coughing)

Case Study

Terms

1. difficult/painful breathing
2. headache
3. shortness of breath
4. spitting up blood
5. deficient amount of oxygen reaching the tissues
6. instrument to measure oxygen content in the blood
7. bluish-looking skin due to lack of oxygen
8. blood in the thorax or lung

Anatomy

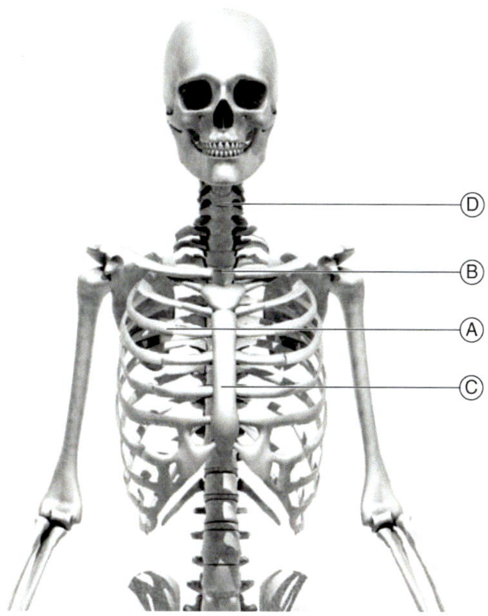

Chapter 8: Neurological System

Self-Assessment

- disc/**ectomy** (surgical removal of a disc)
- cerebr/**al** ather/o/**sclerosis** (fatty plaque in the vessels of the brain [cerebrum])
- neur/**itis** (inflammation of a nerve)
- crani/**otomy** (incision into the cranium)
- cerebr/**al** angi/o/**graphy** (recording the process of the blood vessels in the brain; an x-ray test after contrast medium is injected)
- neur/**ology** (the study of nerves/the nervous system)
- ech/o/encephal/o/**graphy** (the use of sound [ultrasound] to record brain structures)
- neur/o/**pathy** (a disease of a nerve)

A. Label the lobes of the brain from the following list.

1. frontal
2. temporal
3. parietal
4. occipital
5. cerebellum

B. Label the bones of the skull from the following list.

1. frontal
2. zygoma
3. nasal
4. maxilla
5. mandible
6. parietal
7. temporal
8. occipital
9. cervical spine

C. Using this chart, indicate whether each is a sign or a symptom.

TERM	SIGN	SYMPTOM
cephalagia		*X*
fasciculation	X	
neuralgia		X
syncope		X
ataxia	X	
seizure	X	

D. Using your knowledge from previous chapters, separate the word elements and define the following words.

1. cerebral arteriosclerosis (cerebr/**al** arterio/scler/**osis**—hardening of the arteries in the cerebrum)
2. cerebral thrombosis (cerebr/**al** thromb/**osis**—a blood clot in the brain)
3. cerebral aneurysm (cerebr/**al** aneurysm—a dilated/swollen vessel in the brain)
4. neurology (neur/o/**logy**—the study of nervous tissue)
5. arachnophobia (arachn/o/**phobia**—fear of spiders)

E. Matching.

1. d
2. i
3. j
4. a
5. c
6. g
7. h
8. f
9. e
10. b

F. Build the word.

1. **hemi-**
    a. **-paresis** (hemiparesis—partial paralysis/weakness on one side of the body)
    b. **-plegia** (hemiplegia—paralysis on one side of the body)
    c. **par-** + **-esthesia** (hemiparesthesia—numbness or abnormal feeling on one side)
    d. **-ataxia** (hemiataxia—loss of muscle control on one half of the body)
    e. **hyper-** + **-trophy** (hemihypertrophy—enlargement or excessive growth on one half of the body)
2. **para-**
    a. **an-** + **-esthesia** (paranesthesia—numbness affecting the lower half of the body)
    b. **-plegia** (paraplegia—paralysis of the lower half of the body)
    c. **-plegic** (paraplegic—pertaining to having paralysis on the lower half of the body)
    d. **-lysis** (paralysis—loss of motor or sensory function or both)
    e. **-nasal** (paranasal—near the nose)
3. **neur/o**
    a. **-itis** (neuritis—inflammation of a nerve)
    b. **-oma** (neuroma—a tumor in the nervous tissue)
    c. muscul/ + **-ar** (neuromuscular—pertaining to nerves and muscles)
    d. **-plasty** (neuroplasty—surgical repair of a nerve)
    e. **-genic** (neurogenic—pertaining to formation of nervous tissue)

Case Study

Terms

1. loss of consciousness
2. headache
3. pupils equally round and reactive to light and accommodation
4. a muscle or group of muscles innervated by a single motor nerve
5. nerves that carry sensory information, such as touch, pressure, and pain
6. within normal limits
7. vestibulocochlear nerve—responsible for balance
8. ringing in the ears
9. computed tomography
10. rule out
11. bleeding within the brain

Chapter 9: Gastrointestinal System

Self-Assessment

- gastr/**itis** (inflammation of the stomach)
- tonsil/l/**ectomy** (surgical removal the tonsils)
- gastr/o/enter/**ology** (the study of the stomach and small intestines)
- gastr/**ostomy** (creating a surgical opening in the stomach)
- **hemi**/col/**ectomy** (surgical removal of one half of the colon)
- hepat/**itis** (inflammation of the liver)

A. Using the bulleted list of anatomy, list the number on the drawing that corresponds with the anatomical part.

1. gallbladder
2. duodenum
3. transverse colon
4. ascending colon
5. appendix
6. esophagus
7. fundus
8. stomach
9. antrum
10. pancreas
11. small intestine
12. descending colon
13. sigmoid colon

B. Label the salivary glands from the following list of words.

1. parotid gland
2. sublingual gland
3. submandibular gland

C. Matching.

1. f
2. g
3. h
4. j
5. b
6. a
7. d
8. i
9. e
10. c

D. Build the word.

1. **-itis**
   a. cheil/ (cheilitis—inflammation of the lip)
   b. esophag/ (esophagitis—inflammation of the esophagus)
   c. enter/ (enteritis—inflammation of the small intestine)
   d. col/ (colitis—inflammation of the colon)
   e. cholecyst/ (cholecystitis—inflammation of the gallbladder)
   f. ile/ (ileitis—inflammation of the ileum)
   g. hepat/ (hepatitis—inflammation of the liver)
   h. gloss/ (glossitis—inflammation of the tongue)
   i. proct/ (proctitis—inflammation of the rectum and anus)
2. **-scopy**
   a. proct/o (proctoscopy—a visual examination of the rectum and anus)
   b. lapar/o (laparoscopy—a visual examination in the abdominal cavity)
   c. sigmoid/o (sigmoidoscopy—a visual examination of the sigmoid colon)
   d. **endo-** (endoscopy—a visual examination within the GI system)
   e. gastr/o (gastroscopy—a visual examination of the stomach)
   f. esophag/o (esophagoscopy—a visual examination of the esophagus)
3. **-ectomy**
   a. diverticul (diverticulectomy—surgical removal of an abnormal pouch in the intestinal wall)
   b. polyp (polypectomy—surgical removal of a polyp)
   c. uvul (uvulectomy—surgical removal of the uvula)
   d. gastr (gastrectomy—surgical removal of all or a portion of the stomach)
   e. gingiv (gingivectomy—surgical removal of damaged gums)

E. Separate the word elements of the following terms and define them.

1. gastroenterocolitis (gastr/o/enter/o/col/itis—inflammation of the stomach, small intestine, and colon)
2. cholangiogram (chol/angi/o/gram—an x-ray image using contrast medium in the vessels that provides an image of the bile ducts)
3. cholecystectomy (chole/cyst/ectomy—surgical removal of the gallbladder)

F. From the following list, choose the two word elements that match the meaning of the words.

1. mouth (or/o; stomat/o)
2. lip (cheil/o; labi/o)
3. anus (an/o; proct/o)
4. tongue (gloss/o; lingu/o)
5. teeth (dent/o; odont/o)

G. Fill in the blanks.

1. McBurney's point
2. anorexia
3. peristalsis
4. mastication
5. amylase
6. malocclusion

Case Study

Terms

1. indigestion
2. above the stomach
3. watery stools
4. lack of appetite
5. vomiting
6. yellowing of the skin
7. enlarged liver
8. enlarged spleen
9. lower right quadrant
10. pain away from the appendix
11. urinalysis
12. complete blood count
13. within normal limits

14. increased while blood cells
15. a non-invasive test that uses sound waves to see internal structures
16. sudden onset
17. inflammation of the appendix
18. surgical removal of the appendix

Anatomy

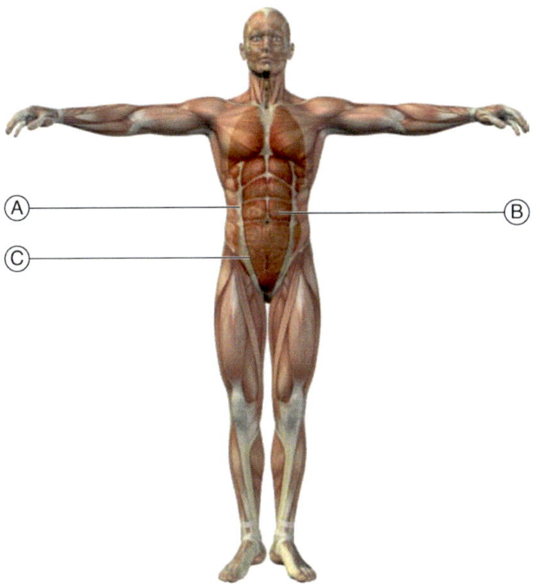

Chapter 10: Integumentary System

Self-Assessment

- dermat/**itis** (inflammation of the skin)
- melan/**oma** (black tumor; skin cancer)
- hidr/**osis** (a condition of sweating)
- scler/o/derm (hard skin)
- **per**/cutan/e/**ous** (through the skin)
- **trans**/derm/**al** (across the skin)
- **hyper**/**plasia** (excessive growth)
- dors/**um** (pertaining to the dorsal aspect or back)

A. Label the aspects of the dermis from the following list of words.

1. hair shaft
2. sebaceous gland
3. arrector pili muscle
4. sudoriferous gland
5. hair bulb
6. subcutaneous layer
7. dermis
8. pore

B. Label the aspects of the fingernail from the following list of words.

1. paronychium
2. nail plate
3. nail bed
4. nail matrix
5. cuticle
6. lunula

C. Matching.

1. h
2. g
3. f
4. i
5. c
6. d
7. a
8. j
9. b
10. e

D. Write the medical word for the following common terms.

1. bulla
2. rubella
3. lentigo
4. acrochordon
5. striae
6. acne
7. varicella
8. urticaria
9. cicatrix
10. comedo
11. verruca
12. tinea pedis

E. Indicate if the word listed is a disease/infection, treatment, or parasite.

WORD	DISEASE/INFECTION	TREATMENT	PARASITE
sclerotherapy		X	
debridement		X	
varicella	X		
fulguration		X	
carbuncle	X		
dermoplasty		X	
scabies			X
rubella	X		
xenograft		X	
Cimex lectularius			X

F. Separate the word elements in the following terms and define them.

1. dermatomyositis (dermat/o/my/o/sitis—a connective tissue disease involving destruction of the muscle tissue
2. melanocarcinoma (melan/o/carcin/oma—a black cancer tumor; malignant melanoma)
3. onychoplasty (onych/o/plasty—surgical repair of the nail)
4. intradermal (intra/derm/al—pertaining to within the skin)

G. Write the medical terms that are used to describe these conditions.

1. stratum lucidum
2. stratum basale
3. thermanesthesia
4. stratum spinosum
5. causalgia

H. Describe what the following medications do.

1. softens the skin
2. anti-itching
3. disrupts activity of the fungi cell
4. inhibits bacterial growth
5. loosens the superficial layer of skin

Case Study

Terms

1. red skin
2. fluid-filled sacs
3. itchy
4. chronic skin condition marked with raised white patches
5. red, itchy, swollen skin in response to an allergen
6. superficial cysts
7. acne
8. localized small infection
9. inflammation of the hair follicle
10. chicken pox
11. without a fever
12. disease of the lymph glands
13. skin infection characterized by crusty vesicles or bullae
14. destroys or interferes with bacterial growth

Chapter 11: Endocrine System

Self-Assessment

- aden/o/carcin/**oma** (cancer of a gland)
- mast/**itis** (inflammation of the breast)
- oo/**genesis** (formation of an egg [ovum])
- gluc/o/**meter** (an instrument to measure sugar [in the blood])
- thyr/**oid**/**ectomy** (surgical excision of the thyroid gland)

A. Label the glands of the endocrine system from the following list of words.

1. pineal
2. thymus
3. hypothalamus
4. pituitary
5. thyroid
6. pancreas
7. adrenal
8. testis
9. ovary

B. Matching.

1. j	6. b
2. e	7. a
3. g	8. h
4. i	9. d
5. f	10. c

C. For each hormone, list which gland is responsible for its secretion.

HORMONE	GLAND
thymosin	thymus
FSH (follicle-stimulating hormone)	pituitary (anterior lobe)
glucagon	pancreas
oxytocin	pituitary (posterior lobe)
melatonin	pineal gland
PTH (parathyroid hormone)	parathyroid gland
calcitonin	thyroid gland
ACTH (adrenocortico-tropic hormone)	pituitary (anterior lobe)

D. Build the word.

1. **aden/o**
    a. **-megaly** (adenomegaly—enlarged gland)
    b. **-otomy** (adenotomy—to make an incision into a gland)
    c. **-oma** (adenoma—a tumor of a gland)
    d. **-itis** (adenitis—inflammation of a gland)
    e. **-oid** (adenoid—resembling a gland)
2. **-ectomy**
    a. oophor/o (oophorectomy—surgical excision of the ovary)
    b. adrenal/ (adrenalectomy—surgical excision of the adrenal gland)
    c. parathyroid/o (parathyroidectomy—surgical excision of the parathyroid glands)
    d. orch/i (orchiectomy—surgical excision of a testis)
    e. thyroid (thyroidectomy—a surgical excision of the thyroid)
3. **menorrhea**
    a. **a-** (amenorrhea—the cessation of a menstrual period)
    b. **oligo-** (oligomenorrhea—scanty, light, or infrequent menstrual flow)
    c. **dys-** (dysmenorrhea—painful menstrual flow)
    d. **poly-** (polymenorrhea—frequent menstrual flow)

E. Separate the word elements of the following terms and define them.

1. adrenocorticotropic (adren/o—adrenal gland; cortic/o—cortex; troph—development; **-ic**—pertaining to: pertaining to the adrenal cortex)
2. orchidorrhaphy (orchid/o—testicle; **-rrhaphy**—surgical repair: a surgical repair of the testicle)
3. somatotropin (somat/o—the body; troph/—development)
4. pheochromocytoma (phe/o—dark; chrom/o—color; cyt/o—cell; **-oma**—tumor: a tumor that is dark in color)
5. adenocarcinoma (aden/o—gland; carcin—cancer; **-oma**—tumor: a cancerous tumor of a gland)
6. parathyrotropic (**para-**—near, beside; thry/o—thyroid; troph—growth; **-ic**—pertaining to: pertaining to growth of the parathyroid gland)

F. Name the gland involved in the following conditions.

1. ovary
2. adrenal cortex
3. pancreas
4. thymus
5. ovary
6. thyroid

G. Using your medical terminology knowledge, write the best medical word for each definition.

1. breast pain (mastalgia; mastodynia)
2. an enlarged thyroid (thyromegaly; goiter)
3. an instrument used to measure sugar in the blood (glucometer)
4. a male born without a testicle (anorchism)
5. the onset of breast development (thelarche)

Case Study

Terms

1. excessive urination
2. increased heart rate
3. beats per minute
4. lack of appetite
5. stomachache
6. gas
7. outward budging of the eyes
8. double vision
9. an enlarged thyroid
10. an autoimmune disorder of the thyroid presented as an enlarged thyroid
11. thyroid stimulating hormone
12. excessive output of the thyroid

Anatomy

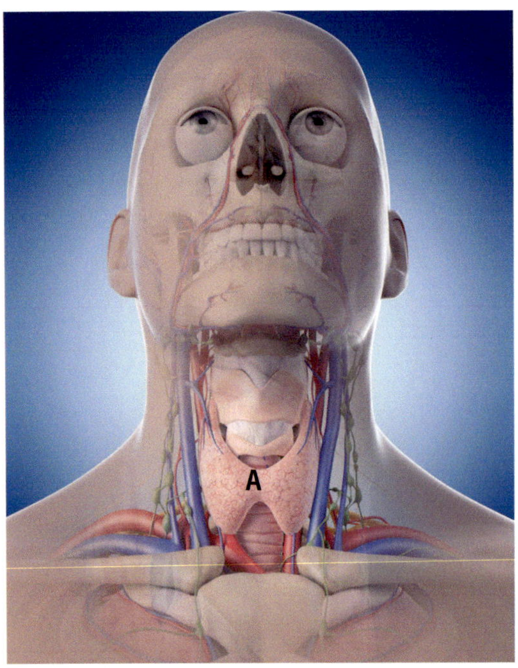

(SciePro/shutterstock.com)

Chapter 12: Urinary System

Self-Assessment

- hemat/**uria** (presence of blood in the urine)
- nephr/**ectomy** (surgical removal of a kidney)
- olig/**uria** (scanty urine)
- **an**/**uria** (without urine, inability to urinate)
- ren/**al** (pertaining to the kidney)
- **supra**/ren/**al** (above the kidney)
- **poly**/**uria** (excessive urine)
- nephr/o/**hyper**/**troph**/**y** (excessive growth/enlargement of the kidney)

A. Label the components of the urinary system from the following list of words.

1. renal artery
2. renal vein
3. ureter
4. major calix
5. renal pelvis
6. pyramids
7. minor calix
8. cortex

B. Indicate the anatomical structures by listing numbers on the figure next to the name listed.

1. ureter
2. trigone
3. urothelium
4. urethra
5. neck
6. bladder
7. apex
8. hilus

C. Match the word element with its best meaning.

1. d
2. f
3. g
4. j
5. i
6. b
7. c
8. e
9. h
10. a

D. Word building: Using the word part, add the other word element and define the new word created.

1. **cyst/o**
    a. **-scopy** (cystoscopy—visual examination of the bladder)
    b. **-ectomy** (cystectomy—surgical removal of the bladder)
    c. **-lith** (cystolith—bladder stone)
    d. **poly-** + **-ic** (polycystic—having many cysts)
    e. **-cele** (cystocele—hernia in the bladder)
2. **nephr/o**
    a. **-malacia** (nephromalacia—softening of the kidney)
    b. **-algia** (nephralgia—kidney pain)
    c. **-pathy** (nephropathy—disease of the kidney)
    d. pyel/o + **-itis** (pyelonephritis—inflammation of the renal pelvis of the kidney)
    e. **-ptosis** (nephroptosis—drooping kidney)
3. **-uria**
    a. **poly-** (polyuria—excessive urine)
    b. **dys-** (dysuria—painful/difficult urination)
    c. **glycos-** (glycosuria—presence of sugar in the urine)
    d. noct/ (nocturia—urination at night)
    e. **py-** (pyuria—pus in the urine)

E. Separate the word elements in the following terms and define each element.

1. antidiuretic: **anti-** (against); **di-** (through); ur/e (urine); **-tic** (pertaining to)
2. polydipsia: poly/dipsia—**poly-** (excessive); **-dipsia** (thirst)
3. hematuria: hema/turia: hemat/ (blood); **-uria** (urine)
4. cystorrhagia: cysto/rrhagia cyst/o (bladder); **-rrhagia** (bursting forth)
5. intravenous pyelography: (intra/ven/ous pyelo/graphy: **intra-** within); ven/o (vein); **-ous** (pertaing to); pyel/o (renal pelvis); **-graphy** (process of recording)

F. Define the word element.

1. **-ectomy** (surgical excision)
2. **-tomy** (incision)
3. **-stomy** (new opening)
4. **-gram** (a record)
5. **-graphy** (process of recording)
6. **-lith** (stone)
7. scler/o (hard)
8. olig/o (scanty)
9. ureter/o (ureter)
10. urethr/o (urethra)

Case Study

Terms

1. visible blood in the urine
2. low back pain
3. scanty urine
4. urinary tract infection
5. sweating; diaphoresis
6. without a fever
7. difficult, painful breathing
8. discoloration, bruising
9. range of motion
10. kidney stones
11. bruised
12. urinalysis
13. computed tomography

Anatomy

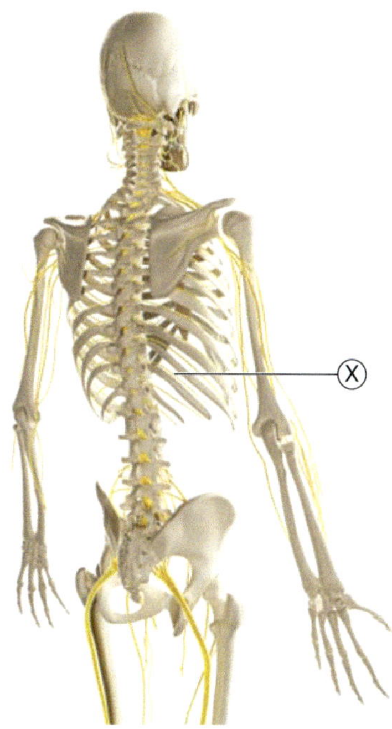

Chapter 13: Reproductive System

Self-Assessment

- orch/**itis** (inflammation of the testes)
- ovar/**ian** (pertaining to the ovary)
- test/**ic**/ular (pertaining to the testes)
- **ec**/top/**ic** (outside of usual position)
- **trans**/cutan/e/**ous** (across/through the skin)
- **multi**/**gravidia** (many pregnancies)

A. Label the components of the male reproductive system from the following list of words.

1. urinary bladder
2. vas deferens
3. urethra
4. penis
5. glans penis
6. scrotum
7. testis
8. epididymis
9. prostate gland
10. anus

B. Label the components of the female reproductive system from the following list of words.

1. fallopian tube
2. endometrium
3. uterus
4. urinary bladder
5. urethra
6. vagina
7. anus
8. cervix
9. ovary
10. fimbriae

C. Match the word element with its best meaning.

1. e
2. g
3. j
4. h
5. b
6. i
7. d
8. c
9. f
10. a

D. Word building: Using the word part, add the other word element and define the new word created.

1. **orchid/o**
   a. **-pexy** (orchidopexy—surgical fixation of the testis)
   b. **-ectomy** (orchidectomy—surgical excision of the testis)
   c. **-plasty** (orchidoplasty—surgical repair of the testis)
   d. **-otomy** (orchidotomy—incision into a testis)
   e. **-pathy** (orchidopathy—surgical removal of a testis)
2. **salpin/**
   a. **-itis** (salpingitis—inflammation of the fallopian tube)
   b. **-cele** (salpingocele—hernia of the fallopian tube)
   c. py/o (pyosalpinx—pus in the fallopian tube)
   d. hydr/o (hydrosalpinx—water in the fallopian tube)
   e. hemat/o (hematosalpinx—blood in the fallopian tube)
3. **-scopy**
   a. culd/o (culdoscopy—visual examination of the retrouterine pouch)
   b. cyst/o (cystoscopy—visual examination of the bladder)
   c. hyster/o (hysteroscopy—visual examination of the uterus)
   d. colp/o (colposcopy—visual examination of the vagina)
   e. lapr/o (laparoscopy—visual examination of the abdominal cavity)

4. **gravid/**
   a. **nulli-** + **-a** (nulligravida—no pregnancies)
   b. **primi-** + **-a** (primigravida—first pregnancy)
   c. **multi-** + **-a** (multigravida—multiple pregnancies)
5. **par/**
   a. **nulli-** + **-a** (nullipara—no births)
   b. **primi-** + **-a** (primipara—first birth)
   c. **multi-** + **-a** (multipara—multiple births)

E. Separate the word elements of the following terms and define them.

1. urethritis (urethr/itis—inflammation of the urethra)
2. panhysterectomy (pan/hyster/ectomy—surgical excision of all the uterus)
3. prostatic hyperplasia (prostat/ic hyper/plasia—excessive growth of the prostate gland
4. sonohysterography (son/o/hyster/o/graphy—using sound [ultrasound] to record the uterus)
5. hyperemesis gravidarum (hyper/emesis gravidar/um—severe nausea and vomiting during pregnancy)

F. Indicate if the word is associated with men, women, or both.

TERM	MEN	WOMEN	BOTH
hysterectomy		X	
phimosis	X		
colposcopy		X	
salpingitis		X	
orchitis	X		
oophorectomy		X	
hydrocele	X		
priapism	X		
BPH	X		
D&C		X	

Case Study

Terms

1. without a fever
2. headache
3. neck pain
4. inflammation of the throat (pharynx)
5. inflamed glands
6. loss of appetite
7. birth control pills
8. absence of a menstrual cycle
9. increase/excessive urination
10. right lower quadrant
11. fainting
12. a group of possible diagnoses that have similar presentations or symptoms.
13. overactive thyroid gland
14. a diagnostic tool that used sound waves to view internal structures
15. viewing into the abdomen

Chapter 14: Sensory System

Self-Assessment

- phot/o/phob/**ic** (fear of light; light sensitive)
- rhin/o/**plasty** (surgical repair/plastic surgery of the nose)
- ot/o/**scope** (an instrument used to look into the ear)
- nas/o/pharyng/**itis** (inflammation of the nose and pharynx)
- dipl/o/**pia** (double vision)

A. Label the components of the eye from the following list of words.

1. cornea
2. anterior chamber
3. sclera
4. iris
5. retina
6. ciliary muscle
7. pupil
8. optic nerve

B. Label the components of the nose from the following list of words.

1. nasal cavity
2. eustachian tube opening
3. middle turbinate
4. frontal sinus
5. superior turbinate
6. naris
7. inferior turbinate
8. nasopharynx

C. Place the following terms for the ear in the proper order, from the external ear inward.

1. pinna
2. external auditory canal
3. tympanic membrane
4. malleus
5. incus
6. stapes
7. oval window
8. cochlea
9. vestibulocochlear nerve (CN VIII)

D. Match the word element with its best meaning.

1. e
2. c
3. b
4. h
5. g
6. j
7. f
8. i
9. a
10. d

E. Word building: Using the word part, add the other word element and define the new word created.

1. **-itis**
   a. scler/o + kerat/ (sclerokeratitis—inflammation of the sclera and cornea)
   b. rhin/ (rhinitis—inflamed [runny] nose)
   c. phot/o + retin/ (photoretinitis—inflammation of the retina caused by extreme light)
   d. conjunctiv/ (conjunctivitis—inflammation of the conjunctivia)
   e. ot/ (otitis—inflammation of the ear)
2. **ot/o**
   a. **-itis** + media (otitis media—inflammation of the middle ear)
   b. **-rrhagia** (otorrhagia—bleeding from the ear)
   c. scler/ + **-osis** (otosclerosis—hardening of the ear, between the oval window and stapes)
   d. **-plasty** (otoplasty—surgical repair on the external ear)
   e. **-lith** (otolith—a stone [calculus] in the ear)

F. Separate the word elements of the following terms and define them.

1. ophthalmalgia (ophthalm/algia—pain of the eye)
2. aqueous (aque/ous—pertaining to water, or water-like)
3. extraocular (extra/ocul/ar—pertaining to outside of the eye)
4. otorhinolaryngology (ot/o/rhin/o/laryng/ology—study of ear, nose, and throat [larynx])
5. corneal (corne/al—pertaining to the cornea)
6. anesthetic ophthalmic solution (an/esthet/ic ophthal/mic solution—pertaining to without sensation [pain killer]; eye drops to relieve eye pain)
7. binaural (bi/naur/al—pertaining to two [both] ears)
8. leukocoria (leuko/cor/ia—condition of white pupil)
9. stapedectomy (staped/ectomy—excision of the stapes of the inner ear)
10. rhinosalpingitis (rhin/o/salping/itis—inflammation of the eustachian tube and nose)

G. What are the medical words for the following?

1. otalgia
2. emmetropia
3. otopyorrhea
4. rhinoplasty
5. otosclerosis

H. Using the medical condition strabismus, what are the terms for the following?

1. esotropia
2. exotropia

Case Study

Terms

1. double vision
2. headache
3. loss of consciousness
4. watery drainage from the nose
5. pupils are equally round and reactive to light and accommodation
6. within normal limits
7. range of motion
8. uncontrollable eye movements
9. ringing in the ears
10. dizziness

Anatomy

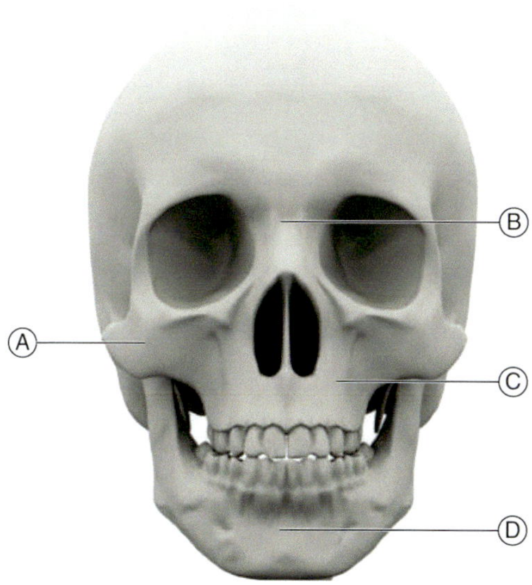

Congratulations! You have learned Medical Terminology!

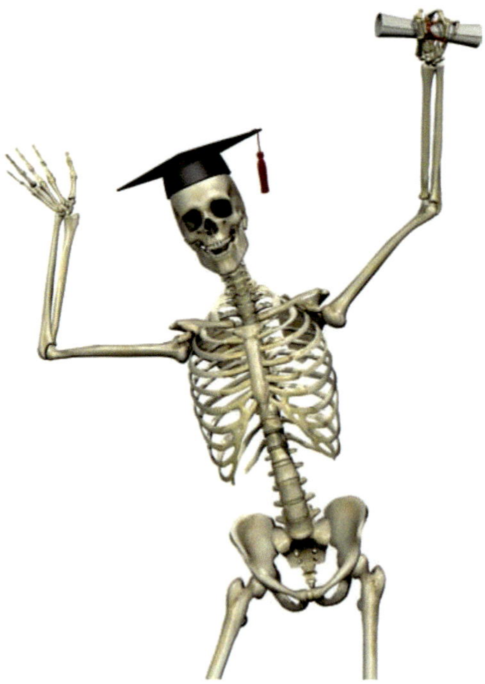

Glossary

PREFIX	DEFINITION
A	
a-	without
ab-	away from
actin-	radiation; ray
ad-	toward; near
allo-	different; other
amphi-	both sides
an-	not; without
ana-	apart; away; up
ante-	before; in front of
anti-	against
auto-	own; self
B	
bi-	two; twice
brady-	slow
C	
caus-	burn; heat
caut-	burn; heat
circum-	around
con-	together
crypt-	hidden
cyan/o-	blue
D	
de-	down; take away; without
dextr/o-	right
di-	two; through; apart; across
dia-	two; through; apart; across
dipl/o-	double
dys-	abnormal; bad; difficult; painful
E	
ec-	out; outside
ecto-	out; outside
em-	in
eme-	to vomit
en-	within
endo-	in; within
epi-	above; upon
erythr/o-	red
eso-	inward
eu-	good; normal
ex-	away; away from; out; outside
exo-	away; away from; out; outside
extra-	outside
H	
hemi-	one half
hetero-	different
home/o-	same
homo-	same
hydro-	water
hyper-	above; excessive; high; increased
hypo-	below; decreased; deficient; insufficient; low; under
I	
in-	not
infra-	below
inter-	among; between
intra-	inside; within
L	
leuk/o-	white
M	
macro-	large
mal-	bad
man-	hand
medi-	middle
medio-	middle
melan/o-	black

(continued)

PREFIX	DEFINITION
meso-	middle
micro-	small
mono-	one
multi-	many
N	
non-	not
nulli-	none
O	
olig/o-	few; scanty
P	
pan-	all
par-	alongside; around; beside; near
para-	beside; near; abnormal
per-	through
peri-	around
poly-	excessive; many; much; over
post-	after; behind
pre-	before
prim/i-	first
Q	
quadr/i-	four
R	
re-	back; behind
retro-	back; backward; behind
S	
semi-	half; partial
sinistr/o-	left
sten/o-	narrow; short
sub-	below; under
supra-	above
sym-	together; union
syn-	together; union
T	
tachy-	fast; rapid
tel-	end
tetra-	four
trans-	across; through
tri-	three
U	
ultra-	excess; beyond
uni-	one

SUFFIX	DEFINITION
A	
-ac	pertaining to
-acusis	hearing condition
-al	pertaining to
-algia	pain
-amnios	amniotic fluid; amnion
-an	pertaining to
-ar	pertaining to
-arche	beginning
-ary	pertaining to
-ase	enzyme
-asthen	weakness
-asthenia	weakness
-atic	pertaining to
-ation	process of
-atory	pertaining to
-atresia	lacking a normal body opening; closure
B	
-blast	embryonic cell
C	
-capnia	carbon dioxide in the blood
-cele	hernia; protrusion; swelling
-centesis	puncture; surgical puncture
-cide	killing
-cision	cutting
-clasia	to break
-clasis	to break
-clast	break
-crine	secreting; to secrete
-cusis	hearing
-cyesis	pregnancy
-cyte	cell

SUFFIX	DEFINITION
D	
-desis	bind; fuse
-dipsia	thirst
-drome	running; to run
-dynia	pain
E	
-eal	pertaining to
-ectasia	dilation
-ectasis	dilation; expansion
-ectomy	excision; surgical removal
-edema	swelling
-emesis	vomiting
-emia	blood condition
-emic	pertaining to blood
-er	one who
-esis	state of
-esthesia	perception; sensation
F	
-ferous	carrying; pertaining to
-fida	to split
-flux	flow
G	
-gen	that which produces
-genesis	forming; origin; producing
-gram	a record of
-graph	an instrument to record information
-graphy	process of recording; the act of recording information
-gravida	pregnant person
I	
-ia	condition
-iac	pertaining to
-ian	a specialist in a particular field
-iasis	condition
-iatrical	related to medical treatment

(continued)

SUFFIX	DEFINITION
-iatrician	one who specializes in a particular treatment
-iatrics	one who specializes in a particular treatment
-iatrist	one who specializes in a particular treatment
-iatry	medical treatment
-ic	pertaining to
-ical	pertaining to
-ics	a medical specialty
-ile	pertaining to
-in	substance
-ine	pertaining to
-ion	process; the act of
-ior	pertaining to
-is	pertaining to; structure
-ism	condition
-ist	one who specializes
-itis	inflammation
-ium	membrane; structure
K	
-kinesia	movement
L	
-lepsy	seizure
-listhesis	slipping
-lith	stone
-logist	one who studies
-logy	study of
-lysis	breaking down; destruction; loosening; separating; to loosen or break
-lytic	destroy
M	
-malacia	softening
-megaly	abnormally large; enlargement
-meter	an instrument used to measure
-metr/o	uterus
-metry	measurement of
O	
-occlus/o	to close
-occult	hidden
-oid	resembling
-ology	study of
-oma	mass; tumor
-opia	vision condition
-opsia	vision condition
-opsy	process of viewing
-or	one who
-orexia	appetite
-ory	pertaining to
-ose	pertaining to
-osis	condition
-osmia	smell
-ostomy	a surgical opening
-otia	ear condition
-otomy	incision; to cut into
-ous	pertaining to
P	
-para	to give birth
-paresis	partial paralysis
-partum	childbirth; labor
-pathy	disease
-peni	deficient
-penia	decrease; deficient
-penic	decrease; deficient
-pepsia	digestion
-pexy	surgical fixation of
-phagia	eating; swallowing
-phasia	speech
-pheresis	removal
-phil	an affinity for; attraction
-phobia	fear
-phonia	voice
-phoresis	migration in a specific manner
-phylaxis	protection

(continued)

SUFFIX	DEFINITION
-physis	growth
-plasia	formation; growth
-plasm	formation
-plasty	reconstruction; repair; plastic surgery
-plegia	paralysis
-pnea	breathing
-poiesis	formation
-porosis	porous
-ptosis	drooping; falling; prolapse
-ptysis	to spit
R	
-r/rrhage	bursting forth; excessive flow
-r/rhagia	abnormal flow
-r/rhaphy	surgical repair; suturing
-r/rhea	discharge; excessive flow
-r/rhexis	rupture
S	
-salpinx	fallopian tube
-sclerosis	hardening
-scope	an instrument used to view or inspect
-scopic	pertaining to visual examination
-scopy	examination of
-sepsis	an inflammatory response to an infection
-sis	condition; state of
-spadias	fissure
-spasm	involuntary contraction

SUFFIX	DEFINITION
-sphyxia	pulse
-stasis	same; still; stopping
-stenosis	narrowing
-stomy	surgical opening
T	
-thelium	specialized layer of cells
-therapy	treatment
-thorax	chest
-tic	pertaining to
-tocia	childbirth; labor
-tome	a surgical instrument used to cut
-tomy	incision; to cut into
-tonia	tone
-tripsy	crushing
-troph	development; growth; nourishment
-trophia	to turn
-trophy	development
U	
-ule	small
-um	structure; thing
-ure	process
-uria	urine
-us	pertaining to; structure
Y	
-y	process of

COMBINING FORM	DEFINITION
A	
abdomin/o	abdomen
acetabul/o	acetabulum (hip socket)
acid/o	acid; acidic; something with a pH of 7 or less
acous/o	hearing
acr/o	extremity
acromi/o	acromion (end of the spine of the scapula)
acu/o	hearing
aden/o	gland
adip/o	fat
adren/o	adrenal gland
aer/o	air; gas
albin/o	white
albumin/o	protein
alges/o	pain
alveol/o	alveoli
ambly/o	dull; dim
amni/o	amnion
amyl/o	starch
an/o	anus
andr/o	male
ang/i	vessel
angi/o	vessel
angio/o	vessel
ankyl/o	bent
anter/o	anterior
anthrac/o	coal; coal dust
aort/o	aorta
append/o	appendix
aque/o	water
arachn/o	spider
arter/o	artery
arteri/o	artery
arthr/o	joint
astr/o	star
ather/o	fatty material
atri/o	atrium

COMBINING FORM	DEFINITION
audi/o	hearing
audit/o	hearing
aur/o	ear
auricul/o	ear
auscultate/o	to listen
axill/o	armpit
azot/o	nitrogen
B	
bacter/i	bacteria
balan/o	glans penis
bar/o	pressure
bas/o	base; bottom
bi/o	life
bil/i	bile
blast/o	embryonic cell
blephar/o	eyelid
brachi/o	arm
bronch/o	bronchial tubes
bronchi/o	bronchi
bronchiol/o	bronchiole
bucc/o	cheek
bunion/o	bunion
burs/o	bursa
C	
calc/i	calcium
calc/o	calcium
calcane/o	heel
calci/o	calcium
capit/o	head
carcin/o	cancer
card/i	heart
cardi/o	heart
carp/o	carpals; wrist bones
caud/o	tail
cec/o	intestine; cecum
celi/o	abdomen
cellul/o	cell

(continued)

COMBINING FORM	DEFINITION
cephal/o	head
cerebell/o	cerebellum; little brain
cerebr/o	cerebrum
cervic/o	neck; cervix
cheil/o	lip
chem/o	chemicals; drugs
chol/e	bile; gall
cholangi/o	bile vessel
cholecyst/o	gallbladder (cyst = bladder)
choledoch/o	bile duct
chondr/o	cartilage
chord/o	cord; spinal cord
chori/o	chorion (outermost layer of the fetal membrane)
chrom/o	color; stain
chromat/o	color; stain
chron/o	persisting over time
chym/o	juice
cirrh/o	orange
claudicate/o	to limp
clitor/o	clitoris
clitorid/o	clitoris
clon/o	turmoil
cochle/o	cochlea
col/o	colon
colon/o	colon
colp/o	vagina
condyl/o	condyle; knuckle
coni/o	dust
conjunctiv/o	conjunctiva
continence	to hold
cor/o	pupil
corne/o	cornea
corpore/e	body
corpor/o	body
cortic/o	cortex; outer portion
cortex	outer covering
cost/o	rib
cran/o	cranium; skull

COMBINING FORM	DEFINITION
crani/o	cranium; skull
crin/o	to secrete
crur/o	leg
cry/o	cold
crypt/o	hidden
cubit/o	elbow
culd/o	retrouterine pouch
cutan/e	skin
cutane/o	skin
cyan/o	blue
cyst/o	bladder; sac
cyt/o	cell
D	
dacry/o	tear; lacrimal duct/gland
dacryocyst/o	lacrimal sac
dactyl/o	finger; toe
dent/o	dental; teeth
derm/a	skin
derm/o	skin
dermat/o	skin
diaphoretic	sweating
diast	to expand
didym/o	testis
dilat/o	to widen
dipl/o	double
dips/o	thirst
dist/o	distal
diverticul/o	small pouch
dors/o	dorsal
duoden/o	duodenum
dur/o	hard
dynam/o	force; energy
E	
ech/o	to bounce sound
electr/o	electricity
embol/o	plug
embry/o	embryo; fetus
encephal/o	brain

(continued)

COMBINING FORM	DEFINITION
enter/o	intestines
eosin/o	rose colored
epididym/o	epididymis
epiglott/o	epiglottis
episi/o	vulva
erg/o	work
eryth/o	red
erythr/o	red
esophag/e	esophagus
esophag/o	esophagus
estr/o	female
excret/o	shifted out
F	
fasci/o	fascia
fec/o	feces; stool
femor/o	thigh bone
fet/o	fetus
fibr/o	fiber
fluor/o	luminous
follicul/o	little bag
fovea	small pit
G	
galact/o	milk
gangli/o	knot; swelling
ganglion/o	knot; swelling
gastr/o	stomach; abdomen
gingiv/o	gums
glact/o	milk
glauc/o	gray
gli/o	glue
glomerul/o	glomerulus; little ball
gloss/o	tongue
gluc/o	sugar
glute/o	buttocks
glyc/o	sugar
glycos/o	glucose; glycogen; sugar
gonad/o	gonad; sex organ

COMBINING FORM	DEFINITION
granul/o	little grain
gravid/o	pregnancy
gyn/o	female
gynec/o	female
H	
halit/o	breath
hem/o	blood
hemat/o	blood
hemorrh/o	likely to bleed
hemorrhoid/o	vascular protrusion through a weakened wall or membrane of the anus
hepat/o	liver
hern/o	hernia; weakened wall/membrane; rupture
herni/o	hernia; weakened wall/membrane; rupture
heter/o	different
hidr/o	sweat
hist/o	tissue
home/o	same
homo	same
hormon/o	to set in motion
humor	fluid
hydr/o	water
hymen/o	hymen
hypophys/o	pituitary gland
hyster/o	uterus
I	
idi/o	unknown
ile/o	ileum
infarct/o	death of an area
inguin/o	groin
infer/o	inferior
ir/o	iris
irid/o	iris
isch/o	hold back; to withhold
ischi/o	ischium
J	
jejun/o	empty; jejunum

(continued)

COMBINING FORM	DEFINITION
K	
kal/o	potassium (the chemical symbol for potassium is K)
kel/o	fibrous growth; tumor
kerat/o	cornea; hard; horn-like
ket/o	ketone
keton/o	ketone
kinesi/o	movement
kyph/o	bent; hump
L	
labi/o	lip
labyrinth/o	inner ear; labyrinth
lacrim/o	tear duct/gland
lact/o	milk
lamin/o	lamina (thin plate)
lapar/o	abdomen
laryng/o	larynx
later/o	side
lei/o	smooth
leuc/o	white
leuk/o	white
lingu/o	tongue
lip/o	fat
lipid/o	fat
lith/o	stone
lob/o	lobe
lord/o	swayback
lumb/o	low back
lumin	light
lun/o	moon
lymph/o	lymph (the watery substance originating in organs and tissues)
lys/o	to break apart
M	
mamm/o	breast
mast/o	breast
mastoid/o	mastoid process
maxilla/o	upper jaw (below the nose)
meat/o	opening
medi/o	medial
melan/o	black
men/o	menstrual
mening/i	membrane; meninges
mening/o	membrane; meninges
menisc/o	meniscus
mens	mouth; menstruation
ment/o	mind
metr/i	uterus; measure
metr/o	uterus
mi/o	smaller; less
micturit/o	to urinate
miliar	tiny
mon/o	one
morph/o	form; shape
muc/o	mucus
my/o	muscle
myc/o	fungus
mydr/o	widen; enlarge
myel/o	bone marrow; medulla; myelin; spinal cord
myos/o	muscle
myring/o	eardrum; tympanic membrane
myx/o	mucus
N	
narc/o	stupor; numbness; sleep
nas/o	nose
nat/o	sodium (the chemical symbol for sodium is Na); birth
necr/o	death
nephr/o	kidney
neur/o	nerve
neutr/o	neutral
noct/o	night
nucle/o	nucleus
nyct/o	night

(continued)

COMBINING FORM	DEFINITION
O	
occlus/o	to close
occult	hidden
ocul/o	eye
odont/o	tooth
olig/o	scanty
omphal/o	umbilicus; naval
onych/o	nail
oophor/o	ovary
ophthalm/o	eye
opt/o	vision
optic/o	eye; vision
or/o	mouth
orch/o	testicle; testis
orchi/o	testicle; testis
orchid/o	testicle; testis
orth/o	straight
osche/o	scrotum
oss/i	bone
osse/o	bone
ossicul/o	ossicle
oste/o	bone
ot/o	ear
ov/i	ovum (egg)
ov/o	ovum (egg)
ovari/o	ovary
ove/o	uvea
ovul/o	ovum (egg)
ox/i	oxygen
ox/o	oxygen
ozot/o	nitrogen
P	
pachy	thick
palat/o	palate; roof of mouth
pallor	pale
palpebr/o	eyelid
pancreat/o	pancreas; sweetbread
papill/o	nipple; papilla

COMBINING FORM	DEFINITION
par/o	to give birth; labor
para	a person who has given birth
part/o	to give birth; labor
patell/o	kneecap
path/o	disease
pector/o	chest
ped/i	foot; child
ped/o	foot; child
pedicul/o	lice (singular—louse)
pelv/i	pelvis
pelv/o	pelvis
peps/o	digestion
pept/o	digestion
perine/o	perineum
perit/o	peritoneum
peritone/o	peritoneum; membrane; to stretch; to stretch over
phac/o	lens
phag/o	eating; swallowing
phak/o	lens
phalang/o	fingers or toes (bones of)
pharyng/o	pharynx; throat
phas/o	speech
phasi/o	speech
phe/o	dark
phim/i	muzzle
phim/o	muzzle
phleb/o	vein
phon/o	sound; voice
phor/o	bearing; carrying
phot/o	light
phren/o	diaphragm
phyma	swelling; tumor
physis	growth
pil/o	hair
pituitar/o	pituitary gland
plasma	the liquid aspect of blood
plegi/o	paralysis
pleur/o	pleura

(continued)

COMBINING FORM	DEFINITION
ply/o	pus
pnea	breathing
pneum/o	lung
pneumon/o	lungs
pod/o	foot
poli/o	gray
polyp/o	a small growth; polyp
poster/o	posterior
praxia	doing; to achieve
presby/o	old age
prim/i	first
proct/o	anus; rectum
prolactin/o	prolactin
prostat/o	prostate gland
prosthes/o	addition
proxim/o	proximal
prurit/o	itching
pseud/o	false
psych/o	mind
pub/o	pubic bone
puerper/o	childbirth
pulm/o	lungs
pulmon/o	lungs
py/o	pus
pyel/o	renal pelvis
pylor/o	gatekeeper; pylorus
Q	
quadr/i	four
quadr/o	four
R	
rachi/o	spine; vertebral column
radi/o	radiation; x-ray
radic/o	nerve root
radicul/o	nerve root
rect/o	rectum; straight
ren/o	kidney
retin/o	retina
rhabd/o	rod-shaped
rhin/o	nose
rhythm/o	rhythm
rhytid/o	wrinkle
rubin/o	red pigment
rubor	red
S	
sacr	connective tissue; flesh
salping/o	eustachian tube; fallopian tube
sarc/o	flesh
scler/o	hard; hardening; thick; sclera
scoli/o	curved
scot/o	darkness
scrot/o	scrotum
seb/o	oil; sebum
semin/i	semen
semin/o	semen
sept/o	wall
sial/o	saliva
sigmoid/o	the letter S
sinus/o	sinus
somat/o	body
somn/o	sleep
son/o	sound
spasm/o	spasm; sudden involuntary contraction
sperm/i	sperm; spermatozoa
sperm/o	sperm
spermat/o	sperm; spermatozoa
sphygm/o	pulse
spin/o	spine
spir/o	breath; breathing
splen/o	spleen
spondyl/o	vertebra
staped/o	stirrup; stapes (third bone in the middle ear)
static	without movement
steat/o	fat
sten/o	narrowing
ster/o	solid structure
stern/o	sternum

(continued)

COMBINING FORM	DEFINITION
steth/o	chest
stigmat/o	mark; point
stomat/o	mouth
strab/o	squinting
stri	line; stripe
strict	contracture; tightening
sudor/o	sweat
super/o	above
syst	contract
T	
tars/o	tarsals (bones of the ankle)
taxi/o	response to a stimulus
ten/o	tendon
tend/o	tendon
tendi/o	tendon
tens/o	pressure; stretching
terat/o	deformity; monster
test/o	testis; testicle
thalam/o	inner chamber; thalamus
thel/e	nipple
therm/o	heat; temperature
thorac/o	chest
thromb/o	clot
thym/o	thymus gland
thyr/o	shield, thyroid
toc/o	labor
ton/o	tension; pressure
tonsil/o	tonsils
top/o	location; place
trache/o	trachea
tract/o	pullling; to pull
trans	across; through
trich/o	hair
trigon	trigone
troph/o	development; growth; nourishment

COMBINING FORM	DEFINITION
tuss/o	cough
tympan/o	eardrum; tympanic membrane
U	
uln/o	ulna (forearm bone)
ultra	beyond; farther
umbilic/o	naval
ungu/o	nail
ur/o	urine
ureter/o	ureter
urethr/o	urethra
urin/o	urine
uter/o	uterus
uve/o	uvea (layer in the eye)
uvul/o	grape; mouth
V	
vagin/o	vagina
valv/o	valve
valvul/o	valve
varic/o	dilated vein; swollen vein; varicose vein
vas/o	vessel; vas deferens
vascul/o	blood vessel
ven/o	vein
ventricul/o	cavity; ventricle
ventr/o	ventral
verm/i	worm
vers/o	to turn
vertebr/o	spine; vertebra
vesic/o	urinary bladder
vesicul/o	seminal vesicle
vestibule/o	vestibule
vitre/o	glassy
vulv/o	vulva
X	
xanth/o	yellow
xen/o	foreign
xer/o	dry

Index

A

B

C

D

E

F

G

H

I

J

K

L

M

R

S

T

U

V

W

X

For Product Safety Concerns and Information please contact our EU representative GPSR@taylorandfrancis.com Taylor & Francis Verlag GmbH, Kaufingerstraße 24, 80331 München, Germany

Batch number: 10745678

Printed by Printforce, the Netherlands